SAFER
VACCINES

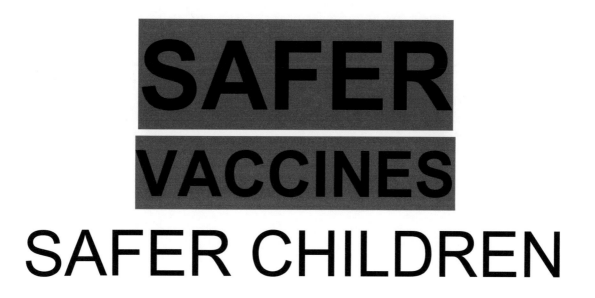

SAFER CHILDREN

Vaccines must not subject children to chemicals that cause abnormal reactions. To subject children to injections that are laced with unnatural to human biology chemicals are a **CHILD ABUSE BY CHEMICALIZATION** and main cause of

AUTISM

There are chemicals in vaccines that are too dangerous and destructive to health.
VACCINES ARE NOT AS CHEMICALLY SAFE AS THEY CAN OR SHOULD BE.
UNNATURAL VACCINE CHEMICALS DOPE BRAIN CELLS
ONLY INJECT WITH CLEANER, SAFER VACCINES

Dr. Robert Caires DC, Esq. inactive

Became inactive in practice to be an advocate of SAFER vaccines

ADVOCATE OF SAFER VACCINES

SAFERvaccines.com = HEALTHYvaccines.com = HEALTHIERvaccinations.com

SAFERvaccines.ORG

SAFER VACCINES, SAFER CHILDREN

iUniverse books may be ordered through booksellers or by contacting:

iUniverse
1663 Liberty Drive
Bloomington, IN 47403
www.iuniverse.com
1-800-Authors (1-800-288-4677)

Because of the dynamic nature of the Internet, any web addresses or links contained in this book may have changed since publication and may no longer be valid. The views expressed in this work are solely those of the author and do not necessarily reflect the views of the publisher, and the publisher hereby disclaims any responsibility for them.

Any people depicted in stock imagery provided by Getty Images are models, and such images are being used for illustrative purposes only.
Certain stock imagery © Getty Images.

ISBN: 978-1-5320-6098-4 (sc)
ISBN: 978-1-5320-6559-0 (hc)
ISBN: 978-1-5320-6099-1 (e)

Library of Congress Control Number: 2018913067

Print information available on the last page.

iUniverse rev. date: 12/19/2018

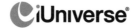

CONTENTS

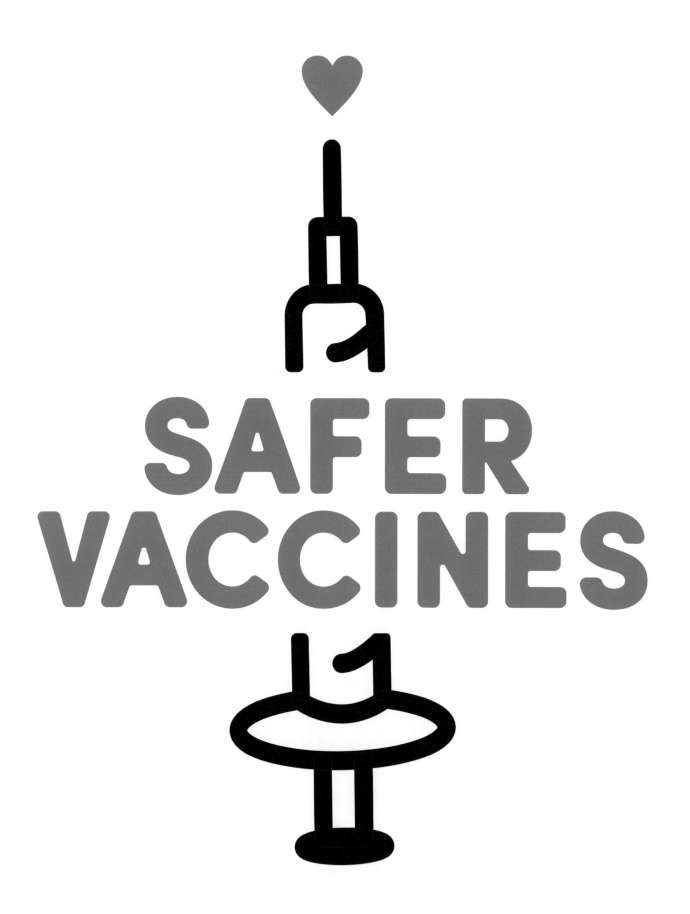

SAFER VACCINES

INTRODUCTION

As a doctor, I witnessed a child become injured after a vaccine chemicalization; I realized we desperately need SAFER vaccines, vaccines with a lot less unnatural to the body and/or biology harmful chemicals. Be cautioned: VACCINATION is the UNATURAL CHEMICALIZATION of blood. This book has the way to SAFER vaccines. Do vaccines cause Autism and/or how many vaccine chemicalizations can your children withstand before AUTISM becomes their reality? I am both doctor and lawyer. As a doctor, let me warn you: for the sake of your child's health and very future, do *not* inject chemicals into the child's blood, musculature, or any part of the body. Injecting unnatural to the body and toxic to the body chemicals are injurious; we must minimize and/or not inject such, chemicals. Good health is extremely reliant upon maintaining just the right chemistry. Vaccine anti-health chemicals are stressful and harmful to the body; cause health degeneration and/ or AUTISM. In order, to best safeguard optimum health please, read every word of this book and do investigate it yourself; do your own research to confirm. Collective ignorance that one can inject unnatural to the body chemicals has majorly contributed in inducing an epidemic of autism. WARNING: vaccines have anti-health, alien to the body, chemicals. PROTECT YOUR CHILDREN; BE EMPOWERED TO PREVENT AUTISM! Anytime you engage in anything that is fundamentally unnatural, expect unnatural results. Unnatural to the body vaccine chemical injections must not be enforced.

Vaccination mandates are mal-law that deny parent's the Constitutional Right to direct children's welfare or healthcare and protect their children. Mandated mass vaccination is child abuse by chemicalization on a mass scale as, it injects chemicals that cause injury and it is repugnant to the Constitution. Blameless parents are deprived of their inalienable Right and/or GOD given Right to decide what is best for their children. Mandated vaccinations violate parent's authority/Right of protecting children; by natural law a parent's Right is supreme. Parents must be FREE to stop children from being chemically infused or chemically exposed. No one should be subjected to CHEMICAL INJECTION SLAVERY. Liberty to protect from CHEMICALIZATION or AUTISM is essential.

Vaccinations do not have the needed safety feature of informed consent/DENIAL and Vaccine Producers wrongfully have impunity from vaccine induced injury litigation; this allows anti-health chemicals to be in vaccines and mass child abuse is the result. Mandated vaccinations promote unsafe chemical vaccines that cause harm; they must not be injected. Injected chemicals are the primary cause of AUTISM. Children are injected with anti-health chemicals often against parents will. Vaccination is mandated, to assure Drug Company profiteering. Prepare to be emancipated from unjust INJECTION SLAVERY.

Programmed people/robots, seeing will see not and hearing will hear not. This book may contradict and challenge your belief that vaccinations are perfect or not in need of removal of anti-health chemicals. Out of fear of being confused you may shut down and not be open-minded to absorb these truths. You likely are programmed to blindly accept vaccine chemical injections and to acquiesce in giving up your Right to protect your children from unwanted, anti-health chemical exposure and/or vaccinations. What you will learn about vaccines and those that supposedly protect you may frighten you and cause you to retract into a denial of the truth or recoil in a psychological defense and stick to the official story, when your belief is so challenged. Do not mentally retreat or cling to a wrong understanding. Learn how to protect your children from CHEMICALIZATION AUTISM. This book is packed with how to achieve optimum health by avoiding chemicals of harm and anti-health choices. Vaccine Producers' puppet government, under a façade of legality, does not protect children; YOU MUST! Pride and blind faith in vaccinations is flawed.

What you are about to read can keep your children healthy; prevent health demise and stop the Autism epidemic. Vaccines will be SAFER if we remove the unnecessary unnatural to the body chemicals; there is an urgent need to do so. Despite strong rational parental objection, children are enforced, coerced and induced to endure injections of anti-health vaccine chemicals. Children are under chemical attack from many sources however, vaccine chemicals are the main cause of the AUTISM epidemic. Victims of AUTISM are the real epidemic to safeguard against; not childhood diseases. The frequency of Autism is constantly on the rise because of the chemicals that our children are exposed to. Vaccine injected chemicals quickly penetrate children's brain cells and is the main etiology of Autism; this book will make that crystal clear. Parent's Right to care for children to the best of their ability and/or their Right to protect children is being grossly violated. A taking has taken place; take your children back and protect them from the vices of chemical injection exposure. The book contains the way to regain or assure your children's well-being and parental authority. It is packed with ways to have control of your children's welfare and assure your children are optimally healthy; without AUTISM. Children's welfare is jeopardized; children are being chemically compromised and medicated more than ever before. Health's number one enemy is CHEMICAL infiltration.

Each chapter of this book gives pertinent information in order, to avoid chemical exposure. Learn how to be protected from injected chemical harm. Children must be under the rightful protection of parents; parents having legal capacity to prevent chemical exposure or unwanted vaccine chemical injections. Become aware of what chemicals are in vaccines and their dangerous propensities. Determine whether to risk vaccine chemical exposure or safeguard the blood of your children. Prevent anti-health vaccine chemicals from being enforced upon your children; do not succumb to VACCINATION SLAVERY.

Vaccine Producers have a liability shield for when their vaccines cause injury; they do not even have to do a cost/benefit analysis in deciding what chemicals to use in vaccines; this liability shield is detrimental to vaccine safety. Be sure that vaccines do not have anti-health chemicals before even considering their injection. Do not stand for your children being subjected to chemical infusions. Decide if vaccines are produced in accordance with rational parental requirements for children's safety. Children's safety is at risk because vaccinations are mandated, and Vaccine Producers are practically impervious to negligence lawsuits. Discover how the prompting of Vaccine Producers not to use certain chemicals and/or prompting production of higher quality vaccines will prevent health degenerating chemistry. It is of extreme importance for parents to decide what is in their children's best health interest, without being over influenced, coerced or enforced to do otherwise. Exercise your liberty to decide what is best for your children; decide if the vaccines are too dangerous to inject and protect your children accordingly.

Each chapter of this book is packed with content that can help prevent chemical exposure of your children and resolve the Autism Epidemic. You will learn how big business pharmaceutical industry has unconscionably positioned itself above your Right to protect your children and how the good standard of product production instilled by negligence law does not apply to vaccine production/safety. This book has TWO STEPS OF CORRECTION needed to clean-up vaccines and curtail the AUTISM epidemic, it is the main content of this book and will allow you to fulfill your parental obligation of protecting your children. Learn how to protect your children by not exposing them to unnatural to the body chemicals especially, injected chemicals. AUTISM may be an injection away! Injecting vaccines by mandate is a desperate measure for only desperate times; it must not be ongoing or in perpetuity. Children must have their caring protection from parents; above government! Learn how to be free to protect your children to the best of your ability; safeguard them from the vices of CHEMICALIZATION AUTISM.

In the best interest of children, vaccination decisions must be made by parents; not government. There is no valid or controlling reason why certain negative to health chemicals are in vaccines. Vaccine producers are in the vaccine money making business; safety of your children is not their number one priority. Certain chemicals in vaccines are not good for you, they cause injury; but are used because they assure higher profits. We need to prompt healthier/safer vaccines for our children through the emancipation of our freedoms of self-healthcare decision, parental protection of children and liberty to litigate directly against Vaccine Producers for vaccine induced injuries. Enforced vaccine chemicalizations cause a detrimental chemical tipping point and are the main etiology of the AUTISM epidemic. It is imperative to the well-being of children to vaccinate with updated SAFER vaccines not laced with unnatural to the biology chemicals and not expose children to abnormal to the body chemicalization.

LET US ABOLISH MANDATED VACCINATIONS AND HOLD VACCINE PRODUCERS LIABLE in order, to have SAFER vaccines and thereby, end the AUTISM epidemic. With what chemicals have been found in vaccines, exposing our vulnerable children to such, "CHEMICALIZATION" has not only violated the circle of trust but has taken those that produce vaccines and mandate vaccines out of the circle of trust. Parents must be in proper control of their children's welfare and completely FREE to protect them from harm! Without question, the contents of vaccines make or break your children's health. As far as, governing what is to be injected into babies' vital systems, the injection of unnatural to human biology chemicals must be considered treason and abuse against our children! Before you make the dreadful mistake of drastically modifying your tiny baby's, little infant's or small child's vital internal chemistry by injecting vaccine chemicalization; learn exactly what chemicals are in the vaccine and make sure you prevent your offspring's unwanted chemicalization. You must take back your rightful control and authority over your children in order, to protect them accordingly and end the perversion of government superseding parental authority! THIS BOOK IS ALL ABOUT ASSURING THAT YOU CAN HELP PROTECT YOUR CHILDREN AND PROCURE SAFER vaccines, FOR ALL CHILDREN! To inject vaccines with unnatural to human biology chemicals is chemicalization madness. Only inject, SAFER vaccines, generated by the TWO STEPS OF CORRECTION of this book.

The charity SAFER vaccines found at SAFERvaccines.org or .com strives to educate all about why the predominate present state of vaccines have become too dangerous to inject because of the chemicals within vaccines and how to achieve much SAFER vaccines. It is the author's hope to give you a good dose of intelligence about what chemicals are in vaccines and what those chemicals are doing to those injected with them. Just as it has become commonly known that chemicals or chemical compounds cause cancer it will soon become common knowledge that unnatural to human biology chemicals that are in vaccines are the cause in fact of the Autism epidemic. Please, do not take my word or words in this book as true; do your own research to determine if it is true and protect your family accordingly. Chemicals are either building blocks of health or stumbling blocks of health; do make sure that what is being injected into your beloved offspring do not in any way jeopardize their vital biochemistry that produces all that is needed for health. Your children deserve only the safest of vaccines so, do consider vaccinating with only SAFER vaccines that obey and/or are ruled by the TWO STEPS OF CORRECTION. Trust in the law of chemistry and parental ingenuity; protect your children!

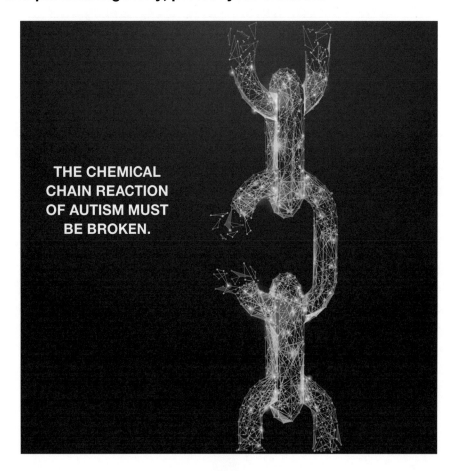

THE CHEMICAL CHAIN REACTION OF AUTISM MUST BE BROKEN.

The below disclaimer is necessary because I am placed under attack for stating that the noxious chemicals of vaccines render children unhealthy and induce **AUTISM** and that it is a ludicrous assumption that injecting unnatural to human biology chemicals is justified and is healthy. I am under attack because I strive for **parents** to have the control whether a vaccination can or cannot take place and that preventing vaccine anti-health chemicalization best **PREVENTS AUTISM** and for revealing that producers of vaccines must be impelled to **GET THE CHEMICALS OUT** of its vaccines to **END THE AUTISM EPIDEMIC**. I am being attacked because I teach individuals to be masters of their body and health, to not be mastered over, and to know that the right chemistry equals health; the wrong chemistry equals **AUTISM**, and the greater threat is not from childhood disease but rather, the injection of vaccines containing unnatural to human biology chemicals and that the number one priority for assuring health of children is the removal of such, chemicals from vaccines. The disclaimer is needed that I may help secure the best interest of children, inform the public about the dangers of the chemicals in vaccines and not suffer for doing this public service. We must live FREE to control what will or will not be injected into our body or blood. Vaccines could be a lot more beneficial and healthier! **I work to assure SAFER vaccines for all children! Visit the SAFER Vaccines' charity website at, SAFERvaccines.org for more vital information and to access all my must read, books!**

DISCLAIMER

This disclaimer overrules and supersedes what is written in this book.
This book was written by a GHOST writer; His first name is HOLY.
All who read any words of this book or learn of this book's contents or recognize it of value, merit or extreme benefit or realize that it will **END THE AUTISM epidemic** must assume it all **no**t true and **no**t at all be influenced by this book and therefore, I can**no**t be successfully litigated against.
Everything in this book is **no**t medical or legal advice and chemicals CAN**no**t cause injury.
Do **no**t read this book without permission from your doctor, lawyer and Indian chief. I only urge you to **no**t read this book and to **no**t rely on it for health and AUTISM prevention.
Vaccine Producers do not **care more for money than safety; there is no conflict of interest.**
THIS BOOK IS unedited, a fabrication, a fiction of my
imagination and mere opinion; it is devoid of FACT.
I do not **claim this book's content has merit and that vaccine chemicals cause AUTISM.**
You have no freedo**m to refuse vaccinations and protect children from vaccine chemicals.**
Being enforced to submit children for unwanted injections is not **VACCINATION SLAVERY.**
Vaccination mandates are not **imperfect law; do** not **refuse vaccine chemicalizations.**
You must give up your liberty if mal-law commands;
you cannot **protect your parental Rights.**
You must **not disagree to chemically exposing your children; even if it causes injury.**
Parents do not **have legal capacity to decide what is best and/or good for their children.**
Parents do not **have mental capacity to decide if chemical injections should** not **be given.**
You need not **to reject vaccine injections of anti-health chemicals; no matter how many.**
I DO not **CLAIM, if you INJECT anti-health vaccine chemicals, AUTISM is likely to occur.**
Vaccine Producers' primary objective is not **to put chemicals for profit in vaccines.**
Vaccine's being chemically safe is not **more important to parents than Vaccine Producers.**
YOU ARE not **FREE TO PRAY FOR HEALTH AND THERE IS** no **FREE**DO**M OF RELIGION.**
YOU CANnot **OBTAIN A RELIGIOUS EXEMPTION FROM VACCINATION.**

CHAPTER 1

VACCINATIONS MUST BE BASED ON FREE AND INFORMED PERSONAL CHOICE

Vaccination is a weapon against disease however, we must assure that vaccines are not rendered a weapon against children by being laced with unnatural to human biology chemicals. We need to assure that vaccines are as safe as possible and unfortunately, that is not the case. There are chemicals in vaccines that are not health beneficial, it is actually health detrimental; these chemicals of harm are in vaccines because it makes more profit. The debate over vaccines causing Autism still is raging on and many hard-streamed vaccination advocates look the other way in order, to assure vaccination compliance. This book gives compelling reasons why injecting unnatural to the body vaccine chemicals are the main cause of Autism. Vaccines can be commanded to be much safer. Reading the contents of this book will help you protect yourself and your offspring from vaccine chemicalization harm. We can and must make vaccines safer; our Right to protect our children and our liberty to litigate for damages caused from vaccinations is required. We must act to secure safety!

The very foundation of parenting is undermined by not being free to refuse vaccinations and children are suffering for it. Parents cannot be expected to allow a vaccination that is an unnatural chemicalization of the blood or if they determine AUTISM may result, despite their being a law to the contrary. Mandated vaccinations are the unauthorized chemicalization of children; it is CHILD ABUSE on a mass scale. My first book, Sting of the Medical Mosquito, 2006, warned, that injected vaccine chemicals was a likely cause of Autism. That book called for the removal of Thimerosal, a mercury derivative preservative and known neuro-toxin, from ALL vaccine production. However, ALL unnatural to the body chemicals must be removed to stop the Autism epidemic. My books stress how important it is for vaccinations to be based upon PARENTAL informed consent/DENIAL, parental freedom and/or parent's prerogative. It is a grave injustice for parents to be enforced to vaccinate. Parents need to be free to protect children from chemicalizations.

Vaccine producers were forced, ridiculed into producing childhood vaccines with LESS mercury however; there remains a host of negative to health chemicals. To end the Autism epidemic, we must remove these chemicals. The united uproar over thimerosal prompted only its partial removal; it is vital to remove all mercury and all other anti-health chemicals. Freedom to protect your children from unwanted chemicalization is imperative to this goal. Empowering parents with liberty to refuse unwanted vaccine chemicals is essential.

A baby today receives more vaccinations by 6 months than the baby's mother did by the time she graduated high school; the chemical exposure is far too great. How many vaccinations or rather, how many injected unnatural to human biology chemicalizations can your baby withstand before abnormality and/or autism is spawned? Chemicals cause Asthma, hyper reactivity, kidney problems and AUTISM, to name a few. Nature's innate intelligence fights off disease and Mother's milk supplements immunity, as an infants' immune system develops; it is very unhealthy to be exposed to vaccine chemicals during this development. Children' best fight off diseases, if they are not vaccine chemically compromised. There must be liberty to not be chemically exposed. In order for vaccinations to be depleted of unwanted chemicals, vaccinations must be based on informed choice, be volitional and Vaccine Producers need to be liable for vaccine injury.

There are TWO STEPS OF CORRECTION required to end the Autism epidemic, which are fully explained in this book. These STEPS will stop vaccination enslavement and GET THE HARMFUL CHEMICALS OUT OF VACCINES. This book reveals how exposure to unnatural to the body chemicals are destroying children's health and how the Autism epidemic will continue until all mercury and anti-health chemicals are removed from childhood

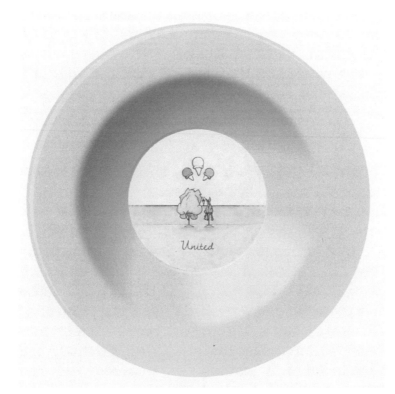

United

Only good can come from making SAFER vaccines so, let us be UNITED to do so.

vaccines. Anti-health chemicals in vaccines serve no health purpose in fact; they cause health problems and exacerbate human weakness. Health status is primarily a matter of chemistry. Once injected with the present state of chemical vaccines; the normal or pure internal chemistry is no longer possible, optimum health is made impossible and Autism becomes much more probable. Vaccine Chemical infiltrations DENATURES children's vital chemistry. Healthcare freedom and/or parental control are essential to prevent unwanted chemical infiltrations. PEOPLE HAVE A RIGHT TO CHEMICAL STABILITY and to remain natural. **ABOLISH VACCINATION SLAVERY** and you stop the mass chemical doping of brain cells and the Autism epidemic will decline.

Vaccinations may be of benefit but have risks and inherent dangers therefore, we must be **FREE** to decide. To mandate vaccination is ludicrous; it perpetuates unhealthy, chemically laden vaccines. Vaccines were once considered by the majority of people to be a panacea and a must however; since the contents of vaccines have slowly become corrupted and are now tainted with chemicals; their injection has become very questionable and intolerable. It is much wiser to vaccinate with vaccines that do not upset the normal chemistry of the body. We must take the necessary steps to purify our children's vaccine supply; **GET THE CHEMICALS OUT.** There are only health positives to be gained by not exposing children to many of the chemicals now found in vaccines. Our children's vaccine supply and/or their production should have the highest level of quality control to assure our children's safety. The chemicals in children dictate optimum health or you are plagued with problems, such as, Autism. We live upside-down if we think injecting children with the present quality of vaccines is health beneficial. The STEPS in this book applied to vaccines and the vaccination delivery system will achieve vaccine chemical quality, our children's safety and establish parental protection of children.

Parents must always be free to question if a vaccine is safe to inject and refuse any chemical injections that they think is dangerous or not in their children's best interest. Parents should be very concerned and cautious about one size fits all, mass medical intervention, such as, vaccination chemicalization by injection or medical intervention that is prescribed for everyone across the board. People do not trust enforced medical intervention especially, since huge profits are being generated from its enforcement. Vaccinations that are enforced upon everyone and has it that everyone gets the same dosage, and all must withstand multiple chemical injections regardless of age, gender, maturity, and health status or health history, are valid reasons to be very leery, very cautious and to refuse the injection. For children to all receive the same vaccine injection is counter productive to health and is not the good standard practice of medicine. Parents should be very leery or rather extremely alarmed about any mandated medical intervention especially, if it is enforced upon children despite parent's objections or desire to refuse the injection for safety reasons. A one dosage size and enforced chemicalization is not the good standard of healthcare in fact, it is the improper practice of medicine and its delivery must be considered negligent. **AUTISM** is an epidemic because of vaccine chemicalization.

The contents of vaccines have chemicals in them that really should not be injected. It is really the worst catch 22, parents are between a rock and a hard place; they would love to protect their children with vaccinations but know to do so exposes them to harmful chemicals. Vaccinations were one of man's greatest gifts to man however, it has become big business, they have ruined the benefit to man by putting chemicals in vaccines for profit not safety; they have commercialized vaccinations to the point of over utilization and/ or to many vaccinations and have made being vaccinated unsafe. It has become a wolf in sheep's clothing. Dirty vaccines can cause **CHEMICALIZATION AUTISM** and cause major health problems. Parents are desperate to take control to prevent injury; the vaccination mandates are extremely disruptive to basic parental protection of children.

Vaccinations are far from being "absolutely safe" as was repeatedly told to the lawmakers when lawmakers contemplated mandating the supposedly "absolutely safe" vaccinations therefore, one is accurate to be leery about laws that were mandated under false pretenses or falsehoods. Vaccinations were only meant to be temporarily mandated during the emergency circumstances of an actual epidemic; we must not live under a permanent emergency state. Unjustly and illegally, vaccinations are mandated forever, in apparent perpetuity, and invasively continue during non-emergency, non-epidemic times.

The fact that vaccinations are a one size fits all intervention and not properly individualized or personalized or that the vaccine chemical content are not geared to the patient's individual intrinsic needs or health circumstances makes mandated vaccinations that much more problematic. Vaccinations administered under such circumstances are an act of negligence. Mandating vaccinations is unjust and menacing to a child's optimum health. Be leery, be wise and be in control of your child's healthcare; demand informed consent/Denial of vaccinations. Every free American must have the right to pursue chemical perfection and prevent unwanted chemical internal upheaval. Parents shall be vested with the Right to self-regulate their child's healthcare. Parents have nothing but love for their children and that is why they are perfectly situated to make the best vaccination decision. Parents are passionate about not exposing their children to chemicals. Preventing chemicalization is the primary directive of parenting not government. Government must not macro or micro regulate personal healthcare.

More and more parents have become logic stricken and now recognize that the injecting and/or exposing of children to chemicals that are not natural or utilized by the body promotes disease, unhealthy children and chemical chaos within. Autism can be a vaccine chemical injection away. We must take the needed STEPS to correct what is wrong with vaccine safety. This book details the TWO STEPS OF CORRECTION needed to abolish vaccination slavery and put an end to the Autism epidemic. Producers of vaccines must be induced to disengage from using anti-health chemicals and we must reestablish the rule of law that dictates that parents REMAIN IN CONTROL, through informed consent/DENIAL of their children's healthcare decisions or healthcare destiny. Vaccine chemical exposure is a danger that parents must be free to protect their children from and in so doing vaccine quality increases and it will become safer for children to receive vaccine injections. Parents require the liberty to concentrate on not exposing their children to unwanted chemicals, that is where the health pay-off is and that is where children's best interest is served. Parents have the highest degree of protection of their children; they distinguish between what is right and wrong for their children.

Present day Injections of vaccine chemicals destabilize the body's chemical homeostasis, throwing the sensitive bloodstream chemical balance into disarray. Parents have to deal with all manner of health issues subsequent to their children being exposed to vaccine chemicals. Excellent health IS RENDERED IMPOSSIBLE and/or the complex systems of the body that are dependent upon proper chemical reactions are compromised. Bio-physical crisis and the dreaded AUTISM result from this lost normal chemical body laboratory. It is a real sobering thought to realize that the mandated vaccination law is enforcing chemical exposure upon children. The insanity of exposing children to all kinds of anti-health chemical inoculations must stop. The People must no longer be enforced by erroneous law to bastardize or compromise their internal chemistry; free citizens must have control of their healthcare and always remain masters of their own internal chemical laboratory. Mandated vaccination law enslaves us to be penetrated by needle and injected with vaccine chemicals. It treats those who do not want to be vaccinated as subhuman, it dehumanizes people to submit against their will for enforced chemical infiltrations; the very essence of freedom is lost because of it. Do not abide the injustice of enforcing unwanted chemical injections; it is an injustice not to be tolerated. Lobbyists have enslaved us to vaccinate; we must ABOLISH VACCINATION SLAVERY and be FREE to protect our children.

Parents have the natural Right and obligation to protect and support their children to the best of their ability. Parents need to be free to do all the right things to protect their children. Parents require the liberty to perform their parenting to the best of their ability. Children require their parent's protection be unhampered or interfered with by law. The People require and their children's survival necessitate that parents be free to be in control of their children's healthcare and/or whether or not vaccine chemicals will be allowed to enter children. In order for children to reach their unlimited potential parents must assure children's chemical perfect balance and thrive to do so. Parents, for the benefit of their perfectly healthy children, must be empowered to prevent any unwanted medical intervention including, but not limited to, vaccine chemical injections. Parents need to take what they think are the necessary steps or preventions to stop the possibility of Autism. All, not just select, adverse events from vaccinations should be required to be given to parents.

It is not a mistake for parents to protect children's natural or perfect chemistry; parents are just mistaken to not protect it. Children's vaccination decisions need to strictly be the territory of parents; parents must determine if vaccine chemical injections are safe and if they are in their children's best interest, instead of government. Families and/or parents and their children must be allowed to be and remain self-organized and self-regulating in reference to their healthcare. Children's health and/or survival are parent's primary concern and the injection of chemicals into their children's blood chemistry is monumental this fundamental parenting concern. The parenting dynamic and equilibrium cannot coexist with a mandated vaccination law. We must not abide by this injustice.

By NATURAL LAW we are endowed to control our very own health or decide if any chemicals will or WILL NOT enter our bloodstreams or that of our children's bloodstreams. A federal or State vaccination mandate is crippling. Mandated vaccination law has perverted what is good and natural, in that it replaces parents, with distant, uncaring, government to decide what vaccine chemicals are to be injected. It is biological and socially accepted that parents be in control of their children and have the Right to protect their children. It is understood by every free minded American that individual's self-govern over their very own being and/or healthcare and that of their children. The decision of whether a chemical vaccine will or will not be injected must legally be for the individual to decide and for the parents of the non-adults. A law is not law if it egregiously violates individual's Rights or health or natural biology. If vaccines have even the slightest capacity to cause harm then vaccinations must not be mandated; law cannot demand self-destruction of one's health. The very essence of freedom is lost and/or violated by enforced vaccinations and the primary quality control for safe vaccines is thrown out the window. The time to act to stop children from being chemically exposed and harmed is long overdue. CLEANING-UP VACCINES IS THE PRIORITY IN PREVENTING AUTISM; ending vaccination SLAVERY AND HOLDING Vaccine Producers LIABLE will do just that.

The seeds that have spawned the Autism Epidemic are the anti-health chemicals of vaccines. Vaccine anti-health chemicals are implanted into the brain cells of children through systematic repetitive vaccinations. Vaccine chemicals injected into children's musculature rapidly penetrate the blood and brain cells; seeding children's brains with the stumbling blocks of health and implanting the building blocks of Autism. The dangerous chemicals you're exposed to when you receive a vaccination are revealed in this book. We must free the People from the oppression of enforced vaccinations and safeguard children's health by seeing to it that vaccines do not harbor negative to health chemicals. There are TWO STEPS OF CORRECTION to end the Autism Epidemic and curtail the needless suffering. The problem of vaccine quality control and the main etiology of Autism will be eradicated once the TWO STEPS detailed in this book are accomplished. There is no neuroanatomic defect when it comes to Autism; it is a chemicalization problem. The etiology of Autism is the destruction of one's pure chemistry, creating biological root disturbances. Vaccine chemical infiltrations are the Autism disorder origins and main etiology of the Autism epidemic. Freedom expressed will save our children from Autism.

The vaccination program has been grossly compromised. Whatever aid to health that vaccination might offer has been severely handicapped and the bad from vaccine chemical exposure now outweighs potential benefit from unsafe vaccines. Children and their families are being harmed by unsafe vaccine production and a mandated vaccination system that promotes less vaccine quality control instead of more. The impurity of vaccines, the anti-health agents that have unfortunately found their way into vaccines have rendered vaccines dangerous. Receiving a vaccination can be health-shattering; vaccines have anti-health chemicals. Hindrances to vaccine quality control should not be permitted and parental Rights must never be ignored. Children should not be exposed to anti-health chemicals; their normal internal chemistry must be safeguarded and properly maintained. Health and sickness are both chemically dependent; everything is chemically related. Parents are properly concerned about the chemicals which their children might be exposed to especially, the chemicals that might be injected. Assuring that vaccines have no anti-health chemicals is paramount. The risks must be minimized, and parents must be free to protect their children efficiently and effectively from chemical injection exposure.

Apathy and/or inactive parental protection have helped degrade the vaccine quality control to the crisis we now are facing. **Parents must be extremely cautious when it comes to injecting chemicals into their children and extra careful not to allow chemicals to enter the vat of their children's blood chemistry that are not natural to that chemistry. Unwanted vaccine chemical injections do violence to those that want to refuse them. Mandated vaccinations violate people in several ways, they alter one's internal chemical integrity and violate one's Right to be left alone and/or the Right to self-regulate what enters one's body. Having no legal ability to refuse unwanted vaccine chemical injections that enter one's internal being is full spectrum dominance over the vaccination recipient and is nothing less than vaccination**

slavery. Making vaccinations mandatory has severely placed unprecedented limits upon parents' ability to protect their children, even if the parents conclude that the vaccine chemicals pose too great of a danger to be injected. It is rather profane that parents voluntarily stand by with no legal ability to protect their children from vaccine chemical exposure or are lulled by an unconscionable vaccination mandate to submit their children for unwanted chemical injections. **Mal-law, which disengages parenting, is an immoral law.**

Follow the money and you will discover why we are enslaved to vaccinate. Who benefits the most financially by keeping vaccinations mandated points to the culprit of our enslavement to be vaccinated and to the orchestrators of AUTISM epidemic? Vaccine Producers and/or Drug/chemical Companies have created a maniac money making market by enslaving our children to be vaccinated. There extreme efforts to enslave children and keep our children enslaved to be vaccinated severely undermine parent's supreme Right and obligation to protect their children from unwanted chemical infiltrations. The vaccine industry will act to suppress anything that might decrease their ability to mega-profit. They have created a monopoly of influence to keep us vaccination slaves. They have spent untold millions to fix our habits of responses to accept mandated/enforced vaccinations.

It is chemical madness and vaccination enslavement to have no legal power to refuse vaccine chemical injections. Lobbyist over influencing law-makers to mandate vaccinations, medical doctors only receiving a single limited course in nutrition to assure doctors are inappropriately geared toward drug prescribing and not natural more conservative means of treating patients, and all the constant commercials that program us into drug taking, have turned us into enslaved robots who to blindly accept the chemicals they profit from and who no longer think independently. This is not democracy; this is corporatocracy gone wild to enslave us for profit. The government, which was meant to serve and protect us, has been hijacked by corporate America. Mandated vaccination laws are the design of vaccine industry's puppet government, under a façade of legality. We are not free to protect our children under this mandated vaccination ENSLAVEMENT mal-law.

Parents must be free to question everything about vaccinations and be empowered to deny an unwanted vaccine chemical injection for their children. We stand at a crossroad, we unwisely can continue to do nothing, allowing the take over of our parental protection Rights of our children, standing idle while government and the pharmaceutical chemical industry unnaturally control whether or not our children are injected, or we can act to protect our children by implementing the TWO STEPS OF CORRECTIION detailed in this book. Doing nothing has already lead to the current vaccine quality crisis and the health demise of our children. The delicate balance of children's blood chemistry must be under parental control and not under governmental control, regulation or rule. We can take back what is naturally ours to have and control; our children and/or the decision as to whether the chemicals of vaccines are really safe or are actually too dangerous to inject. Parents are the primary and supreme protectors of their children; vaccinations must be allowed to be refused. Release parents' protection of children and health will take care of itself.

It is cognitive dissidence and reduction in absurdum to continue along the same unhealthy path of injecting chemicals into the immature and chemically sensitive bloodstreams of

children. It is willful ignorance to mandate injection of anti-health chemicals. Exposing children to the onslaught of multiple vaccine chemical injections has headed our children into uncharted unhealthy territory. Of course, parents are and should be concerned about what chemicals are affecting or infiltrating and causing autism. Make no mistake: unnatural to the body vaccine chemicals play a major role in poisoning your baby's, infant's and children's once perfect blood chemistry. The fact that they inject chemicals that are in vaccines which, have no health benefit has become of major and utmost concern to parents. The People do not want their children's vaccines tainted with chemicals that are unnatural to fast growing, maturing fragile chemically perfect bodies. No chemical or vaccine must be coerced or forced; parents must be free to protect their children from conceived of chemical dangers.

We must act to make vaccines clean and end the degradation, of our children's health and that of our Rights. We must initiate the **TWO STEPS** detailed in this book to prevent unnecessary suffering and to restore our Rights. The improper vaccination mandate makes parents spineless, it has taken the very backbone out of parenting; making it incapable for parents to prevent children from being chemically exposed by vaccine chemicals. It causes multitudes of heartaches when people are dominated to inject or when children are injured. No longer should the vaccination erroneous law sever parent's protection of their children. Vaccine industry's puppet government, under a façade of legality, dominates us; makes us **vaccination SLAVES**. Parents must be in control of children's welfare and that control empowers you to refuse unwanted, conceived of too dangerous to inject vaccine chemicals. To be chemically infused by vaccination is no slight detour; too many children are caused **AUTISM**.

To not have your healthcare under self-control is so wrong that it must be made right. It is of core value to decide upon your own healthcare. For government to command parents to submit their children for vaccinations is outlandish. People have become logic stricken; determining many of the chemicals in vaccines are much too unhealthy to inject. **Vaccine chemicals are not indigenous to the natural chemistry of the body; they pose an ominous danger to children.** We must be free to deny chemicalizations. Law commanding you to submit your children for unwanted vaccinations is cruel and unjust. Enforcing exposure to anti-health vaccine chemicals is beyond what government can ask of citizens. Citizens require the common decency and respect of their healthcare decision, we must not be enforced to inject; to do so enslaves us. Parents do not want to be enslaved to vaccinate their children; they want liberty. It is improper law, illegal and unjust law that mandates vaccinations. **The TWO STEPS OF CORRECTION of this book will terminate being mastered over and enslaved to vaccinate. ABOLISH VACCINATION SLAVERY AND YOU END THE AUTISM EPIDEMIC.**

Parental freedom to protect children from unwanted medical intervention and/or unwanted vaccine chemical exposure must win over medical tyranny and/or mandated vaccination slavery. Your perfectly healthy children are for you to protect; government must not overpower parent's decisions. Government must not violate the sanctity of your privacy and/or your parental decisions. Healthcare freedom is an essential; it must be vigorously safeguarded. Police Power of the State is limited; it goes beyond its authority, permanently dictating that children must be vaccinated and often against parent's will. Moreover, government must not demand citizens to inject chemicals into their children. Parents recognize that the vaccine chemicals can cause their children side-effects or injury or Autism. Parent's

primary directive of protecting their children cannot be set aside by law, for to do so, the law would be erroneous, and parents and their children would be violated by such, mal-law. Mandated vaccination law, better known as vaccination enslavement law, is erroneous law come to fruition. The People must act to correct this injustice. It is high time for parents to take back their power and be properly empowered to protect their children the way they were meant to and to the best of their ability.

Parents would be remiss to allow chemicals to enter their children that are not harmonious with health. Parents' protecting their children from vaccine chemical exposure is about as basic to proper parenting as parenting can get. To be forbidden to refuse injections of vaccine chemicals is opposite the good standard of parenting and deflates and/or eliminates parent's primary directive of protecting their children. The mandated vaccination law enforces the piercing of skin with needle and injecting of chemicals. We must restore the blessings of liberty to ourselves and our posterity with freedom to refuse vaccination. Freedom to refuse the unwanted medical intervention of vaccination is required to assure safer vaccines. It is a most basic freedom to decide what goes into our bodies; we need the TWO STEPS OF CORRECTION to secure this freedom.

Government commanding healthcare is destined for problems. Government has major difficulty in doing what it was meant to do let alone what is vested for parents to do. Government is constantly making mistakes and it extremely slow and/or incompetent in recognizing and correcting its mistakes. Thomas Jefferson said, "If the people let the government decide what foods they eat and what MEDICINES THEY TAKE, their bodies will soon be in as sorry a state as are the souls who live under TRYANNY." Autism is a result of living under the tyranny of mandated vaccinations. Thomas Jefferson would stand for not mandating vaccinations; he would recognize it as tyranny and the demise of our basic freedom of healthcare choice and the eventual degradation of our health. The reason why vaccines are in a sorry state is because they are mandated, and Vaccine Producers cannot be held accountable and liable when their vaccines induce injury. The AUTISM EPIDEMIC is a result of tyrannical enslavement of our children to be vaccinated. The mandated vaccination enslavement law plunders parent's protection of their children. Parent's primary directive to keep their children out of harms way has been compromised.

Mandated vaccination is government out of control, controlling what WE THE PEOPLE must be in control of. The People have a Right to decide their healthcare. Mandated vaccinations function autonomously, with no accountability to the people. There power over us is unchecked while the People's powers, vested by our Rights, are being nullified. The Right to decide healthcare is supreme. The FDA sensors and suppresses natural healthcare and health ingenuity that cannot be patented or profited from; they are toothless when it comes to vaccines/drugs. Freedom in healthcare is under siege; there is enslavement to vaccinations. We require control of our internal chemistry. We must not be dictated to in the sacrosanct area of our internal chemistry. Be FREE to reject, injections.

The main etiology of Autism is vaccine chemicalization. The normal chemistry of the body is altered by the chemicals of vaccines. Normal chemistry promotes good health and prevents most, if not all, disease. If you want to safeguard against Autism and cancer do not inject the obvious anti-health chemicals of vaccines. Seniors in their 70's or 80's state, "only old people got cancer; not children". We are chemically poisoning our children. There must be unfettered freedom for every parent to strive for the living chemical geometries or chemical coherences of health. Control your chemistry; health is dependent upon the right chemistry. Children must not be injected against their parent's will. Vaccination enslavement must end. Parents must control the vaccination decisions.

The mandated vaccination mal-law is a theft of parenting and/or the parental protection of children. For Vaccine Producers to claim that children are not injured by the chemicals of vaccines or that no harmful chemicals are in vaccines is willful ignorance and an affront on intelligence. People must be enabled to practice the healthcare that they think is best. Patriotism does not mean not asking questions or remaining silent when government misappropriates what yours is rightfully or wrongfully commands you to submit for healthcare that you do not want. Patriotism means protecting freedom or the very idea of liberty. A patriot takes a stand for the American way of life and will not acquiesce to what does violence to their Rights or what subverts or controverts the meaning of the supreme law of the land, our Constitution. Free People can sift through the pros and cons of vaccinations; they can decide if it is in their children's best interest. What special interest groups conjure is good for all is most likely not good for you. Drug lobbyists dictate to government to mandate vaccination. **Be FREE** to follow what you think is best; decide if vaccines are worth injecting. **Be FREE** to reject injections.

There is no history of parent population neglecting their children's vaccination verses best health interest and yet parents have been stricken from deciding what is in their children's best vaccination healthcare interest. **No blameless parent should be denied the direction of their children's vaccinations. Parents are baffled why they have been cast out, stripped of their seated power of control over their children's welfare**. There is no evidence that even a small number of parents are neglecting their children's welfare therefore, government has no valid reason to make healthcare decisions that parent's normally and traditionally make. **There is no need for government to intrude and command what parents are not negligent in doing.** It is the general rule in healthcare that parents control their children's healthcare. Government continues to mandate vaccinations because of pharmaceutical lobbying. **Drug manufacturers use government as their puppet to assure their vaccines are mandated; an endless supply of children to needle for endless profiteering. We need optimum chemical biological coherence and we must be free to pursue it. We must have freedom to reject injections and in that liberty of healthcare decision have strength in being obedient to keeping one's children's internal chemistry free of unnatural to human biology chemicalization. Being obedient to purity of blood chemistry keeps your children healthy and safe from Autism.**

CHAPTER 2

TWO STEPS OF CORRECTION

TWO STEPS OF CORRECTION can end the systematic chemical doping of children's brains and STOP the Autism epidemic. Children's welfare needs to be protected with basic parental informed consent/DENIAL of vaccinations and negligence law must be properly applied to vaccinations. The TWO STEPS OF CORRECTION are the solution to the Autism epidemic and vaccine safety crisis; it will repower parent's parenting authority to best protect children from AUTISM. Chemicalization of children's blood is extremely, dangerous and disruptive to health.

STEP ONE: Demand your informed consent and/or INFORMED DENIAL of any proposed vaccination. This Self-Preservation Right in healthcare allows you to self-govern what if any medical intervention will be permitted. Informed consent doctrine is a legal concept that demands that you be informed, educated about the pros and cons of the vaccination and thereby, alerting you about the contents in the vaccine, including but not limited to all of the CHEMICALS in vaccines; it ultimately requires you the patient to determine whether or not the vaccination will be given. STEP ONE requires there be 100% volitional permission from parents for a vaccine to be administered and this will control if a vaccination will or will not be delivered. This will prompt vaccine producers to produce vaccines that parents will be more likely to approve of; which are vaccines without potentially harmful chemicals. By making vaccinations strictly a matter of PARENTAL INFORMED consent/DENIAL, the vaccine industry will NOW have to satisfy parental safety requirements and thereby, prompt the elimination of unnatural to the body chemicals in vaccines. Normally concerned parents or rational thinking people do not want anti-health agents or chemicals in vaccines. Parents will likely not give consent for suspect and/or chemically laced vaccine injections whereas; parents will be more rational to give their consent to vaccines that have no unnatural to the body vaccine chemicals thus, bolstering compliance. Vaccination will rightfully only be given with PARENTAL REPRESENTATION and TRUE PERMISSION. Vaccinations based upon informed consent or DENIAL will GET THE UWANTED CHEMICALS OUT of vaccines and end the pernicious system of healthcare liberty oppression thereby, instilling SAFER vaccines.

STEP TWO: As is the universal and traditional rule of law dictates, there must be freedom to litigate against the negligent party. Before considering vaccination make sure you can litigate directly against the Vaccine Manufacturer in the unfortunate event that the vaccine chemical injection causes injury; making absolutely sure you can seek damages against the very source of your child's vaccine induced injury if it occurs. Prior to you agreeing to allow the vaccination of your child assure being able to seek compensation from the actual maker of the vaccine if any injury occurs otherwise, you are defenseless. This will instill a need for greater vaccine quality control in the producers of vaccines, further prompting them to **GET THE CHEMICALS OUT.** This traditional liberty of lawsuit will rightfully establish that vaccine companies defend and pay for their vaccine production negligence; the wrongful use of tax dollars to pay for vaccine production negligence will stop. STEP TWO ends the improper and unwise protection of Vaccine Producers; no longer will the big business of vaccines be impervious to the results of its own negligent vaccine production, negligence will no longer be protected or promoted. The safety of our children and the Rights of the People will now come first, trumping the mega-lobbying efforts or over influence of Vaccine Producers. The unfair and unwise protection of Vaccine Producers and the wrongful profiteering from any negligent vaccine production will end. Vaccine producers or the big business of vaccines will not be permitted to hide behind bargained for inequitable legislation or induced government covered negligence. Moreover, this step will wisely, prompt vaccine manufacturers to produce safer vaccines that are not laced with chemicals for strictly profit and not safety. Manufacturers' will begin to produce vaccines that are not prone to cause injury or bear the burden of consequential negligence litigation and pay out compensation to the vaccine injured. Children's best interest will be secured instead, of vaccine profiteering!

Expose the Vaccine Producers to vaccine induced injury lawsuits and our children will no longer be exposed to anti-health, harmful chemicals that have been found in vaccines. The alien to the body chemicals, anti-health agents, found in vaccines make vaccines dirty; making vaccines dangerous. Vaccine Producers need a carrot and stick approach to assure vaccines are safe; greater sales if vaccines are safe and litigation and resultant expense when vaccines are not safe. Just as the threat of a speeding ticket acts as a major deterrent not to speed, the defending of litigation and paying out of awards due to vaccine induced injuries will act as major deterrents, inducing or promoting safer vaccines and/or an important reason to be more safety vigilant. This will prompt producers of vaccines not to use harmful chemicals in their vaccines. We need more deterrents not less, to assure children have safe vaccines or are not exposed to or injected with, unnatural to the body chemicals. To not grant parents the right to refuse vaccinations or give Vaccine Producers a liability shield is the reckless endangerment of children! To mandate vaccination or not punish negligent vaccine production results in mandated mass child abuse and/or the exposure of children to unnatural to the body chemicals.

There are two primary purposes for posing lawsuits or litigating against manufacturers for their negligence or production of negligent products which cause injury. One purpose is to attempt to compensate the person who received an injury due to the negligence. The other reason is to punish the negligent manufacturer enough that they cease and desist in being negligent. This assures that the company's future production is safe. Sometimes very large awards, known as treble damages are given to the injured party to not only compensate the victim but rather, to send a strong message not to consciously produce products negligently. In the case of anti-health chemically laced vaccines a treble damage award to the injured party sends the right message, a needed message that this type of malfeasance and/or gross negligence will not be tolerated and will be severely punished if it occurs. Children's welfare can be severely, negatively impacted by negligently produced vaccines therefore, treble damages should be applied. The possibility of litigation and paying out damage awards will instill Vaccine Producers not to place anti-health chemicals in vaccines. Being allowed to litigate against producers of bad vaccines means the prevention of future bad vaccines. Litigation against Vaccine Producers must be allowed, and parents must be free to refuse vaccinations that they conceive as too dangerous or are not determined safe; to do otherwise is sheer lunacy!

Vaccine Producers whom produce a harmful vaccine and/or vaccine with anti-health chemicals need strong deterrents otherwise, poor vaccine production remains a threat. Because Vaccine Producers hold our children's health in their profit minded hands they must be made to suffer majorly when their vaccines cause injury. Right now, they do not suffer at all; Vaccine Producers must at minimum be made to reasonably suffer if they produce vaccines with harmful chemicals. Vaccine Producers should be freely litigated against by the public, without undue burden, cost or procedure. When parents claim their children were injured by a vaccine it should not be so difficult or next to impossible to litigate against the producers of injurious vaccines. The concept and theory behind vaccinations is to supposedly grant the vaccination recipient some level of immunity it is not to grant Vaccine Producers certain immunity from litigation. Vaccine Producers of negligently manufactured, chemically laced vaccines have for all intensive purposes an absolute immunity from being sued and not held liable for their negligence. Vaccine Producers must not be immune for it is counter intuitive or counter-productive to vaccine quality control/safety and terribly unjust to do so. Unwarranted liability immunity for Drug Companies means needless injuries will continue. Parents are disarmed from preventing chemicalization of their children because of this liability shield and no informed consent/DENIAL. Protect your children with these TWO STEPS OF CORRECTION.

Parents of Autistic children who claim that their children were injured (caused Autism), by negligently produced chemically laced vaccines, must be entitled to have their day in court against those that are accuse of causing the injury, just like anyone that is injured by any other kind of negligent behavior can have their day in court. It is an injustice that Vaccine producers skirt their liability; it makes a mockery of the judicial system, undermines the legal system and treats those injured by vaccine prejudicially and/or inequitably. Vaccines impact children's lives it must be much easier to hold Vaccine Producers accountable; to have government pay for vaccine induced injuries is a tremendous distortion of accountability. Vaccine Producers need to worry; they need the hammer of negligence litigation in order to best secure a safer vaccine supply. Granting a liability shield is counter-productive to securing safe vaccines. THERE MUST BE NO LIABILITY SHIELD FOR PRODUCERS OF UNSAFE VACCINES; producers of chemically laced vaccines MUST NOT BE immune from liability lawsuits. Vaccine quality is reliant upon keeping Vaccine Producers vigilant about what they put in their vaccines; the possibility of litigation does just that, it enroots safety conscientiousness. A good standard of production, a safe vaccine production, is secured by traditionally holding negligent Vaccine Producers accountable and liable and by granting parents the ability to refuse unwanted vaccination. There must be no chemicals that mainly assure profit in vaccines such as, but not limited to the preservative mercury or aluminum etc.!

The multitudes claiming injury from the chemicals of vaccines must be permitted to seek 100% **LEGAL LIABILILITY REDRESS** against the producer of the claimed injurious vaccine; vaccine safety and children's health is at risk if we do otherwise. A liability shield undermines children's safety, the legal system and sense of fair play; it allows negligence to go on unpunished, promoting non-safety. The whole concept or purpose of negligence law is being thrown out the legal window by continuing to wrongfully grant Vaccine Producers their unprecedented liability shield. To not be free to seek damages against Vaccine Producers is a gross injustice. Tax dollars should not be spent footing the bill for the negligence of Vaccine Producers; Vaccine Producers must pay for their negligence. If the public were to become aware of this anti-safety total liability shield that Vaccine Producers carved out for its self-serving profiteering interest, the public would not put up with it; the public would think it insane to protect corporate profits instead, of children's welfare.

Our children's vaccine supply is in desperate need of allowing the highest of treble damage awards to assure that vaccines are produced with our children's safety first and foremost. Mere profiteering cannot come before children's best interest. The second purpose for being free to litigate against Vaccine Producers is to compensate the injured party that suffered because of the negligence and to allow the injured to seek retribution against the actual party that caused the injury. Without this ability to litigate against the causer of the injuries, the injured are frustrated and safety will take a back seat to profiting. Vaccine Producers must be adjudicated into submission to produce vaccines with safety first instead, of profit first. Parents must not be deterred from litigating against vaccine companies in order for the safety measure of taking the chemicals out of vaccines to be paramount and/or optimally prompted. Vaccinations are groundlessly enforced upon the public, not giving parents the common decency and major life responsibility of the well-being of their very own children. Vaccinations inexplicably stand as the only exception to the informed consent golden rule in healthcare. Mandated vaccinations unnecessarily, unjustly and disproportionately reduce children and their parents to vaccination slaves. Self-healthcare and/or self-determined healthcare is at risk.

Both **CORRECTIVE STEPS** are essential to clean-up vaccines and to secure parental protection of children. Both **STEPS** are required to best serve the health interest of all of our children and in so doing put an end to the Autism epidemic. Our children's welfare is far too important to leave their safety merely to the whim of profit minded Vaccine Producers and/or to happenstance. Vaccine Company's primary directive is to maximize profits, they currently have no down side in producing harmful vaccines that are laced with alien, foreign to the body chemicals or that parents fear and should mistrust. The vaccination mandate holds us captive to vaccinate and we basically have no recourse or can be recompensed when vaccines do injure our children. The companies must be prompted by parental potential refusal and by responsible liability. Their primary directive must be the production of vaccines that have no anti-health chemicals and/or harmful chemicals. Parents must be completely free to deny an unwanted vaccine injection and Vaccine Producers must be held liable otherwise, Vaccine Producers will continue doing what is not in the best interest of children. There is an overall distrust of the American people towards mandated vaccination enslavement laws and in the safety of vaccines. The overwhelming power of the truth, that health is reliant upon proper chemistry and that vaccines have unnatural to the body chemicals, is all one needs for one to become an activist of change for the better; the implementation of the **TWO STEPS OF CORRECTION.**

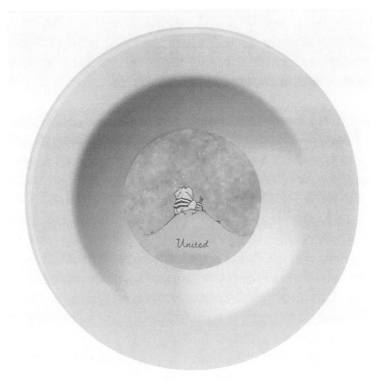

The achievement of **SAFER** vaccines is possible if we are **UNITED** to make it so.

Together, we must make vaccines safer, much safer than they presently are. The vaccine industry neither has the integrity or the capacity nor the predilection to make vaccine safety their priority. Remember, absolute power corrupts absolutely, therefore, it is imperative that Vaccine Producers not be in absolute control of vaccine contents; parents being the decision makers, as to whether, a vaccine is content safe enough for injection will safeguard children and prevent absolute power in Vaccine Producers. Unfortunately, we have been victims of those that have absolute power over our children's vaccine contents and consequently, we now face an Autism epidemic; parents must be the main reason for its ending. The pyramid of vaccination decision authority must be capped by non-other than parents of the children to be considered for vaccination. Parents will assure the safety of their children, always taking into consideration their children's best interest, as their highest priority and parents will see to it that vaccines do not harbor anti-health agents or harmful chemicals. Parents must be empowered to deny vaccinations.

Parents protecting their children from unwanted chemically laced vaccines and holding Vaccine Producers accountable and liable for the chemicals they place in vaccines will put an end to the Autism epidemic. Children's blood must no longer be denatured by the chemicals presently in vaccines. Children's brains are being infiltrated by chemicals that cause Autism and it up to parents to stop it. This book is about ending the Autism epidemic. United, parents by having the Right to refuse unwanted vaccinations will induce the responsible production of safer vaccines. The TWO STEPS OF CORRECTION will leave Vaccine Producers no choice but to produce vaccines in a toxin free way. Parents must be assured vaccines will not cause injury. There can be no limit placed upon parent's love of their children and/or limit on parent's protection of their children from harm. Logic stricken parents require proof that vaccinations do not injure and/or do not have anti-health chemicals. Before they even consider vaccinations, they need to be convinced it is safe. Demand that vaccinations strictly be voluntary and not enforced by law upon children. Parents are naturally skeptical about anything that is going to be injected into their children and by Right must be enabled to refuse chemicalization.

It is scarcely debatable that free people are entitled to decide just what is best for their body or healthcare and it is consonant with the highest idles of human dignity and the moral law of the universe. Parents deciding not to vaccinate because they have determined vaccine chemical injections pose a very real danger is justifiable and must not be annihilated by unjust and immoral law. We do not have to abide by immoral law or bad law that is contrary to the just law of the land. Unjust law is not law at all; the mandated vaccination law enslaves children to be vaccinated and unlawfully annihilates parent's protection of their children. Of all things we hold most sacred, is for parents to freely protect their children and to do so without government interference or permission. Government and/or Vaccine Producer's puppet government must be brought inline with life's supreme concept or controlling rule of law that the People must be in control and remain in control of their body, internal being, blood chemistry and that of their children's. They must know and act in accordance that no one can tell individuals what is right in this most private area; it is only for the individual to control their life and body; people must not be enforced to inject unwanted chemicals.

Law must not violate the protective requirements that treatment has to be directed by the doctor - - not the insurer or by government – and that THE PATIENT HOLDS THE DECISION POWER as to whether any proposed care will or will not be delivered. The patient is required to be in command over his or her body and/or healthcare and this health care safeguard is supported by the legal/health care delivery protective requirement known as informed consent and/or INFORMED DENIAL. You the patient hold the key to either unlock the door for health intervention, so it can be delivered or keeps the door locked; DENYING its delivery. This golden rule of self- determined healthcare protects the People from unwanted or tyrannical medical intervention and generates quality healthcare. Without the patient's ability to self-determine their own healthcare or being empowered to refuse unwanted intervention the quality of healthcare is quickly lost. The erroneous mandated vaccination law enforces vaccinations; not giving the People the common decency and SELF-PRESERVATION RIGHT TO REFUSE. The negative consequence of this bastardization of the healthcare tradition has degenerated vaccine quality, allowing unwanted CHEMICALS to be in children's vaccine supply; the main cause of CHEMICALIZATION AUTISM.

Health is reliant upon the proper chemical configuration within the body. Good health depends upon maintaining the right amount of natural to the body chemicals and assuring that no unnatural to the body chemicals find their way into the body. Keep your internal chemistry as pure as possible and you will be as healthy as possible. Parents are perfectly capable of deciding if a chemical is good or bad for their children. Chemicals that enter the body particularly, those chemicals injected into the body, can devastate health. The chemicals within resonate health or sickness. Exposure to chemicals that are not native or natural to the body or needed for proper function and development; the higher the probability of illness is. Let natural chemicals be your medicine and your medicine be natural chemicals. Fundamental to generating good health and proper development; you must not be exposed to chemicals that are not utilized by the body or that have propensity to degenerate health or cause harm. There are chemicals in vaccines that never should be injected. There are chemicals in vaccines that when injected are the main cause of Autism in children, Alzheimer's in adults and a host of health degeneration that comes with altering the normal chemistry. The natural chemical equilibrium or chemical ecosystem is rendered unhealthy by the injection of vaccine chemicals. GET THE CHEMICALS OUT of vaccine production and it safeguards the health of children and will prevent AUTISM.

Health and disease prevention are mainly about maintaining the proper chemistry within your body; vaccine chemicals disrupt the chemical harmony. You must enjoy the basic liberty to deny unwanted chemicals. You must be completely free to accept or not accept medical treatment chemicals. Chemicals that are not the natural flora of the body will cause health issues and be refused without legal or negative consequence. UNWANTED chemicals must not be injected. Whatever is disturbing the normal chemistry must be eliminated. Freedom to refuse unwanted chemical injection infiltrations is the freedom to be healthy and live undisturbed. The pursuit of chemical perfection or optimal chemical balance is a very reasonable goal. Mandated vaccinations are exploiting children's health, leaving the vaccine recipient no legal choice but to be exposed to the chemicals inherent in vaccines. We must resist the degradation of our children's blood from vaccine chemical exposure. Parents must regain their freedom to protect their very own children and/or direct their welfare; your children's survival depends on it. No one but you the parent holds your children's best interest at the highest priority and no one but you should have the decisive control or the ultimate decision power to accept or refuse healthcare particularly, vaccinations. Vaccines will become safer through parental liberty to refuse vaccines, children will be a lot less chemically exposed and autism will decline!

It is not necessary to render children's chemistry impure with injections of vaccine chemicals instead, let us act to clean-up vaccines by making them void of anti-health chemicals. Vaccine chemicals cause the brain/neurological system to not function normally. The fine-tuned chemical balance required for normal neurological function can be tipped too far when vaccine chemicals circulate into the brain. I call this "the vaccine paradox". The public is in a quandary, there is the theorized good that can come from being vaccinated and the definite bad from injecting vaccine chemicals. We need to purify the vaccine production and parents having the Right to refuse vaccinations in combination with holding Vaccine Producers liable for the chemicals that they place in vaccines will GET THE CHEMICALS OUT of vaccines. The entire concept of injecting vaccines is unnatural and must strictly be done with parental permission. Chemical vaccine exposure is a very real danger that parents must be able to avoid and/or refuse.

Parents cannot help but be parents. Parents must be free to be parents and, in that freedom, have the unfettered liberty to stop or prevent what they think are unhealthy injections or chemicalizations. Certainly, we must vest parents with the power to protect their children; fundamental to this power is to allow parents to decide if vaccines pose a danger for their children and/or are too toxic to inject into their children. The public expects government to allow parents the common decency to decide what is best for their own children and decide for themselves if the chemicals of vaccines are to dangerous to inject. These most reasonable expectations in our free minded society will assure vaccine quality, prevent unwanted vaccine chemical exposure and curtail runaway numbers of vaccinations. Parents require their basic freedom of healthcare decision for their children to protect them from unwanted chemical infiltrations. Comparatively, government is inept at protecting children; parents are naturally the best protectors and must be free to do so.

With Vaccine Producers being so unwisely and unfairly protected from viable lawsuits, involving children that have been injured by chemical vaccines and with vaccinations being illegally mandated, to be injected into children despite parent's objection, is it no wonder vaccine quality has dwindled. Is it any wonder Vaccine Producers are left only having to concentrate upon maximizing profits and not our children's best interest? Is it any wonder vaccines have chemicals in them that assure Vaccine Company profiteering instead of children's safety? Is it any wonder a vaccine related Autism epidemic has ensued? Is it any wonder that parents must take action? Trust that parents are the best at deciding if vaccinations are in their children's best interest. Do not leave your children's fate in the hands of strangers such as, puppet government or money hungry Vaccine Producers. When it comes to children parents do not make rapid fire decisions or decisions that take anything else but their children's welfare into consideration. Anything but parents deciding is a distortion of what is good for children. The family running the risk of problems from vaccination or the remote or unlikely consequence of complications from childhood disease for not vaccinating should determine if a vaccination is or is not to be given.

The FDA finally banned the use of BPA (plastic), also known as, Bisphenol A, in baby bottles and sipping cups; it waited much to long. Neurological development issues, cancer, obesity and thyroid problems have been linked to BPA. Here we can see how anti-health chemicals can be destructive; it has been discovered that BPA chemicals destroy health. This chemical upset indicates how chemically intolerant our health is. We really need to remove BPA chemicals from all our food packaging. The FDA has irresponsibly allowed BPA to remain in canned foods such as, canned soups, vegetables and fruits. If you want to assure the reduction of BPA exposure, it would be wise to only eat foods that are not canned. The FDA inaction and its failure to alert the public, tell Parents that they are best protecting their own children and are wise to protect their own children from chemical exposure. Although, our bodies have a chance, through digestion and elimination processes, to rid the body of BPA to some degree, you should avoid BPA. BPA (plastics) is a contributing cause of Autism. Vaccine chemical exposure is more unhealthy because it is injected, a direct hit; its chemicals pass thru the blood-brain barrier and penetrate brain cells.

PROTECT YOUR CHILDREN FROM VACCINE CHEMICAL EXPOSURE. The protective system has been corrupted and is broken, for it will not protect your children from chemical exposure in fact; the erroneous vaccination mandate law sees to it that children are exposed to vaccine chemicals. Parents must demand their parental protection Rights for their children. Parents must see to it that their children are not exposed to vaccine chemicals and demand that if their children are injured by chemical vaccine injection exposure that they can seek damages against the Vaccine Producer. Vaccine chemicals pose the greatest hazard in that they are injected directly into the bloodstream to take their toxic toll. We are dependent upon a chemical balance or proper normal chemistry to be healthy; vaccines disrupt the needed normal chemistry of the blood, the BRAIN and the body. INFORMED DENIAL OF VACCINES IS FREEDOM TO REFUSE CHEMICAL EXPOSURE AND THIS IS ESSENTIAL FOR SAFETY. Parents and freedom minded individuals need to come together in a critical mass action to prevent children from suffering a vaccination resultant critical mass syndrome and/or Autism by seeing to it that the TWO STEPS OF CORRECTION implemented.

We are being exposed to untold amounts of toxic chemicals from all kinds of sources. Whenever, you manipulate the natural chemistry of the blood it will tend to cause health problems. Chemicals injected directly into children's bloodstreams ARE THE MOST DANGEROUS TYPE OF CHEMICAL EXPOSURE. Vaccine Producers are hell bent on pumping and dumping our children's bloodstreams with their vaccine chemicals. Parent's authority to decide not to expose their children to vaccine chemical injections is commonsensical; parents must be free to be parents. Government must NOT prevent parents from protecting children; parents need to maintain consciousness protection of their children from chemicals. The mandated vaccination law is for the benefit of Vaccine Producers and not children ; it is not fair or square. It was enacted by Vaccine Producer's puppet government.

Chemical toxins cause sickness. Parents need to be free to prevent unwanted vaccine chemical injections. Making vaccines that have no unnatural to the body chemicals or unwanted chemicals is paramount. The chemical broth which promotes health is the chemicals that are natural to the body; they are the building blocks of optimum health and needed by the body. Many vaccine chemicals are stumbling blocks of health. It must be an absolute rule not to produce vaccines with anti-health chemicals. We cannot live free of harmful chemical contact because of vaccination law mandates injections. It is most reasonable to save your children from chemical exposure. Informed consent/DENIAL is the shield which, defends our children from unsafe vaccines and being freely enabled to litigate against Vaccine Producers is the offensive spear, the instrument for punishing those that produce vaccines that harm our children; together they instill positive changes that assure safer vaccines and protection of our children. IT IS RECKLESS ENDANGERMENT TO NOT REQUIRE INFORMED CONSENT/DENIAL OF VACCINATIONS. It comes down to balance of power; apparently, Vaccine Producers have been putting what they want in vaccines; for far too long, to keep vaccine contents in check, parents need to be free to refuse unwanted vaccines; this will best keep children safe.

An in-depth, double blind study about Autism and vaccination was never done. There needs to be a study comparing the health status of those children who were not vaccinated to those children vaccinated. Compare the children's health history and/or health status. It is important that all the children were healthy at the time the children either did not receive the vaccination or did receive the vaccination and then begin to look for differences in health. The study would reveal that children who are healthy remain healthy if not vaccinated compared to those children vaccinated. I am not just talking about proximate in time to vaccination; the overall health status throughout the children's early years to teen years will be most revealing. The study should evaluate how many visits to the doctor, how many diagnoses were given, how many times antibiotics were prescribed, how many missed days of school and an analysis by parents of their children's energy, astuteness, ability to engage and overall health status. Is this not the most obvious study that needs to be done or released and ask yourself why it has not been done? Children exposed to chemicals especially, injected chemicals cannot be as resilient in health as children that were not chemically exposed; any chemist or doctor or parent will agree. An honest and properly performed study will evidence what is common sense; injected unnatural to human biology chemicals are the main etiology of Autism and health problems.

A free People must be armed with the Right to be informed about the contents and controversy inherent with being vaccinated; have sufficient arms and ammunition to maintain a status of independence from any who might attempt to abuse them with unwanted medical intervention, which include their own government. Being armed with informed consent/ DENIAL and having the ammunition of freedom to litigate directly against Vaccine Producers who cause children injury, are essential to maintaining the status of independence and/or the liberty to protect oneself and one's children. Parents must be free to reject injections as part of their main protective objective of children.

THE TWO STEPS OF CORRECTION ARE THE STEPS TO FREEDOM AND SAFER VACCINES. Parents should not have an uphill battle to protect their children. Vaccines that are recommended for injection must be devoid of chemicals that cause harm. If there is debate about the chemicals in vaccines causing health problems; it is always better to side on the side of caution and safety and/or safer vaccines. Whenever, children are not optimally healthy the first suspect should be the chemicals that children are exposed to especially, the chemicals that are injected. To ASSume vaccine chemicals, play no role or to make it the last suspect of causation is negligent and places children at risk. ABOLISH VACCINATION SLAVERY by ending vaccination mandates and the chemicalization crisis will stop; vaccines will be made cleaner.

Law must allow parents to decide if vaccination is in their children's best interest. Parents Right to protect their children is a most basic human Right. Stripping parents of this human Right is inhumane. Healthcare decisions are very personal and are at the heart of individuality and independent thinking. Enforcing everyone to become vaccinated slaves is much worse and much more unsettling than how the millions of Chinese are all induced to walk around dressed alike, in the same dark blue Mao suit. We need the liberty to live unvaccinated, non-chemically exposed, lives. Enforced conformity in healthcare is loss of the basic liberty to self-govern oneself; it is medical intervention tyranny and is extremely dangerous. We have been enslaved to vaccinate our children. The TWO STEPS will resurrect our lost freedom and end the ongoing, ever growing, Autism epidemic.

Obviously, there are unnatural to the body chemicals in vaccines that may have to remain in order, for a vaccine to be a vaccine. However, it must be up to the potential vaccine recipient or parents of the potential child vaccine recipient to decide whether to allow the vaccination otherwise, it will spawn chemicals for mere profit in vaccines. Please, notice that the mission statement of SAFER vaccines, the charity is to GET THE CHEMICALS OUT does not state "ALL" the chemicals. A primary goal is to remove those chemicals most concerning like mercury and aluminum or other known harsh or toxic chemicals. However, if we do not implement the **TWO STEPS OF CORRECTION** vaccine producers have and will continue to put **CHEMICALS FOR PROFIT and not safety in vaccines, chemicals that do not have to be and should not be in vaccines.** In order, to achieve **SAFER** vaccines, **SAFER VACCINES THE CHARITY,** is making the public aware of the pertinent fact, that unnatural to human biology chemicals are in vaccines and that it is very unhealthy to inject such, chemicalization. There are chemicals in vaccines not for our children's welfare but rather, to generate or assure maximum profits and parents and the public should be proactive to have these chemicals removed. Our precious freedom to decide what will or will not be injected into our very own children is essential to secure **SAFER** vaccines for our children's welfare. Being **FREE** to hold vaccine producers accountable and liable for vaccine induced injury is another vital **STEP OF CORRECTION** in the securing of **SAFER** vaccines and our children's health. **You do not want strangers or vaccine producers to have the ultimate control as to what will or will NOT be injected into your children's delicate and susceptible systems; you the parent must be FREE to protect your children from what you consider a too dangerous to inject, vaccination. Vaccine safety and/or quality control can only improve by this basic liberty!**

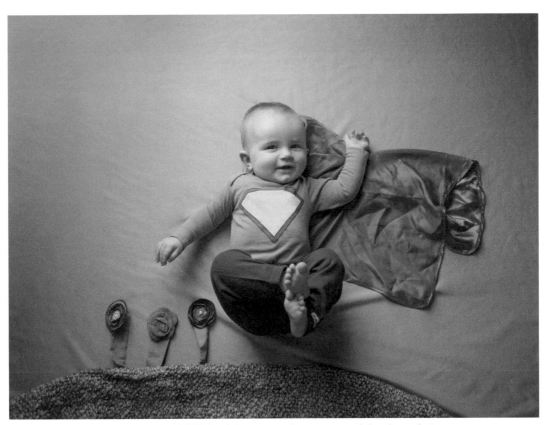

Healthy SUPER babies require a pure biochemistry.

CHAPTER 3

VACCINATION SLAVERY

Slavery is grave injustice that should befall none.
Abolish vaccination slavery and the Autism epidemic ends.
Stop mandating vaccine chemical exposure and THE EPIDEMIC WILL END.

A wise man will be a master of his own mind/body and internal chemistry; a fool will be a slave of unwanted vaccine chemical injections. It is all important for the health of children that their parents believe in their hearts and minds that vaccination is in their children's best interest; for belief translates into positive or negative results. When parent's hearts/minds are not convinced that vaccine chemicals are safe or in their children's best interest the vaccination must NOT BE GIVEN. Belief translates into physical results. Parents must feel it in their hearts that vaccination is the right choice; the heart magnetic field is about 5000 times stronger than that of the brain. The brain and heart must come to the same conclusion before vaccination can be given. It is health detrimental to go against parent's wants. Vaccination independence assures vaccine quality, safety, self-preservation, autonomy, parental healthcare control and the best results. To an all-important degree, reality or results exist only where the mind is focused. Government enforcing citizens to submit their perfectly healthy children for unwanted medical intervention and/or what is conceived as chemical injection exposure is extremely disruptive and is characteristic of ENSLAVED people; not a Free People or Free America.

Slavery is domination over another. **The enslaved have been substantially deprived of free will in some aspect of their life and/or their body has been made to undergo or endure something that they did not freely choose.** You can consider yourself enslaved if someone commands or acts with dominion over your body, mind or spirit, not allowing for independence and/or freedom in one or more of these areas. **A law that commands that your child must be vaccinated despite your parental objections, a law that demands parents to stand down not being able to protect one's child from an unwanted vaccine injection is slavery, VACCINATION SLAVERY.** The degree of slavery is rising higher the more it impacts your life or health. A slavery surrounding a fundamental Right violation or domination is a highest degree of enslavement. Erroneous laws that mandate vaccinations severely impact the lives of those injected, grossly violating and dominating; the People are denied their Right of self-preservation. **If there were no profits from vaccinations, you would see mandated vaccinations disappear in the blink of an eye; it is all about securing mega-profiteering and keeping children enslaved to be vaccinated secures Vaccine Producer's huge profits.** There is nothing wrong with profiting the free-market way, the American way, however, enslaving children to be vaccinated in the wrong way to make profits, the un-American way, the illegal way.

The People need to be in self-control of their body chemistry; armed with informed consent/ DENIAL. People require unfettered freedom, the ultimate control over their very own health destiny. The People must be totally free to deter, prevent and out right refuse chemicals especially, chemicals pointed at their children's circulatory systems in the form of vaccine injections. Freedom of self-preservation, the liberty to be in self-control over what will or will not be injected into one's very own body is fundamental and absolutely, necessary to assure that an individual's decisions in healthcare are not disregarded or disenfranchised. Parents are vested by a higher authority to care for their very own children the way they think serves their children's best interest. Man-made laws must not interfere with this vested high authority. The mandated vaccination enslavement laws grossly and blatantly violate the People's freedom to direct their own healthcare and/or basic Right to live undisturbed and free from unwanted chemical infiltrations. There is a tendency to abuse the People or their health for mere profit; to prevent it we must assure self-control authority in the People and protect the People from unwanted chemicalization.

We will celebrate the production of SAFER vaccines if we are
UNITED to implement the TWO STEPS OF CORRECTION.

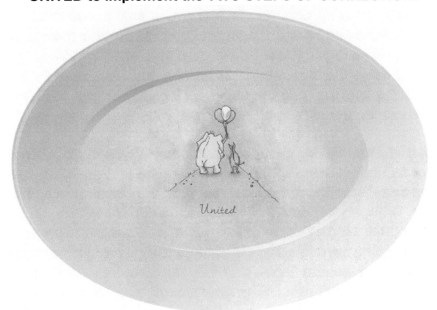

Republicans and Democrats, need to be UNITED to implement the TWO STEPS
to achieve SAFER vaccines because it means SAFER CHILDREN.

All competent individuals should have complete control over their very own health. The People are vested with the absolute power to safeguard their health the way that they individually think best. Vaccinations are an influx of chemicals and it must be up to the individual to accept or deny any chemical. The decision to accept or deny a vaccination is matter of personal healthcare choice that must be treated with utmost respect and privacy. Parents hold their children's healthcare decision power until their children come of competent age. No adult's personal health care decision or parent's health care decision for their children should be ignored, unrecognized or made insignificant. Law must be promulgated with these essentials intact otherwise an erroneous regulation results that cannot be considered law. The mandated vaccination law tramples upon the People's freedom to decide and live by what the individual determines is best for their health or their children's welfare. This basic freedom abolishes vaccination slavery!

Determining your own healthcare destiny is an essential natural Right; this liberty enables you to protect your children from unwanted vaccine injections and prompts better, cleaner vaccines. We have a supreme Right to control and protect ourselves and/or what is done with our own body. The People must not be shackled by law to not fully express the protection of their children; parents must have an inexhaustible power to prevent unwanted vaccine chemicalizations. Parents must be free to resist and/or refuse chemical injections for their children without prejudice or punishment for doing so. Moreover, the mandated vaccination law that enforces the injection of unwanted chemicals is an immoral and erroneous law. Law must not cause individuals or parents to submit their children for unwanted injections that penetrate the body with unwanted chemicals. The strong hand of the law must not take part in reducing parental authority or enforce the defiling, degrading or contamination of one's sacrosanct bloodstream. Mandated vaccinations in perpetuity are an unwarranted jurisdiction over our personal health and family decisions. The firmness of the mandate coerces parents into submitting their children. Not allowing school entrance and the threat child services unfairly accusing parents of child abuse sole purpose of fatiguing parents into vaccination compliance with these measures prevents parents from protecting children from unnatural chemicalization. Parents are deprived of being parents; their parental right to protect their offspring is ravaged, plundered and destroyed by this unwarranted jurisdiction over us. Parents must be the supreme judge over their children's welfare and freely decide upon vaccinations!

Parents must not be forced by law or vaccination compulsion to go against their decision not to vaccinate or relinquish their Right to self-determine their child's health care. Parents must not be asked or expected to obey a law that commands them to submit their child for vaccinations when doing so forces parents to disobey their primary parental directive of preventing injury to their child. Parents must not be coerced or enforced into submission to accept vaccination or be subdued to go against their prerogative or determination of what is in their child's best interest. Parents should not be manipulated or made to lay down their protective shielding of children; parents must be free to deny an unwanted, conceived of as, too dangerous to inject, vaccination. Parents agree that preventative health care decisions are all within the confines of parental jurisdiction and is not for government. Parents almost unanimously agree that being free to refuse unwanted vaccinations is an essential and fundamental freedom. Parents expect the common decency and liberty to prevent unwanted chemical exposure. Parents are perfectly capable of deciding what is in children's best interest. REDUCED CHEMICALS IN VACCINES will result in cleaner vaccines that are a lot less harmful. The AUTISM EPIDEMIC WILL SUBSIDE and CHILDREN'S BEST INTEREST WILL BE SERVED. Injected chemicals upset the natural health generating chemical ecosystem. Mandated vaccinations are insidious, entrapping the public to forever be enslaved to vaccinate under the guise of public good.

Parents by natural supreme law are the ultimate authority when it comes to the welfare of their children no mal-law should divest parents of their God given supreme right. The mandated vaccination mal-law violates this right not only temporarily but rather, in perpetuity.

Either from instinct, knowledge or legitimate, heartfelt, corporal caring a parent knows just what is right and best for their children's welfare. Parents are the only ones with the qualifications needed for an unbiased vaccination decision; they truly have their children's best interest as the priority, parents are genuinely properly concerned. Parents must be the controlling authority to decide as to the worth of the vaccine chemicals proposed for injection. Parents legally must be free to decline a vaccination in the best interest of children. Mandated vaccination laws invade the province of parents and/or parenting. This invasion is unwise and cause for unneeded child injury. Parents have a supreme Right to protect their children from unwanted chemical infiltrations or vaccine chemical injections. Parents must have the unfettered liberty to preserve the purity of their children's blood or bloodstreams, to be the decision makers and not be enforced to submit their children for unwanted injections or chemicalizations. Accordingly, parent's written consent must be first obtained and parents for the sake of safety itself have liberty to refuse vaccine injection. Parental disengagement in the protection of children must not be commanded by mal-law; no mandated vaccinations!

Historically, we always have trusted that parents will do what is best for their children. Parents are one with their children and children are one with their parents; there is no vast separateness like that of government making vaccination decisions. The principle of parents taking care of their children is so perfect that it must not be replaced or usurped by government or any other foreign entity. Parents must no longer be forced to place their children's survival or health in the hands of corporations or corporate know how or greed. To hold that government must step in and make mandated vaccination laws because parents do not know what is best for children is absurd. There is no good reason why parent's authority to decide what is best for their children does not control vaccination! The main reason why vaccinations are now mandated is to really only assure profiteering for the drug industry. If there were no mega-profits to be made by mandating vaccinations, there would be no mandate enforcing parents to submit their children. Parents must always be vigilant in the protection of offspring from toxic chemicalization. Indeed, parents must remain sober; never embroidering the truth about vaccine contents.

Parents traditionally can block any medical intervention; vaccination should and must not be the exception. Vaccinations surround merely preventative healthcare and are administered to perfectly healthy children with no required immediate need of medical intervention therefore, it is that much more apparent that the golden rule of healthcare requiring obtaining parents non-coerced informed consent control vaccinations; parents must be free to decide whether to accept or deny the vaccination. Parental decision for their children must be respected. Government has no jurisdiction to enjoin, interfere, ignore, disregard or over-power parents' refusal of vaccination especially, in perpetuity or during non-emergency situations. Profiteering, Vaccine Producers' with their cohorts of lobbyists that have wrongfully spawned sanctioned government mandated vaccination laws must not be permitted to disregard the mass of parents who long to protect their children from unwanted chemical vaccine injections. Law that commands exposure to unwanted chemicals or medical intervention is grossly flawed and must be stricken! Parents must have their highest degree of protection of their children especially, if a vaccine needle is being pointed at their tiny baby, very small infant or immature child.

Toxins in the food we eat and in the air are causing disease however, nothing is more horrific for health than injecting chemical toxins into our children's bloodstreams. Always remember, what is injected into the blood quickly circulates, unimpeded, into the brain; doping the cells of the brain with whatever chemicals are in the vaccine. We have been told repeatedly that there is no harm and they are safe however, let me warn and assure you that disrupting the natural chemistry within is a sure recipe for health disaster. The fact that injected vaccine chemicals entering vaccination recipient's upsets their normal chemistry is unimpeachable! The truth is a vaccination of today is a blunder into the unknown, the void of anti-health realm and is chemical Russian roulette. Abnormally high levels of Autism mainly result from exposing children to multiple injections of vaccines that are laced with unnatural to the body chemicals. These harmful chemicals quickly enter the brain after injection into the bloodstream, doping the brain with interfering and life altering chemicals. Parents need to be aware of the contents and dangers of the chemicals delivered by vaccine injections. Take back the control that wrongly has been taken from you; regain your children's healthcare welfare, do not let erroneous government vaccination mandates interfere with your parental obligation and responsibility of protection of your children! Liberty to be in command of your own health and that of your family is at stake. Fundamental freedom of self-preservation, self-determined healthcare and self-regulation must never be taken from the People! Law must not diminish parent's capacity of protecting children; it must only support or bolster it.

Voluntary vaccinations will have individuals empowered to refuse unwanted vaccine injections; this will promote safer vaccines and a needed trust in the vaccination program perpetuating improved vaccination compliance. The violence being perpetrated upon individual's Rights and parent's Rights will end. This will establish a moral vaccination program and proper vaccination system, creating needed trust and better attitude about vaccinations and thereby, effectuate an efficient and effective vaccination program. People must not be enforced/enslaved to vaccinate but rather, allowed to discern the pros and cons of vaccination and determine for themselves and their children if it is safer to accept or deny vaccination. Knowing just how much chemical exposure is involved is vital to the vaccination determination or whether vaccination is or is not in one's best interest. We need an honest voluntary vaccination program that boasts freedom to choose, freedom to deny unwanted vaccine chemicals. Mandated vaccination is an abuse of our dynamic freedom and results in chemicalization child abuse on a mass scale. The People require the freedom to individually determine if the offered vaccine is of benefit or detriment to health or if the injection will or will not spawn autism! Parents must have liberty to protect their children from vaccine chemicalization harm. Vaccines have chemicals or molecular compounds that are toxic to the body such as, glutamate, aluminum and still to this day mercury to some degree etc. People who would refuse vaccination suffer an assault and battery when enforced to endure unwanted vaccination; this mal-law affliction and madness must be stopped by abolishing vaccination slavery!

Free people are not demanded by law to submit their children for unwanted vaccine injections in perpetuity; only an enslaved People are under such oppression. Through coercion, fear or fraud parents have been made to give up their **essential natural Right of self-determined health care**. Emancipation of self-determined vaccinations is required to clean-up vaccines and to live free. **We**

are enslaved to inject vaccines into our children. This is a case of undue influence, a coercing of unwanted, suspect vaccinations, an inappropriate governing and penetration of our internal being, a slavery of the worst magnitude and kind, an obstruction and taking of parental Rights. Government has no jurisdiction over our internal being or personal health care decisions and/or health care choices. The sphere of influence of proper government does not extend into whether or not our children will or will not receive vaccinations. **Your health decisions are yours alone to make and you have a right to left alone. People must be free to pursue their healthcare, to follow their own beat of their very own health drum. The monopoly of influence, which enforces parents to have their children submit for unwanted chemical injections, abridges parental Rights; it must no longer be permitted.**

Human Rights protect us from what would violate, without permission, our body integrity. Forcing children to be injected is inhumane. Vaccinating children against their parent's will is un-American and uncivilized. Parents have a **GOD** given responsibility and **GOD** given Right to protect their children; when parents determine that a vaccine chemical injection is too dangerous to inject, there decision not to inject is **SUPREME**. The law assuring parents that they can protect their children from unwanted vaccine chemical exposure or unwanted medical intervention is not only very reasonable, it is down right American, civilized and in accordance with the **NATURAL ORDER**. Parents and their children are **bonded into vaccination slavery** because of an erroneous vaccination law that coerces parents, leaving them no choice, but to submit and endure unwanted, suspect vaccinations. **Unwanted injections are taking place even though parents determine the vaccinations are not in their children's best interest.** In addition, parental informed consent to inject is never really given or legally obtained; the spirit or intent of informed consent and/or volitional acceptance of vaccination is being skirted, ignored or made a moot point. Forcing parents to submit their perfectly healthy child for unwanted vaccinations is slavery of the worst degree; it violates the Constitution and the **Right to Self-Determine one's health care**. Mere vaccination profiteering must not trump basic liberty; we must break the chains that keep us shackled to mandated injections of vaccine chemicalization.

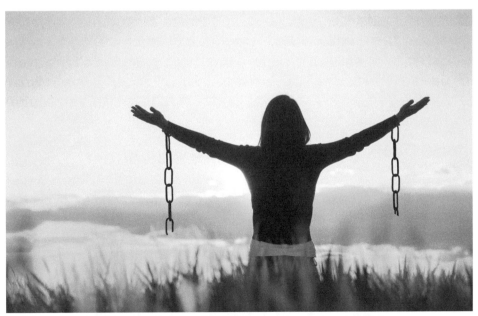

FREE not to inject; FREE to protect your children.

Fundamental to liberty, essential to parent/child autonomy, imperative to vaccine purity and vital to freedom of choice in health care, parents require the decision authority, the power of vaccination control. Parents naturally and traditionally hold the highest degree of decision control over their children's health care. This same degree of parental decision control must steadfastly apply to vaccinations. When it comes to protecting one's internal chemistry or contemplating vaccinations, freedom minded individuals say, "this is my life, no one is going to tell me what is right" and the parents say, "this is my child, no one is going to tell me what is right; no one is going to tell me that my child must be vaccinated. If I do not think it is in my child's best interest to be vaccinated, end of story; do not enforce me to vaccinate my child or interfere with what I think best for my child. Please only suggest or educate me; do not command me into vaccination or coerce vaccinations by shouting you must vaccinate it's the law. **The People hold that Parents are free to protect their children and within the purview of this protection, are enabled to refuse unwanted medical intervention such as, vaccine chemical injections, as a self-evident truth. Law cannot be based upon mere conjecture or fiction and it is a complete fiction that perfectly healthy children somehow pose an ominous threat to others therefore, the unvaccinated can enter school without pressure to be vaccinated.**

Government, drug industry or doctors must not enforce injections; it is dehumanization. Parents should not be made **subjects of a master** that commands their children undergo vaccination. Our Rights as parents, empower us to deny unwanted injections for our children. The legal controlling decision of whether or not a child is to be vaccinated must rest with the child's parents. Parents hold their child's best interest; they know what is best for their children. This will prompt Vaccine Producers to not use anti-health chemicals in children's vaccines and end the Autism epidemic. **Parents must have the liberty to prevent any and all kinds of chemical dumping into their children's bloodstreams especially, injected vaccine chemical dumping**. Children must not to be enforced by law to endure vaccine chemical injections, they must not turn pure healthy bloodstreams into chemical dumps; "no dumping" without permission, and permission will rarely be granted until vaccines are **CLEANED-UP**. Vaccine chemicals do cause health problems and parents must be free to stop an unwanted vaccine chemical exposure, infiltration or dumping. Remember, vaccine chemicals are alien to the body, have anti-health propensities and some of the chemicals used in vaccine production are very toxic. These injections will cause chemical alterations in your children. Remember, your child's life stands in the wings; their health can be severely negatively impacted by such chemicals if injected. There is a huge economic incentive to keep children enslaved to be vaccinated however, the child is yours and you must be empowered to protect your child.

YOUR CHILD = YOUR DECISION!

Your children are for you to cherish, have, hold and care for. Nothing must stand in the way of parent's decisions of what is in their children's best interest. No law or entity should prevent parents from protecting their children from danger. Parents have a liberty from a higher authority than man-made laws and a natural instinctive Right to protect their children. This omnipotent Right empowers Parents to say "NO" to unwanted vaccine chemicalization. Children's vaccination destinies are for parents to decide. Recognize the consequences of injecting vaccine chemicals. Realize that Vaccine Producer's puppet government enforces vaccination, forbidding parental protection of children from an

unwanted injection of chemicals; inducing a chemicalization of the blood, exposing children to all kinds of chemical hazards. Chemicals cause tectonic health problems.

The People must have healthcare dominion over themselves and their children; not being overruled by government. Man must control his internal-self, never to be internally regulated by government or by others. Mandated vaccination and/or VACCINATION SLAVERY are ONE AND THE SAME, an unauthorized taking, A TOTAL TAKING CONTROL of our children's vaccination health care. This is done despite the cosmic fact that vaccine contents have been and continues to be the CAUSE IN FACT of significant known adverse side-effects and are the highly probable cause of many told and untold injury. Government that was meant to serve the People must not rule over the People; it must not enslave us. Government has enslaved us to be injected with chemical toxins; there is no free will when it comes to vaccinations. The People are awakening to the realization that they are enslaved. The conscious understanding that we are not free is causing mass stress and depression. The fact that enforced vaccinations expose children to chemical toxins has People in rational fear of Autism and in fear for their children's very lives. Patriotism to the Constitution and the true principles of what America was founded upon is rising among the People to recapture our lost freedom and end our enslavement.

Family freedom, family autonomy and the ability to protect your very own children demand that vaccinations be completely voluntary. The People are not fundamentally free if they do not have the liberty to refuse unwanted chemical infiltrations such as, unwanted vaccine chemical injections. Chemical injections must no longer be coerced or forced upon the People. Mandated vaccinations are a plight upon the People and an abomination to all that is proper in health care. Self-determined health care is an essential freedom. Human bondage to vaccinations which can cause injury is inhumane and being free to exercise one's self-determined health care is an essential freedom. Parents should have unabashed insistence that they be empowered to refuse unwanted vaccine chemical injections. Being enabled to protect children from unwanted chemical infiltrations is fundamental to being a caring and responsible parent. The present vaccination delivery system overwhelms and overcomes the parent's freedom of objection, coercively discharging their decision not to have their children vaccinated. It is a transgression against parent's protection of their children.

The mandated vaccination law does violence to the Constitution; in many ways it eviscerates the Constitution. The mandate violates the People's Right to be left alone and not chemically injected, it also, violates parent's right to protect their children to the best of their ability and violates one's Right to travel freely between the States. Just how the vaccination laws interfere with one's Constitutional protection of traveling freely between the States will be explained in more detail later but for now a brief understanding follows.

The violation occurs when one State that has a forbidding law, a law that does allow the People their basic freedom to decide against vaccinations, disallows unvaccinated State's citizens to FREELY ENTER the prohibitive State which burdensomely requires all to be vaccinated. Because the mandated Vaccination State forbids the People's fundamental freedom of health care decision, not to be vaccinated or to live by their philosophy not to be injected with unwanted chemicals, (commonly referred to as a "philosophical exemption") individuals Right to travel freely between the States is overburdened and thereby, violated. The unvaccinated individuals, attempting to freely travel from a non-mandatory State into a mandatory vaccination State are overburdened and/or blocked from freely traveling because of having to become vaccination compliant. The amount of vaccinations and their quick timing; amplifies the danger of vaccination placing the traveler in a further untenable position. Unvaccinated individuals seeking to travel into States that strictly mandate vaccinations would be majorly deterred from entering a strict Vaccination State for fear of being enforced to suffer multiple chemical injections. The length of time before you must become vaccinated in the mandate Vaccination State may vary however, the result is the Peoples' Constitutional liberties to travel freely from State to State are being violated. The States cannot be divided when it comes to vaccinations; they all must allow for refusal and/or parental refusal.

The next time someone insists that you or your child must be vaccinated, if your a freedom minded citizen or an individual who does not want to live under the oppression of Vaccination Slavery, take rightful control of yourself or child by saying "excuse me this is my life, my body and my child; no one can command me or my child to inject chemicals, no one else but myself can dictate what is best for my child's health; no one but me will decide whether or not a vaccine chemical injection shall or shall not be administered." Control your children's and your own health care destiny. Let no one dictate or enslave you or your children to be vaccinated. Let no one force you to go against your belief of what, you as parents think are best for your children and never be coerced to vaccinate. Live free to decide what is in your own and your children's best health interest. Parent's ideas of what is proper and in line with being health logical, health wise or having health sense must be respected and control preventative, non-emergency, health care decisions.

Do not be foolish or act like mere SHEEP-PEOPLE by throwing away your fundamental freedom of health care decision or by being herded to receive mandatory vaccine CHEMICAL injections. Stand up for what you think is best and right for your child; do not throw away your parental responsibility of protecting your children. If you conclude that a vaccine chemical injection is dangerous to inject then demand to be free to say "NO"; insist upon the liberty to protect your children from unwanted chemical vaccine exposure. Nothing should vaporize your protection of your children from chemical toxins. Always remember that health is reliant upon having the proper chemistry in the body and that it is your child; your decision. Be free, not enslaved into vaccinations. Of course, if you determine, not someone determining for you giving you no choice, that the vaccine injection is in the best interest of your child, then, you are free to give your informed consent and do receive the vaccination. Either way, the decision must be only for you to make and live by; this must be to consider yourself autonomous and/or a FREE citizen.

Recognize the high degree of violation that is be perpetuated upon you and your children when you have no choice, no freedom, no realistic ability to refuse an unwanted chemical vaccine injection. Remember that altering the natural chemistry of your child is destructive to their health. Note how frequent Autism has become and do what you think is best to prevent your child from becoming a victim of chemical infiltration. You of course have the power and the responsibility to decide just what is best for your child. Ask all the questions you reasonably feel that you need to about the vaccination in order to make the right decision for your child. Be the parent that you were meant to be and let no one deter you from doing what you think is in your children's best interest. Although, there are democratic principles that are at the root of our country it however, is not a Democracy; it is a Republic and a Republic purposefully limits the size and power of government. Regulation of healthcare, as is the instant case of mandating vaccinations, is not a Republic but rather, a dangerous enslavement of children to submit to chemical injections. To establish justice and protect Americans from an all-powerful government we must abolish vaccination slavery. Freedom depravation of parents protecting children must end.

They have managed to dull our senses, to perversely become complacent in surrendering our children to outside authority rule, enforced by invasive law to submit our children for chemical infiltrations, which a free-spirited individual would not stand for. They have spent millions to assure we have no choice but to submit our children. They have used every media possible to program us all to except in the pervasion that injecting chemicals into our children's delicate and susceptible bloodstreams is expected, the right thing to do and to accept that there is absolutely no choice in the matter. I am here to inform you, to alert you and to awaken you that mandated vaccination enslavement laws abuse your children with chemical exposures and that the chemicals that have been found in vaccines are insanely dangerous. We pollute the planet and we pollute our children with vaccine chemicals; parents are waking up to the fact. Parents are finally taking a stand, shouting out "enough is enough"; parents now require their natural controlling authority of their children and healthcare. The public is finally recognizing that to be left no realistic choice but to submit your children for chemical vaccine injections is really outrageous, a violation of the worst kind. Commanding all children MUST be vaccinated, despite parent's objections, is nothing less than tyrannical MEDICAL INTERVENTION ENSLAVEMENT.

Individuals find that they are powerless, coerced and enslaved to submit their children for unwanted chemical injections. There is an answer; the People do have Rights protect them from tyrannical MEDICAL INTERVENTION ENSLAVEMENT. Mandated vaccinations has crossed the line of proper ethical health care and has entered a realm of enforced health care which is not ethical and does not grant the decency of informed consent and/or INFORMED DENIAL of vaccination chemical infiltrations. This gross manipulation or twisted medical intervention has unleashed an Autism epidemic. Because the Vaccine Producers operate their business with unprecedented dictatorship authority and know that the public is enslaved to be vaccinated and that they cannot be held liable for vaccine induced injuries, vaccine safety has plummeted. Vaccines have been found to contain chemicals that you would not want to put on your child's skin let alone, inject the chemically lace vaccines into your child's susceptible bloodstream. The TWO STEPS OF CORRECTION give parents their children back; parents can protect their children from unwanted chemical impurities, they can refuse unwanted vaccinations. Chemicals are the enemy to health and parents must be free to protect their children from the chemical exposure enemy. The renegade law of mandated vaccinations must be corrected through our natural Right to protect our very own children by instilling the TWO STEPS OF CORRECTION. Parents must have dominion over their children's vaccinations.

Chemical infiltration of children is the cause of the Autism epidemic. Vaccine injected chemicals enter the bloodstream and quickly bombard the brain cells. The erroneous mandated vaccination law has prompted less vigilance to secure children's well-being and allowed Vaccine Producers to place chemicals in vaccines that secure profit instead, of safety. The sorry CHEMICAL state of vaccine safety and the related Autism epidemic has made parents outraged; no longer are parents complacent with being enslaved to vaccinate their children. Parents will no longer be fooled. The chemical formula of vaccines does not coincide with the natural chemistry of the body. All parents need to be alerted, through the desired informed consent/DENIAL requirement of the chemical composition of vaccines and decide if the vaccine injection is safe. Vaccines must be manufactured with the understanding and strict rule that they must not have chemicals which are not intrinsic to the body or have anti-health properties. The TWO STEPS will instill the cleaning-up of vaccines; prompting GETTING THE CHEMICALS OUT.

All vaccinations are dangerous and for this reason by itself must be voluntary. Let us briefly look at the adverse reactions from receiving just one of these chemical concoctions, the MMR vaccine chemicals. Although, the adverse reactions seem to keep changing over time you can expect signs and symptoms alerting you to the fact that you have chemically insulted your body. For example, the MMR vaccine causes a fever up to 1 person out of 6, a rash in 1 person out of 20, swelling of the glands in the cheeks or neck in about 1 in every 75 people, seizure (starring or jerking) in about 1 out of 3,000 doses given, low platelet count, which can cause a bleeding disorder in about 1 in 30,000 doses given. Although, not as frequent many other very severe problems can occur such as serious allergic reaction, deafness, lowered consciousness, long-term seizures, comas and permanent brain damage or even death. Let us not be negligent and add Autism to this long list. This list indicates how dangerous it is being exposed to the chemicals of vaccines. This list includes problems that are too frequent or too severe for reasonable parents to risk injecting their children with the chemicals that cause harm. Vaccines are laced with anti-health agents such as but not limited to aluminum, glutamate etc., all of which, cause brain inflammation and malfunction; excellent reason to refuse vaccination.

Bad law and bad acts against the People can be stopped. Involuntary sterilization was performed and funded by the same powers that have perpetuated many other afflictions upon the People and they and/or the involuntary sterilization was stopped and declared illegal. In 2007 California activists succeeded in stopping the spraying of a toxic spray designed to destroy the Light Brown Apple Moth (LBAM). The spraying was commenced because the government declare there to be a "state of emergency" because moths were damaging agriculture crops. People claimed they were getting sick from the spray and began to organize themselves as collective activists against the spraying and the result was they stopped the spraying. Similarly, parents are claiming that their children are being injured by vaccine chemical injection exposure. Together, parents and concerned freedom spirited individuals can become activists against vaccination slavery.

The People do not want enforced vaccination slavery; they want to decide for themselves what vaccine will be accepted or denied and if the risks commensurate with being exposed to vaccine chemicals is to great a risk to take. Perhaps individuals might want to wait till their children are stronger before vaccinating and/or their systems are more mature or wait till their children are old enough to readily clearly communicate an adverse vaccination reaction if it occurs. Certainly, there must be latitude and choices permitted and not treat children like cattle being branded with vaccination slavery. A probable reason why Vaccine Producers insist that infants be vaccinated at such a young age is that infants cannot communicate aches and pains or express in detail how bad they are feeling after injection making it more difficult to detect adverse vaccination reactions.

To be enslaved to vaccinate children is extremely egregious and totally improper. Our sense of being free is lost if we cannot care for our children the way we as parents deem best. To be blocked by an erroneous mandated vaccination law, to not be free to care for and protect your children the way you personally think is best, not being properly empowered to refuse vaccine chemicals and/or to protect your very own children from chemical exposure by injection is so wrong that it must be made right. Parents cannot be made to stumble around in the dark or have no say in the matter or no power to refuse. Parents must be free to question everything about vaccinations and have the ultimate power to refuse injections. We hereby, declare to ABOLISH VACCINATION SLAVERY and the TWO STEPS OF CORRECTION will do just that. Live free to reject vaccine chemical injections and protect your children from vaccine chemical exposure if you think it wise to.

The level of importance of parental protection of children from unwanted chemical exposure is of the highest magnitude. Parents' being free to protect their children is almost assumed in a free society. If a parent is against a vaccine injection being administered, then the law must support that parent's decision. Children's welfare has and always will be best served by allowing their parents to safeguard them and/or decide what is best. The mandated vaccination law is an enslavement of children to be injected with vaccine chemicals. Let us abolish vaccination mandates and/or abolish vaccination enslavement. There is nothing wrong with parents seeking advice about vaccinations or someone helping parents do all the right things for their children. Parents should be able to seek advice and/or learn all the pros and cons of vaccination however, the ultimate decision to vaccinate or not vaccinate is for non-other than the parents. Parents must not be over-influenced; the decision must be theirs and the decision must not be coerced or made for them. Parent's children must remain parent's children and protected accordingly.

Our children's well-being is in jeopardy because informed consent/DENIAL is not in control vaccinations; the vaccination mal-mandate prevents parents from refusing unwanted vaccinations. Since parents cannot refuse vaccination, unhealthy preservatives are in vaccines to give vaccines longer shelf-life; this wrongfully assures greater profits at children's expense and is being done without parental consent or knowledge. Keeping one's body free of unnatural chemicals is ESSENTIAL TO GOOD HEALTH; the vaccination mandate forbids this most basic health essential. United States history has shown that corrupted or mal-government has experimented on citizens and outside the U.S. people have been made victims of covert experimentation that put toxic chemicals in vaccines. Informed consent steadfastly applied to vaccinations will safeguard against the placement of unwanted chemicals in vaccines in that no vaccination can take place without first giving the knowledge of everything that is in the vaccine and then asking the patient's or parents' permission. In addition, the makers of vaccines must no longer be wrongfully sheltered from negligence lawsuits; when their foul chemical vaccines are proven to cause injury they must be punished and pay. When producers of any consumer product are impervious to irresponsible negligent production litigation it opens the door to negligent production, actually promoting it; an attitude is created of profit first not safety first.

The for profit chemical industry and their puppet government have design to chemically infiltrate us, to manipulate the very nature of us, without our consent or knowledge, through the means of vaccines such as, Gardasil vaccine but also, through genetically modified food. They have spent the time, energy and huge outlay of money to produce a spermicidal genetic strain of corn that promises to render males infertile when consumed. The fact that they would produce infertility generating corn signifies that there is design to chemically alter us, manipulate our biology and force unwanted changes upon us. The vaccine chemical content and/or the history of vaccines are testament to how abusive these companies can be and how our Rights are being violated and our precious children's health placed in jeopardy. What continues to precipitate mandated vaccination during non-epidemic, non-emergency times is not really children's need or best interest but rather, vaccine chemical industry greed, self-serving interest and to increase profits.

We are losing the power of our Rights because they happen to be in the pathway of corporate profiteering and those who want to control and dominate us. Rights are precious so whenever, laws are passed that place limits or decrease our Rights; those laws must be viewed in the most negative of lights when determining if they are legal. There are now free speech zones or First amendment zones or Free speech cages instead, of the true American way of free speech being throughout the land. These limited areas of allowable free speech are for so called, political activists. Government has limited your free speech by regulating its time, place and manner. Your Right to self-determine vaccinations has been taken; in fact, the unjust vaccination mandate gives no freedom to refuse. True freedom is strategically being limited for the sake of controlling our actions or choices in order, to secure monopolized profiteering. They dilute evidence and downplay facts and are hiding the horrific truth that VACCINE CHEMICALIZATIONS CAUSE AUTISM.

There is a concerted effort on the part of puppet government and the FDA for the benefit of Drug companies to stamp-out competition or what might threaten the financial welfare of the chemical industry/pharmaceutical industry. If nothing is done to reverse the onslaught against our freedom of healthcare and information about the benefits of products of health, there will soon be no choice in healthcare. Producers of natural health products such as, walnuts, prunes, pomegranate, cherries, oregano have been fined or stopped from informing the public of their benefits. All-natural products will soon not be able to be told to the consumer and current or newly discovered health benefits will be suppressed; bargained for lobbyist made mal-law and/or FDA will see to it. Once again lobbyists for the benefit of corporate greed and monopoly agenda are depriving the public of essential information and natural cures and/or natural healthcare choices. People have a Right and need to know of proposed benefits of natural remedies and make the decision for themselves if the product is worthy of use; they must not need the permission of the FDA or puppet government to use a product and do not want to be ruled over; enslaved.

We will soon have no independent health decisions; we are swiftly becoming totally dependent upon medicine and at the mercy of the profit based pharmaceutical industry. The FDA has taken unprecedented and uncalled for measures to force natural products for weight loss, dietary supplements and practically all-natural remedies to go through a negatively slated, totally unneeded, approval process that is meant to over burden and cause undue expenditure; resulting in the suppression or elimination of the drug company's competition and thereby, assuring pharmaceutical dominance, monopoly and profiteering. This unjust action is costing a tremendous loss of health for Americans in that viable health promoting or lifesaving sources will either be taken off the market or will never even reach the market. Vital health or lifesaving discoveries and innovations will resultantly not be bestowed upon the public. The FDA's approval process is not making natural products safer; they already are very safe especially when compared to drugs. On the international level in Europe, Codex Alimentarius, a global agency, is destroying the efficiency and effectiveness of vitamins and minerals by limiting the formulas to very, very low dosages; these low dosages defeat the reason to take them. The FDA has said they intend to align or HARMmonize our laws with Codex here in the U.S., to coincide with their content amount regulations or requirements.

Freedom of choice in healthcare is becoming non-existent. We need to stop the lunacy and madness of eliminating our freedom of choice in healthcare; if you want a high dosage of vitamins or minerals you must be free to buy it and vendors must be free to sell it. Please, be acutely aware that the pharmaceutical industry sets the agenda for Codex, to eliminate natural medicine. Our parental right to care for our children to the best of our ability has been taken and our right to a free and competitive American market is being destroyed. Take back what has been wrongfully taken from you; demand to refuse unwanted chemically laced vaccines and protect your children by deciding what is best! We absolutely need to make sure both natural products and drug products are not harmful however, all drugs have negative to health side-effects whereas, natural remedies all do not. Is it not then obvious that it is drugs and not vitamins or minerals that need to be more difficult to come to market or really scrutinized before doing so? Just look at the Cialis or Viagra commercials that we are constantly being bombarded with and you can readily recognize that it is such drugs and not natural products that really need to put a lid on it or be suppressed to at least some reasonable or tolerable degree.

A limiting and restraining approval process for drugs, which have propensity to cause harm is a proper standard however, for natural based essential food sources and their derivative products that have comparatively, miniscule propensity to cause harm and are intrinsically benign products it is not needed and will only serve to eliminate natural healing sources from the market place and thereby, solidify a healthcare monopoly and dependence on drugs. Drugs and vaccines are intrinsically harmful and must be treated and analyzed according to their dangerous propensities whereas, vitamins, minerals, herbs and nutrients must be treated essentially as food, without propensity to cause harm and without need to be proven safe or FDA approved in order to be sold. If the People are not made aware of the benefits of natural remedies the market for natural remedies that has been steadily growing will practically, cease to exist. A mere statement that a natural product is beneficial to health automatically categorizes it as a drug that is unauthorized for use;

illegal. These actions are another form of censored speech, which is unconstitutional and therefore, illegal. If they succeed in this dastardly plan, the public will not hear, read or learn of the benefits of natural remedies and will fall further into an ever-growing dependence and enslavement upon drugs, unnatural to the body chemicals and/or injected vaccine chemicals. The FDA does not so much serve the People as it serves to assure drug use. The FDA and pharmaceutical industry ties are much too close! There is an obvious bias for drug taking and bias against natural product taking.

The proper taking of natural supplements does not cause injury and even the improper consumption rarely induces injury and yet these comparatively natural health aids are too often attacked or restricted. Meanwhile; drugs that all have side-effects, have caused too numerous iatrogenic diseases and too numerous deaths are rarely restricted or inexplicably allowed to stay on the market. FDA too often has turned a blind eye when it comes to their conflict of interest partnership with the pharmaceutical industry and is purposely, toothless against harmful vaccines. Yet, they have a long history of bias to restrict access to natural products and what can be said about them. We should not be at the mercy of the pharmaceutical industry or be manipulated to take drugs and/or be enforced to be injected with vaccine chemicals. The supposed drug policing agency that is more of a drug protecting agencies should be placed in check. The harmful drugs should be placed in check whereas; natural remedies that have no track record for causing death should be liberated and unshackled so that the public can freely exercise their freedom of choice in healthcare and benefit from doing so. The FDA is doing the public a disservice; the public's health is suffering because of it. Even though, what is in a dietary natural supplement is completely found in the food that we eat; the FDA would make it go through the FDA's nonsensical approval process, which the FDA will more than likely disapprove. This nonsensical approval process regulation of the New Food Safety Modernization Act (FSMA) of 2007 is almost as dangerous as mandated vaccination enslavement laws and cause for major alarm; our Rights are under major attack prompted by greedy corporations.

The FDA's unprecedented power to ban needed natural remedies and to remove choice for consumers must be curtailed. The public should be able to rely on safe, low cost, natural, remedies and not be handcuffed to rely on the much more dangerous, patented for major profit, pharmaceutical drugs. Natural remedies are not patented and therefore, they will never generate unconscionable profits however, the powers that be are hard at work to restrict their use and wrongfully categorize them as drugs in order, that the pharmaceutical industry can obtain a new source of unconscionable profiteering. As far as the dangers of monopolies goes; restricting access to healthcare and/or enforcing certain or any healthcare (vaccinations) is by far the most dangerous and egregious of monopolies. Furthermore, there is intent to label and categorize any natural product that claims to have a health benefit as a "new drug" and is now under the testing and scrutiny of the FDA and will now require a PRESCRIPTION for its use; this will result in the suppression of its use, restrict it as a monopoly for the Drug industry, allow patents or increased prices and make the public have to visit a doctor to get a prescription in order to obtain natural, non-invasive, generally non-harmful natural remedies.

We must have legal standing to pursue litigation against the FDA and for our children's sake, against the Vaccine Producers of negligently produced vaccines and/or for the injuries that their negligently produced vaccines cause. Without legal standing or legal recourse, we are left naked, defenseless and with no viable offense. We must not be so blind, deaf and dumb to leave our children are at the whim of Vaccine Producers, who can and will put any agent and/or chemical in vaccines that turn a profit because of their liability shielding. If there was ever a purpose or directive to apply negligence law to producers of consumer products certainly, its application should and must be applied to the producers of our children's vaccine supply. In addition, for the sake of children's best interest parents should and must be enabled to refuse unwanted vaccine chemical injections. TWO STEPS of CORRECTION must be taken otherwise; chemical hell will continue to break loose within our children's injected bloodstreams. The dark ages of blindly, venerating vaccination chemicalization is over and our freedom is renewed.

The parent and child bond must never be weakened or severed by law. Parents deserve their freedom of care for children the way they think best, and children need parent's optimum protection; it is perfectly natural for this autonomous relationship. Government making personal healthcare decisions for the People is totally inappropriate, alien and destined to cause problems. Only during emergencies government can act for our safety however, any long-term mandated intervention must be banned. Any law that replaces parenting Rights and skills is suspect and must be viewed in the must negative light. There must never be long-term governmental healthcare intervention; mandated vaccinations in perpetuity must be stricken. PARENTS ARE CHAMPIONS IN KNOWING WHAT IS IN THEIR CHILDREN'S BEST INTEREST; government should keep a healthy distance from dictating healthcare. Parents must be free to be parents by being protectors.

Abolishing vaccination slavery will not only free People from the oppression of injecting chemicals but will align vaccination healthcare with the tradition of all other healthcare. People are generally free to decide what medical intervention will or will not be given. Parents are generally free to decide what is best for their children. Nowhere in healthcare can you find this differential treatment that vaccinations wrongfully have; it is an enigma; the mandate vaccination enigma must be corrected. Parents are astounded to learn what is in vaccines. Parents that are opposed to injecting their children with these vaccine chemicals find themselves in a quandary; placed in an untenable position. It is unfair and obscene to enforce parents into injecting unwanted chemicals into their children. No one should MASTER another's health or healthcare decisions; that is slavery. No parent should be placed under duress to lay down their parental protection of their children. No parent should be turned into a law breaker for refusing to inject their children with unwanted vaccine chemicals. Do not be enslaved to vaccinate! Exposure to chemicals must be freely avoided and the law must never controvert such basic ambition.

On April 6, 2000, Mary Megson, M. D., testified at the House Government Reform Committee affirming: "The segment of children with 'regressive Autism,' the form where children develop normally for a period of time then lose skills and sink into autism most commonly at 18-24 months of age, is increasing at a phenomenal rate. I am seeing multiple children in the same family affected, including in the last week four cases of 'autistic regression' developing in four-year-old children after their MMR and DPT vaccination. In the past, this was unheard of. …I think we are staring a disaster in the face that has affected thousands of Americans." Avoid exposing children to the anti-health chemicals of vaccines by abolishing vaccination slavery. Do what is needed to prevent chemical exposure. Clean vaccines will result from the **TWO STEPS OF CORRECTION! It an absolute abdication of responsibility and accountability to not hold vaccine manufacturers liable when their vaccines are chemically impure or the cause of injury! There is no greater parental need than to prevent injury to children; parents by the most fundamental and supreme right are and must be free to refuse an unwanted or perceived of as too dangerous to inject vaccination. Safervaccines.org can help you protect best!**

Fundamental liberty protects us from the vices of monopolistic healthcare or tyrannical mandates that demand vaccination enslavement. The public should and must be free to seek natural means of healthcare; to pursue what is naturally good for health and decide just what is best for oneself and for one's offspring. Be free to surround yourself with layers of natural protections from disease. Take natural health measures and prevent exposure to unnatural to the body chemicals; build layers of natural protection. Similar to the cumulative benefits of adding air bags, seat belts and fog lights in a motor vehicle; you are building protection and reducing risk of injury by assuring you have the natural to the body building blocks of health and not the unnatural to the body chemicals that are the stumbling blocks of health. The chemicals found in vaccines are anti-health agents. Parents are naturally vested to control their children's chemistries; all States must conform to this MASTER concept-rule, natural order or plan. Slavery of the worst kind is currently in existence today and is growing with each new vaccine chemicalization mandate; we must abolish vaccination slavery by freeing up our God given right to protect our offspring. The TWO STEPS OF CORRECTION will set you free and end the autism epidemic. Be free to reject unwanted chemical injections; protect children accordingly!

It was claimed that a child was injured by a vaccine chemical injection after the parent witnessed their child very quickly degenerate and fall victim to its unnatural to the body chemicalization. It needs to become widely known that unnatural chemicalization is the enemy of good health and the promoter or cause of non-optimal health and/or health problems. Autism is among the results of abnormal infiltration of these very bad chemicals. It is known to many who understand the physiological connection of how these alien to the body chemicals can and do take their toll or rather, how the introduction of such, chemicals destroy health by interfering with the normal everyday every minute and every millisecond reaction within the body. The why it happens is because the natural reactions of the body are completely dependent upon having only the natural chemicals of the reaction present during the time of the reaction and injecting chemicals that are alien to this natural chemical makeup changes reactions; stopping needed reactions and create renegade abnormal reactions, all of with is unhealthy or is causation of ill-health, creating or setting the stage for health problems such as, but not limited to inability to relax when one wants to or is supposed to, lack of proper nerve flow, developmental problems, attention problems and abnormal conditions too numerous in number to not destroy health and/or the life of the child you once knew. Both parents were first baffled over how our government could MANDATE A LAW THAT SUBJECTS ONE TO INJECT their baby with such chemicals or why

VACCINES HAVE UNNATURAL TO THE BODY CHEMICALS. The parents felt they were made to be part of their child's health demise; enforced to do it.

Once the parents became educated as to what chemicals were in vaccines or are still in vaccines they became sick to their stomachs', rightfully; extremely concerned and upset. Both parents were brought to tears and one parent wanted to punish the maker of the vaccine and even do harm to them for not just allowing these chemicals in the vaccines but being part of system that enforces injections with these chemically laced vaccines. When one of the parents found out that they could not seek damages or traditionally use the courts of law to seek redress that parent wanted and still wants to do violence to anyone who knowingly acted or even allowed their child to suffer a vaccine chemicalization with chemicals of mass health destruction. The madness and lunacy of injecting **CHEMICALIZATION AUTISM** will stop; but not until the **TWO STEPS OF CORRECTION** rule over the vaccination system.

Your children should not, must not be subjected to withstand injections of any kind let alone, injections that are vessels for unnatural to the body chemicals. The one most important and extremely positive thing that you can do to prevent autism is to keep your quickly developing baby's clear of alien to their body chemicals by injection or otherwise. Know that injected vaccine chemicalizations that harbor unnatural to the body chemicals quickly circulate to the brain doping the brain cells; abnormal to the natural physiology chemicals enter into the highly sensitive and fragile brain cell biochemistry. Do not risk exposing your offspring to any array of chemicals that are for profit or chemicals that are put vaccines by sheer negligence and/or stupidity. All other freedoms fade or pale compared to liberty of self-regulated healthcare or the freedom to determine one's very own blood chemistry or maintaining and protecting the natural internal chemistry of one's children when you realize your child has been injured by an enforced by mal-law an injected, man-made, chemically engineered, vaccine chemicalization injection. Do not wait till an injury occurs to you or your loved ones; make sure they **GET THE CHEMICALS OUT!** Think of all the things that you can do in the best interest of your children! Certainly, assuring children are not chemically compromised or their health's placed in unnecessary jeopardy is part of proper parenting and **THE ONE MOST IMPORTANT ACTION** for parents!

If a child tests positive for any unnatural to human biology chemicals that maybe laced in vaccines, after vaccination, then the parents of that child must be **FREE** to pursue litigation against the vaccine producer and/or doctor for suffering the child with such, chemicalization and/or for the imperfection of the child's perfected natural chemistry. However, if the doctor made it known to you about all of the chemicals in the vaccine and also, received your informed consent then you have no meritorious case because you ASSumed the risk and agreed to suffer your child with whatever, chemicalization that is in the vaccine unless, the doctor coerced you to inject thereby, nullifying informed consent. You want what is best for your children and need to be **FREE** to make sure they have the best and not be injured or chemically compromised! Health does not come in a needle! Health comes from the inside-out and is totally dependent upon proper chemistry. Do not adulterate your children's chemistry! Natural biochemistry equals optimum health.

The chemicals within us dictate our level of health.

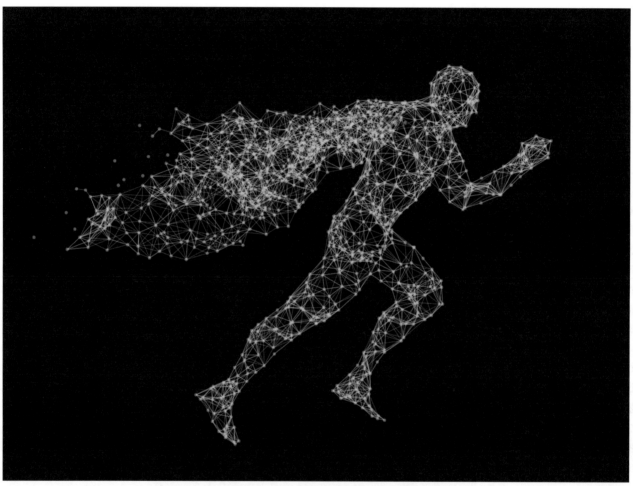

Super health requires a normal biochemistry.
Inject only **SAFER** vaccines.

CHAPTER 4

AUTISM AND VACCINE CHEMICALS

Vaccine chemicals are alien to the body.
Vaccine chemicals are anti-health agents.
AUTISM IS COMORBID WITH VACCINATION

There is an unprecedented urgency to GET THE CHEMICALS OUT of vaccines; the chemicals that are in vaccines for profit and not health, must be removed. It is becoming abundantly clear that the greatest affliction we face today or conflict we must combat is the result of chemicalizations; the unhealthy consequences of being infiltrated by unnatural to the body chemicals is being proven to be our greatest advisory. Injecting such, chemicals through vaccination is an actual attack upon our children and their well-being. Chemicalization needs to be stopped right now, not later; for doing so is essential for the preservation of your children's normal level of health. In order, to prevent a well-being demise or health degeneration the single most important action and/or inaction is to not inject your children with vaccine unnatural to the body chemicals. Chemicalization of our waterways, soil, food and air are grave problems however, the injection of unnatural to the body chemicals that are in vaccines is enemy number one; it is a direct hit with no ability to lessen its impact, it is an immediate blood chemistry alteration, manipulation or distortion. To put unnatural to the body chemicals in our children's vaccines and inject these harmful toxins or unnatural to the body chemicals is madness to the millionth, billionth and zillionth degree. The harm that is taking place to tiny babies, very small infants and immature children when they are chemically compromised by mandated mass vaccine chemical folly is extreme and beyond any other danger. Make no mistake, children require optimum chemistry for optimum health and Autism requires abnormal chemistry!

People are rightfully concerned about the pollution in the air, soil, food and water! Do you think we should be concerned about polluting baby's blood by injecting unnatural to the body chemicals? You should be extremely concerned about injecting unnatural to the body chemicals because all hell breaks loose when you do. Of course, we are rightfully cautioned not to ingest food that has foreign to the body chemicals or breathe in air with such, chemicals or drink dirty chemicalized water however, we must be extremely concerned to the highest degree, to the zillionth degree, when a vaccine needle is pointed at a child is about to be injected with a vaccine having unnatural to the body chemicals. There may be unhealthy consequences whenever we are exposed to pollutants but be warned: injected pollutants penetrate the blood, there is no buffering; there are negative to health impact such as, what results from quickly doping the brain with whatever chemicals happen to be in the vaccine. Autism is more a chemical manifestation than anything else or another comorbid factor. To mandate injections of anti-health chemicals is to mandate child abuse on a mass scale! Save your children from a life that is not chemically optimum; do not be coerced, subdued or enforced to inject, do not be a vaccination slave! For the sake of safety and self-preservation you must be perfectly free to reject vaccine chemicalizations! If you determine vaccination is not in the best interest of your children stand strong; do not submit to vaccination enslavement, protect your children! Protect children from chemicalization autism by not injecting unnatural to the body chemicals!

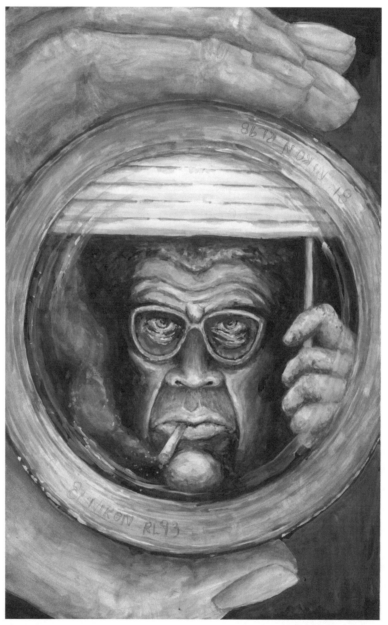

Focus on the unnatural to human biology chemicals that are in vaccines. These chemicals are too dangerous to inject and cause harm to your children.

It is a false assumption that you can inject vaccine chemicals and not disrupt the vital internal chemical matrix or that AUTISM cannot occur. Autism is mainly a chemical manifestation. Chemical stability is lost if vaccine chemical exposure occurs; the chemical web of abnormal reactions takes place. The following is only a partial list of the anti-health chemicals, which have been found in vaccines: Aluminum, known to be associated with Alzheimer's disease and seizures and is cancer producing in lab mice, aluminum phosphate, aluminum hydroxide, formaldehyde (a known cancer causing agent), polysorbate 80, polymyxin B, Neomycin, Streptomycin, 2-phenoxyethanol, Monkey Kidney Cells, Newborn Calf Serum, Ethylene glycol (antifreeze), Phenol also known as carbolic acid (this is used as a disinfectant, dye), human diploid cells (the dissected organs of aborted fetuses), chicken embryo, Formalin, gelatin, Amino Acid, Soy Peptone, Yeast extract, embryonic guinea pig cells and glutamate. Exposing children to such chemicals is the reckless endangerment of children! These chemicals are anti-health agents; contaminants that cause bio-physical crisis. Before the vaccination boon cancer afflicted mainly the old; not the young. Parents' must stop chemical exposures. It is not just the singular exposure; it is multiple vaccinations and combinations of chemicals that are extremely dangerous. It is no wonder that childhood cancer and Autism have rapidly increased. The Autism epidemic is primarily the result of the anti-health chemicals of vaccines; they are the building blocks of Autism. Having chemical clarity and being free to decide your chemical destiny is imperative to your health. Vaccine chemicalization is comorbid with AUTISM. Injecting all the antigens of vaccines also creates a health crisis.

Enforcing unwanted chemical injections is the callous and wanton disregard for the public's safety and violation of personal Rights. The present chemical state of vaccines DENATURES the recipient's blood chemistry. Impure vaccines are disruptive to health; they need to be produced in a way that does not expose children to UNWANTED CHEMICALS. Put abnormal to the body chemicals into rapidly developing babies expect abnormal results. When unnatural, alien to the body vaccine chemicals are PLUNGED INTO THE BLOODSTREAM via injection needle; parents are PLUNGED INTO UNCERTAINTY about the health of their children and the likelihood of resultant chemicalization autism. Vaccination mal-law place parents who have determined a vaccine is too dangerous to inject or that the vaccine chemical concoction will place their children into health uncertainty, in an untenable and intolerable position.

Law has no proper jurisdiction, no business or permanent legal power to enforce chemical infiltrations into perfectly healthy children. Parents find themselves in bondage to this inescapable evil; having to submit their children against their will and better judgment. We must rid parents and their children from this cruel bondage by redeeming children in the safety of their parents! Parents require the freedom to decide what if any medical intervention will be accepted. Parents rightfully must control the vaccination decision. Parents need ultimate authority of decision; deciding to keep their children's chemistry pure or bastardize their chemistry with the mongrel chemistry of vaccines. The mission is to obtain vaccines that are safer; free of unnatural to the body chemicals.

Exposing children to multiple vaccines not only dopes their brains with harmful chemicals it also causes an overstimulation of the brain immune response. Vaccines that enter the brain stimulate a brain immune response that is injurious to the brain. When you massively stimulate the immune system systemically by vaccination you massively activate the immune system of the brain. The microglia cells of the brain are induced to continually respond and for an indefinite period due to the vaccine chemicalization exposure. Microglia cells act as phagocytes cleaning up the CNS therefore, an auto-immune problem result. At the immature age, when most vaccines are injected, the brain is highly susceptible. Cultures that do not vaccinate as much are generally healthier. Unvaccinated children are infinitely healthier than vaccinated children. The unvaccinated have less Autism, less cancer, less frequency of being on antibiotics, less likely to suffer from infections or asthma or allergies. Look at the Amish People or cultures that do not vaccinate and the truth be told that chemicalization of tiny babies is the cause of many health problems. Most vaccines are laden unnatural to the body chemicals, creating chemical warfare within the vaccinated; plundering the vaccinated health's into disarray and spawning Autism. We must act to stop the unlawful mandated chemical infiltration of our children! Over exposure to ever growing numbers of multiple vaccines must also end.

The rate of autism has been skyrocketing as the rate or number of vaccines have increased. The national number of children afflicted with autism has grown to a staggering 1 out of 62 children. However, there is a revealing fact that each States' autism rate is markedly different; the rates are closely related to the rate of vaccination compliance and/or the rate of non-compliance. Why is it that they do not break down the autism rate among the States and give each state's vaccination compliance rate; are they hiding something? States that have the highest vaccination compliance rate have the highest autism rate. States which have higher non-vaccination compliance records or numbers of children whom are not at all vaccinated have less frequency of autism. This reveals that the epidemic of autism is primarily induced by vaccine chemicalization or that if you are not chemicalized with vaccines you stand a much better chance of not having a child with autism. Once unnatural to the body chemicals enter the brain cells it becomes something insidious and autism becomes more a possibility; it is the culprit of the epidemic. Injection of vaccine chemicalization takes its unhealthy toll at the cellular level. Abnormal chemicalization of the brain places a child in grave danger of autism. Do your own research and conclude about vaccines and the autism causation. The truth allows you to make an informed decision and liberty to self-regulate your health allows you to act on your decision. Parents must not be commanded to inject chemicals into their children! Your children need and deserve their optimum natural chemical environment; our children must not be enslaved to be chemically compromised! BE FREE TO REJECT, INJECTIONS!

In addition, the laws of chemistry points to what is spawning autism. The laws of chemistry or the rules of chemical reactions apply to the chemistry within children's brain cells; when vaccine chemicals strike into the reactive mixture the homeostasis is lost. Chemicals govern reactions and toxic cells which are infiltrated with alien chemicals dictate abnormal reactions. Toxic cells do not survive well or not at all; the inherent intelligence of cellular functioning or cellular creation is interfered with. The penetration of unnatural to the body chemicals found in vaccines bastardize, alter and manipulate the internal chemistry of the brain cells. Once normal reactions are disrupted, and abnormal reactions begin perfect health is impossible or rather, autism can occur. Vaccine chemicalizations short circuit a healthy happy life. When unnatural to the body vaccine chemicals are injected it enters the child's brain cells; not only disrupting the normal reactions of the brain but also, creating renegade, completely alien to the body reactions. We need to live free, empowered to keep our children's blood chemistry naturally pure. Reject injections of unwanted chemicalization and GET THE CHEMICALS OUT of vaccines!

The rule of chemical engagement is when an unnatural to the body chemical, one that is alien to the normal reactions of the body and foreign to natural chemical constituents is that abnormality will occur. Vaccine' chemicals such as, aluminum or a mercury derivative, is not an essential or needed chemical or one of the normal chemicals in making biologically required or needed products that produce optimum health; chaos or abnormal reaction products occur. Production of normal products that generate health are curtailed, interfered with and made impossible. What is perhaps more disconcerting being that abnormal production of totally unnatural to the body chemical reactive concoctions are spawned into existence. The injection of chemical A produces renegade abnormal reaction after reaction; resulting in abnormal B, C, D, E or F abnormal chemical molecular structurers that are alien to the once healthy body. All the inability to produce essential products needed to generate optimum health and the production of unnatural products, alien to the body or that are not part of the natural metabolism act to destroy health; allowing autism to become a nightmare reality.

Only a fool would say that a mere unnatural chemicalization of tiny babies, little infants and small children is okay or will not impact their health or contribute to or cause autism! Those who knowingly place unnatural to the body chemicals in vaccines which, by their very nature, cause health problems are considered madmen by the rationally health minded and certain individuals who insist upon its injection especially, over the objection of parents are not only madmen; they are guilty of child abuse by chemicalization and must be considered criminally insane or at minimum found to be guilty of gross negligence for the reckless endangerment of our offspring whom are all naturally sensitive to the chemicals that have been found in vaccines. Like vultures they prey upon our children in order, to make obscene profit. They manipulated for their self-serving benefit the twisted concept that vaccinations are mandated over parental objection and when their negligently produced vaccines cause injury the makers of the hurtful vaccine have seen to it that they cannot be touched or made to pay for causing the injury. The mighty wave of public opinion is that parents, not government, must be empowered to control whether a vaccination will be delivered or if it is in the child's best interest. In addition, society expects that when a vaccine is accused of causing an injury; the injured party must be legally enabled to bring the vaccine manufacturer to a traditional court of law to seek justice and hold accountable the maker' of the vaccine. It is a heinous crime which has been committed upon society; the exposure of the masses with such, chemicals for profit and not safety and the wanton disregard of the parental right to protect children by mandating vaccine injection over parental objection, has perpetuated and advanced the autism epidemic etc. The blatant disregard for parental authority and child abuse by vaccine unnatural chemicalization must not be left unpunished!

Mandated vaccination laws are BAD LAWS, mal-laws which are NOT constitutional and that MUST NOT CONTINUE TO REMAIN AS LAW. Mandated vaccination laws reduce our children to MANDATED VACCINE INJECTION ADDICTS that are ENSLAVED TO SUFFER INJECTIONS OF VACCINE CHEMICALS. The worst drug addicts are those which inject, quickly penetrating their bloodstream and brain with all of the chemicals injected and thereby, causing perpetual listlessness; vaccines that are laced with anti-health, unnatural to the body chemicals can cause perpetual listlessness, like an injecting dope addict. The abnormal neurological listlessness and AUTISM SPECTRUM can result from ENFORCING VACCINE CHEMICAL INJECTIONS, ENSLAVING CHILDREN TO BE VACCINATED AND MAKING CHILDREN VACCINE INJECTION ADDICTS. We must take measures to GET THE CHEMICALS OUT. The regulatory agencies have corrupted the system that it is in desperate need of repair, there are TWO STEPS necessary to begin the uphill battle of needed reform; this book is all about the TWO STEPS OF CORRECTION.

My proverb to live by is, "if you face the risk of childhood disease or the risk of AUTISM it is much smarter to face childhood disease". Make no mistake, chemicals in vaccines are harmful to vaccine recipients; chemically laced vaccines are a realistic threat. Vaccine Producers must be made to take prudent safety steps to make vaccines devoid of anti-health chemicals. Vaccine contents can even be life threatening. There must be transparency in what chemicals are in vaccines. There must be full disclosure of all the contents of vaccines, there must be full disclosure of what chemicals are used in the production of vaccines and what the vaccines are cultured in. If there is not transparency or full disclosure that means they have something to hide. If there is not full disclosure the Vaccination recipients are not being adequately informed, making the informed aspect of informed consent/DENIAL a sham. Without transparency or full disclosure, it not a legal or moral informed consent/DENIAL and fraud is perpetuated upon the People. There is no legal requirement of consent or denial because the law abdicates one's Right to refuse.

Ask yourself, how many chemicals can my child's body handle until AUTISM? The chemicals of vaccines can cause a critical mass syndrome and/or AUTISM. So why do they put such chemicals in vaccines and why are animal tissue remnants found in vaccines? The main reason why preservative chemicals are used is to secure profits; they give the vaccine greater shelf-life thereby, preventing returns and inducing stock piling. Tissue remnants are found in vaccines because the process of making the vaccines requires them to be cultured in live cells. When parents are informed of what chemicals are in vaccines, or what is used in the vaccine production or what the vaccines are cultured in it is then that they realize vaccines are too dangerous to inject, are not in their children's best interest and are the greatest health threat to children. Informed consent emancipates our decision over vaccinations and promotes vaccine quality, instilling that there will be no anti-health chemicals in vaccines. Informed consent assures that parent's childrearing health decisions are neither ignored nor deprived. Informed consent is required for self-preservation and to assure we can self-govern our very own health care.

What is of concern other than health problems and/or genotoxicity or DNA damage that can stem from the injection of anti-health or unnatural to the body chemicals is the fact that all vaccines have antigens that are foreign to the body DNA, RNA and proteins that cause allergic reactions and could cause a genetic problem. In addition, there are yeast, bacteria and other foreign to the body biological entities in vaccines. The world's leading vaccine expert, who was Chief of the Merck pharmaceutical vaccine division, Maurice Hillemen said there were problems with the agents in vaccines "tumors popping out in

these hamsters" when referring to those hamsters injected with vaccines. He also said that he "had a feeling in his bones that the viruses in vaccines could have some long-term affects" when asked what long-term affects he responded "cancer". About the claims of vaccine success or that vaccines were being taunted as successful he said that there was, "too much of a show, too much Hollywood, too much exaggeration." He also, said that the science of vaccinations was a "crude science." It is of ultimate importance that people be given the naked truth about vaccines and be given the knowledge of these entire negative to health facts and be given their freedom of healthcare choice and/or self-preservation Right. Enforcing, injection of vaccine chemicals violates people. People must have the Right to be in self-control! The wall of protection that best protects children is parents being free to refuse unwanted chemicals and liberty to litigate against vaccine producers when vaccines are accused of causing injury.

Informed of the pros and cons of vaccination you then can make an educated decision and exercise your Right of decision. The sorry state of vaccines has occurred because informed consent/ DENIAL is not in control of whether a vaccine will be administered; the mandated vaccination law makes it so. In addition, it is because Vaccine Producers are not held accountable and liable for vaccine induced injuries. Vaccine Producers must be prompted to a higher level of vaccine quality safety control. This is accomplished by allowing those injured by a vaccine to litigate directly against the vaccine companies for compensation; making Vaccine Producers pay when their negligently produced vaccines cause injury to our children and by applying the traditional healthcare requirement of informed consent/**DENIAL**.

There is a continuum of undue influence upon our legislators to inappropriately protect or benefit Vaccine Producers at the detriment of our children's safety. Aggrieved parents of children injured by the chemicals of vaccines have been precluded from seeking damages against vaccine producers. Due to the heavy bombardment of lobbyists doing Vaccine Companies bidding they have manipulated the Legislature to not only impede citizens' right to access the courts for injuries that have been perpetrated by the vaccine chemical industry but have unjustly blocked victims right to have recourse against the overly self-serving Vaccine Producers that were the cause of injury. Society has reflexively been programmed into vaccination and mal-law has it that all parents must have their children vaccinated; we are enslaved to be vaccinated. All the above is counterproductive to vaccine safety; it allows runaway negligent vaccine production. The public can greatly benefit from a just vaccination program that is based upon full disclosure of vaccine contents, freedom of decision or being enabled to refuse a vaccination and being free to bring vaccine producers to court to be held accountable and liable and pay for injuries their vaccines cause. We must take the steps necessary to make vaccines reasonably safe. This book will repetitively point out the need to hold Vaccine Producers accountable and liable for the dangerous chemicals that they continue to place in vaccines; chemicals that are for profit and not safety. Vaccines and/or its producers' must be brought under proper standards of negligence law and there must be liberty to refuse unwanted vaccine chemicalization; the result will be cleaner, safer vaccines. **Mandated vaccinations render the Constitution and Bill of Rights worthless.**

Energy or magnetic fields rule the interaction of chemicals and therefore, have control of reaction outcomes and health itself. Health has a certain energy vibration and autism has a distorted energy vibration. Every chemical that is injected into tiny babies has a magnetic

signature and is this magnetic/energy that is extremely disruptive. The injection of alien to the body chemicals wreaks havoc with the magnetism or energy fields within babies quickly developing bodies and/or brain cells. Unnatural to the body energy fields or magnetic signatures forms alien matter or non-essential molecular structures or foreign proteins or abnormal constituents that are destructive to health and/or interfere with normal brain function or development. Whether it is the physical presence of the injected chemicals with its negative to health propensities or the quantum physics or magnetic properties of the alien to the body injected chemicalization; one thing is certain and that is that no one should be enforced to undergo mass chemicalization child abuse or be enslaved to be vaccinated! Adults must be responsible for our own health and parents for the health of their offspring; the fundamental liberty of self-determined healthcare or self-regulation of what will or will not enter our very own bodies protects us from healthcare dictatorship!

Vaccines must not be injected if they contain ANTI-HEALTH CHEMICALS. Anti-health chemicals are those chemicals which are alien, foreign to the body that are not naturally found in the body. The presence of such chemicals causes abnormality. The normal reactions of the body cannot freely take place and abnormal reactions are catalyzed. ANTI-HEALTH CHEMICALS are synonymous with ANTI-HEALTH and/or AUTISM; their presence does not have benefit, only detriment. These chemicals interfere with the normal biochemistry, causing renegade biology. It certainly does not serve or stand for truth, justice and the American way to not adequately inform the public about all the chemicals in vaccines and to not be enabled to seek justice when injured by vaccination or wage a lawsuit against Vaccine Producers when vaccines cause injury. To not allow parents their basic protection of their children or to forbid parents to refuse unwanted vaccine chemical injections or not allow the decency of the vaccination healthcare decision is egregious. There is a cascade of immune response to being vaccinated, not just the desired antibodies; the chemicals are destructive to health.

Anti-health chemicals must be removed from the vaccine production. Through the repeated practice of satisfying the demands of parents whom insist upon chemical free vaccines and/or to obtain parent's true informed consent, a point where there are minimal chemicals in vaccines will be reached and minimal disturbance to the vaccine recipient's chemistry will thereby be achieved. There is no health benefit to having ant-health agents in vaccines, only health detriment. The chemical constituents of vaccines have a direct impact on the health of the injected hence, vaccines must become clean.

We the People need the autonomy of vaccination decision for ourselves and our posterity. Informed consent and holding vaccine companies liable will remove unwanted vaccine chemicals. Autism frequency will decrease when all the **dangerous chemicals** are removed from **vaccines**. Vaccination compulsion must end, and **PARENTAL DECISION COMPULSION and PARENTAL SATISFACTION COMPULSION** must begin. Americans look forward to the time when there is **FREEDOM OF SELF-DETERMINED VACCINATIONS AND ONE CAN REFUSE BEING INJECTED.** There are few things worse than losing your freedom to protect your child such as, not being able to legally prevent your child from receiving, a conceived of as to dangerous to inject, vaccine injection. To pollute a child's chemistry is wrong period.

Democracy and vaccination slavery cannot coexist indefinitely; we must make a choice to achieve healthcare freedom by putting an end to vaccination SLAVERY. Government is not meant to dictate what will be injected into children's bloodstreams by subcutaneous or intramuscular injection or tweak or fine tune blood chemistry or enforce the risk and shock of vaccine CHEMICAL injections. We must secure our natural Right of self-determined healthcare and be free to make the conclusive decision to vaccinate or not. PARENTS ARE NATURALLY EMPOWERED TO DECIDE for their children if vaccines are to be injected. Chemicals can be the building blocks of health or the stumbling blocks.

Premise: It is much smarter and healthier to not expose your children to alien to the body chemicals. Exposure to unnatural to the body chemicals can only have negative impact upon one's health. The present state of vaccines has unnatural to the biology or physiology chemicals and therefore, should be avoided. By avoiding such, vaccines the production of safer vaccines will be stimulated. Parents must be free to prevent their children from chemicalization. Parents must no longer be made or enforced by mal-law to gamble with their offspring's health or compromise to any degree the chemical well-being of their children. All children are chemically sensitive to unnatural to the body chemicals. Before considering vaccination make sure you know what is in the vaccine; be absolutely, positive that there is no alien to the body chemicals! While it is true that certain children, because they already have a distorted chemical make-up prior to being exposed to a vaccine chemical injection are more vulnerable to vaccine chemicalization; the fact is, vaccines have unhealthy chemicals that need to be avoided. The chemical toxins of vaccines take their unhealthy toll on everyone, just more so in individuals who are already chemically compromised or that have a higher foreign to the body chemical exposure level previous to the injections. Avoid chemicalization; demand safer vaccines; demand the TWO STEPS OF CORRECTION to GET THE CHEMICALS OUT!

Good health, excellent human physiology and bodily functions are all dependent upon a proper chemistry. Upset the natural chemistry of the body or brain cells or homeostasis brings on autism etc. We are chemically dependent and must have certain chemicals to survive. On the other hand, outside the realm of the chemicals that we need to sustain optimum life there are those chemicals that are a burden to a healthy existence and are so unnatural to the body that they destroy health and cause abnormality; they are the stumbling blocks of health. Each one our cells have a permeable membrane that protects each cell; it allows entrance into the cell and exit out of the cell. Unnatural to the body chemicals distort or abnormally manipulate membrane permeability causing dysfunction on the cellular level. Some natural to the body chemicals are absolutely required for the proper physiology and function of the cell membrane and the cell itself. Unnatural to the body chemicals are anti-health chemicals that cause our cell's membrane to malfunction, this jeopardizes the integrity, health and life of our cells. Toxic chemicals are the enemy and must not be in vaccines! Injections of such chemicals are the main cause of the autism epidemic. Prompt the removal of such, chemicals, by being free to reject injections!

We are dependent upon the proper chemistry to be optimally healthy and to prevent Autism; this optimum chemistry must not be disturbed. The injection of anti-health chemically laced vaccines sets the stage for abnormality and the critical chemical mass syndrome. **Proper human physiology and biological functions are completely dependent upon marinating just the right chemistry.**

We must maintain this delicate balance of proper chemistry otherwise abnormality and/ or Autism can take place. Your child's bloodstream chemistry must be safeguarded; chemical exposure destroys health. The law should not invade individual's privacy to the extent that it not only demands vaccination records but also, dictates that your children must be vaccinated. A law which demands its citizens or its citizen's children to be chemically exposed and/or be injected with vaccine chemicals is **BAD LAW**.

How dependent we are on the normal chemical composition or rather how our millions of cells existence is completely dependent upon just the right chemistry and/or chemical configuration can be realized by understanding what is known as the Sodium/Potassium pump, a physiological mechanism responsible for transporting chemicals in and out of each one of our cells. This pump mechanism of the cell is just one example of just how dependent we are upon the natural chemistry of the body. Chemicals such as potassium, an electrolyte mineral, are natural and needed to be healthy whereas, vaccine chemicals are unnatural to the body and only serve to interfere or harm the natural processes. The present chemicals that can be found in vaccines alter the chemistry in and out of the cells. Exposing cells to such anti-health chemicals can interfere with the needed sodium/ potassium pump, normal biological reactions and render the individual health compromised. Mandating the present state of chemically laced vaccines is like **MANDATING VACCINATION OF POISON** and/or is a law or **ENFORCEMENT OF VACCINE CHEMICAL POISONS**. Will you demand to be free to refuse? Being chemically compromised is synonymous with being health compromised; protect your children accordingly!

This same pump system keeps cells healthy by taking what needs to be removed from inside the cell to the outside of the cell thereby, keeping the cell clean from **unwanted chemicals**. This transport takes place at the cell membrane and is totally dependent upon the **proper level of just two (2) chemicals, Sodium and Potassium**. Sodium and potassium act like guards escorting chemicals in and of the cells. Without the adequate amount of these needed chemicals or if anti-health chemicals are present the physiological pump breaks down; cells malfunction and die. **Vaccine's anti-health chemicals interfere with the normal biochemistry of the body, producing abnormal physiology that can escalate to Autism. A proper functioning brain is reliant upon the proper sensitive chemical environment; brain cells malfunction when saturated with blood that has anti-health vaccine chemicals. Vaccine chemicals are the main cause of Autism; we must rid vaccines of their harmful chemicals.**

People have a Right to be left alone and not have their bloodstreams defiled by unclean fluids and/or vaccine chemicals. The chemicals of vaccines are unclean in fact; they are dirty and harmful. The purity of the bloodstream is destroyed or rendered abnormal by the injection of vaccine chemicals. Man cannot be permitted by law to defile his fellow man and/or make one subject to unwanted injections of chemicals. The law must not require children to be exposed to chemicals. Parents must be allowed to secure chemical stability for children.

Adults are cautioned to not subject themselves to vaccine chemicalization of unnatural to the body chemicals otherwise, health can readily be lost. If adults that have mature systems, with everything on line and functioning optimally are much better off not being exposed to chemicalization by injection then babies, must be saved from the abuses of vaccine chemicalization of unnatural to the body chemicals. The early in life multiple assault and battery of mandated vaccination chemical abuse is taking its toll on children; parents are warned to make sure that there are no chemicals for profit in vaccines. In this book I will state many times that the autism epidemic is caused by unnatural to the body vaccine chemicalization and Alzheimer's in adults is caused by such, chemicals particularly, when adults are injected with a Flu shot that still has its full dosage of thimerosal, the mercury derivative preservative. Know what you are getting into to when you are contemplating vaccination and never let anyone decide for you or force you! It is not merely gambling with your offspring's life or health; it is an actual chemicalization insult! The time to act, to be proactive for your children's welfare, is prior to injection chemicalization, post injection the harm is done; there is no turning back once the chemicals are injected!

Vaccinations can be modern medicine's gift to mankind however, vaccines have anti-health chemicals and to blindly accept them turns the "gift" into a **health hazard**. The mandate and no legal recourse turn the gift into a wolf in sheep's clothing, **a plight upon mankind (AUTISM)**. Being enslaved to vaccinate and no negligence applied to vaccination has caused anti-health chemicals that are for profit, not safety. Medical intervention should always be questioned or sought to be determined if there are any adverse consequences from its administration; it needs to be regularly analyzed to be improved upon and be safe. Vaccine chemicals are a problem that must be resolved. The common cause of the Autism epidemic has a common denominator that being; common vaccine chemical injection exposure of the masses. **There are dangers in mandating (enslaving) vaccinations such as**, **the runaway number of vaccine injections** with its prolific harmful list of chemicals for profit instead, of safety.

The chemical content within your children's blood and/or body dictates whether they are healthy or not; chemicals influence upon health supersedes genetics and chemicals can command or trigger genetic expression. You can have the best genetic of possibilities but still; if unnatural to the body chemicals or anti-health chemicals are present it may cause disruption of health and even eventually precipitate genetic changes. The mind can visualize or believe in optimum health however, what the mind conceives and believes is not necessarily achieved in the presence of unnatural to the body chemicals. You can consider that chemicals take on a life of their own since, chemicals influence reactions and all its end products. Enforced injection of vaccine chemicals manipulates the particles and/or natural chemistry of the bloodstream; manipulation of one's homeostatic chemistry perpetuates Autism. The familiar particles and/or normal ingredients of the body begin to be altered and a new class of particles and ingredients ensues, the changes are difficult to detect; they are on the molecular level. A resultant gateway of abnormal/alien reactions occur, and normal reactions may not take place. One just cannot totally anticipate the harm from injecting the chemicals that have been found in vaccines.

Parents are unwise to submit children for vaccine injections without knowing just what chemicals are in vaccines. It is presumptuous and is so very naive to repetitively inject chemicals into children and think that children are better off for it. **Chemicals must be eliminated from vaccines** to protect our children and end the Autism epidemic. Parents' having freedom to prevent their children from being exposed to unwanted chemical infusions is crucial to securing health and **ENDING the Autism epidemic**.

Freedom of choice in healthcare is extremely important. People naturally require choices in healthcare and the **LIBERTY to decide what is best for their body and/or health**. For example, if a female child did not naturally get chickenpox because they were vaccinated with Varicella vaccine for chickenpox; the vaccination induced immunity will wane over time allowing the now adult the risk of chickenpox. If this adult becomes pregnant and gets chickenpox it can cause a spontaneous abortion. **People need to be told the risks of vaccination and have the choice to refuse those risks by choosing not to be vaccinated. If you limit the public's choices in healthcare a monopoly forms with absolute power over you and/or over your choices; absolute power corrupts absolutely. The People's Right to Self-Govern their bodies is violated by MANDATED VACCINATION ENSLAVEMENT CHEMICALIZATIONS. The liberty to self-govern over your health and for parents to govern over their children's health or healthcare is natural law, fundamental law and understood as, sacrosanct!**

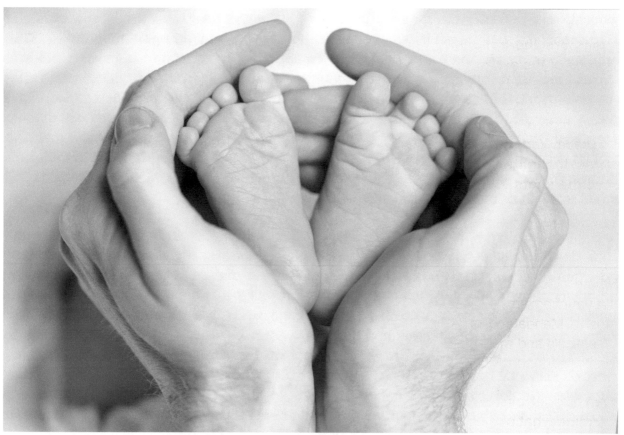

**YOUR CHILDREN = YOUR DECISION
BE FREE TO REJECT INJECTIONS!**

CHAPTER 5

CHILDREN NEED THEIR PARENTS' PROTECTION

PARENTS NEED TO PROTECT THEIR CHILDREN

Parents are the natural custodians of their children. Parents must always remain the keystone of the arch of protection for children; having supreme power to protect. Inherent in parents is the innate ability and caring to decide what is best for their children. Under GOD's law children must be secure in their parent's protection. It is imperative to children's welfare that parents are emotionally okay with vaccination otherwise, no vaccination should take place. Vaccinations can be bad or good depending upon their chemical content and parents' thoughts and/or heart felt emotions. In the best interest of children, parents need to call the shots. Children are emotionally, spiritually and physically anchored, in their parents' care for them and/or protection and parents are anchored in protecting their children to the best of their ability. Parents must have the **DECISION POWER, the control** over whether a vaccination will or will not be administered. No law should overrule parent's preventative healthcare decisions for their children or overpower parent's Right to protect their **PERFECTLY HEALTHY** children from unwanted vaccine chemical exposure. Children need their parents to protect them by securing their optimum chemistry of optimum health. Any government control of children's health is extremely offensive. Mandated vaccinations are an outrage, an affliction, an ongoing, ever growing exposure to chemicals and major violation of human Rights. Government control over people is especially, wrong when it comes to our children's healthcare!

Do not be controlled instead, have control over your children's internal being and welfare; you determine what chemicals, if any, are to be injected. The erroneous mandated vaccination law replaces parents with government, dismisses parents from performing parenting, it puts parents out of commission; and wrongfully commands that children will be vaccinated over parent's objections. We must build a greater sense of children being anchored in their parents; protected by them. The mal- vaccination mandate forbids parents' from refusing vaccination even when parents have done their research and determined that the injection of vaccine chemicals is not be in their children's best interest or plunges their children into health uncertainty. The growing continual increase in the number of chemical vaccine injections that government enslaves children to withstand is beyond reasonable; it is preposterous. The faulty mandated vaccination law cuts parents' off from protecting their children, it wrongfully prevents parents from saving their children from unwanted chemical exposure; it annihilates parenting. Children need their parents' protection and parents need to protect their children. Parents need to be free to protect their children from the vices of overly zealous medical intervention or unwanted chemical exposure. **Parents must be free to protect their children from unwanted, vaccine**

chemical injections and/or stop what they think causes autism. Your children need to rely upon your judgement; not government's!

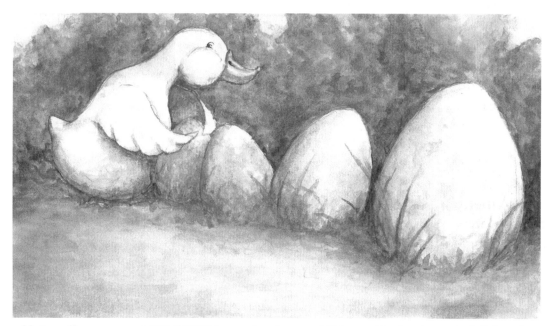

Naturally we must BE FREE to protect our children. Protect your children's vital blood and body biochemistry by only considering SAFER vaccines.

It is unconstructive suffering to place chemicals not natural for the body in vaccines and inject them. Not giving parents the basic Right to refuse chemicalizations is insane. It is not the first time the understanding that exposure to anti-health chemicals cause health crisis has been passed down to the intelligentsia. Too much chemical exposure, too many vaccinations, too much medical interest impedes your existence, rather than enhancing it. The least amount of chemical exposure from vaccine's the better! Making vaccinations a mandate is the practice of neurotic vaccination intervention and is slavery! People must be free to pick and choose their own health care destiny and not be forced to follow one pathway or another's decision of what healthcare is best. The risks inherent with each vaccination decision must be born by the family therefore, it must be up to the family; not the law. No matter how insignificant or severe the risk of receiving or not receiving preventative healthcare and/or vaccinations; parents must hold the power to refuse or allow the medical intervention. Preventing unwanted chemical infiltrations is a primary directive of parenting. Freedom to reject injections promotes safer vaccines and thereby, protects children; to advocate otherwise, is to advocate chemicalization child abuse that perpetuates the **AUTISM EPIDEMIC**. Your children should not be stripped of your vital decision protection role by mal-law!

There are important to life and health consequences to the vaccination decision and therefore, must be decided by parents; not government. Being made dependent upon government in the course of how we live in a society or what is permissible or not in society under rules and regulation is one thing however; government making our healthcare decision or ruling upon our internal well-being or deciding upon just what healthcare shall or shall not be accepted or denied is quite another thing in fact; it is a violation upon our core right to be left alone or in control of our very being. People must not be dictated to in decisions about their healthcare such as, preventative healthcare vaccinations. People are vested with a fundamental right to be in control of their person or personage. For

government to dictate one's healthcare decision of vaccination is not only an affliction upon one's right to be left alone and is immoral and illegal; it is a command affliction to health by chemicalization injection that has spawned the autism epidemic. No one can rationally argue that mandated vaccination is not an unnatural to the body chemicalization. Parents must live in the freedom of caring for and protecting their children to the best of their ability; free to keep children from such, chemical infusions and out of the reach of reach of overly zealous medical intervention or mandated vaccine chemicalization child abuse. Parents' be free to reject unwanted vaccine chemicalization!

Many are awakening, becoming aware of what has been taken from them and are recognizing mandated vaccinations for what they are. Recognition that your children's vital blood chemistry is being manipulated by enforced vaccination is hard to reconcile or differ to or acquiesce to when you learn that vaccination is an industry that is based upon profit and not necessarily safety. Make no mistake, the contents of vaccines too often are formulated not for your children's safety but rather, to maximize profits. Putting preservatives in vaccines is just the tip of the iceberg when it comes to unneeded unnatural to the body chemical exposure. What has been taken from parents is not mere money or possessions; what has been taken is the primary reason for being a parent and that is to care and protect children to the best of one's ability. Parents' that do not agree with all these mandated vaccinations or have determined that the multiple chemical vaccine injections are health degenerating or cause autism etc. are forbidden to refuse; this is so, so wrong, that it must be made right. Be free to reject unwanted injections!

A major threat to those children who are injected with the chickenpox vaccination is that it does not give lifetime immunity; superior lifetime immunity only comes from naturally getting Chickenpox. If a pregnant woman was vaccinated as a child the pregnant woman can get shingles from the vaccination or worse, can get chickenpox because the vaccine waned over time; this could cause her pregnancy to end in a spontaneous abortion. The impact of Chickenpox vaccination can be severe; parents must be free to decide! The audacity for government to decide such, life decisions is beyond reasonable and/or legal. Parents need be told of this horrific possibility before allowing their child to be vaccinated and is obvious reason that the choice to be vaccinated or not be vaccinated must be up to the parents; not government or Drug companies that profit from it!

No other than parents should decide if their children should face the immediate perils inherent from injecting the chemicals of vaccines along with the horrific possibility of losing a pregnancy because of not naturally getting the childhood disease. There must be freedom for parents to way out the risks and decide what is best for children. Families must not be forced to jeopardize their health or a future pregnancy because they were enforced to vaccinate. People must be given freedom of healthcare choice and not made to suffer the consequences of Varicella vaccine chemicals or be made to rely upon waning vaccination immunity. Parents should not have to endure their children being **stuck** with a vaccination needle and then be **stuck** with the risks inherent or negative consequences. **The risks of vaccine chemicals causing health problems and vaccines leaving you susceptible to problems later in life must not be forced upon the People. Problems such as, loss of pregnancy if the vaccine wanes, must not be coerced, enforced or forced upon free citizens otherwise, we are not fundamentally free.** The People must decide what is best for their very own healthcare, based on an individual basis. Mal-law must not prevent parents from being efficient and effective protectors of their children; **parents must be free to prevent vaccine chemical injection exposure.**

If you are vaccinated for chickenpox you become susceptible to painful Shingles later in life. In addition, natural immunity to chickenpox is better than immunity from a series of vaccinations. Natural immunity can have its rare risks of shingles however, the decision whether to vaccinate must be yours and you should not be blocked by an erroneous vaccination mandate to decide what is in your or your children's best interest. **The People must have the Right to decide what is best for their children and not be forbidden by the puppet governmen If a child tests positive t which is bent on assuring Vaccine Producers' profiteering.** Whose choices are these anyway, whose body is at risk and who should be entitled to make the healthcare decision; **individuals' must choose, not government.** The short-term, mid-term and long-term health consequences are ours to bare. It is a matter of personal healthcare choice and mandated vaccinations **obliterate those choices,** enslaving us to be vaccinated with all its negative results. **LIVE FREE TO PROTECT YOUR CHILDREN; BE EMPOWERED TO REJECT VACCINATION. ALLOW YOUR CHILDREN TO LIVE A CHEMICALLY FREE NON-AUTISTIC LIFE. LIVE UNDISTURBED IN THE CARING OF YOUR CHILDREN; DECIDE WHAT IS BEST FOR THEM.**

We must right the wrongs of enforced vaccinations. **Vaccines are not wholesome with their current state of chemical contents.** A new standard of vaccine quality that has no alien to the body chemicals must be achieved. We must assure this standard, having production as close to this good standard as possible. **Nothing should champion the defeat of parent's** protection of children from chemically laced vaccines or deter the pursuit of this desired vaccine quality good standard. Children do not need a nanny government dictating vaccinations; what are needed are the unfettered natural protections afforded by parents. To postulate that parents are incapable of making the vaccination decision or that government is a better vaccination decision maker is the height of human arrogance and an act of **over paternalism** on the part of **nanny government.** **Children need their parent's protective decisions adhered to such as, the decision that a vaccination is too chemically unsafe. Make sure you protect your children properly.**

Picture what likely occurred in a pharmaceutical company board meeting when they chose to put unnatural to the body, chemicals for and not safety in vaccines that would eventually be injected into your baby. One person seeking a pay increase and promotion calls out that he has a method of increasing profits by approximately 40 million. The master or head person of authority said qui5e everyone; let this bright person have the floor please, do tell us how! This is how; we put a preservative in the vaccine, a chemical concoction known as thimerosal, a mercury derivative. This will give the vaccine longer shelf-life and because of the increased shelf there will be less vaccine returns and our sales reps will only have to go to the doctor's office once a year instead, of four times which, represents a 75% savings. The money we save from returns or from spoilage will make us or save us mega-millions. One supposedly, caring board member meekly raises her hand and then states, "but mercury is a known neurotoxin ..."; the money crazed head says "sit down and shut up, the 40 million has it, it will assure our jobs and bonuses." It matters not why they have breached our confidence and placed our children in jeopardy; what matters is that there are unnatural to the body chemicals in vaccines and what we are going to do about it!

Know every chemical that is in the vaccine and then decide yes or no; be free to say "NO" and protect your children to the best of your ability. Imperial government or puppet government of drug companies or their lobbyists must not discount parental authority or disavow what parents think is best for their children; parents' must have the basic and most precious liberty to refuse unwanted medical intervention and readily refuse unwanted vaccine injections or chemicalization, if they deem it in their children's best interest! Mandated vaccination is slavery of the worst kind and it is chemicalization child abuse on a mass scale. If we are not free to decide what will or will not be allowed or not allowed to be injected into our blood vessels or body, then we are not free; we are enslaved to be vaccinated, enslaved to suffer the consequences of chemicalization.

Vaccination laws treat parents as if they have a history of being negligent parents or were pre-determined to be feeble minded without the basic ability to discern the vaccination question. Parents for the sake of their children need to be their **legal** vaccination decision makers'; this will also propagate safer vaccines that parents' will be more likely to approve of. Parents commonly make all health-related decisions for children; it is as a matter of fact that parental informed consent is required for all medical intervention. **Vaccinations are an enigma, the WRONGFUL exception to the golden rule that parents control their children's healthcare. Every chemical used in the vaccine's production should be boldly informed to parents and parents who think that the chemicals are too dangerous to inject must be free to refuse the vaccination. The least chemical exposure the better! Injected chemicals quickly circulate to the brain; can pass the blood-brain barrier and chemically dope brain cells. Yes, there are other causations of Autism but, injected vaccine chemicals are the main etiology that has spawned the autism epidemic. BOYCOTT or refuse dirty vaccines! Your baby, infant or child is dependent upon you; do not let them down, properly, protect them! Do not let the vaccination monopoly or paid for government law deter you from your mission to protect!**

You want the most competent chemistry for your children that assures their optimum health! You want SAFER vaccines; not unsafe vaccine chemicalizations. An all-important reason why parents must be free to say "NO" to a vaccination is that it prompts, stimulates or induces safety, in that safer vaccines that do not contain unnatural to the body chemicals will always be produced. Parents freedom to protect their children gives them the complete liberty to refuse an unwanted vaccine chemicalization thereby, instilling safer vaccines that parents may consider for injection. CHILDREN NEED THEIR PARENTS' PROTECTION and PARENTS' NEED TO PROTECT THEIR CHILDREN!

The negative impact of infusing brain cells of tiny babies, little infants and small children with unnatural to the body vaccine chemicals is immeasurable. A vaccine chemicalization attacks quickly and there is no defense or buffering its impact whereas, if you eat an unnatural to the body chemical, the body can at least to some degree, deal with it to eliminate it by either vomiting, urinating or defecating it out. Parents should be on high alert; making it their highest protection priority not to expose their offspring to such, alien chemicalization which, are injected, bypassing the natural elimination systems!

Parents are encoded to care for their children optimally. Parent's brains are hardwired with certain instinctual behavior patterns, being predisposed mentally and physically to respond to their environment in ways that will enable their children to best survive and be optimally healthy. Parents have no conflict of interest when it comes to securing their children's health; their allegiance is only to their children. Nanny government and Vaccine Producers at best have comparatively sporadic moments of clarity in caring for our children and certainly, are guilty of gross conflict of interest. We live in the age where lobbyists self-serving agenda or profiteering rule decision making. The fact that certain chemicals have been found in vaccines rebukes any trust that we have blindly put in Vaccine Producers. Parents must hold the vaccination reins, having total control of the decision of whether to vaccinate. Being enabled to refuse an unwanted vaccine injection is essential to vaccine quality and in the best interest of children and parents. Children need their parent's protection and parents need to protect their children. Reduce your risk of Autism or cancer; be free to avoid toxins or chemicals!

Parents must be free to cultivate safety for their children and do everything to prevent their children from becoming a statistic or victim of the Autism epidemic. Parents have a Right to be proactive in the prevention of injury of their children. Please help children have a full spectrum healthy life! P**arents need to assure that Vaccine Producers avoid indulging in producing unwholesome chemically laden vaccines.** Vaccine Producers do not have the requisite inner discipline that leads to safety first in vaccine production. Bringing about safety first in the minds of Vaccine Producers is generated from parental informed consent/**DENIAL**. Vaccine Producers business sense is to make a profit whereas, parent's primary directive is children's safety. **There are destructive consequences to mandated vaccinations. We must instill for children's welfare the vaccination safety safeguard of TRUE informed consent/DENIAL. No longer should vaccination be mandated; it is mandated madness, mandated chemicalization child abuse that causes biological entropy! There is no predictability of good health when you penetrate immature, developing systems of children with unnatural to their body chemicals; there is only unhealthy certainty. Parents protect your children!**

Autism is spawned by the unleashing of harmful chemicals into the bloodstream of children. The anti-health chemicals of vaccines, once injected, quickly flood the susceptible immature brain cells of children. The chain reaction of negative to health events that ensue leads to the destruction of children's well-being rendering children Autistic. Each alien to the body chemical that is injected can be considered a building block of Autism. The People must not be enslaved to inject their children. The People need their fundamental freedom to refuse chemicals or any medical intervention posed. Parents most essential liberty is the freedom to protect their children from perceived of threats. When you weigh out the risk of the vaccine verses not being vaccinated recognize that not only does the vaccine chemicalization spawn autism as a major concern; the vaccine may not even work and therefore, may not be worth the risk. Government policies enforce 69 doses of vaccines before the age of 18 is way too many chemicalization particularly, since just one chemicalization can cause health decline. This book will not give an in-depth analysis of just how inefficient or ineffective vaccines are instead, the concentration is on how to make vaccines safer however, please know that vaccines are far from a panacea.

Many parents are repulsed that Vaccine Producers are using certain chemicals in vaccine production. Parental informed consent/**DENIAL is vital to assure the successful removal of**

such chemicals. Parents must have prestige and influence in the protection of their children; vaccination delivery must reflect this. Informed consent applied to vaccinations will lead to the resolution of the problem of chemicals in vaccines. It is fundamental to human nature for parents to protect children. **Injecting vaccines** with their chemicals into delicate bloodstreams of children is risky and/or a danger that parents may not want to risk. **We are forced to live under a vaccination dictatorship, having no viable avenue to refuse injection.** It is apparent that whenever you manipulate the natural chemical composition of the blood chemistry health problems will develop. **True informed consent** will end such oppression and prevent injury. Children need a greater sense of security and safety.

William Thompson, a CDC scientist and whistleblower said that the CDC removed data in its final report about the MMR vaccine and how it was causally linked to autism. There is definite agenda to keep us in the dark about autism causation and there is suppression tactics constantly being used to prevent the truth about vaccines or that they cause autism. Look into what have happened to the Robert De Niro's film about vaccinations and the film entitled VAXXED. Children need their parents to become educated or informed so that parents can adequately protect them. Keep in mind that this censorship, misinformation and the outright deceit and cover-ups'; along with the mal-law vaccination mandate are obstacles to being enabled to protect your children. Be safe, not sorry; make sure that your children are not defiled by vaccine unnatural to their body chemicalization. The laws of chemistry apply to your children's welfare; so, let us act to **GET THE CHEMICALS OUT** of vaccines! This book offers **TWO STEPS OF CORRECTION** to do just that.

In accordance with nature and assuring health generating chemistry we must be free to refuse unwanted vaccine injections especially, those vaccines that pose a threat of being chemically laced. A predominate feature of parenting is to protect children from conceived of dangers such as, a vaccine chemical injection infusion infiltration and/or a vaccination induced harm. This protection is most basic and an underlying nature of parenting. Parents' guide their offspring and make children's life decisions until they are old enough to do so; the vaccination decision is under the umbrella of parenting; government overstep its authority or jurisdiction when it positions itself to make the vaccination decision or command it. The fact that mandated vaccinations have no sunset or date certain of ending or that for all purposes, the vaccination of all our children is permanent; makes it that much more egregious and illegal. Parents require their full expression of parenting when it comes to protecting their children. They need to be enabled to fully engage their protection of their children and not be hindered by an erroneous vaccination mandate. Children need their parents to be fully empowered to protect them. People want to be in control of their children's health destiny or decisions. **We must be free to live a chemical free life and not be violated by unwanted injections. The mandated vaccination law violates essential parenting and our Right to be left alone or in full control over our internal being.**

Each unnatural to the body chemical that penetrates children's highly susceptible systems is like a tiny chemical bomb going off within. The delivery of a vaccine unnatural chemical injection is like the delivery of an "A bomb"; it devastates health. A vaccine chemical injection is an "A" bomb = AUTISM BOMB. The present chemical laden state of vaccines is an "A**utism bomb**" waiting to be set off by injection, this "**A bomb" obliterates children's health** and **creates Autism**. The chemicals within vaccines are menacing to our children, a chemically laced vaccine is like a menace looking for a place to happen. Although, Vaccine Producers may merely have the seed of compassion for our children they are prevented from germinating and cultivating this seed of compassion because of their overwhelming commitment and agenda to secure profits for their company and/or stock holders. Vaccine companies are publicly held and therefore, not the optimal environment for securing children's safety. The reduction of chemicals used in vaccine production must first pass a cost/benefit analysis in order, to satisfy their **OBLIGATION** to stockholders. Vaccine Producers pay close attention to any number of things besides vaccine safety and are not solely committed to our children's vaccination safety and best interest. **Live free not to inject CHEMICAL-A-BOMBS**!

In comparison to vaccine producers or its puppet government law makers; parents have no mixed singles, no diverse obligations. Parents' primary mission and foremost desire is to do only what is in the best interest of their children. A parent in control of whether or not a child is to be vaccinated is proper and is generally in the child's best interest. Parents should choose wisely; know what chemicals you risk exposing your child to. Vaccination must only take place for proper cause and with safety first. The vaccine should not have unnatural to the body chemicals or chemicals for profit and not safety! ALLOWING FOR VACCINATION REFUSAL IS THE MASTER KEY TO THE SECURING OF VACCINE QUALITY AND THE SAFETY OF CHILDREN. PARENTS CONTEMPLATING THE INJECTION OF A VACCINE, NEED TO BE ENABLED TO REFUSE IF THEY ARE NOT CONVINCED THE CHEMICALS IN THE VACCINE ARE SAFE TO INJECT AND/OR IF PARENTS DO NOT THINK THE INJECTION IS IN THEIR CHILD'S BEST INTEREST. Parents' refusing unwanted vaccine chemicals, to protect children, is an essential freedom. Absolutist thinking that vaccinations are for all or enforcing unwanted vaccination is dangerous. Your children must be yours to protect and yours to decide what is best!

It is bad enough that drugs are constantly over prescribed; to mandate or force mass vaccination of all children is not only an over prescription; it is the improper practice of medicine; it is tyrannical enslavement of our children to undergo vaccine chemicalization child abuse. The chemicals of vaccines have anti-health properties and propensities that destroy the health of children, denying the underlying gentle nature of children and/or their optimum health. **It is hostile to children and their parents to be held hostage to enforced vaccinations.** For children's best interest their parents must be permitted to regulate their children's vaccination healthcare, being endowed with the power to deny unwanted vaccinations. **Parents need to be allowed to direct Vaccine Producers attention through informed DENIAL of unwanted chemical laced vaccines.** This will turn Vaccine Producers and their chemical laced vaccines from being a hostile environment to a helpful one that is devoid of unnatural to the body chemicals. Children must be able to rely upon their parent's in order, to be adequately protected.

In order to conquer the Autism epidemic parents must be enabled to refuse any vaccine chemicalization. The risk of an Autism reaction from chemically laced vaccine injections is a risk that parents must be free to refuse; be free to self-determine and be in control of whether the risk is worth taking. It just makes no sense to have certain chemicals in vaccines; there are no health benefits, only health risks; there are chemicals that only serve to profit from in vaccines serving no health benefit. Parents must counterbalance the greed and/or profit first mentality of Vaccine Producers. The TWO CORRECTIVE STEPS (explained later) will establish a good standard of vaccine quality control and the production

of vaccines that do not endanger our children with toxic, unnatural to the body chemicals. Having vaccines that must pass parental scrutiny will lead to improved vaccines, health promotion, prevention and wellness strategies.

Make no mistake, Vaccine Manufacturers are in it just for or more for the profit and have one burning or concrete concept to make the maximum profit and if that means using chemicals that parents do not think are health wise then that it just too bad; it is business as usual. It is the business of Vaccine Producers to see to it vaccines are sold and find its mark into children. They make sure vaccines are mandated or enforced upon the public in order, to assure drug company's profiteering. As for parents' it is inborn and business as usual to see to it that their children are healthy and safe; not exposed to chemicals and/or unwanted vaccine injections. **Parents must be free to be parents! Preventing an unwanted or conceived of as too dangerous to inject vaccine, is primary to parenting and required for a parents' to be considered FREE TO BE A PARENTS.** The Vaccine Producers put whatever they want in vaccines; this must be counterbalanced by parents having the unfettered capacity to **refuse vaccines**. When a parent determines injection is not in their children's best interest there can be no injection otherwise, we are **ENSLAVED** to be vaccinated. Vaccines have become tainted and its quality has become corrupted. Vaccines have chemicals that parents do not want injected and this must be corrected. **Parents must be free to assure chemical stability for children.**

Allowing the natural and fundamental protection of children, through the enabling of parents to refuse unwanted chemical injections, will arrest the vaccine quality corruption; safer vaccines result. Also, the prompting of Vaccine Producers to produce safer, non-unnatural chemical vaccines, through the holding of Vaccine Producers accountable and liable for vaccine induced injuries will triumph the end of vaccines being produced tainted with disruptive to health chemicals. These common ground, most reasonable safety generating actions will result in no more vaccine injection slavery and the end of the escalating Autism epidemic. Parents realize that their children's well-being is under attack when they learn what chemicals are in vaccines. The People understand that the mandate of vaccinations have caused less health for children because of unnatural to the body chemicalization. Unsafe vaccines are the result of inability to refuse vaccinations and no accountability on the part of vaccine producers. Vaccine producers have no controlling reason to keep vaccines chemically safe. Chemicals that assure greater profit but not health are in vaccines. Parents that recognize the threat are often subdued or coerced into submission. The suppression and coercion must end! Freedoms bell must ring loud and clear; vaccination slavery must be abolished, empowering parents with liberty to protect their children through refusal to inject unwanted chemicalization!

Parents have the best vantage point to detect whether a vaccine injection caused their children injury and/or Autism. Parents also have the best vantage point to determine if the chemical exposure of vaccinations are in the best interest of their children and the law must recognize and support this truth and the aforementioned truth. Parents observe and know their children constantly, day in and day out; they readily recognize any changes in children's behavior or level of health. In general, parents are the authority or greatest detectives as to when children are caused an injury; they know the timing of the injury and what caused the injury. The multitudes of parents reporting vaccine induced injuries has been callously ignored or belittled by the powers that want vaccines to sell. The mandated vaccination law disregards these truths and insists that we have no legal choice but to endure the risks incumbent with being vaccinated. This is not only counterproductive to assuring vaccine purity and/or quality but also, is counter to the goal to best protect children. People need their healthcare freedom of decision and to be enabled to self-regulate what is allowed or not allowed to enter their very own bloodstreams. Mandated vaccination enslavement mal-law expects parents to sit on their hands, doing absolutely nothing to protect their children from unwanted, conceived of as too dangerous to inject, vaccine chemical injections. The freedom bell is sounding very loudly, calling all to stop the injustice especially, when children are being injured from unwanted, enforced, vaccine chemicalization injections!

The child is yours to have, hold and raise therefore, the vaccination decision must be yours! It cannot be argued with any true validity that, government should make the decision for all children to be or not to be vaccinated! The one obvious fact is that parents not government hold children's best interest. Parent's primary mission in life is the caring for their children. The very concept that government can intrude upon this personal parental space, violating parents God given Right or supreme primal Right is so off base that it is grossly improper. The chemical industry and/or pharmaceutical industry must not be permitted to trample upon parent's right to be in control of the welfare of their very own children. Government swayed by the strong arm and deep pockets of Vaccine Manufacturers no longer should do Vaccine Producers' bidding or continue to enforce for profit vaccination slavery. If there were no profits in mandating vaccination there would be no vaccination mandate and parents would have their childrearing freedom! Parental vaccination decision or choice is an essential parental freedom!

The likes of big business have been methodically chipping away at our rights in order, to achieve a surer but, unethical and un-American, torturous pathway to unworthy profiteering. They will stop at nothing in their pathological striving and put our children's lives in risk for doing so. The chemicals for profit in vaccines and the autism epidemic is an end result of this madness. We have been asleep or way too complacent in the taking; too many people have acquiesced in letting big business for profit or its puppet government mandate vaccine chemicalization. They have methodically dictated that our children be injected, despite our reservations or absolute concern that it is unhealthy for our children to be so exposed. Our right to protect or direct our children's welfare is under fire and has been severally compromised. We need to regain our children's welfare or the right to direct or protect our offspring. We should spend all our energy protecting our right to say "NO" to unwanted vaccine chemicalization. Fighting for it. Working so hard not to spill one single drop of the precious right to protect our children or ability to keep children's blood pure and clean from unnatural to their body, vaccine chemicalization. You must never stop believing. Why or how could our control to protect children or our liberty to refuse unwanted chemicalization have occurred? It is the fundamental lack of understanding of what is taking place as parents are replaced, set aside, or completely disempowered by lobbied for government 's demands, commands and enslavement of our children to be injected for big profit.

Follow the money or ask just who is making the money and you will know who is making the policy or is behind the scenes assuring things get done in a self-serving policy that makes it the law of the land. Stealthily, more vaccines have been added to the list for mandate. Children are the pincushions for the multiple vaccine chemicalization injections not because good Government is listening to the voice of the people but rather, due to the insistence

of lobbyists that strictly serve big business pharmaceutical industry. Our children are in chemical jeopardy; used to use up vaccines in order, to attain ever increasing profits. They have devised every way possible measure to assure children have no way around being vaccinated to reap profits. Remember, chemicals combine in our children's highly sensitive bodies, but are rarely tested that way. Children need their parent's protection and parents need to protect their children! Fundamental parenting must be protected and not be violated by mal-law. Enforcing vaccinations, when parents determine the vaccine chemical injection is harmful and/or injecting children against parent's will, creates acrimony, loathing and aversion toward the vaccination program. In fact, it creates bitterness, antagonism and hostility toward those that are involved in or responsible for the mass hysteria of enforced injections, tyrannical medical intervention and injection enslavement. Children need their parents to be free to refuse vaccine chemical injections; to shield them or protect them from vaccines which their parents determine are not healthy to inject or are not in their best interest. Vaccine chemicals do cause injury; so, protect your children with liberty to refuse unwanted chemicalization!

We need a vaccination program that is volitional, one that creates good will, with an affinity toward both respecting self-determined health care and the Right of parent's to freely and fully protect their children from unwanted chemical injections. Institute a vaccination delivery system that does not insight unrest or turmoil and does not dispirit parenting or disenfranchise, reduce and subjugate parenthood. Parents must always be activated to be parents; empowered to fully protect their children. It is a universal truth that parents genuinely want and know what is best for their children; the vaccination mandates are opposite of this truth. Parents not only have the right heart in caring for their children, they also have an intuitive sense of what is best for their children. Vaccination compulsion must end; PARENTAL DECISION COMPULSION and PARENTAL SATISFACTION COMPULSION must begin. We require the liberty to decide what is best.

Parental power to refuse medical intervention or vaccinations must not be reduced, stifled or eliminated. The potency and effectiveness of parents, in the protection of their children, are essential to the securing SAFER VACCINES and is children's best interest. The vitality, muscle or spirit of parenting require that parents be endowed with refusal of unwanted vaccinations. Without parents holding the keys to vaccination acceptance or denial children are unwisely left to the vices of medicine or the uncaring, non-diligent imperfection of strangers who care far, far less than parents' care and that are too far removed from any harm from vaccine chemical injections such as, Autism. Moreover, vaccine safety needs and requires parental input and/or parent's demands for quality control; rendering vaccines to no longer be laced with anti-health chemicals. Claiming vaccines do not harm is fraudulent whereas, parents' protecting from real harm is valid.

A law that interferes with parent's determination of what is best for their own children must be considered automatically suspect and flawed. The amplitude and magnitude of parent's responsibility, authority and relationship with their children must never be subjugated or diminished by law. **The mandated vaccination enslavement law eviscerates parent's protection of their children, it attenuates their parenting authority; it enervates or disables parents' obligation to prevent unwanted, injected chemical exposure.** If anything, law should be promulgated to enforce parents to be responsible as parents. Parents are vested to take care of their children by a higher authority than manmade law; they naturally are expected to be the decision makers. Parents must be free to be parents and the mandated vaccination law grossly violates this essential. Parents perception, judgment and intuition about taking care of their children or deciding best whether a vaccine injection should be accepted or refused is next to none. Law should not intrude upon parental protection; children need parents to freely protect.

The People never really sanctioned government to abridge or regulate one's internal being or command all children to be suffer injections and be pumped with vaccine chemical content. Freedom's core is close to being empowered to having control over one's very own blood chemistry and that of one's children. **Securing of our vital or core freedom and assuring that vaccines are being made responsibly and/or safer; having no unnatural to the body, anti-health chemicals is crucial. Cleaning-up vaccines is imperative to the prevention of vaccination induced injuries such as, Autism.** This will serve to prevent vaccination recipients from suffering a **critical mass, chemical episode** and thereby, decrease the prevalence of Autism and other vaccination related health problems. What we need is a **critical mass** action by parents and freedom minded individuals to instill the **TWO STEPS OF CORRECTION** of this book in order, to prevent **critical mass** chemical episodes from vaccine chemical injections.

The Merriam -Webster dictionary defines freedom as, "1: The quality or state of being free: as (a) **the absence of necessity, coercion or constraint in choice or action** (b) **liberation from slavery or restraint or from the power of another: INDEPENDENCE** and (c) the quality or state of being exempt or released usually from something **onerous**." The **mandated vaccination law defies** these very definitions of **essential freedom**. Parents must be free to control and protect children; this includes the vaccination situation or dilemma. If we are not free to do so and are enforced to suffer unwanted vaccine chemicalization then we are being oppressed to the point of slavery; enslaved to suffer vaccination. Live free to reject injections!

The vaccine Autism connection is apparent to multitudes of parents who have witnessed their children fall victim to vaccine chemicalization autism. There are multitudes of doctors and scientists and chemists concluding that the increase of vaccine unnatural to the body chemicalization has spawned autism. Those not coming to this obvious connection are those that practice hysterical use of vaccination or those that have something to financially gain from it. We need to come the realization that the mass use of vaccination or to mandate mass vaccination is to mandate mass child abuse by mass vaccine chemicalization. **THE RATE OF AUTISM IN THE VACCINATED POPULATION IS CONCLUSIVELY HIGHER THAN THE RATE OF AUTISM OF THE UNVACCINATED POPULACE.** The prompting of vaccine manufacturers to become vigilant, to not place foreign to the body chemicals within vaccines, is one of this book's primary directives. All health issues from being exposed to the chemicals of vaccinations will markedly improve **once vaccinations are based upon informed consent/DENIAL and Vaccine Producers are held accountable and liable; no longer oblivious to lawsuits**. Vaccine companies need to be driven to rise to a reasonable level of vaccine production quality control and this is best achieved through liberty to refuse vaccine chemicalization and **negligence law**. Vaccine Producers must be **held accountable**; made **liable to pay victims** when their negligent vaccine production is the cause in fact of injury. Absolute power corrupts absolutely; there must be a balance of power.

If Vaccine Producers are made to be reasonably vaccine content responsible by having them pay out compensation when their vaccines cause injury and grant potential recipients

of vaccinations their reasonable human dignity to refuse an unwanted vaccination, then healthier vaccine production will be produced. Better vaccine quality production control will be stimulated resulting, in no harmful chemical contents in vaccines; effectuating a reduction in Autism, healthier children, a higher confidence level in vaccinations and therefore, increased voluntary vaccination compliance. The people are vested with an inalienable Right to preserve their very own blood chemistries or health and preserve the same for their children; individuals must have the decisive control over whether a vaccination will or will not be injected into their personage.

Diligent parents who properly spring into action to stop their children from being infiltrated by the unnatural to the body chemicals in vaccines are held to a different standard; they are wrongfully singled out for prejudicial, negative treatment. There can be no differential treatment for those that decide not to vaccinate; no coercion to vaccinate, nor constraint in healthcare choice. The range of tactics to enforce vaccination must be stopped and only proper education or healthcare advice be permitted. Stopping the perfectly healthy unvaccinated from entering school or bringing down the wrath of child protective service to bear must no longer continue. Perfectly healthy children must always be treated as perfectly healthy! People must be treated equally, equitably; not be held to a different standard for merely remaining unvaccinated or not have been subjected to vaccine chemicalization. The only thing parents are guilty of is being educated about chemicalization harm and caring enough about their children's well-being to refuse the unnatural to the body chemical infiltration or exposure. Live free to reject, injections!

The morbidity from vaccine chemicalization will diminish as vaccines are cleaned-up. Granting people their liberty of decision or vaccination freedom of choice and holding vaccine makers' accountable and liable for vaccine induced injuries will **GET THE CHEMICALS OUT** of vaccines; vaccines will be clean with no harmful unnatural to the body chemicals. The fall-out from giving people the choice not to vaccinate induces a safer degree of vaccine production and holding vaccine producers' liable when their negligently produced vaccines cause injury also, achieves better/higher quality control. Vaccines are a gold mine for its producers and a poor bargain for those that receive vaccines that have chemicals for profit, not safety. This books' **TWO STEPS OF CORRECTION** will legitimize the profits gained from vaccine sales and make vaccines safer by **GETTING THE CHEMICALS OUT**.

Chemicals in vaccines are poisoning our children. They know vaccine chemical injections cause health problems and Autism but will deny any implication of the fact and keep injecting and profiting for as long the public sleeps on their rights and allows it. The standard procedure for Drug Companies is to keep dangerous products on the market in order, to make unearned profits. Just like they allowed Vioxx, Triazolyl, Lipitor, Avandia, Zocor, Bextra, Ketek, Paxil, Accutane, Zoloft and Atorvastatin to remain on the market; they are wrongfully continuing to use harmful chemicals that secure profit, not safety in vaccines. The present state of anti-health, chemical vaccines stay on the market. Children need their parents' protection and parents need to protect their children; hold your children close and do not put them in chemical harm's way! Recognize that Autism can be one unhealthy chemicalization injection away!

Vaccines are minimally studied for their harm potential and not studied for their cumulative harm from multiple injections and/or over the prolonged period of the multiple injections. Toxins accumulate and interact with each injection, taking their negative to health toll. Vaccine chemicals cause chemical malformation, leading to biological malformation and Autism. Analyze the chemical content for yourself and decide if you want it injected into your tiny baby, little infant or small child. Do not be mastered or made subject to unwanted dangerous vaccine chemicalization; protect your children properly! Demand clean vaccines that are not laced with unnatural to the body chemicals!

I cannot stress just how important it is to health, how important it is to secure your child's life as a productive, achieving, healthy successful individual that your child is protected by none other than you, not ill-seated government, from a vaccine chemicalization. A harm that is devastating to health, happiness and fulfillment; that harm comes in the form of a vaccine injected chemicalization, an exposure to unnatural to the body chemicals. In life your priority is as your child's protector, should be to analyze what the puppet government of vaccine producers are enforcing into your child's vital blood and biological system. If you learn that the vaccine they are pointing at your child does in fact, have unnatural to your child's blood or body chemistry then act. you do not allow a vaccine injected chemicalization of their body and brain.

Be aware, they may have averted you from concentration on keeping your children safe by seeing to it that you place blind trust in the vaccination for profit industry; by droning in you that your child will not or cannot be injured by vaccination. They also, arrest your parenting by making you think you have no choice or that it is not your concern because your child must be injected, it is the law. Basically, they have targeted children to be inoculated in order, to secure increasing profits. However, become acutely, aware that vaccines do cause health problems! The media blitz has flooded the market place; there is no escaping drug companies' barrage of, "take this drug and be vaccinated". Pay close attention to the ads, since, mandated vaccinations are their way to be assured of mandated profits you will never see or hear in any of their commercials a single word about side-effects or signs or symptoms from vaccination; this illusion gives the false sense that none exist. Government has been taken over by the droves of drug and vaccine lobbyists; government has been hijacked, it is the puppet of vaccine manufacturers and is used to support drug/vaccine profiteering. If there were no profits to be made from mandated vaccination there would no vaccination mandates! Know what chemicals are in vaccines; never allow unnatural to your children's body chemicalization!

They have induced many to give them all the reins of vaccination and have one blindly close their eyes and deafly close their ears to the valid understanding that chemicals do injure and that vaccines are carriers of chemicals not part of the human condition or belonging in one's natural biological reactions or configuration. In fact, they have managed through the constant siege of media blitz to arrest parents will to even look into whether vaccines are safe or NOT. Too many parents have either surrendered to having their children's safety or welfare be dictated to by others; they have instigated parents to allow the drug companies to one-sidedly decide what is what chemicals children must endure. We have methodically been indoctrinated in the enslavement of mandated vaccine chemicalization that is mandated mass child abuse by chemicalization. Drug company's puppet government demand by mandate that your child suffer many injections of vaccine chemicals. They have programmed people that the vaccination decision is not theirs to make. People look in the mirror of reality and fail to see that their children are enslaved to undergo vaccine chemicalization. They downplay or censor any risk factors or any voice that warns or cautions the public about the absolute risks or real dangers of suffering a vaccine unnatural to the body chemicalization. Children need their parents' protection and parents need to protect their children; so, start protecting! Vaccine chemicalization autism is the main cause of the autism epidemic.

We are lulled to ASSume the vaccine is only good or is worth the risk of injection. What if you became aware that vaccines are NOT ALL HEALTHY FOR YOUR CHILDREN AS YOU WERE DUPED TO BELIEVE? The truth will set you free; vaccines have been found to harbor unnatural to the body chemicals. Chemicals cause injury in the form of symptoms and signs; these reactions to the chemicalization can cause sickness in fact, the signs and symptoms is a level of sickness or health problem. Look closely at the signs and symptoms caused that are known adverse reactions already listed on the information insert and you will recognize they are many of the same signs and symptoms of autism. They purposely do not put a diagnosis to it; however, a diagnosis that is spawned from vaccine chemicalization is merely, a name. A diagnosis may or may not be known but none the less; it is unhealthy to suffer unnatural to the body chemicalization. As free Americans, we cannot live under rule of mal hijacked government that assures or supports drug company's profiteering agenda and enforces vaccine chemicalization against parents' will or better judgement. The fact that vaccines are the primary cause of autism makes it that much more egregious however, the too long list of adverse effects from vaccines which are inconspicuously listed on the vaccine information sheet is more than reason enough to not be forced to vaccinate or be placed under duress to vaccinate. Parents' must be free to access the vaccination situation and determine what is best! Do not be burdened with unnatural vaccine chemicalization unless you decide for it! This book elucidates the dishonesty, greed and deceit of vaccine chemical mandate madness.

It must not be up to distant strangers to decide or dictate what is best for your children or decide their vaccination fate; there must be no commanding of healthcare or disrupting parental health preferences! The decision must be for only parents to decide! Make no mistake, they have perverted what is the natural order of things; a taking has taken place. They have dared to take your vital decision authority about your child away from you; in that you do not control whether it is in your child's best interest to be vaccinated and they have actually been completely calloused as to, enforce vaccine chemicalization; even when you disagree or think it harmful. Mal-government has no valid jurisdiction to take over core parental territory or command that parents submit their children to suffer unwanted vaccination or induce child abuse by chemicalization injection! The essence of parental freedom has been lost because of permanent vaccination mandates. We are enslaved when our perfectly healthy unvaccinated children are forbidden their school entrance; it is a whip that enforces vaccination compliance.

If vaccination were worthwhile or not harmful people would readily, volunteer children for it. There would be no need to mandate vaccination if it were truly based upon need and vaccines were not harmful. The truth is that vaccination is mandated because it fills the greedy pockets of drug companies and that people are commonly injured by vaccine chemicalization and would freely choose not to vaccinate. Vaccines are much more dangerous or have more unnatural chemicals because vaccination is mandated. Money crazed drug companies are behind the mandate in perpetuity; to assure more their profits than the welfare of children. **BE FREE TO PROTECT** your children by being **FREE TO REJECT INJECTIONS**; execute the parental right of protection! People are responsible for their own journey in life and must be free to decide what is best for their children or decide whether their child should or should not be vaccinated. There is an ecstasy of unity between parents and their offspring, there is a natural intelligence and connectedness which, allows parents to know what is best; a visceral feeling that combines with learned intelligence that makes parents far superior decision makers'.

Walk with me for a few moments to experience the truth or the true situation. Yes, you want your child to possibly be vaccinated to hopefully receive health benefit however, you first and foremost want your child not to be poisoned at the same time for doing so! You are unpleasantly surprised to learn that there are unnatural to the body **CHEMICALS IN VACCINES** and that there is a crazy law that your children must be vaccinated. This book will guide you and free your parental authority to decide what is best for your children. This book has the **TWO STEPS OF CORRECTION** that will not only help you have your proper protection of your children but also, secure their safety or health by prompting vaccines to be made without chemicals that a reasonable responsible parent would not want injected into their tiny baby, little infant or small child. So, if you think vaccination has benefit do you think it should not also have health detriment? What parents need to protect against is the infiltration of their children with unnatural to the body chemicals that can lead to chemicalization autism.

Be a proponent of much safer vaccines! Vaccinations that are strictly voluntary, based upon informed consent/DENIAL brings about the result of SAFER vaccines. Individuals must always maintain dominion over themselves and/or their healthcare decisions to secure freedom and prevent medical intervention tyranny and to prompt proper vigilance in healthcare quality control. Be an advocate of eliminating all the foreign to the body chemicals found in vaccines and inspire extreme caution and/or discourage the continuing use of present toxic chemicals in vaccines. Promote the vindication of those injured by vaccinations by holding Vaccine Producers liable; prompting safer vaccines and/or a reasonable standard of production. Be free to directly litigate against negligent Vaccine Producers in Civil Supreme Court and thereby, prompt a reasonable degree and much needed higher degree of vaccine quality control. **No more special legal treatment for negligent vaccine companies, no more foreign to the body chemicals in vaccines and no more forced vaccination slavery. The best interest of children will be served, and/or the best protection of children will be attained by GETTING THE CHEMICALS OUT of vaccines; informed consent/DENIAL of vaccinations and making Vaccine Producers pay is a must. Children need the ever-watchful eye and vigilant decision control of parents to be safe. Be in control of your children's healthcare destiny.**

Each unnatural to the body chemical that is injected has its propensity or energy field that disrupts the normal or homeostasis of the vaccine recipient's bio physiology. Each alien to the body chemical takes on a life of its own; altering the internal bio-mechanics or production. Vaccine chemicals can combine in reactions with the normal chemistry of the body and with other unnatural to the body injected chemicals to distort what was once the normal biochemistry of creation or production. Rapidly developing babies, infants and children are rendered not optimally healthy with such, manipulated or distorted internal chemical stumbling blocks of health and life; autism can be spawned. Quantum science and the laws of chemistry indicate that if the purity of the blood is distorted the end results will not be the same or will be unknown. Children need their parents' protection! Be free to keep your children secure from unwanted chemicalization!

For the sake of children's well-being parents should attempt to grasp just what is going on when an injection of alien to the body chemicals is injected to circulate within the blood. The infiltration of these chemicals disturbs or disrupts the health of the vaccine chemicalized recipient; this disruption takes place at the physical chemical reaction level and at the electromagnetic field level; this formulates autism. Chemicalization autism creates a sea of motion of abnormal bio physiology. The laws of physics and chemistry rule biology! The properties of optimum health have a chemical and magnetic signature. This health signature is negatively, influenced by the internal exposure to unnatural to the body chemicals; it is fluctuated, disrupted, distorted and altered. The normal energy field of reactions within the body are caused a ripple of unharnessed abnormality.

The particles, molecules or chemicals of the body are attracted or repelled by the alien to the body vaccine chemicals. The negative or positive charges of these unnatural to the body chemicals are intrinsic to the spawning of autism. Electricity and magnetism influence chemicals and the reactions and products that result. Brain cells are highly susceptible to the physical presence and to the electrical or magnetic fields of vaccine's alien to the body chemicals. There is region of influence where ever these abnormal to the body chemicals flow; it perturbs health and can degenerate it into autism. Brain fogging or malfunction in the hive of activity of the brain results; autism is spawned. There is an uncertainty principle whenever you inject such, foreign chemicals that you should consider when determining if vaccines are good or bad. Vaccines need to come clean; GET THE CHEMICALS OUT, in order, for parents to rationally approve of it!

If you think that vaccines have chemicals that do not pass your test for safety, then you have the God given authority and responsibility to do something about it. If you want the benefit of vaccination but, do not want any negative to the health consequences then REFUSE THE UNWANTED CHEMICALIZATION AND DEMAND that they GET THE CHEMICALS OUT! The law of chemistry and that of physiology make it certain, that injecting unnatural to the body chemicals into a baby, infant or child has negative to health consequences. If you do not agree with an injection of unnatural to the body chemicals, you have an obligation to not let your offspring become a victim of it; do not let it befall them. For if children cannot rely upon their parents for protecting them against chemical exposure or suffering an internal chemicalization and chemical doping of the brain then who can they rely upon; certainly, not money-making vaccine producing drug companies or their puppet government law makers. Parents are the only ones to be trusted with such, all-important obligation and responsibility.

People must be free to be parents, free to decide after careful analysis of what is in the vaccine if it is worthy of injection or in our children's best interest. If it does not meet our standard of excellence, we must not be subjected to it or enforced to do what vaccine producers' or puppet governments' think best. People must not be mastered over or given no realistic choice but to vaccinate. Parents have been rendered useless or unable to protect their offspring against unwanted vaccine chemicalization. Parents must be made whole again by having their parental protection of children set free with liberty to say "NO" to vaccination; free to refuse unwanted vaccine chemicalization for their children. Vaccines are guilty of having chemicals that are unnatural to the body, chemicals that are not part of the normal bio physiology. Vaccine chemicalization has been proven to cause signs and symptoms that indicate the body is stressed or injured. Autism could be a vaccine chemicalization away! Vaccine chemicalization autism is enemy number one.

Parents must stand in the way of all enemies, always answering the call; the call to prevent actual harm or possible harm or conceived of harm to their offspring. All people must be free from being commanded or humbled to submit to healthcare especially, healthcare that is unwanted or thought of as harmful. Parents that feel, think or conclude or know for a fact that injected vaccine chemicalization of tiny babies, little infants and small children is injurious must be free to refuse, say "NO" or REJECT INJECTIONS. This freedom of rejecting any proposed vaccination must be afforded whether the potential injury is to lesser insignificant degree or to a greater infinite degree. Do not surrender your will or power of decision! Unwanted injections of substances or chemicals must never be jammed down our throats or jammed by needling into our babies' bodies or blood. Mandated medical vaccinations are a blemish on America, an actual violation of our most precious right to be left alone, undisturbed. It is a taking of our freedom to care for our children the way we think best. Do not submit to mandated vaccine injected chemicalization child abuse. Do not surrender your babies for unwanted pricking by needle to suffer vaccine unnatural to the body chemicalization. Free people are not enforced to have their children injected or chemicalized. Law must be enacted that supports parents' protection of children from what parents conceive as too dangerous to inject vaccination; enabling parents' to be the very best parents that they aspire to be!

There is a pattern to autism. The one consistent theme is that children are being injected with unnatural to their body chemicals and proximate to the chemicalization they show signs and symptoms indicating a direct adversity to being exposed to the chemicals of vaccines. Biological chemical reactions become abnormal as the unnatural to the body vaccine chemicals infiltrate the cells of the body and/or brain. Chemicals or molecules speak to each other through waves of its electromagnetic signatures. Just as drug chemicals make changes within; unnatural to the body vaccine chemicals have cause and effect. Each alien to the body vaccine chemical has its propensity and unique frequency; polarizing the spawning of autism. Chemicals or molecules communicate with the living cells in an exchange of chemical information, encoding bio-production creating a cascade of electromagnetic impulses that resonate autism. Chemicals dictate to the cells or to the DNA to produce or not produce proteins etc. **Cellular manipulation by chemicalization spawn autism. Alien to the body vaccine chemicals encode and carries information that impact biology, bio-balance, biochemistry and/or human physiology. An imbalance of energy and equilibrium, a trembling of motion of molecules disrupts optimum health and the delicate equilibrium of life. GET THE CHEMICALS OUT of vaccines!**

The harm that **forced** vaccinations cause to our children's health, the imbalance in the bloodstream created by the chemicals of vaccines and its violation to our parental Rights are excellent reasons for unwavering laser focused determination to correct, what so desperately needs correction to vaccine manufacturing and its administration. No longer can it be generalized that vaccines do no harm; it is only the matter of the degree of harm. How best to assure the reduction of harm? Parents are the answer; the safety requirement of having parents first giving their true informed consent/DENIAL is the key to inducing vaccine purity and/or safety. The central point is to allow parents to secure what parents conceive of as the best possible health choice for their children and thereby, alien to the body chemicals in vaccines will be removed and consequently Autism will decrease. **Parents making vaccination decisions that are in the best interest of their children is the bread and butter of parenting and will sunset the Autism epidemic.** Parents deciding whether to vaccinate will promote chemical free vaccines and no injected chemicalization means; **the epidemic of autism will begin to subside. Mandating vaccination is the antithesis of parental freedom and is the opposite of being in the best interest of children. Children need their parents' protection and parents need to protect!**

Mandated vaccinations and all its enforcement measures are far too draconian. It is an onerous intrusion into one's personal space and private healthcare affairs; it is far too great of an intrusion, far too reaching governmentalizing. Parent's fundamental responsibility of caring for their children and/or protecting them from unwanted medical intervention is grossly being interfered with. The erroneous mandated vaccination law annihilates an adults individual Right to decide what healthcare is best for her or himself and totally disrupts a parents Right and/or prerogative to decide what healthcare shall or shall not be accepted for their children. The mandate is an attack on human dignity and a perversion of the natural order. The staggering amount of mandated vaccine chemicalization is escalating at a breathtaking pace. We must not turn a blind eye nor be complacent about these violations of our Rights and bodies. Vaccination slavery must be abolished. Vaccine safety and our children's best interest are not served by a mandated vaccination system. Enslaving children to be injected is outrageous in a FREE America. Despite the fact that vaccines have chemicals or that parents do not want their children to undergo vaccine CHEMICALIZATION; vaccination is enforced upon a ONCE FREE people.

For government to even temporarily make healthcare decisions for our children such as, enforcing vaccinations down the throats of once free Americans, is revolutionary and cause for great alarm; to do it in perpetuity is an outrage and cause for revolution! **Drug big business is bent on making sure vaccination is forever enforced upon us, not a matter of freedom of choice; they strongly lobby to keep vaccinations mandated and our children enslaved to suffer unwanted vaccine chemicalization. Drug lobbyists have assured mega-profiting by assuring vaccinations will continually be enforced-mandated. The habit of government enforcing vaccines upon us is a bad habit that was very easily acquired but very difficult to cure.** This bad habit keeps expanding with more and more mandated-enforced vaccinations, with no end in sight; guaranteeing **billions** in profiteering. Vaccine Producers are like a grossly, engorged, fat, bloated, profiteering tick on the hide of America; that needs to be removed by our laser FOCUS ON LIBERTY. The **TWO STEPS OF CORRECTION** is required for positive vaccine content safety and freedom. **Children's safety must come first** before corporate profiteering.

No one other than the individual himself and/or the parent for their children must have the profound command over what will or will not be injected and/or what medical intervention will or will not be administered. Government and its laws must be of the People, by the People and for the People; enforced vaccinations are not wanted by the People and therefore, must end! The fact that mandated vaccination laws are attempting to **permanently** make our health care decisions for our children is an atrocity of the greatest magnitude and **must not be tolerated**. There is no end in sight for enforced vaccinations, there is no intention to end mandated vaccination **SLAVERY**; there is only profiteering agenda to enforce more and more vaccine injections in order, to attain more and more guaranteed profiting for Vaccine Producers. Parents must become proactive to take back what is rightfully theirs; take the protection of your children back from the vices of profiteering, be your children's healthcare decision makers. A**bolish vaccination slavery** and restore parental caring control over your children. **Vaccination mandate is more for the benefit of profiteering Vaccine Producers than children's welfare**. If it were not so profitable to mandate vaccinations, they would not mandate vaccinations!

Parents must be free to protect by deciding whether or not vaccines are safe enough to inject into their kids. Parents cannot rest upon the mere representation that vaccinations are safe. Injection of alien, unnatural to the body, vaccine chemical is a sure recipe for health disaster. Truly, the fact that Vaccine Producers do not adequately protect our children from vaccine chemical exposure strongly indicates that the vaccine production **engine is running with no one adequately caring at the wheel**. Parents naturally must be entitled to **safeguard their children** by **refusing unwanted vaccine injections**; this will prompt cleaner and/or uncontaminated vaccines. **Parents' must be FREE to be PROTECTIVE parents**.

The sheer numbers of vaccinations being enforced upon our children today is major reason for concern. In your first few years of life you can be enforced to receive 26 inoculations and as many as 5 shots at once; exposing children to too many vaccine chemicals by injection. Each unnatural to the body chemical presence has disruptive reaction propensity and has an emission magnetic field signature that is an encoding and carrier of information commands; all of which, set abnormality in motion and can spawn. These chemicals propel and attract abnormal biology. There must no longer be chemicals for profit and not safety in vaccines and/or unnatural to the body chemicals; we need to GET THE CHEMICALS OUT! Parents are being forced to gamble with the welfare of their children. The People must be in charge of their health and/or of the healthcare of their children; there must be no enforcing of such an onerous amount of chemically laced vaccines. No one should be ENSLAVED to vaccinate; abolish vaccination mandates!

While it is true that a child may already have a distorted chemical make-up prior to being exposed to vaccination and therefore be somewhat more chemically susceptible; the enforcing of vaccine chemicalizations is a distortion of one's natural chemistry that

can further disfigure those already chemically compromised readily, exhausting their optimum health chances and escalating autism to be spawned. The autism epidemic is a chemicalization manifestation and its main causation is the multiple unnatural to the body vaccine chemicalization exposures. Children are in desperate need of their parents to be free to refuse unwanted vaccine chemicalization injections. Be free to deter chemical exposure from vaccine injections! The fact is that the chemical toxins of vaccines take their unhealthy toll on everyone, just more so in individuals who are already chemically compromised. Freedom to reject chemical exposure must be considered a dynamic freedom that must never be violated or abridged to any degree by vaccination mandates.

Those who do not want Autism and/or ADHD (attention-deficit hyperactivity disorder) which is comprised of problematic symptoms such as distractibility; impulsivity; restlessness; poor tolerance of frustration; poor time management; poor organization skills; anxiety and depression; moodiness; poor socialization and a tendency toward inconsistent performance must be free to point a finger at chemical vaccine injections and have liberty to refuse any vaccination. Self-determined vaccination, voluntary vaccination and self-preservation are consistent with dynamic freedom. Be free to reject, injections!

Placing unnatural to the body vaccine chemicals in children's bloodstreams violate several basic concepts of maintaining optimum health. The influx of vaccine chemicals destroys the normal chemistry and the capacity to maintain homeostasis. The normal range of chemical reactions is disrupted by vaccination. The shortsighted, ill-advised injection of vaccine chemicals is a risk parents must be enabled not to have their children take. Injecting unnatural to the body chemicals into children is a recipe for health disaster including, but not limited to, Autism. People have the SUPREME RIGHT to disallow vaccine injection medical intervention and/or parents have the right to protect their children from chemicalization. The vast numbers of vaccines and/or vaccine chemicals, slated for injection, is controlling reason to be in control over your vaccination destiny.

Vaccines enter the body via the bloodstream, they can be injected into a vein, artery, intramuscularly and subcutaneously. Vaccines are also introduced into the body orally and by nasal spray. If it is intramuscular or subcutaneous, the VACCINE WILL QUIKLY GET INTO THE BLOODSTREAM VIA TINY BLOOD VESSELS IN THE MUSCLE OR SUBCUTANEOUS TISSUE. A vaccine that sprayed into the nose can be absorbed into the bloodstream from the nasal mucous membranes. The chemicals of vaccines pose an ominous threat because they enter the bloodstream QUICKLY, with no filtering or buffering to reduce the strength of their impact. The important fact is that after vaccines enter the bloodstream, without reduction, they penetrate the brain cells to dope the cells with chemicals; it is a CHEMICALIZATION. Vaccines are usually injected into muscle however; their chemicals QUICKLY/DIRECTLY enter into the bloodstream. Chemical brain doping and/or CHEMICALIZATIONS ARE SOMETHING THAT PARENTS MUST BE FREE TO STOP. DO NOT BE ENSLAVED TO INJECT VACCINE CHEMICALIZATION.

Each cell of the body undergoes an average some of 100,000 reactions per second. When a vaccine is plunged into a baby to surge through their bloodstream and penetrate the cells of the brain a wave of interference ensues. This disturbance to health wave builds and become a tsunami of abnormality. The old concept of sticks and stones causing injury needs to be advanced to the deeper level understanding that injury or health disharmony is created by chemical physical presence with its chemical impulses and wave interference: language of phase, amplitude and frequency spectrum. We resonate and get in sync with the chemicals we absorb or that are injected into us. Wave interference spawn autism in the electro-chemical circuits of the brain, transforming us to resonate and/or produce autism. Vaccine chemicalization tunes us to the frequency or mechanism of autism. At the ends of every neuron, the basic unit of the brain are synapses where CHEMICAL charges build up triggering electric firing across these spaces to other neurons thereby, commands or bio- instruction occur. An abnormal cascade of ceaseless scramble of electromagnetic impulses or wave collision formulates autism.

Perhaps it is the degree of harm that can come from being vaccine injected that you feel is important which, makes the decision more readily decided upon by you. If one chemical of a vaccine cancels out one reaction or causes an abnormal reaction is that enough to convince you to decide against the clericalization? At what point of chemical chaos, turmoil or interference is it intolerable to you; at what degree of chemicalization do you decide against the chemicalization by vaccine injection? The breaking point or rather, the determination turning point for many parents is the fact, that vaccines do have any degree whatsoever, of unnatural to their children's body chemicals! Is it not vital to you that it be your parental decision or that you can say "NO" to unwanted chemicalization?

Should you be made to surrender your children to suffer any chemicalization or consequence from vaccine chemicalization? Make it your decision! Protect your children the way you think best! Make no mistake, what is important is not about how much the vaccine costs or does not cost; what is important is that the vaccine be made in accordance with the highest degree of safety for children! There must be an option to receive a vaccine that does not have chemicals for profit or chemicals that do not need to be in the vaccine. In order, to affect the safety of your children; make sure the decision whether to vaccinate is for you to decide. Most people did not even know that there were vaccines that did not have mercury; so that choice was not even given or afforded most people. Most people did not know there was a decision to be made. To this day most people still do not know that there are unnatural to the body chemicals in vaccines; chemicals that have propensity to cause health problems. For the sake of your children's safety, health and lives; make sure the vaccine does not have any chemicals that can be a causation of negative health and/ or autism. Be free to protect your children! Children need parents' protection and parents need to protect their children; so, do protect them.

In order, to prevent autism there must be no break in wholeness or loss of global coherence of brain function. Abnormal chemicalization of the brain from, doping brain cells with unnatural to the body vaccine chemicals is destructive to the quantum normal function of the brain and disrupts the retrieval and read-out mechanism of the brain or the way the brain coordinates and directs al functions of the body; this inducing a disruption of coherent emission of brain signals, no global coherence results. The implications of doping brain cells with vaccine chemicalization are something that parents should become aware of and must for the sake of children safeguard against. If an adult with a mature online system are infiltrated with vaccine chemicals it is destructive to optimum health whereas, if a baby whose systems are immature and not functioning 100% the infiltration of vaccine chemicalization is devastating; setting into motion the spawning of autism. Know what chemicals are pointed at your baby for injection; do protect them! Be chemically safer; consider only chemically SAFER vaccines!

We frown upon drug users and we consider the drug addict that feeds his addiction through the use of needles as the worst type of drug user. The drug addict that injects his poison into their bloodstream is considered the lowest form of drug addict. The very idea that we inject children repetitively in life is considered by many an atrocity. The fact that we are injecting innocent children with vaccine **chemicals** that are unnatural or alien to their body violates the injected victim and repulses parents who recognize the harms associated. Vaccine Producers are considered drug-makers and the mandated vaccination law and/or enforced delivery system are considered drug-pushers bent on inducing innocent children into **shooting-up users of vaccines**. The sadness or feeling of sickness that people experience when viewing a person shooting up drugs is comparable to what many parents experience and/or feel when seeing their **children shooting-up vaccine chemicals.** When a parent has no legal choice but to submit their child for unwanted injections they are wronged and are **enslaved** to stand by and witness their children shot-up with chemicals; suffer chemicalization. Vaccine chemicals alter the natural chemistry of the injected victim. **Law must not enforce people to submit their children to undergo unwanted chemical injections or be forced to endure the putrefaction of their children's blood. Vaccinations are so profitable they have seen to it that we are enslaved.**

The distaste that the public has for drug addicts shooting-up pales compared to parents' distaste about their children being injected with unwanted vaccines or against parents' will; making children vaccine chemical addicts. For those parents who agree with administering a vaccination or determine that the vaccination is in their child's best interest administer the vaccine however; when parents do not want the vaccine injection then no vaccine injection should be given! Law must not hinder parents' natural Right of protecting their children; nor should mal-law enforce the DENATURING of children's blood chemistries. Law should not render parents powerless or cause them to have decreased parental authority, directive or drive. Parents must not be enforced or made to surrender children for needle injections of chemicals that parents do not want their children exposed to. The vaccination mandate enslaves children to be VACCINE INJECTION ADDICTS. Without legal refusal of injections; we are ENSLAVED to vaccinate!

Parents influence the path their children take or what they experience and must be free to do so. How far parents' sphere of influence is should not be limited by a mal-law vaccination mandate. If parents are not in sync with or on the same page with having their children undergo vaccine chemicalization then it must not be done. For if it is done over-ruling parents the conflict is damaging. A parents' anxiety or understanding or visualization that the vaccine will harm their child can remotely influence what their child experiences; it is of course negative to the health of the parent to witness their child be injected with chemicals that the parent thinks can injure or have researched as harmful. Consciousness creates order; the mind influences matter. If parents are convinced or expect negative results from vaccine chemicalization injections there must be no vaccination. How far the mind or body

extends out is unknown however, it is known that the mind can influence the outcome. The physical presence of the unnatural to the body chemicalization is destructive to health, the electromagnetic alteration is destructive to health and the psychokinetic influence that is also, problematic! What one conceives and believes it tends to achieve thus, if you're not on board with the vaccination or think it harmful; it is not recommended your children suffer undergoing it. Enforcing unwanted chemical injections is an abomination that negative consequences are imponderable!

Here is a thought that nobody thinks about but, really should, the brain runs on energy; without energy the brain cannot function in fact, nothing can. So, what makes this energy or what type, or level of energy is of outmost importance. If you inject chemicals that are not part of the normal CHEMICAL EQUATION, then the energy is rendered abnormal. We are like a great big electric circuit board; all our cells run on energy and all our function is directed, coordinated and influenced by energy. Let us assure that children have the normal energy required to be healthy and not be negatively impacted by what produces abnormal energy. Chemicals and thoughts control our energy! Every chemical has an electromagnetic field or energy signature. Make sure the chemicals in your baby have the chemical electromagnetic signatures that spell health; not autism! Injecting vaccine unnatural chemicals is grossly incoherent with optimum health!

There is more reason not to mandate vaccination or be mastered over by vaccine producers or their puppet government! Electric activity within the hemispheres of the brains of parents and their children are synchronized. Strangers and/or vaccine producers' or its puppet government yes men, are not naturally wired to best serve the best interest of children therefore, the decision to vaccinate or not vaccinate must be for parents to decide. What parents radiate for their children carries essential encoding or information that is predominately geared to help optimize health and/or human potential in their children; and parents' directional energy is far more influential than that of strangers. Unfortunately; at times this energy can be induced to be destructive as a negative frequency as when parents are under the stress of their children suffering an unwanted vaccine chemicalization by injection. The idea of their children suffering an altered reactive state as a direct result of a vaccine chemicalization creates unhealthy parental visualization and/or unhealthy magnetic vibration waves.

The atrocity of enforcing unwanted vaccination or its negative ramification is difficult to fathom; vaccination slavery or any slavery must never be tolerated! If the vaccination occurs voluntarily when it is understood as harmful that is tragic however, the act of actually enforcing vaccination against parental will, misgivings or understanding that the vaccination is to some degree harmful or is going to be injurious has additional, exponential harm. There is negative impact caused to the mind and/or made to be produced by the traumatized mind by mandated vaccination. Mandated vaccination is an over burdensome regulation and is a stress that is beyond mere legal mishap; it is sanctioned slavery. We are given no realistic or legal chance to not comply; we are corralled, coerced, forced to submit, surrender for vaccine injected chemicalization.

Do super radiate health in your children and/or restore them to an ordered coherence of health; never infiltrate them with unnatural to their body chemicals! Children as compared to adults are an open book, children are more readily affected by unnatural to their body chemicals and are more easily influenced by what or how their parents' think. Adults can inject their thought waves into children to influence children's biology and parents have more affinity to do so for their children. Know that as a parent you can influence your child's state of health by super radiating your child with positive goodness or optimum health thinking. However, the physical presence of unnatural to the body vaccine chemicals has its severe negative to health propensity and will tend to a predominate or negate moderate positive parental projection. When parents have actual fear of vaccination or absolute knowledge that the vaccine chemicalization is causing degeneration to their children's well-being then the mental saturation can increase the negative to health consequences of vaccination. When parents are enforced by a mal-legal vaccination mandate to vaccinate their children despite their rational fears or absolute understanding of harm the consequences are exponentially harmful to both parent and to their children. Vaccinations should never be enforced especially, upon those that are afraid of the vaccination or are educated that vaccine, unnatural to the body chemicalization is strongly potentially harmful or have negative to health propensity.

Adverse reactions proximate to vaccine chemicalization strongly indicate declining health. Fever, inconsolable crying, staring, sleep pattern disturbance and convulsion are some indications that an unnatural to the body chemicalization has begun to take its unhealthy toll. More abnormal behavior like running into walls, continually walking around or spinning in circles, no eye contact and/or eyes often being extremely fixated to the side, lack of socialization or a marked decrease in the normal love and affection for their parents and siblings are just the tip of the iceberg of the signs, symptoms and degeneration are the aftermath of chemical vaccine injections. Parents should not wait with baited breath for the vaccine industry to act to remove unnatural to the body chemicals; parents need to protect their children. Demand informed consent or rather, INFORMED DENIAL of vaccinations to prompt increased vaccine safety and bring about NO CHEMICALS IN VACCINES. Parents reserve the Right to preserve children's chemistry.

Since children are one with their parents and their parents are without question, responsible for the upbringing and safety of their beloved children, parents are best to control whether a vaccine is or IS NOT injected; NOT GOVERNMENT. Parents' being vested with control of their children and/or their health is the natural order of things; this promotes vaccine safety by prompting a needed reasonable level of vaccine quality control in order, satisfy parent's expectations. Parents do not want, nor do they expect, any alien, unnatural to the body chemicals in vaccines. In order, to be considered for injection vaccines must not have unnatural to the body chemicals. The realistic way to assure vaccine safety and that no chemicals sliver their way into vaccines is to give PARENTS their natural Right to REFUSE for their children any unwanted CHEMICAL vaccinations. Parents protecting their children from medical intervention dangers particularly, unnatural to the body VACCINE CHEMICALIZATIONS best protects children.

Take every factor into account when determining if vaccination is in your children's best interest become aware of what chemicals are in vaccines. Know what vaccine options are available. Recognize that parents have purity of heart and on target conscientiousness concentration on doing what is in the best interest of their children. Strangers to your children will have strong tendency to do what is in their own best interest that not necessarily coincides with your children's best interest. Personal of drug companies will do what makes the most money, securing their jobs; they have a different set of values or priorities than parents. Do not be so foolish as to leave your children's health decisions to others; take rightful control, authority and command! Be aware that unnatural to the body chemicals do not belong in the formulation process of needed proteins or other biosynthesis. Know that when vaccine chemicals combine with other unnatural to the body chemicals it is even more harmful. Make sure they GET THE CHEMICALS OUT of vaccines; only then consider the pros and cons or possibility of vaccination! Do not be made to throw the dice with your children's health! Protect your children to the best of your ability! A baby's health is not sustainable if injected with alien to the body chemicals! By divine law, natural law or man-made proper law you can refuse unwanted chemicalization; you have the liberty to protect your children from denaturation!

Make the offeror of the vaccination satisfy your rational and reasonable level of safety. The injection of a vaccine is perhaps the most important decision that parents' make for their children. Be sure that the vaccine is not laced with chemicals that could or do cause internal chemical upheaval or dope the brain cells of your offspring with abnormal electromagnetic signatures. Make sure the chemical propensity is health generating. Your input or ability to refuse vaccination is essential to assure vaccines are made as safe as possible. Make no mistake, the present state of vaccines does indeed have chemicals that are alien or unnatural to the potential recipient; making it unworthy for injection! Once your child receives an injection there may be no turning back; make sure autism is not an injection away or is being chemically spawned!

The chain of transmutations or spiraling abnormalities due to the introduction of alien vaccine chemicals into the once pure chemistry of a child is analogous to the spinning of a bicycle's pedals giving rise to the turning of its wheels – with the chain representing the varying alien vaccine chemicals that comingle with the natural chemistry of the body, connecting the two in abnormal reactions. Vaccine chemicals denature the once normal chemistry and is negative to health. **Let me be crystal clear; you cannot chemically adulterate children's blood without causing health problems. Some of these health problems may not come to the surface or show itself as a diagnosable health problem with obvious signs and symptoms however, be assured the harm to health is the reality. This is analogous to people that smoke; not all get lung cancer, but you can be sure, it is not good for you to smoke; it is causing health degeneration. Children are sicker than ever; vaccine chemical exposure is a cause. The reason why autism has risen as the number of vaccinations has risen is because of the increased exposure to unnatural to the body vaccine chemicals. It is prudent for parents to be sure that vaccines are safe and refuse injections that they are not convinced are safe.**

The **GREAT and GOLDEN RULE** of health care, known as **informed consent,** dictates that the patient always **BE IN CONTROL** of their very own health. Informed consent/**DENIAL** grants us the **Liberty** to deny unwanted vaccinations and saves us from unwanted chemical injections. Our liberty to decide upon our very own healthcare or health is supreme. Words are not enough; there must be strong initiative or action on parent's part in order to take back their rightful control and/or protection of their children. People must take a stand against the abuses of overzealous medical intervention. **There must be liberation from vaccination slavery. There must be vaccination independence. Healthcare decision power must be vested in parents. This essential freedom of self-governing one's very own blood chemistry or blood content gives parents the collective capacity to secure SAFER vaccines; GET THE CHEMICALS OUT! The collective capacity to instill the need for vaccine producers to achieve safety. Parents authority to control their children's vaccination is imperative for children's safety! In making the vaccination decision always remember that we are indivisible from the chemical constituents within us; chemicals drive health or sickness. The epidemic of chemicalization autism can be curtailed by minimizing or eradicating the unnatural to the body chemicals in vaccines. Be informed of what is in a vaccine and decide accordingly!**

Government serves us, it is only meant to assure our Rights are preserved; seeing to it that we enjoy the basic freedom to self-care of our bodies thereby, providing that we can freely deny unwanted medical intervention. The mandated vaccination law is an enigma that defies this core principle and most basic freedom. It is an erroneous outcast law which stands so far to the left that it drops off the platform of what is legally proper or just; it is not a constitutionally permissive law. This illative unjust law continues to grossly infringe upon our basic freedom to control what enters our bloodstreams or that of our children's blood. This ill law is in perpetuity and/or with no deadline to discontinue; it has no sun set clause or contemplated regulatory end and this further its non-legal status. The erroneous mandate continues out of greed to mega-profit and out of force of habit; enforced chemicalization is not in the best interest of the People. The law violates the People causing chemically induced Autism. Vaccination **slavery** is taking place in all States to a greater or a lesser degree; we must **ABOLISH** slavery!

The never-ending vaccination mandate reminds me of another antiquated mal-law which is erroneously still on the books to this day. It is law that was put on the books during WW TWO when syphilis was prevalent; this intrusive antiquated law wrongfully still requires all newborns to have Silver Nitrite or an antibiotic put in newborn's eyes just in case the mother has syphilis. Most if not all parents are unaware that within the very first seconds of a newborns life this intrusive medical intervention is perpetrated upon our babies. It is a terrible eye-opening experience that newborns are forced to be welcomed into the world with, a beginning of life enforced invasive medical intervention that also, needs to be remedied by being eradicated. Once the drug/chemical industry sinks its very long fangs into securing profit it never lets its profiteering prey go; once it has a profiting by law scenario they see to it that it continues in perpetuity even though, there is no longer valid reason for it. Today, hardly anyone has syphilis, there is no emergency, but children still are mandated to be abused by having this garbage put in their eyes. Parents be aware, as soon as your baby is born this eye clogging violation occurs without your permission and usually without your knowledge. Analogously, there are no childhood disease epidemics of today or emergency that might require the quasi legal reasoning for a vaccination mandate and yet, injection of vaccine chemicals is still mandated and in ever increasing numbers. No imminent threat or epidemic means no more pathological mandates of mass vaccinations; to continue mandating vaccination is just chemicalization child abuse on a mass scale. The chemical/drug industries are strong lobbyists.

Vaccines are big business. Be discerning about the chemicals in vaccines and demand liberty to refuse unwanted chemicals!

Authority wrongfully claiming that vaccines are safe to inject must not be granted license to force inject our children and/or enslave families into their mandated vaccination way of life; they are not our masters! No intelligent, fair minded person can make such a blanket **ASS**umption of safety or that we must be injected for our own good or societies benefit especially, with the intolerable number of vaccines being forced upon children that are laced with alien, unnatural to the body chemicals. It is indisputable that vaccines currently have unnatural to the body chemicals that have biological impact. Parents are the proper authority to make the vaccination decision. Vaccine Producers, mega-profiting from vaccine sales creates a mega-conflict of interest; their ludicrous blanket claim that vaccines are all safe to inject should be dismissed and/or not trusted. One individual's idea of what is safe may not be another individual's idea of what is safe or rise to the level of what loving caring parents' think safe. **We are enslaved to vaccinate; compromising our children's natural internal chemistries and jeopardizing our children's health. The People must be free to decide on an individual basis if a vaccine is worthy and/or safe enough to inject into the delicate and susceptible bloodstreams of their children. Who decides what vaccine or chemicals may be injected must ultimately be up to the potential vaccination recipient adult or by parents for their dependent children!**

If someone said to you, "your child must be vaccinated by law" or if you do not vaccinate child services will be called and your child may be taken from you in order, to be injected with a vaccine that you have concluded too dangerous to inject; what would you say or what would you do? What is important is that you realize that your rights are being violated and perhaps most importantly, what chemicals are they threatening to enforce upon your tiny baby! It is justifiable civil disobedience to refuse a vaccine that you deem unsafe or not in your child's best interest.

Children need their parents' protection and parents need to protect their children! By knowing what is in vaccines and by knowing your rights you are armed to protect them accordingly. This book has verse after verse of protection please, use it wisely! Save your children from what must be considered the worst chemicalization that they will likely ever face. Vaccine chemicalization upsets the natural chemistry and magnetic signature of health with resultant destruction to one's biological mechanics or productive existence. Be free to ward off vaccine chemical attacks, be free to stop needling and injection of vaccine chemicalization by being free to refuse unwanted shots! As a parent you have the right to refuse what you consider not in your child's best interest by God given law, by the natural order of things and/or by unadulterated, pure parental superior authority! Know that your body is 75% water, but your brain is 85% water. The increased percentage of water in the brain is due to the amount of communication taking place in the brain; the water is required for the communication to take place. Chemicals present encode messages or allow messages to be signaled, a form of chemical communication that requires water to radiate the messages and coordinate everything. Ask yourself this question, "does the vaccine have chemicals that impede, pervert, alter or render abnormal the mass amount of communication taking place"; then protect your children accordingly!

There is a perfect balance in nature, a perfect chemistry that perfects health. It is not by happenstance that the brain is 85% water; the percentage is required for health and/ or homeostasis. In fact, there is a balance or chemical configuration certain in order, to be healthy or even alive; to manipulate or alter the natural chemical make-up by injecting unnatural to the body chemicals creates disharmony, degenerates' health and/or can spawn autism. The entire chemistry of the brain is configured to allow for health and/ or homeostasis. To be optimally healthy make sure the chemistry in your infants' brain is perfected with its natural, normal chemistry and not distorted with unnatural to the brain chemistry' chemicals. As a parent' make sure the vaccine is not going to upset this perfected natural balance of chemicals otherwise, reject the injection! Put all your power into protecting your children from unnatural chemicalization! We the People' must be free to decide what is best for our children and protect them from unwanted vaccine chemical exposures; our government must secure this parental freedom of protection!

Let us assure that SAFER vaccines are made to a standard to satisfy parent consumers of vaccines; making absolutely, sure that the injection of the vaccine does not distort in anyway the contents of the highly perfected chemistry of the brain. Traditional consumer rejection of what that consumer concludes as inferior or too dangerous to inject vaccines must rule the vaccination delivery system. Freedom to refuse under informed consent/ DENIAL and liberty to seek damages under traditional negligence litigation against vaccine manufacturers, efficiently and effectively secures SAFER vaccines and the safety of our children. Protect babies' perfect chemistry with freedom to reject injections! As parents we are vested with supreme authority and power to make sure the vaccine will not subject one's offspring to actual or potential harm and/or manipulate the natural chemistry or cause chemical reaction abnormality, upheaval, chaos or happenstance. Any degree of chemical change to the natural chemistry should not be tolerated; any vaccine chemicals for profit that do not support or aide the body most not be allowed in vaccines!

There is a guiding principle of health that keeping one's internal chemistry pure will keep one optimally healthy and that to deviate one's internal pure chemistry causes health problems. Not living by this life and health principle will lead to disaster. The idea of a threat from vaccine chemicalization is so opposite of what is ingrained or what has been repetitively programmed into us that this very real threat to many cannot be perceived and yet, others have been restored to self-thinking individuals or have regained their ability to recognize a truth or threat that exists. Open your mind and put aside false assumptions to recognize the disharmony and danger of chemicalization! The act of injecting unnatural to the body chemicals against the will of parents is an act of terrorism against children's health! We need to regain parental control over what may or may not enter children's blood or vital chemistry; preventing acts of chemicalization warfare upon offspring. Be free to be the parents that you aspire to be and safeguard your children with liberty to refuse unwanted vaccine chemicalization? Be free to protect your children to the very best of your ability! Government should and must secure this fundamental freedom by granting parents their basic liberty to say "NO" to vaccine chemicalization. Whether it be refusing any vaccination or forbidding injection of chemicals that have no biological advantage or that cause biological disadvantage; we need to decide what is best for our children with unfettered refusal freedom!

The disadvantage of being exposed to chemicals that interfere, adulterate, manipulate or make abnormal the natural biorhythm or biological functions must be freely avoided by parents. Mother and father must be fully empowered to protect their children from chemicalization and an integral part of this protection is to decide if vaccines are safe or not. The enforcement of the mandated vaccination law **shuts down parenting!** Parenting is impinged upon by not allowing parent's their essential refusal of unwanted vaccine chemical injections. Parents must be in control; parents need to determiners of whether vaccination is to be administered. There is no question that parents are their children's supreme guardians however; the mandated vaccination law dictates otherwise. **You might as well ask a parent not to breathe than ask them not to protect their children from a danger or vaccination harm**.

Parents aware of what chemicals are inside vaccines are astounded; they must not tolerate being forbidden from stopping such injections. Parents' under their God given Right of procreation and/or parenthood must be allowed to protect their children from unwanted or thought of as too dangerous to inject vaccinations. Parental protection of children from potential vaccination harm or impending actual harm is a protection parents must not stand to be interfered with; **children need their parent's unbridled protection to prevent abuse from tyrannical enforced vaccine chemicalization. It is a violation of mega proportion to enforce vaccine chemicalization upon children of parents that do not agree with the vaccination. To unleash vaccine chemicalization by needle and injection into innocent offspring of parents' that do not want to expose their offspring to such, chemical folly is an offence that must no longer be permitted; it is an offence of vaccination slavery!**

Parents have by divine law and require by man-made law to be empowered with the authority supreme when it comes to the health or welfare of their children or whether or not a vaccine chemicalization by injection shall or shall not take place. Parents must have the ultimate power of decision; being free to determine if the vaccine has negative to health propensity and therefore, must be disallowed from entering one's tiny baby, small infant or immature child! History has always shown us that parents are the best decision makers; know and rely upon the fact that parents are the best decision makers for their children's welfare.

Parents have purity of heart and no conflicts of interest, they will decide what is in the best interest of their beloved children; deciding just what is right by their very own flesh and blood. To place anyone else other than parents in control is ludicrous and dangerous to the welfare of all children; not having parents in control is a major reason why health problems are caused in children. The sum of the total numbers of people realizing vaccine chemicalization has been causing health devastation is staggering and is ever growing. Parents' for too many years have been clearly reporting that their children are being caused vaccine induced injury in the form of pain, stiffness, spams, fever, convulsion and autism to name a few. To state that vaccine chemicals are safe to inject is ludicrous and controverts parents' observations of what has befallen their children. To not grant the essential freedom of personal or family health decision is inconsistent with the basic premise of what law is or supposed to be enacted for.

Energy of parents is focused upon their children's well-being and/or best interest. How many seconds of the day or how many hours of the day or years spent dedicated or devoted to children's welfare is indicative of who must be entrusted with the vaccination decision. That being said; parents are naturally vested to be children's vaccination determiners. Importantly, only parents' have either the heart, energy or time spent in doing what is in the best interest of children; only parents have the focused energy for the welfare of children. Vaccine Producers or its puppet government do not have the requisite mind set or purity of action. Vaccine producers have removed themselves so far from the results of vaccine induced injuries that they are not even held accountable or liable or made to pay for the injuries that their negligently produced vaccines cause. Focused energy allows you to learn everything, including but not limited to professional skills, getting into shape, learning to play the piano; it also allows to keep your child safe, healthy and happy. Parents are so powerful when it comes to children's best interest and/or welfare that no one or thing must replace or rule the vaccination decision. Do not undergo infiltration by injection of unnatural to a human's biology and/or physiology chemicals; do not risk chemicalization autism of your children!

The Ninth Amendment of the Bill of Rights was added to the Constitution to protect all the rights of the People that are not memorialized in writing in the body of the Constitution but are nonetheless vested in the People. The right to decide upon what will or will not enter one's bloodstream or children's blood does not have to be mentioned in the body of the Constitution to be in fact, protected by the Constitution. Protecting one's children from unwanted vaccine chemicalization is a natural or inalienable right; it does not have to be written in some man-made law for it to be law, it is understood under the umbrella of the Ninth Amendment. Vaccination is a sacrosanct personal decision that children need their parents to make and that parents need to make for their children. It is automatically understood and a supreme rule that parents determine if any preventative healthcare will or will not be given. What an individual allows to be injected into their bloodstream does not get more personal.

The truth that vaccines have unnatural to the body contents has made parents wide eyed and made them no longer sleep on their rights and properly step up to the plate of parenting; parents are no longer putting their blind trust in Vaccine Producers or those who blankly or falsely state that vaccinations are safe. Parents are now initiating the changes needed to protect their children. Always remember, Vaccine Producers have a deep-seated conflict of interest in that they are loyal to their stockholders and profit comes first not safety; they are posed to put profit ahead of our children's safety. Vaccine producers' function to serve what makes the most profit; they do not get paid or receive bonuses to keep your children safe or assure your children are not in any way chemically compromised. They have a propensity, proneness, inclination and/or weakness to place chemicals in vaccines that will maximize profit. If it is more profitable to use a chemical or if you dangle enough cash in front of those that decide; the chemical will be in the vaccine. Parents are incorruptible when it comes to their children; they do the right thing; so, do not blindly trust vaccine producers!

Since Vaccine Producers have unfairly and wrongfully been enabled to produce vaccines without the worry of liability, a floodgate of vaccines without due diligent safety care has resulted. Unwisely, they have a liability shield and consequently, do not have to do a cost/benefit analysis or must concern themselves with negligence law suites; they merely concentrate on maximizing profit. This promotes careless production and corners cut when it comes to safety. There is a marked proclivity to put chemicals in vaccines that maximize profits and not safety. There must be no **ANTI-SAFETY VACCINE LIABILITY SHEILD for Vaccine Producers; the survival of our children depends on it**. There needs to be condemnation and punishment for negligent production of vaccines; **GET THE CHEMICALS OUT**. There must be **PUNITIVE DAMAGES** for purposely producing chemically laced vaccines particularly, when Vaccine Producers are found to have knowledge that the **CHEMICALS THEY USE IN VACCINE PRODUCTION ARE DETRIMENTAL TO HEALTH**.

Vaccine Producer's must have stringent production parameters to best safeguard our children. There needs to be accountability and answerability to parents. A reasonable constraint upon what is used in vaccines is necessary and there must be recourse against the producers of vaccines if their vaccines cause injury. Producers of vaccines should not be exempt from parents seeking justice and compensation for vaccine induced injuries. There needs to be obligations for safety. Vaccines must not have unnatural to the body, anti-health chemicals. **THERE SHOULD BE NO LIABILITY SHEILD.** There must not be undermining of our legal tort system; vaccine negligence actions must be enabled to seek damages from the source of the negligence, in the instant case; Vaccine Producers. Compensation must only be paid by non-other than the negligent party; not government spending tax dollars when the fault is upon Vaccine Producers. Injured vaccination recipients must rightfully burden negligent Vaccine Producers and not drain tax dollars.

Vaccine Producers know there is no harm going to come their way, no judicial hammer going to slam down upon them if they cause children injury. They manufacture vaccines with chemicals that should not be injected into children and will not be punished for doing so even if the vaccines induce injury. When you know that you cannot get hurt if you cut safety corners, the tendency is to cut safety corners; concentration on safety becomes less imperative and even unnecessary. Often manufacturers place profit ahead of safety, even in the face of negligence liability; you can imagine the increased propensity to place profit ahead of safety, how it escalates when the manufacturers have a liability shield and/or cannot be hurt when they produce products (vaccines) negligently. Do not entrust your children's safety to the frailty of profit minded businessmen that have a liability shield. Informed consent/DENIAL of vaccine injections is also required for safety.

When it comes to the welfare of your child do not blindly trust that there is nothing bad in vaccines or allow an injection uninformed. Be in control of your health and that of your child's health by demanding informed consent/DENIAL. The mandated vaccination law threatens the very foundation of proper parenting and primary parental responsibility. Law must not disembowel citizen's healthcare control or take over children's welfare decisions. It is not within the jurisdiction of law to sacrifice the health and/or lives of some for the theoretical well-being of others. Vaccine chemicals do cause health problems and that makes their enforcement that much more impermissible and unjust. The People must be in control of their health and healthcare destiny. Children's vaccination decision must rest with the children's mother and father; for the best interest and/or health of children.

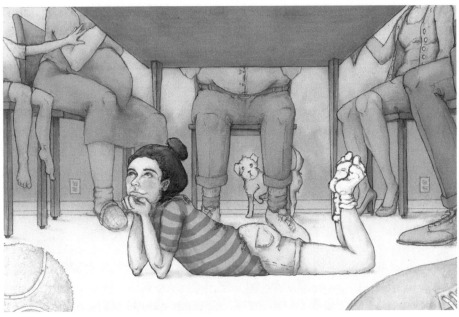

Vaccination is a family decision. Government must not dictate or intrude upon it.

It can be rationally considered the waging of chemical warfare upon our children to be overpowered or enforced to inoculate children, against parental will, with vaccines that have chemicals that are unnatural to human biology and/or physiology. The waging of this chemicalization warfare directly causes signs and symptoms and/or health problems and there is collateral damage incurred. Parents have been disarmed through the takeover of our government by special interest groups or lobbyists that see to it that chemical for profit bombs reach its target; our children's vital blood chemistries are under attack. Our right of informed consent/DENIAL has been sidestepped or taken out by the money crazed vaccination mandates. The Second Amendment secures one's right to bear arms and/or protect oneself, certainly; the liberty to refuse vaccine chemicalization arms parents with the ability to prevent chemicalization by needle injection which, falls under the Second Amendment. The faulty and callous vaccination mandate severs the parent and child connection, disarming parents from defending their children or preventing unwanted vaccine chemicalization. It disallows refusal of vaccination under the legal concept of informed consent/DENIAL and thereby, allows chemical warfare to lay siege into unprotected children. Children are without their parents' protection and fall victim to unwanted medical intervention. Children need their parents' protection and parents need to protect their children from unwanted vaccine chemicalization or chemical warfare! Parents' must not be disarmed from protecting children by mal-law mandates! No one should feel safe with what chemicals are in vaccines or if, we remain legally unable to refuse vaccination! It is high time parents are set free to protect their children!

Human physiology and/or biology is dependent upon the range of reactions of required chemicals but also, the energy charges that arise from the chemicals or molecules. There is a coalescence of energy, an information source that guides and coordinates in order, to be optimally healthy. Chemicals and its energy signatures are the language of the cells. For example, the Limbic system of the brain which has to do with our emotions and perceptions responds to chemical communication signals allowing one to experience sensations and/or sensations that can be experienced by all the cells of the body. Nerve cell membranes have receptors that are designed to respond to the presence of chemicals and chemicals coordinate signals in these neural receptors that are in all cells. BE ACUTELY AWARE THAT THE CHEMICALS INJECTED INTO YOUR OFFSPRING TAKE ITS TOLL. It is unimpeachable that chemicals can make or break health and the orthodox community needs to acknowledge, respect and revere this biological truth. SAFER vaccines do not have unnatural to the body chemicals! Just as it is now known that the earth is not flat; the injection of unnatural to the body vaccine chemicals is now known that it is not harmless and is in fact, detrimental to health and is the cause of chemicalization autism. Do not allow your children to have their perfected natural chemistry to be compromised or bastardized with vaccine injection chemicalization! Be free to reject the injection of chemical chaos; have authority over your children's welfare!

Trust in the safety of vaccinations has all but vanished and rightfully so. It is outrageous that unnatural to the body chemicals are in vaccines and it is incredulous that parents are mandated by mal-law to have their children stuck with vaccination needle and plunged with vaccine chemicals. This is about chemical insult after insult by vaccination. There is rational fear of Autism brought about by enforced unwanted vaccine chemical exposure. Make no mistake; vaccine chemicalization brings about reactive AUTISM. Of course, it is true that chemical infiltrations cause health problems and that injected unnatural chemicals are extremely hazardous. It is the impermissible enforcement of vaccine chemical injections and the divesting of our Right to self-determined healthcare that has led to children's health demise. The long list of chemicals found in vaccines such as, aluminum, glutamate etc., is more than ample reason for parents to take back the control of their children to secure their safety. Live FREE to REJECT INJECTIONS to protect your children and/or prevent dangerous internal exposure to vaccine chemicals. If vaccines were so good they would not have to be mandated; they would sell themselves. Vaccinations are a big business that has lobbied long and hard to keep us enslaved to be vaccinated. Distrust any healthcare that is mandated! Always avoid chemical adulteration of your children's blood! FREE Americans must not be ENSLAVED TO VACCINATE!

Chemical injections are the worst form of chemicalization because the chemicals directly enter the bloodstream to quickly penetrate the brain tissue; doping the brain cells. Only crazoids, crazies, idiots or madmen put unnatural to the body chemicals in vaccines. Chemical injection exposure circulates unchecked into the brain to take its unhealthy toll. Vaccine chemical exposure is an unhealthier chemical exposure because the chemicals are injected. We can and should take the TWO STEPS OF CORRECTION to resolve the vaccine quality issue and thereby, GET THE CHEMICALS OUT. Vaccination slavery, submitting children out of coercion or legal threat or glacial compliance, does not best serve the public. A better way to achieve vaccination compliance and a way to safer vaccines is the TWO STEPS OF CORRECTION way.

Children need their parents to be free to protect them from all danger and unnatural to the body chemical injections is such, a danger that parents need to be free to protect against. Obviously, parents want what is best for their children and generally will decide what is in their children's best interest. For law to step in and upset this natural order of things is uncalled for and unwarranted. The entire population of parents have not been found grossly negligent to have necessitated mandated vaccination in fact, it is grossly negligent to mandate that all children be vaccinated with unnatural to their body vaccine chemicals. There is no history of parents in general not doing what is right for their children therefore, parents must be free to determine just what is right for their children; unimpeded by government and/or not commanded to do otherwise by mal-government mandates. Free America needs to count on parents to decide what is in their children's best interest; not big government. It is an intrusion beyond reason to mandate vaccinations. For parents to decide what is best for their children and/or whether or not children will be injected with chemical vaccines is part of parental Rights and/or authority. Vaccination has tremendous impact on children's lives; parents' must have the decision!

Since, the injection or non-injection of vaccine chemicals have major impact upon health and/or life, the vaccination decision must only be made by those who must live with the results of the healthcare decision. Parents must live with the results of the vaccination decision and therefore, it is for parents to make the vaccination decision. Government or the puppet regulators of drug companies are much too distant from the health impact of the vaccination decision; it does not have to live with the consequences of the decision. Wayward, governing or intrusive mandates over the People must not be tolerated; the mandated vaccination law is wayward governing and operates to enslave people into vaccine chemical infiltrations. In addition, mandated vaccination has given less reason for assuring vaccine safety and thus, unnatural to the body chemicals or chemicals for profit not health is now found in vaccines. Healthcare freedom requires parental freedom of decision! Children need their parent's protection and parents need to protect their children; the erroneous vaccination enslavement mandate violates these intrinsic needs.

People are passionate, religious and absolute about their health. Some dictate their devotion or religious conviction of health on others; frantically trying to make others follow what they think is right and do not let individuals bask in their own glory of healthcare decision. Some lobby, form groups and associations to enforce their ego-maniac healthcare convictions; as is the case of mandated vaccinations. They coerce and enforce their health religion on you. They condemn all differencing healthcare decisions. Adhered to healthcare conformity allows for mega-profiteering. Mandated healthcare is a dangerous loss of healthcare liberty. Mandated vaccinations dictate what is right or wrong for everyone; a totalitarian rule. Some who dictate, do it automatically and do not realize how obnoxious it is or how obtrusive and yet some revel in condemning the healthcare decisions of others. The over-reaching mentality, of tyrannical medical intervention, has spawned an ENSLAVEMENT of children and parents to suffer enforced chemicalizations. May each free person be considered a sovereign State with vested control over what chemicals can enter his or her body or borders; may no one dictate, command or control another person's internal being, health or healthcare. We hereby, ABOLISH VACCINATION SLAVERY and FREE our children from the vices of profiteering medicine. By law one must not be enforced to defile or denature one's blood, body or brain cells! FREE people are not mandated to be injected or must submit their children for unwanted vaccination in perpetuity or otherwise. FREE people live unmolested and undisturbed by preventative healthcare; deciding for themselves and for their children what healthcare is accepted.

CHAPTER 6

MANDATED VACCINATION IS MANDATED CHILD ABUSE

CHILDREN ARE BEING EXPERIMENTED ON, USED AS CHEMICALLY INJECTED GUINEA PIGS

Attention: Government must not command by mandate the defiling, denaturing or reconfiguring of children's blood, body or brain cell chemistries. Warning: a vaccine is a biological and unnatural to the body chemical complexity therefore, much harder to produce and test for its safety; **WHEN RELEASED UPON THE PUBLIC THERE IS NO TELLING WHAT HEALTH PROBLEMS MAY OCCUR.** Because of the complexity of vaccine manufacturing the level of health problems are extremely difficult to determine or pinpoint. One thing is certain; there are chemicals in vaccines that cause health problems! **The unnatural to the body chemical character of vaccines denatures the vaccine recipient victim and increases the probability of health problems or likelihood of health degeneration. Autism in children and Alzheimer's disease in seniors are primarily a consequence of chemical exposure. The chemicals that we foolishly inject into our delicately balanced internal chemistry are the stumbling blocks of health and the building blocks of Autism in children and Alzheimer's in seniors. Mandated vaccination is mandated child abuse on a mass scale; it is chemical uncertainty, chaos and/or induced chemical reaction happenstance! Parents must not be made by mal-law to surrender their offspring to chemical reactive uncertainty and/or health uncertainty! Chemicals dictate if one is healthy or autistic! One must not be enforced to surrender their offspring to become chemicalization guinea pigs!**

When we are callously enforced to submit our children to be injected with unwanted vaccine chemicalization, we are submitting our children for an internal chemistry experiment; they become CHEMICALLIY INJECTED GUINEA PIGS. Mandated vaccination law is misguided law; it tramples our Rights and is the mishandling of children's welfare. Regulating that Vaccine Producers are not to be held liable and accountable for vaccine induced injuries promotes negligence and parents unable to protect their children from unwanted chemical exposure are the reckless endangerment of our children. Vaccination is such, an inexact science that children are being used as guinea pigs and with its array of injected chemicals children are being subjected to chemicalization child abuse. The unvaccinated are often healthier and more robust; the vaccinated are more often plagued with health problems, are more dependent upon medications and autistic. Every vaccine is not just a dire experiment when injected but rather, it is an act of chemicalization child abuse; having grave health consequences. The unnatural to the body chemicals in vaccines have chemical propensity that generate abnormality, and/ or the alien chemicals have signals that direct to create abnormality.

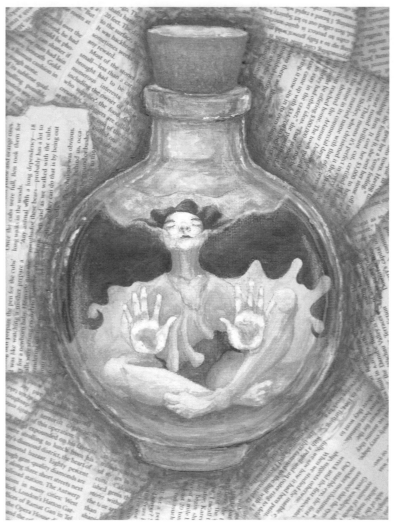

Children are trapped by vaccination mandate to suffer an unwanted vaccine injection which, contains abnormal to the body chemicals that stress the body and cause abnormality. Many scholarly articles warn how dangerous it is to be injected with unnatural to human biology chemicaliztion.

There are a great deal of unanticipated health problems and anticipated health problems because of injecting children with unnatural to the body chemicals. There are signs and symptoms that indicate chemical insult and there are known diagnosis such as, intestinal intussusceptions, cancer and Autism that spawn from alien chemical infiltration. It is no coincidence that we are now faced with mass Autism at an epidemic proportion as vaccines have become laced with alien, foreign to the body chemicals and as the numbers of CHEMICAL vaccination insults have drastically increased over time. The People must be free to decide what is best for their very own children, free to police their very own bloodstreams; and not be enforced to endure unwanted, injected chemical infiltrations. Americans, living in a free society demand to have such basic liberty. Parents have the supreme freedom of protecting their very own children from what parents conceive is a chemical threat to health. The vaccination program is a mass experiment upon our children and a definite unhealthy chemicalization. Freedom requires that parents can refuse to have their children injected with vaccine chemicals; to not be enslaved by mal-law to have their children's delicately balanced bloodstream chemistry or brain cellular chemistry denatured, disrupted, altered and/or violated. The basic understanding of the laws of chemistry and human physiology tell us that it is extremely, unhealthy to inject chemicals that are unnatural to the normal chemistry of the body. There are caustic chemicals in vaccines, having severe anti-health properties, propensities and/or electromagnetic signals. There is a NATURAL CHEMICAL GEOMETRY of good health; vaccine chemicals distort this geometry and is the predominate cause in fact, of Autism.

Frankly, vaccines are really tested on the public as they are mass injected, a type of wait and see process; you could call it an experiment in process. Our children are being forced by a legal mandate to be used as human guinea pigs in an uncertain, non-exacting, enforced medical intervention project. In that most adverse reactions from vaccinations are not reported by doctors, the public is further being blindsided about the problems inherent with injecting vaccine chemicals. Even with the diminished reporting or improper observation or lack of statistics there are still so many reported adverse reactions that the powers that be are well-aware that vaccines cause much harm. Parents have been long reporting that vaccinations do cause problems; reports have been ignored or suppressed. Children are our future; they desperately need empowered parental protection from unwanted vaccine chemicalization. There is a huge amount of money just waiting to be deep pocketed by injecting these vaccine chemicals. Mega money making has corrupted the safety first above all manufacturing concept. Children are being exploited, pushed into taking part in nothing less than a chemical experiment; often causing children's internal chemistry to generate Autism not health. What is being unleashed through the infiltration of anti-health chemicals no one can be sure. Parents must not be enforced (ENSLAVED) to sacrifice their children's chemical integrity or be made to suffer or live with the results of chemicalization. We need to be FREED, emancipated from mandatory chemical injections.

Modern vaccine guru, Maurice Hillemen, who developed NINE of the vaccines that are currently used today said, "I never breathe a sigh of relief until the FIRST 3 million doses are out there." Apparently, even the head authority of vaccine production is worried, skeptical and not sure how much injury will result until at least 3 million are experimented on; and then they can only hazard a guess. Vaccine injections are the systematic chemical doping of children's brains. The level of chemical upset prior to being vaccine chemically infiltrated can be a significant AUTISM factor. However, multiple vaccine chemical exposures set the chemistry toward AUTISM. WARNING: vaccinations swing the pendulum of internal chemistry much too drastically. Vaccines contain chemicals that must not be injected. Enforced vaccination is enforced CHEMICALIZATION OF CHILDREN ON A MASS SCALE AND IS CHEMICAL CHILD ABUSE ON A MASS SCALE. Vaccine producers are morally bankrupt for placing chemicals for profit and not safety in vaccines and for insisting that vaccines which, have unnatural to the body chemicals are to be injected especially, when the parents of the child are against it! Indeed, those placing chemicals in vaccines which, absolutely have nothing to do with the health of the child but everything to do with making lots of money are morally bankrupt and guilty of profiteering. Devoid of the requisite level of caring, consideration and intelligence vaccine producers or its puppet government must not dictate or command parents to vaccinate; it must be for parents to make the vaccination decision, determining if injection is in the best interest!

No one takes into consideration your child's health status or if your child has already been chemically compromised; they just command that all children be injected with the one size fits all vaccine. Since the mandated vaccination poison law cares not or does not take into consideration a children's health history, weight, maturity level or age, gender or chemical make-up they are dangerously injecting their chemical vaccine concoctions; there is no concern about your child's individual health status or specific needs or sensitivities. This is not the practice of proper healthcare! It is a strike against your child's good health to be exposed to the chemicals of vaccines especially, without taking the child's individual health into consideration. Parents' may want the sort after immune response brought about by vaccination, but they do not want their children exposed to harmful chemicals especially, chemicals that are in vaccines for sheer profiteering. If this injected chemical doping exceeds the chemical tipping point, a chemical critical mass syndrome can occur and thereby, sets the course for Autism. Certainly, parents must be free to refuse this systematic chemical doping and/or not have their children undergo injections of unknown consequences or be experimented upon or face any probability of chemical upset or disruption. Of course, all parents must be free to do what they think best for their children. Parents need to prevent children from becoming an Autism epidemic statistic. Even if vaccines were absolutely safe, and they are far from it in fact, they are absolutely unsafe; it would be unjust, immoral and unconstitutional to enforce vaccination over parental objection. **PARENTS LIBERTY TO PROTECT CHILDREN ENDOWS YOU WITH THE POWER TO REFUSE VACCINE CHEMICALIZATIONS!**

Parents are best positioned to determine when a vaccination has negatively impacted a child's health; not doctors or Vaccine Producers. Adverse reactions from vaccinations are best told by the parents of children injected with vaccine chemicals. Parents are best situated to witness and observe the vaccination crime scene, as the negligently produced vaccine takes its unhealthy toll. Parents are constantly near their children and are extremely familiar with their children's health and behavior therefore, are the most credible assessors of changes in their children. Parents can best observe short and long-term reactions from vaccinations; parents, first hand, document adverse reactions due to vaccinations. Parents have long been reporting post vaccination health problems; do not be fooled by the profiteering vaccination industry. It is sheer poppycock that parents are not observing vaccine induced changes. In addition, parents do have the best capacity to decide if vaccinations are or are not in their children's best interest; not government Vaccine Producers. No one is better than the parents of the child for determining if a vaccination injury has occurred or if a vaccine is too dangerous. It is common sense that children must not be exposed to minute dosages of harmful chemicals; to expose them to multiple vaccine chemicals is sheer stupidity. To enforce vaccine chemicalizations is the enforcement of children to be human guinea pigs.

We should bring every resource to bear to make vaccine's safer however, parents being free to refuse what they consider unsafe vaccines is one of the most important if not the most important way to assure SAFER vaccines. Mandated vaccination, all but obliterates

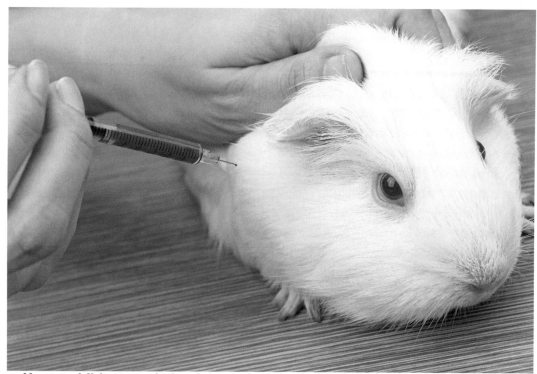

If your children are being injected with vaccines that contain unnatural to human biology chemicals they are being treated like human guinea pigs.

parents' ability to refuse a bad vaccine and/or protect children from unwanted vaccine chemicalization injections. Producers of vaccines using government as their puppet implementers are cause for alarm and great concern. It is consummately wrong to induce vaccination slavery and unjust that Vaccine Producers are not subject to litigation or economic harm when vaccine chemicalization injury occurs. Profiteering Vaccine Producers and their cohorts conspire to mandate vaccinations and induce vaccination slavery. Vaccines are fraught with chemical harm but, they bloviate that vaccine chemical infiltrations are safe or do not cause Autism. Over the sorted history of vaccination, the contention that vaccines are not harmful have been proven utterly and completely wrong. Their pompous pontifications of falsehoods allowed an AUTISM epidemic to spawn and rapidly grow. At the conception it was declared that vaccines are "absolutely safe"; this misleading and deception allowed the vaccination mandate to become law and continues to do so still to this day. Vaccines are NOT absolutely, safe; they cause signs, symptoms and/or countless injuries. Human bondage to vaccination is inhumane; we must ABOLISH VACCINATION SLAVERY, all root and branch of it!

Those who claimed that vaccinations were "absolutely safe" and the government officials of today who have been induced to blindly be resolute that vaccine chemicals are good for children are placing our children's health and very lives in jeopardy. Virtually all the evil committed in this world is by people or government who are so certain they know what they are doing. Those who allow unnatural to the body vaccine chemicals in vaccines and those that insist vaccines be injected by mandate against the will of the child recipients' parents, are morally bankrupt. Parents must be free to discern the vaccination question, to agonize over the question as they ponder a decision. Parents deciding whether a vaccination is in their children's best interest can prevent their children's health demise from chemicalization. The mandated vaccination law takes away a person's healthcare decision, granting absolute power over us. We are commanded to vaccinate because they, not us, are erroneously certain vaccines are safe and must be injected. Many know very well that vaccines have unhealthy chemicals and others have willful ignorance of it and some dare to purposely hide or suppress the fact. Children are enforced to be chemically injected guinea pigs, experimented on; causing untold injuries.

Vaccinations are far from being "absolutely safe" in fact, vaccines are chemically dangerous and in desperate need of quality safety control generated by parental ability to refuse an unwanted vaccine chemicalization. If a toxic vaccine is pointed at your child's blood vessel for its injection, are you going to let your child be chemically exposed? Vaccine chemicals circulate through the blood disrupting and manipulating the natural chemical homeostasis. Your Right of healthcare decision is violated, and you have lost control over your health. Our collective action in the implementation of the TWO STEPS OF CORRECTION is required to remedy the situation. Together, let us demand informed consent/DENIAL; safer vaccines will result. Holding Vaccine Producers liable for vaccine induced injuries is the second needed STEP OF CORRECTION. Venerate the idea of collectivism to abolish vaccination slavery, in an associated awareness of our interdependence and interrelatedness with one another we will put an end to vaccination slavery. One by one; refuse unwanted, unnatural to the body, chemical exposure; insist upon protecting your children. Self-regulated vaccinations and healthcare justice can and must be accomplished. Children must be afforded the protection of their parents and parents' being free to refuse vaccine chemicalization is paramount to this protection. People must speak their minds; remember, the squeaky wheel gets the grease. Demand SAFER vaccines with no anti-health chemicals; shout-out your refusal of chemicalization! Ask safety questions! Your child is yours to protect! Your child means; it is your decision!

There is an underlying collectivism in everyone's goal for safety in healthcare. There is also a collectivism born out of the mass desire for healthcare autonomy and/or self-regulation. Individualism, a sense of independence, self-regulated healthcare, independent vaccination decisions, self-reliance and self-preservation; lead to a collectiveness or greater sense of community. All working together for the greater good of our children and securing of volitional vaccinations are paramount. The dangers of extremism in mandating chemical injections must be eliminated by having liberty of decision in healthcare. We must have autonomy in healthcare to combat the oppressions of being mastered by another or by narrow-minded or short-sighted healthcare socialism. It is not narrow-minded individualism or shortsighted for parents to be free to refuse chemical injections. Billions of dollars are being made through mandated vaccinations and yet Vaccine Producers are unsusceptible, unaccountable, unchangeable and unanswerable when their vaccines cause injury; they have an ill-conceived liability shield. They have breached our trust by seeking profit before safety; they placed a too long-list of anti-health agents in their vaccines. History will reflect that it was extremely wrong for parents to be enforced, coerced or forced to submit their children for unwanted vaccine chemical inoculations. History will signify that the underlying reason for continual vaccination mandates was to guarantee profiteering; not children's safety. Vaccination would not be mandated if there was no profit to be had because of its mandate. Mandated vaccination is vaccination SLAVERY and mass child abuse by unnatural chemicalization!

Drug Company's long history of being misleading and misrepresentative continues; now they are purposely misleading the public about the cause of autism by wrongfully stating that vaccination it is not at all the cause of autism but rather, it is certain children's unique sensitivity. This is hogwash and is a misleading distraction technique; vaccine chemicalization autism is the reality! Many of the chemicals in vaccines are anti-health chemicals; vaccine chemicalizations are the main cause in fact, of the Autism epidemic. It is an incalculable evil to knowingly induce parents to unknowingly chemically derange or denature their children's internal chemistry through the submission to vaccine chemicalization. Injected, unnatural to the biology and physiology vaccine chemicals bombard the brain cells of children, chemically doping brain cells thereby, spawning Autism. Multitudes of observant parents have witnessed health deterioration after vaccination. Parents know their children so very well, they know if their children's nature or health is altered or caused injury; parents are the most credible assessors of vaccine induced harm! All the wiggling and denial and damage control by the vaccine industry serve to assure the continued mass profiting from mass vaccination enslavement; all at our children's health detriment. Do not be so easily mislead or deterred from the truth of the fact that injected CHEMICAL vaccines cause injury. Until the TWO STEPS OF CORRECTION produce SAFER vaccines; REJECT, RECONSIDER, REFUSE! You have been stripped of your basic Right to decide what will enter your bloodstream by an ill-conceived vaccination enslavement mandate. Injected vaccine unnatural chemicals spawn CHEMICALIZATION AUTISM and is the main etiology of the autism epidemic!

Think about the disharmony caused from vaccine chemicals when they flow through your tiny baby's blood and penetrate their highly sensitive brain cells. When the injected chemicals of vaccines rage through the bloodstream it carries with it a stream of information and wave of energy, this frequency or vibration is alien to the body; thereby, spawning abnormality and/or autism. The chemicals in vaccines and the adverse reactions from vaccinations indicate that children are being experimented on; used as human guinea pigs. Parents have long been reporting their children's regression and/or health problems proximate to vaccinations however, it has been ignored or suppressed. There is a definite gamble, a hazard, a peril, an inherent risk and/or danger with receiving each vaccination chemicalization. Every chemically laced vaccine injection incrementally raises your body's chemical imbalance; manipulating the needed perfected chemistry. Today, with children facing the increased number of vaccines injected, it is imperative we implement the TWO STEPS OF CORRECTION to prompt SAFER vaccines. The alien, foreign to the body chemicals of vaccines is a danger that Americans must be free not to be subjected to. The unvaccinated populace's lack of Autism as compared to those vaccinated is revealing. The idea that injecting chemicals is counter to health is logical. Be in harmony with the natural chemical balance of biology and/or physiology; to be healthy!

Warning: this next bundle of words is emotional. When a parent unfortunately, witnesses, observers or begins to see their child quickly or slowly go into a deep under-spiraling in health; this can destroy one's life, both child's and parent' life. Too often after vaccination a vaccine chemicalization recipient too often presents with fever and often very high fever, sleeplessness, starring at the ceiling, lack of the child's normal abilities both mentally and/or physically or shows signs of not being biologically or physiologically enabled to look into your eyes to have that special contact between parent and child and then you witness a convulsion or shrill inconsolable crying or your child begins banging its head into your chest when you hold her or him when the baby, infant or child should actually be sleeping it tells the parent or kicks the parent in the head that something has gone wrong and the only crazy think your offspring has had is a vaccination or better understood as, exposed to unnatural to their body chemicals; it becomes obvious that the child's health demise was spawned by vaccine chemicalization by injection. Parental enslavement to vaccinate must be abolished! Parents' who have not been found guilty of child neglect most have unfettered freedom of vaccination decision; parental decision must be unmitigated, unmediated and unlimited! "NO" to vaccination must be respected!

You would think that vaccine makers would have come to the inescapable logical conclusion that vaccines must be void of anti-health chemicals and taken safety measures in order, to protect our children long ago. Because it makes profit sense to use certain chemicals that does not mean it makes health sense; unfortunately, it is what makes the most money that makes policy as to what chemicals are in vaccines. How do you prove that one is guilty of putting profit first above our children's safety or chemical purity or chemical bio integrity? All you must do is show that chemicals exist in vaccines that are unnatural to the body or have mere profiteering purpose and not safety. Unnatural to the body chemicals are inherently dangerous; it is not in harmony with health. Unnatural to the body chemicals cause signs and symptoms and/or autism. There are chemicals in vaccines that assure profit not health and yes; these chemicals are unnatural to the body and cause disharmony or denatures one's vital naturally perfected chemistry. Check out what is in vaccines; what chemicals lay in wait to be injected to take its unhealthy toll! Unnatural to the human body chemicals destabilize one's biology and/or physiology. Let my words be your words in your stand to protect against vaccine chemicalization abuse!

To maximize profits, Vaccine Producers put in chemical preservatives, assuring longer duration shelf-life such as, but not limited to, thimerosal a mercury derivative. This stops costly returns from vaccine spoilage and prompts greater profit because doctors can now stockpile vaccines that may never expire; such unnatural to the body chemicals places children's health in grave jeopardy. Vaccine producers would not dare defend by saying they did not know that mercury is a neurotoxin; of course, they know the propensity of the chemicals or molecules or compounds that they use in their vaccines; they are in the chemical business and but not necessarily, in the good health or safe vaccine business. Do not be so gullible to think that Vaccine Producers will sacrifice profit for safety! When mega profiteering occurs from having vaccination mandated and if lacing vaccines with chemicals will in some way pump up profits then despite illative health results vaccination will be mandated and bad chemicals for profit will be in vaccines. Big monetary gain is why vaccination is mandated and why chemicals for profit not safety is utilized in vaccine production! Corporate ethics, honesty or integrity are hard to come by in publicly traded companies; so, do not trust that your children's health come first with these money makers. Parents protect your children from unwanted chemicalization, do not let your child be experimented on; demand freedom to REFUSE vaccine chemicalization!

There were and remain much SAFER options when it comes to preservatives. NATURAL TO THE BODY SALT should be your choice as a preservative; if you need one! For centuries non-toxic to the body salt has been known to be a preservative and since; salt is naturally found in the body it should be used as a preservative in vaccines. Just because mercury gives greater shelf-lift than salt it is not health wise to use it in fact, it is health unwise. Why increase shelf life at the health expense of our children? Profit must not come before SAFETY; parents being free to refuse any vaccination that they do not agree with and holding vaccine producers' rationally accountable and liable is are needed deterrents from utilizing unnatural to the body chemicals in vaccines. Vaccine producers will continue to use whatever chemicals that bring their greed before safety mega-dollars until and unless, the TWO STEPS OF CORRECTION make it otherwise! Children's safety comes first for parents and we must make it so with those that make our children's vaccines; so, let us act to GET THE CHEMICALS OUT of vaccines that are unnatural to the body. Take back your rightful protection of your children; protect your offspring always!

Statistics, the ratio of numbers, strongly point to vaccine chemical infiltrations causing the Autism epidemic. The increased number of CHEMICAL injections, with their chemical onslaught gave rise to the Autism epidemic. Logically the more chemicals that your children are injected with the greater the chances of Autism or becoming unhealthy. The laws of chemistry apply to vaccine chemicals entering the body; the laws tell us that injecting multiple vaccine chemicals not native to the normal chemistry of the body will cause unhealthy renegade reactions; spawning AUTISM. The seeds of Autism are not just mercury but rather, all the anti-health chemicals of vaccines; together they are the main etiology of the Autism epidemic. It is outrageous that parents are enforced by mal-law to expose children to such chemicals and/or to become unwilling participants and victims of a VACCINE CHEMICAL EXPERIMENT. It is obvious how bad mercury is for children, in that all cells die in its presence! Vaccine Producers' or its puppet vaccination mandates must not command the undermining of children's blood chemistries. Warning: mercury is just the tip of the iceberg when it comes to chemical manipulation or chemical destruction of the normal chemistry! Children are exposed to all kinds of chemicalization however, to best stop the Autism epidemic; STOP VACCINE CHEMICALIZATION!

It hits parents like a ton of bricks when they see their little girl or boy falter after a vaccination that they trusted in. It is the ultimate bedrail; to give your child up for vaccination and end up with lifetime health problems and/or autism. The key to autism prevention is for parents to open their ears and eyes prior to vaccination; become acutely aware of what chemicals are in vaccines and the dangers inherent with receiving a vaccine by needling and injection. Recognize that you as parents are ultimately responsible for the well-being of your offspring and that no one should be allowed to dictate what if any vaccine chemicalization shall or shall not occur. Do not hesitate; the time to protect your prodigy is now not later; protect them before the vaccine chemical injection, not after! Do not let them turn your child into a vaccination slave or be coerced to submit or take part in a mass chemicalization experiment and/or be used as human guinea pig participants. Keep your children out of chemicalization harm's way!

You would not want the chemicals that have been found in vaccines in the food or in the water that you or your children drink; so, do not stand for it being injected into your tiny babies, small infants or immature children! Open your eyes to see, open your ears to hear; unnatural to your offspring's' body chemicals should not and must not be injected. To inject such, chemicals is to distort the needed perfected chemistry that rules health. Apply the basic principles or laws of chemistry to recognize this monumental truth! Always remember, that when you eat unnatural tom the body chemicals your design is that your elimination system will to a large extent rid your body of those alien to the body chemicals whereas, when such, chemicals are injected there is no buffering its harm or negative to health effect; there is no elimination, it already has penetrated deeply and circulates freely throughout your body. Therefore, a vaccine chemicalization is so much more of a dangerous chemicalization and is why it must be the priority to guard against! The full quantity of vaccines' unnatural to the human body chemicals circulate in the blood to quickly penetrate the cells of the body. Do not let unnatural to the body chemicals dope the brain cells of your tiny baby, small infant or immature child; protect them from it! The danger from the chemicals of vaccines is more dangerous than that of childhood disease! Humans have a natural defense system against childhood diseases; there are killer cells that attack viruses, so the dependence upon vaccination may not be so needed. Vaccine chemicalization can be an unhealthy occurrence; be safe not sorry, vaccinate only with SAFER vaccines.

There is another side of the equation to cleaning up vaccines and/or to making vaccines much safer. Besides prompting SAFER vaccines through freedom to deny unwanted vaccination and holding vaccine companies liable for vaccine induced injuries; those that deliver the vaccine injection need to get a good dosage of ethics. Doctors, physician assistants or nurses or anybody that holds the vaccination syringe and whose job it might be to administer a vaccination must never deliver a vaccination to someone who is against it or is not sure or has not given their unadulterated informed consent to have the vaccination. To violate someone's body in an enforcement of vaccination is morally reprehensible; it is an abomination, an act of assault and battery and should be considered criminal besides unethical. Refusal to enforce vaccinate because either the potential vaccine recipient does not want it or because the deliverer of the vaccine does not think it safe, prompts the manufacturer to heighten quality control and/or make SAFER vaccines. So, besides the TWO STEPS OF CORRECTION; those who deliver vaccination need to only administer the vaccination under ethical circumstances and that means obtaining TRUE INFORMED CONSENT. Under no circumstance should someone deliver a vaccination if the potential vaccination recipient gives their INFORMED DENIAL or if there is no obtainment of TRUE INFORMED CONSENT. In addition, never give a vaccination if you the deliverer of the vaccination do not think it is in the best interest of the individual or if you know that the vaccine has unnatural to the human body chemicals in it! All who deliver vaccination do not be a hired gun for Big Pharma or be a patsy for mal-law vaccination mandates; do only what is right and ethical for the patient and yourself!

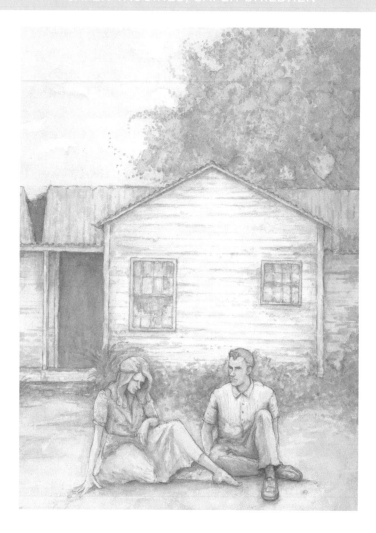

Be safe, not sorry by only injecting SAFER vaccines. The consequences of injecting an unsafe vaccine that contains unnatural to the body chemicals can be devastating.

One of the most important realization is that a child's parents must be in protective control of the child's welfare and/or health; parents must be the determiner' of what is in a child's best interest. It could never be wrong to make a general rule of law that parents are free to do what they think right for their children. Natural law dictates that parents' have the power of decision over vaccination. For government to even temporarily supersede parental authority in this area is grossly wrong; for government to permanently do so, as in the case of mandated vaccination, is most egregious and is an act of tyrannical medical enslavement. To hold that government can supersede parents' wants and/or healthcare determinations which, are determinations of what is or is not in the child's best interest, is a violation of natural law and an affliction of the natural order of things. Parents' are not a mere member of the decision team; parents are the one and the only team; when it comes to deciding what is best for children nothing should supersede parents. For government to even premise or act as if they are on the decision team is a legal misconception and is too controlling; to supersede or by-pass parents is outrageously illegal, unnatural and is evil.

Vaccination remains controversial and there is no unanimity of decision pro or con for vaccination however, for liberty to ring out loud and clear there must be no vaccination enforcement against parents' directive and/or no vaccination slavery. It is of mega-importance that parents be free to do what they consider their very best for their offspring.

Do not let lobbyists who act for special interest groups and who have ill-conceived ground worked mal-law vaccination mandates, break essential parental caring for their children and/or eliminate parental vaccination decision authority. Do not let Big Pharma dictate or have control over your children's vaccinations; taking control of your health decisions or placing your children's health in its highly incapable, greedy hands. Stay in control of your offspring's lives or life effecting decisions, always maintain the supreme authority over your children's vaccination welfare, be FREE to refuse unwanted vaccines! Determine if your child shall or shall not be injected with unnatural to the human body vaccine chemicals or any vaccination! Demand the option of a vaccine that has no unnatural to the body chemicals for consideration. Always protect and preserve decision control. Live under the 14th Amendment liberty to pursue health and/or happiness! In addition, if you cannot refuse vaccines; vaccines will tend to become even more unsafe!

Let us be very cautious about the all-important healthcare decision of vaccination. One must agree that only a person who is ignorant of the law of chemistry and lack of knowledge of human biology would use unnatural to the body chemicals in a vaccine and/or think it is good to be injected. That means those who have done so have too much control over us. If we are under this misguidance or led by ignorance it is extremely vile and outrageously wrong that it is illegal one to refuse vaccine chemical concoctions or chemicalization injections. To be doomed to suffer a vaccine chemical distortion and/or undergo chemical manipulation or be made to absorb any of the negative consequences from an enforced vaccination is an atrocity and is enslavement! Mandated vaccination is mandated child abuse; it is mandated participation as human guinea pigs in a chemical experiment, injecting unnatural to the human biology chemicals.

If vaccination was not so unconscionably profitable then vaccination would not be mandated, and vaccines would never have chemicals for profit not safety. When it comes to publicly traded companies everything is always about money or rather, what makes the most money; vaccination is no exception. Parents are smartly advised to not let money mongrel's make you vaccinate your children unless, you determine it is in your children's best interest to do so. Do not let Big-Pharma control what vaccine chemicals will infiltrate your children or rage through your children's bloodstreams to dope your children's highly susceptible brain cells. Know what chemicals are in the vaccine that is being pointed at your baby; always be absolute sure you control if it is to be or will not be injected!

The array of chemicals that children are exposed to through enforced vaccine chemical injections must stop! It is not just each molecule of mercury that needs to be removed, it is all the anti-health chemicals of vaccines that must stop being injected. Unnatural to human chemicals in vaccines is ludicrous and extremely harmful. Those who violate our offspring with such, alien to the human physiology chemicals must be stopped from doing so! It is an act of chemical warfare being waged upon our children. We need to go to war to stop it and take back the control over our children's internal being and/or welfare; resurrecting liberty of parental protection! The battle to stop mercury in vaccines has been partially won in that there is now supposedly a lot less mercury in childhood injections however, autism will continue at epidemic proportions until vaccines are totally cleaned-up; we must prompt the cleanup. GET THE CHEMICALS OUT! Concentrating on just the mercury aspect of vaccines is very revealing but again, it is all the chemicals in vaccines, which in combination, denature the internal chemistry and therefore, must be eliminated, until then, vaccines are anti-health chemical time bombs and too injurious. Between 1988 and 1992 mercury exposures from childhood vaccines more than doubled and exposure to all kinds of anti-health chemicals is markedly increasing; these chemicals interact. Parents must not be demanded or enslaved to inject chemicalizations; parents must be free to preserve their children's chemistries. The best way to prevent AUTISM is to prevent the unnatural chemicalization of children's internal systems and in order, to do so the TWO STEPS OF CORRECTION need to be implemented.

Before the marked increase of chemical exposures from the marked increase in numbers of vaccinations CHEMICALIZATION AUTISM Spectrum Disorder was uncommon; not at an epidemic proportion. The incidence of Autism began to skyrocket from a much lower frequency level of 1 in every 10,000 births in the 1980's to 1 in 500 in the late 1990's to 1 in 250 in 2000 and now to the crisis level of 1 in less than 68 and rising. Vaccines contain unnatural to the body chemicals. Toxins that cause abnormality and the increase in number of vaccinations is the cause in fact, of the autism epidemic. Statistics' do not lie; the Autism incidence increases strongly indicate that vaccine chemicals are the enemy. The very nature of vaccines and its chemicalization effects makes it the culprit.

There are some 250 types of cells and approximately 37.2 trillion cells in the human body; amazingly, they all come from but one single cell. All these cells coordinate, and this coordination is dependent upon having the right chemistry; the natural chemistry. Cellular function is completely dependent upon chemicals; natural to the body chemicals are the building blocks of health and unnatural to the body chemicals are the stumbling of health. THE EPIDEMIC WILL NOT SUBSIDE TO A MAJOR DEGREE UNTIL THE HARMFUL, ANTI-HEALTH CHEMICALS ARE NO LONGER IN VACCINES AND CONSEQUENTLY NOT INJECTED INTO CHILDREN. THE TWO STEPS of CORRECTION must be implemented to prompt SAFER vaccines and thereby, END THE AUTISM EPIDEMIC.

The purpose of vaccination is to attempt to keep your children healthy by inducing an immunological response to attenuated viruses (viruses that cause childhood disease). In doing so there are some risks just from the attenuated viruses and from the needling itself however, what is not bargained for, what is not anticipated by the vaccination recipient is unnatural to the body chemical exposure. This chemicalization was never part of the equation of risks to be taken or part of what most parents are willing to allow their children to be subjected to. There are chemicals in vaccines that are not in children's best interest they primarily are in vaccines to obtain further unconscionable profiteering; it is chemicals for profit, not safety! These chemicals for profit have no benefit for the vaccination recipient; only health detriment. In addition, there are chemicals in vaccines that are unnatural to human biology, physiology and have nothing to do with the concept and/or goal of keeping children healthy. To inject tiny babies, small infants and immature children with alien to the body chemicals is not only an experiment upon children; it is child abuse by chemicalization, a denaturing of the normal health generating chemistry that causes signs, symptoms and/or health problems. Mandating the injection of vaccine chemicals is causing chemicalization autism and has spawned the autism epidemic crisis!

Autism is mainly a brain and/or neurologically based disorder caused by chemicalization. Vaccine chemicals reach the brain fastest when breathed in or injected in; making vaccine chemicalization much more deleterious than other forms of chemical exposure. Induced brain dysfunction and/or neurological breakdown result from chemicalization; this spawns AUTISM. Vaccines are injected, pumped in by syringe, into children's delicately, sensitive blood chemistries; this chemicalization attacks the central nervous system quickly, with full chemical strength. Brain cells are chemically doped from circulating unnatural to the body vaccine chemicals; resulting in chemicalization autism.

Just as concerned parents would not want their children to be given any pain; parents do not want their children to be given any unnatural to human biology and physiology chemicals. Vaccines most not have such chemicals, GET THE CHEMICALS OUT of our children's vaccines! Parents are wise to be very cautious about vaccine CHEMICALIZATION. Vaccine chemical injections are the major causes of the Epidemic whereas, other types of chemical exposures do not so penetrate the brain to so commonly affect the masses. The erroneous mandated vaccination law sees to it that mass injections take place under rule of vaccination enslavement; enforcing children to suffer multiple chemical infiltrations. In countries that are more conscientious about not exposing children to as many vaccine chemicals the rate of Autism has not exploded into an epidemic. In cultures that do not vaccinate Autism is almost non-existent. There must be liberty to refuse chemicalization; freedom to keep children's blood natural and pure!

If you are going to consider vaccination, then at least make sure the vaccine does not have toxic chemicals otherwise, it is far safer not to risk chemicalization especially, if you want to prevent chemicalization autism. Cultures or religions that do not expose their children to vaccine CHEMICAL injections are not plagued with an AUTISM EPIDEMIC. A visit to certain large groups of people that do not embrace invasive medical intervention of vaccination such as, the Amish People, who rarely vaccinate, sheds light on the fact that chemical laden vaccinations are indeed the major cause of Autism. Populations that are vaccination compliant and/or are enslaved to vaccinate have higher rates of Autism. Upon visiting the Amish, you will be hard pressed to find a child or young adult with Autism. If you visit the Amish of Pennsylvania, you will not likely even find one child that was either diagnosed with Autism or displays objective signs of being Autistic; there is no epidemic. Injections of anti-health chemicals too often, destroy the chances of health perfection certainly, it must be up to parents to decide upon vaccination not wayward government! Vaccine chemicals absolutely cause perturbation to the normal brain or body chemistry. No one should be enforced to be experimented on as a vaccination human guinea pig!

Why not live with the freedom and/or the basic dignity afforded the Amish who are not enforced by mal-law to be vaccine chemicalized and therefore, are not plagued with Autism? Amish' rarely vaccinate and therefore, are not exposed to injected chemicalization; their children are not enforced to suffer as CHEMICALIZATION HUMAN GUINEA PIGS. It is much worse than chemical experimentation since, vaccines definitely harbor unnatural to the body or toxic to the body chemicals, it is an enforced unnatural chemicalization that is child abuse and/or mandated health degeneration. If the vaccine industry is blind to the fact that the chemicals in vaccines cause injury; it does not mean, we must suffer because of their neglect or purposeful blindness. Lobbyist's antics or special interest Big-Pharma must not shackle or handcuff us into vaccination SLAVES!

Logic, common sense and/or understanding the laws of chemistry; all tell us that children's health is placed in harm's way if unnatural to the body chemicals are injected. Children are far better off not suffering chemical injections; do not be forced to throw the chemical dice! The major cause of most diseases is exposure to chemical toxins and these chemicals have been found in vaccines. Chemicals of vaccines are not part of the needed natural chemical makeup; it is stumbling blocks of health, it is toxic! Toxic to the body chemicals cause Autism. Injected toxic vaccine chemicals quickly dose the brain tissue; doping brain cells. Injected chemical exposure is the most dangerous, it is the worst kind of toxic/chemical exposure. Do not let them subject your offspring to an unnatural to the body vaccine chemicalization or be enforced to take part in a **CHEMICAL INJECTION EXPERIMENT;** live free as parents to decide what is best for your children! Vaccination is all about big business; it is mandated because it is so profitable to do so. Many politicians hand in lobbyist versions of a Bill or those that write vaccination regulation are not your true representative but rather, are the hired guns of Big Pharma. Liberty to keep your offspring's blood clean of toxins and steer clear of Autism, is a must!

VACCINE CHEMICAL INJECTIONS BREACH THE CHEMICAL INTEGRITY OF THE BLOODSTREAM, ALTERING THE NATURAL REACTIVE ELEMENTS; RENDERING ONE SUBJECT TO AUTISM AND INDUCING A HOST OF HEALTH DETRIMENT. It is wrong that Vaccine Producers and their puppet government law makers can denature or manipulate children's internal chemistries through vaccination mandates! Parents are vested by natural law to care for their children to the best of their ability; this gives parents supreme power to decide if vaccine chemicalization is to be or not to be. Supreme law and consistency of law require that parents be free to protect children. Unwanted vaccination is a chemical assault and battery; it must be forbidden! **THE PEOPLE WANT FREEDOM FROM ENFORCED VACCINATION SLAVERY!** Chemical exposure is the enemy and vaccine chemical/toxin exposure is enemy number one; the main cause of the Autism epidemic.

America spends the most on drugs and yet we rate low in health. The idea of fighting off disease or staying healthy by taking drug or vaccine chemicals is not the wisest approach. Keeping a natural chemistry best assures good health. Having anti-health chemicals in vaccines is just ludicrous. Ingesting toxic drug/chemicals or injecting unnatural to the body vaccine chemicals is fraught with problems. The body is ultra-sensitive to chemical exposure and we really must take heed to this obvious understanding. Doris Rapp, M.D. who is Board Certified in environmental medicine, allergies and pediatrics wrote the book "Our Toxic World". In the book she continually references that practically all of man's modern-day afflictions is caused by chemical exposures. Dr. Rapp gives a good example of how sensitive the body is to even slight toxic/chemical exposure, for example: a pregnant woman who uses flea soap or a pest collar on her dog, her unborn child has a fourfold to six-fold increased chance of developing a brain tumor, leukemia, or lymphoma by the age of six years. One can hardly imagine the magnitude of health damage from injected alien to the body vaccine chemicals. Parents need to be on the alert to **PREVENT CHEMICALIZATION.** Lack of vitamins or minerals, spinal distortion and poor genetics, all cause ill-health however; chemicalization is a more common cause and vaccination is the primary cause of autism.

Those who profit from vaccine sales agenda is to keep us enslaved to vaccinate by inducing **VACCINATION SLAVERY** mandates. Vaccination needs to be strictly voluntary, based upon informed consent/ **DENIAL** in order, for there to be freedom and prompt **SAFER** vaccines. People have an urgent need and fundamental Right to live naturally, free from involuntarily pierced by needle and pumped with vaccine **CHEMICALS**. Children need and deserve the full protection of their parents and **PARENTS MUST BE FREE TO SECURE THEIR CHILDREN'S SAFETY**. When parents deem vaccine injections unsafe, the unwanted vaccine must not be injected. You are born free to decide upon you and your children's healthcare. You must not be criticized or mistreated for your personal vaccination decision and your health decision and/or vaccination status must remain private unless you dictate otherwise. There must be unfettered liberty to live by your private health decisions and/or life choices and not have your right to privacy violated. People of each State need to act to **ABOLISH VACCINATION SLAVERY**; allow liberty of health decision!

According to the CDC, as of March 27, 2014, one in 68 U.S. children has an Autism spectrum disorder, with 1 in 42 boys' and 1 in 189 girls' have autism spectrum disorder (ASD). Look to the chemicals that are being injected as the main cause. The statistical fact that the general population of children within the United States have an off the chart much higher rate of Autism when compared to the Amish community's much lower rate of Autism is revealing; it is the **SMOKING GUN** of causation. The vaccination compared to non-vaccination aftermath is evidence that the vaccine **SHOTS** are indeed the major material cause of Autism. More revealing is the fact of what unnatural or alien to the human biology and physiology chemicals are in vaccines; you cannot expect to remain healthy or autism free if these chemicals are injected to dope the brain cells. Furthermore, among the Middlefield, Ohio Amish, Dr. Heng Weng, the medical director, at the DDC Clinic for Special Needs Children, reported that the Autism rate was only 1 in 1,500. Children of Christian Scientists or Chiropractor's families etc. are not plagued with high numbers of Autism; revealing much lower rates of Autism for those children not exposed to the barrage of vaccine chemicals. Chemically laced vaccines are the problem! Parents do not have to be hit by an oncoming train to know when to get children out of harm's way. Parents do not require absolute proof one way or the other in order, to decide to protect. Parents' require being given the information and that **PARENTS BE FREE TO DECIDE WHAT COURSE OF ACTION IS BEST**, these are after all; parents' children and parents live with the aftermath of the vaccination decision. Be not **ENSLAVED** to vaccinate; **BE FREE!**

You are not free if an unjust mal-law enforces you to submit your children for unwanted vaccine chemicalization. It is inhumane for children to be used as guinea pigs in a mass chemicalization experiment! More and more parents and doctors are convinced vaccine chemicalization are presently too dangerous to inject. Some doctors choose to either not vaccinate their own children or do not vaccinate according to the recommended schedule; they do not want the chemical exposure. Doctors are reporting that children not vaccinated are healthier; with no Autism, as compared to children vaccinated. Autism escalates as the number of vaccinations and/or the number of chemicalization increases. The rate is now 1 in 68 chances of Autism and that signals parents to protect their offspring from vaccine chemicalization; it shakes sense into them or hits them like a bolt of lightning to do so. According to my analysis, the Autism rate of the fully vaccination compliant is alarmingly, even higher, than the epidemic general population rate. However, parents do not need statistics to recognize they need to protect their children from vaccine chemicalization; all they need is basic understanding of chemistry and/or that chemicals impact human biology and/or physiology. Medical and natural healthcare doctors agree that the least exposure to unnatural, alien, toxic to the body chemicals the better we are all off. Anti-health chemicals in vaccines is wrong but yet it exists because it makes more money to do so, vaccination is mandated, and we cannot seek damages against vaccine producers for doing so when its vaccine chemicals cause injury. Doctors' agree, the decision to vaccinate must rest with the parents of the child!

The public is strongly urged to recognize the pertinent fact that unnatural, alien, toxic to the body chemicals in vaccines are a plight on children; when injected they are the major etiology of Autism. Almost all doctors interviewed agreed that there should be no enforced preventative healthcare; there must be self-dominion over healthcare. Vaccinations must not be mandated or enforced upon the public and no healthcare should monopolize the healthcare field as does, mandated vaccinations. Refusal, of unwanted or conceived of as too dangerous to inject vaccination, must be the rule. Children are not in better hands or more capable hands when government decides what healthcare is best; parents must decide children's vaccination future! In general, children are far better off with parents being their protectors and making the decision to vaccinate or not vaccinate. Vaccine Producers or their puppet vaccination mandate must no longer dictate healthcare! Children are being experimented on, used as chemical guinea pigs. There is design to inject children without parent's permission or knowledge. Do protect your children!

Religious like belief or trust in vaccination or that vaccines are safe is wrong. To blindly trust those whom make profit from vaccine sales has helped allow the poor safety state of vaccines to come into existence and placed children's lives in grave danger of chemicalization autism. Parents must always be legally enabled and/or empowered to refuse all preventative healthcare; this assures children's protection from unwanted or conceived of as too dangerous medical intervention and keeps the formulation of vaccines to a safety standard that parents will be much more likely to approve of for injection. Taking away parental refusal takes away perhaps the single most safety promoting prompter that needs to always be in place and instead, leaves children's safety strictly in the money crazed incapable hands of non-parental Big-Pharma. The unconscionable liability shield that was carved out for Big-Pharma makes vaccines less safe, allowing chemicals for profit and nor safety in vaccines; no longer should there be this shield. Parents must be completely free to seek damages from producers of vaccines that injure. Do know what chemicals are in vaccines or have been used in its production and always be in control. Never blindly trust that vaccines are safe to inject! When it comes to anything that enters or is injected into your tiny baby, small infant or immature child be safe not sorry; make absolutely, sure your offspring are not being violated!

Sometimes the slightest mistake can have dire consequences and almost always gross negligent mistakes have horrific results. The fact that vaccines have been found to have unnatural to the human body chemicals is not a slight mistake; it can be considered either, gross negligence or criminal in nature especially, since, vaccine producers willfully and/or knowingly utilized such, chemicals. Parents that would purposefully expose their children to some of the chemicals that have been found in vaccines would be accused of child abuse; vaccine producers should at least be held to the same standard. Taking the mal-legal restraints unfairly placed upon parents of not being free to refuse vaccination or not being enabled to protect children from what parents know as too dangerous to inject vaccines or being legally disabled from preventing what parents determine is an actual threat to the welfare of their children into consideration; we must take it as a most egregious offence that unnatural to the body chemicals are in vaccines. It is a violation of severest magnitude! Therefore, we must apply the severest restraints upon what is allowed in vaccines and the heaviest hand of the law to the perpetrators of this chemicalization orchestrated offence. Runaway chemicalization by vaccination must end!

Hold those who dare put unnatural to the body chemicals in vaccines accountable and liable. Punish the willful and knowingly utilization of such, chemicals in vaccines; assign punitive monetary damages for those injured and prison sentences for those guilty of the offense. Any degree for the doping of cells of our offspring to any degree including all important brain cells with such, chemicals most be dealt with extremely, harshly. Vaccine producers not only showed and still show great carelessness in allowing unnatural to the body chemicals in vaccines but rather, it can be considered being engaged in gross negligence for willfully and knowingly doing so. There is strong evidence that vaccine manufacturers possess criminal intent to impute mens-rea for using unnatural to the body chemicals in vaccines or causing children harm and/or a wanton disregard for securing the chemical welfare of vaccine recipients. To impact children's lives with unnatural to the body chemicals is at minimum experimentation upon those injected by chemical reaction uncertainty however, to do so causes injury by abnormal to the body chemical reaction certainty! They have breached the trust we placed in them! Be free not to be experimented on and have liberty to choose not to suffer chemicalization!

Parents liberty to make life's major decisions for their children especially, those that have the most impact upon their children's lives such as, vaccination is paramount. This essential freedom of decision must be without government interference, direction or issue. It must be required by law to obtain parent's TRUE INFORMED CONSENT before giving vaccinations. Freedom in healthcare assures quality of healthcare and optimum health. Parents must not merely bemoan the fact that their children are by erroneous law being made to endure unwanted vaccine chemical injections; parents need to demand their Rights and be advocates of the TWO STEPS OF CORRECTION. Your children are yours to have, hold and protect! Parents must be free to follow their own path of decision. Droves of parents are crying out, screaming out, that their children's health disintegrated after vaccine chemicalization. Parents' witnessing children's health annihilation proximate to being vaccinated is more relevant, more revealing and more precise of an account of the truth than what profit based corporate Vaccine Producers attest to, falsify or purposefully cover-up. The burden of proof must be upon vaccine advocates to show vaccines are not harmful; with what chemicals are in vaccines it is presently impossible!

Certainly, we want to do as much as possible to deal with viruses and other pathogens however, let us not poison our children in the process. Vaccine chemicalization is a greater threat! An unnatural to the body chemicalization is a poisoning, toxic chemical exposure or manipulation of the normal chemistry. Assure that your offspring are not being subjected to unnatural to human biology or physiology chemistry and/or molecules or compounds that are alien to the body's natural, homogeneous or normal chemistry! Do not give your children up for enforced vaccination slavery or be made to suffer unwanted chemical infiltration. Take a stand as protective parents; do not bow under the pressure of the over burdensome, callous and inequitable command to inject your children with chemicals that you determine are too unhealthy to be injected or are not convinced the vaccine chemicalization is safe! Parents priority in life is to protect their children to the best of their ability. You must be free to protect your children from vaccine chemicals!

Do not succumb to mal-law mandates that enforce suffering your offspring with unwanted injection or needling which, infiltrate children with chemicals that have nothing good for human biology or physiology; it is inconsistent with the goal of being healthy and free. Mandated vaccination slavery has rendered vaccines not safe! Be a hero to your children, protect them from chemical injury; step in to do everything you can to prevent them from being a statistic of unnatural to the body chemical infiltration and becoming another unfortunate statistic of the autism epidemic. Do not be a victim of chemicalization autism! It is ridiculous and grossly wrong that parents are prevented from being protective parents by a mal-law vaccination mandate which, only really serves to secure money interest of Big-Pharma. In making your vaccination decision remember, if vaccines were not mandated they would not be as chemically dangerous and the main reason vaccines are mandated is for profiteering. Protect children from chemicalization!

Yes, it is very important to have the vaccination option to assure health. However, it is vastly important to not jam it down our throats or rather, inject it into our cells unless we agree to the vaccine chemicalization. It is also, imperative that if are to consider it for injection or penetration into our brain cells or any cell that it not be harmful or have chemicals in it that are unnatural to the body! We the People must no longer be enforced by vaccination mandates to surrender our children to endure, suffer or have mandated vaccinations! Yes, I want vaccines to be available for myself or offspring but in no way should I be enslaved and/or commanded to do so especially, if it is against one's free will and/or judgement. Right, wrong or indifferent it must be so that vaccination must not be mandated otherwise, all is lost; our freedom to not be violated, our liberty to decide what is best for oneself or child and the self-control or self-governing of one's vital health is lost, it is grossly violated and is unconstitutionally taken.

Bacteria, viruses and/or bugs that are virtually ubiquitous can exist in children without harm and yet destroy health in others. The reason for disease is not the mere presence of bugs but rather, the lowering of one's resistance and/or the deviation from one's optimum health chemistry. The best way to combat health demise is to keep one's resistance at optimum level by securing one's internal natural chemistry. To infiltrate a tiny baby, small infant or immature child with unnatural to the human body chemicals upsets and distorts the needed natural chemistry required for health perfection and thereby, sets in motion the spawning of autism. Parents by natural law and supreme parental authority must be free to protect their children's naturally perfected chemistry of health and not be coerced and/or forced by mal-law to manipulate or imperfect the vital to health chemistry! Fundamental to liberty and parenting; there must be power to protect!

People must be free to naturally bolster their immune system and/or resistance against opportunistic pathogens and pursue health resilience without being enforced to inject vaccine chemicals; this healthcare liberty is perhaps our most basic and essential freedom! Chemical infiltration is the root of most health problems and/or health degeneration; and being exposed to the chemicals of vaccines which, are injected directly into children, is the main etiology of Autism. For the most part, the Autism epidemic is due to the anti-health chemicals within vaccines that should not be in vaccines. We must GET THE CHEMICALS OUT of vaccines before we even consider its injection! Chemically induced Autism will begin to subside by implementing the TWO STEPS OF CORRECTION. CLEAN-UP VACCINES by giving people the power of choice or freedom of decision not to be vaccinated and rationally punish makers of vaccines that are injurious and/or contain unnatural to the body chemicals with possible criminal charges and litigation for damages.

Parents' for the sake of their children's health need liberty to REFUSE UNWANTED TAINTED VACCINE CHEMICALIZATION! How long the deception goes on about enforced vaccination depends upon how long it takes to become aware of the deception or that the chemicals that we inject that are unnatural to human biology are harmful. The chemicals that we ignorantly inject into tiny babies that are alien to the natural and/or normal blood chemistry create abnormal chemical reactions and of course negatively impact the brain and/or the body. This understanding or negative to health truth is all parents' really need to know to step up to protect children from unnatural chemicalization! To have unnatural to the body chemicals in vaccines is an affliction upon the welfare of children and is a greater threat than the threat of what vaccines are designed for. To enforce or mandate vaccine chemical injection is an atrocity, an affliction upon good health, is child abuse and is a gravest violation upon our rights and body.

Freedom in healthcare is essential to assure the most beneficial healthcare and that it is safe. All healthcare; must be voluntary and predominate solely based upon consumer satisfaction. Healthcare, including vaccinations, must never be enforced upon the public by a mal-legal mandate. There must be no medical intervention enslavement; no command to submit to another's healthcare viewpoint or be subjected to any tyrannical medical intervention. The People must be free to choose what is best for their individual healthcare needs and not be chemically experimented on human guinea pigs. Parents for the sake of their children best interest must be enabled to enjoy their liberty to choose what if any healthcare shall or shall not be administered and if desired, choose the less traveled healthcare path. It is the natural order that parents' control their offspring's healthcare destiny and that parents can decide upon vaccination. Yes, doctors or government can educate, advise or even lightly remonstrate with parents about the pros and cons of vaccination or other healthcare however, the decision must be parents!

Many healthcare experts are now advocating to only NATURALLY bolster children's health and resistance to childhood diseases; citizens who determine this is the best for health must be free to do so and not be condemned or whipped with legal action for doing so! As

FREE American parents, we require this basic LIBERTY OF HEALTHCARE CHOICES and LIBERTY TO SELF-DIRECT CHILDREN'S VACCINATIONS! No one should overpower or limit one's personal or parental healthcare decisions. To be enforced to not live under your own health decisions or to be commanded to be standardized under another's health standard or healthcare decisions is HEALTHCARE SLAVERY! Government must assure that over reaching or overzealous medical intervention does not tread upon parental rights and/or our freedom of health decision. Health and healing come from within and our chemistries are vital to healing. Parents must be free to determine if vaccine chemicalization is too great of a threat and be completely free to protect their children accordingly! Be empowered with healthcare choice; do not be enslaved!

If someone aspires to do better or live differently or strive to live a chemical free and/or healthier lifestyle they must have the liberty to do so; if someone wants their children to not be exposed to vaccine CHEMICAL injections, they must have this most essential liberty to do so. We must not stand for mal-law or mal-government interfering, limiting or superseding one's healthcare prerogatives or choices. People who are free can exercise the way they want to live, eat the way they choose and determine for themselves to accept or deny any healthcare; this means postpone vaccination, limit vaccine chemical exposures or opt not to face the dangers of vaccinations. People must be free to eliminate or prevent disease the way they individually think is best. People need the basic ability to mitigate what they want, limit what they want, eliminate what they want and introduce what they think is in their best health interest. Government or rather, lobbyists must not set the criteria for our healthcare or command it especially, in non-emergency situations, nor should it enforce any preventative medical intervention such as, vaccine CHEMICAL injections. At most, government can highly recommend or make it financially possible to be vaccinated. Government must not cross the line by enforcing vaccinations. We must be free to SELF-DETERMINE OUR VERY OWN AND THAT OF OUR CHILDREN'S HEALTHCARE; this includes vaccination. People have a Right to make health choices; to determine if vaccination is or is not in their best interest. Be an advocate of natural living!

We need the option of vaccination to be as safe as possible and in order to achieve safety we have to make sure vaccination recipients are not exposed to unnatural to their body chemicals. Assure health by not injecting anti-health, toxic chemicals into children's bloodstreams. Pursue optimum chemical biological coherence and you assure health! The building blocks of health are the chemical flora that the body utilizes in order, to produce optimum health whereas, the stumbling blocks of health are unnatural to the body chemicals. Do not have chemicals in vaccines which, produce abnormality and/or abnormal reactions. Vaccines have chemical stumbling blocks of health that will no longer be in vaccines after the TWO STEPS OF CORRECTION! Assure your child's vaccine safety! Do not make the tragic mistake of leaving vaccine safety strictly up to others or be subdued to inject what you have discovered as unsafe vaccines; be in control!

Be free to pursue less invasive healthcare and not be enslaved to vaccinate with unwanted vaccines or chemicalizations. Excellent nutrition, intelligently designed vitamins and mineral supplements, disease preventative sanitation, drinking and bathing, clean water, regular exercise, opening the body's pores to perspire profusely to rid the body of toxins, utilizing natural herbs and remedies, acupuncture, regular chiropractic adjustments are just some of the pillars of health that are of great value in securing health preventing Autism or recovering from Autism. Adequate, clean hydration is a pillar of health worth highlighting; dehydration causes widespread major health problems and is a primary cause of numerous health problems including, stroke; so always stay properly hydrated. It is best that the People have the liberty to decide for themselves what healthcare is best. Parents' protect your children from receiving a vaccine injection which, you determine can lead to autism or increase the chances of autism or cause any harm whatsoever. Medical tyranny or vaccination ENSLAVEMENT is a crime not to be tolerated!

Mandated vaccination law is the epitome of over governing our lives! Free minded Americans' do not want to be told what medical intervention they must have or be told they have no choice in the matter as is the unfortunate case of the mal-law vaccination mandate. Parents must not be forced or coerced to sacrifice their children to unwanted medical intervention or throw the dice of unnatural chemicalization especially, if it might turn up Autism. No one should be enslaved to face post vaccination health uncertainty! No free person can be made to suffer as a human guinea pig experimental subject! Free people are in control of their health destiny and/or self-regulate what healthcare will or will not be administered! Parents must not be placed in a quagmire as they attempt to best protect children; they must have unfettered liberty to decide if vaccination is or is not in their children's best interest. The mandated vaccination law creates a quandary for parents who do not want the risk of exposing their children to chemical injections but want to obey the law even if it is mal-law; their paternal obligation conflicts with the burden of vaccination submission in order, to be law abiding citizens. Mandated vaccination place parents in an untenable position, law that is equitable or just does not!

Doing what parents think best for children's welfare must always supersede fulfilling wayward legal vaccination requirement. Parents finding themselves in this dilemma should not be deterred; always do what is best for your children! Parent's primary concern is to protect their children to the best of their ability and manmade mal-law must never interfere with this parental obligation, responsibility and/or instinct. There must be no prejudice or legal consequence for not being vaccinated or for not submitting children for injections. Parental integrity, efficiency and effectiveness are reliant upon being free to make children's healthcare and/or life decisions; without stumbling blocks or government input. Chemical excellence is needed to be healthy and parents' priority is to assure it! See to it that your offspring's internal chemical homeostasis is well maintained!

According to Dr. Mayer Eisenstein, Homefirst's medical director and 1973 founder said "We have about 30,000 or 35,000 children that we've taken care of over the years, and I don't think we have a single case of autism in children delivered by us who never received vaccines." These doctors are in the know; their vital statistics of frequency of autism as compared to non- vaccination status point to what is causing the autism epidemic. Homefirst' has five offices in the Chicago area and six doctors. This doctor (director) report of lack of autism should alert parents that enforced chemicalization is the main cause of Autism; mandated vaccination law is a dangerously, injurious mal-law. More professionals and parents are realizing that when children receive chemically laced vaccines Autism is a much more likely event and when no vaccines are injected Autism is a highly unlikely event! It does not take a rocket scientist to realize that the chemicals found in vaccines are a sure recipe for disaster. Informed consent/DENIAL needs to protect us; any mortal, when they are informed of what chemicals are in vaccines can determine if the vaccine is or is not in their children's best interest. Unbiased, honest, loving parents best protect children; parents must control. Parents have no conflict of interest in their assessments whereas; those that make money, have jobs or benefit from VACCINATION ENSLAVEMENT do. No unnatural to human biology chemical exposure equals NO AUTISM EPIDEMIC!

It is in children's best interest to GET THE CHEMICALS OUT OF VACCINES. The chemicals in the drugs prescribed and, in the vaccines, injected perpetuate problems. CHEMICALIZATION of young children has no positives; only negatives. Healing comes from within and chemistry is vital to healing; so, keep a near normal chemistry! Informed consent and/or informed DENIAL of vaccinations will best prompt getting the CHEMICALS OUT of vaccines. In addition, holding Vaccine Producers legally liable for vaccine induced injuries will promote SAFER vaccines. Instead, of inexplicably allowing producers of harmful chemically laced vaccines to escape all responsibility, accountability and/or liability we should put their feet to the fire of quality control reasonable standards; this will prompt the removal of toxic to the body CHEMICALS. There is no health benefit for having unnatural to the body chemicals in vaccines; only health detriment. Our trust has been breached; we need to take affirmative action by never allowing such chemical folly.

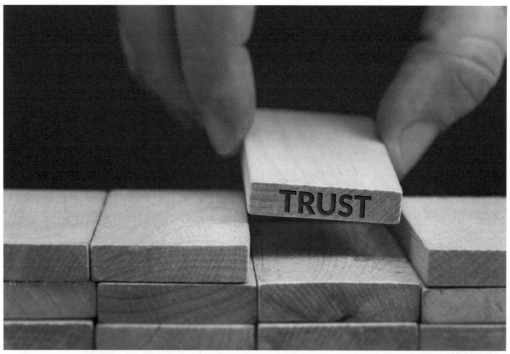

We need SAFER vaccines that we can trust in. Build trust by making sure vaccines do not chemically compromise; do it, one vaccine at a time.

You hope and pray that your children are safe; because vaccines are money making it too often dictates that chemicals for profit and not safety are in vaccines. Misplaced trust that vaccines for profit are safe jeopardizes the health and life of your offspring. Unwanted vaccine CHEMICAL injection administration is a violation that the law should protect

against instead of promoting or enforcing. Children must be secure in the protection of their parents. When a child's parent decides that a vaccine is unwanted and/or too dangerous to inject; the protective parental decision must be respected and be controlling. Government must recognize this universal rule and not allow a profit based pharmaceutical industry to dictate to free thinking Americans. The People require the fundamental freedom of caring for their children without government interference; people do not want to be violated by unwanted medical intervention. Mandated vaccination laws are wholly inconsistent with this most basic freedom and desire. Parental liberty to protect children is the freedom to reject unwanted vaccine CHEMICALIZATION injection. Do not allow your children to be part of a vaccine chemicalization experiment; keep them safe!

The only thing needed for the mal-law mandate to continue or for vaccines to remain polluted with chemicals or for the triumph of evil, is for good people and/or mothers and fathers to do nothing. The decent people of our society need to stand up for parent's Right of protection of children and for what is in the best interest of children. The **TWO STEPS OF CORRECTION** is our children's salvation and ours as well. Vaccination slavery must be abolished; we must take rightful control of the vaccination decision, be liberated to follow one's very own decision **to be or not to be vaccinated**. Vaccine Producers' must be litigated against for placing harmful chemicals in vaccines that can and do injure; liberty to seek damages is a needed safety prompter.

Parents must be free to address the court system to seek damages and to seek an injunction to stop the use of anti-health chemicals in vaccines. The long arm of the Drug Company and monster monetary influence must not abate or divest parents Right to protect their children or derail the proper seeking of compensation from Vaccine Producers for vaccine induced injuries. The system has been manipulated to the point that meritorious lawsuits against vaccine makers cannot be heard in a Civil Court. We live under martial law to have children vaccinated and yet cannot bring equitable litigation for injury from enforced vaccination. Corruption and the best interest of Vaccine mega-profits have inappropriately been secured instead, of our children's health safety. **Take the profit out of negligent vaccine production and actually make it cost prohibitive and vaccines will become safer**! Parents, who cannot stop vaccination are reduced to being hollow parents and are ENSLAVED **to vaccinate**.

Under the cloak of darkness, in the midnight hour, buried deep within the pages of the Homeland Security Act, they conspired that the Vaccine Compensation Bill be included as a Rider to the Homeland Security Bill. Wrongfully, it made it that our tax payers' dollars are used instead of properly expending vaccine manufacturers' dollars to cover all the injuries caused by vaccine chemicalization. In appropriately, it protects producers of vaccines that cause the all these injuries and perpetuates runaway negligent vaccine production. The result of the Bill is as if a dagger has gone ever deeper into to the heart of children's safety and blocks parent's from seeking compensation from the entity that induced the injury. Nothing happens to vaccine producers when children are injured by bad vaccine chemicals or vaccine production negligence. In addition, it is extremely unjust and makes a mockery of our law-making system to secretly attach a Rider to a Bill in the midnight hour or late in the evening, the day before the vote. It mocks the procedural process and reeks of impropriety in that the last-minute attachment could not be scrutinized or properly analyzed and does in fact, result in Representatives not even looking at or consider it for its' merit. Most of the law enactors did not even know that it was part of the long and lengthy Bill.

Proper law making requires that a proposed Bill be properly analyzed, scrutinized and mulled over to assure its contents are understood and that the law is beneficial for the People; only then can it be considered for enactment. To do otherwise is a sham, a mockery of justice and is underhanded; it is un-American and places children's welfare in jeopardy.

Homeland security has nothing to do with vaccine producers having a liability shield. A law that is voted on and passed (the last-minute Rider) without the enacting voters' being given time to adequately decipher the Rider's contents is really lawlessness or unjust law and considered not to be law; non lex injusta non- ex lex (a law that is unjust is not law). The Vaccine Producer's liability shield was snuck in the Homeland Security Bill without congressional consideration; it violates **DUE PROCESS.** It also violates Due Process Right of those claiming injury from vaccines. Parents for their children are unjustly and completely blocked from litigating or having a jury decide if Vaccine Producers are responsible for their children's injuries; this severely limits one from obtaining justice. This unprecedented protection of Vaccine Producers allows these multi-billion revenue companies undeserved financial security; no liability for vaccine production negligence. **There must be justice** and enough punishment to **DETER negligence**. In the best interest of children; producers of injurious vaccines must be held accountable and liable. In fact, those who put unnatural to the human chemicals in vaccines should be made to pay treble damages in order, to stop continual utilization of such, chemicals and/or negligence! This type of chemicalization not only is an experiment on the recipient; it causes injury.

Frist, a Senator from Tennessee, drafted the Vaccine Compensation Bill but, **it did not pass**. An ill-conceived plan was devised to get the failed Vaccine Producer's liability shield passed under the radar. It was incorporated into the enormous Homeland Security Bill to go unnoticed. Homeland Security has nothing to do with protecting Vaccine Producers from liability and yet; it was included in the Homeland Security Bill with almost the identical language of the Bill that was voted down. They knew politicians would only keep their eyes or concentrate on the big ball (Homeland Security) and not scrutinize the fuzz on the ball (the Vaccine Compensation Bill) especially, if it were to be stealthily put in as a mere Rider, purposefully not drawing any special attention to it or its inclusion and done at the very last minute; just before the vote. In this way, the extra baggage Rider (liability shield) became mal-law. Falsely, under the call to secure America they conspired to secure the profits for Vaccine Producers; **compromising child safety. First, vaccine producers have breached the public trust by allowing unnatural to the body chemicals in vaccines and second, they and their puppet politicians have breached the public trust for wrongfully protecting vaccine makers at the expense or detriment of the public when vaccines cause injury and the public is totally blocked from litigating against vaccine producers that orchestrated or caused the vaccine induced injury. This denaturing of children's internal chemistry and travesty of injustice by not bringing negligent vaccine production to bear the full brunt of negligence law must be stopped and be corrected!**

The verbiage in the Homeland Bill and/or the effect of the added Vaccine Compensation Bill destroyed parent's Right to litigate against Vaccine Producers for vaccine induced injuries such as, mercury poisoning and/or Autism. **However, it is all of the anti-health chemicals that are still in vaccines that is still the main etiology of Autism that need to be removed. ALERT, the language in the Bill is specific just for mercury thus, lawsuits against Vaccine Producers for other chemicals might be viable.** The language of the Homeland Security Bill can be

narrowly construed thereby, limiting the liability shield to only those injuries induced from vaccine mercury exposure. **They left the door wide open for litigation over the rest of the anti-health chemicals in vaccines that cause injury and/or Autism; so, if you litigate it will cause the removal of these chemicals! THE TWO STEPS OF CORRECTION WILL GET THE CHEMICALS OUT!** Children are used as **chemicalization guinea pigs! The affliction upon the People due to enforced vaccine chemical injections will be lifted through the TWO STEPS.**

Bill Frist weakly defended the inclusion of the Vaccine Anti-Liability Rider, "The threat of liability should not become a barrier to the protection of the American people." This Frist' statement is nonsensical in that, honest lawsuits surrounding unsafe mercury chemicals or other anti-health chemicals can only work to protect people from future injury whereas, granting Vaccine Producers a liability shield from all CHILDHOOD disease vaccine related injuries only works to allow and promote negligence. The cloak is seen here since, anthrax or smallpox vaccines (vaccines against bioterrorism that protect Americans) have absolutely no mercury and have nothing to do with all the childhood vaccines that do cause injury. There is no realistic safety purpose for including the Anti-Liability Rider which, wrongly protects villains of negligence. It was slipped into the Homeland Security Bill, at the last minute, in a cloak of darkness, in the midnight hour. Reportedly, most **Congressmen were not even aware of its last-minute inclusion when they voted YES** in the heated rush to enact the cumbersome but needed Homeland Security Bill.

It appears that the extent of assuring Drug Company profiteering and wrongfully protecting Vaccine Producers from lawsuits has no limits and is pervasive at all levels. The Vaccine Producers will stop at nothing in assuring their **profiteering. Vaccine/Drug companies consistently make the most money or are among the top money-making businesses, so it is commensurate that they not only pay for their negligence but rather, be made to pay treble damages for it; they certainly can afford to defend or pay for their negligent production of vaccines. Whereas, parents having to foot the costs associated due to vaccine production negligence and/or their child being vaccine injured and/or becoming Autistic can devastate a family both financially and emotionally. It is most equitable, and justice is best served if Vaccine Producers are held accountable and liable; they must NOT be granted a negligence promoting liability shield. Best protect children not Drug Makers!**

The Vaccine Producers and their puppet advocates secured the liability shield in a Federal Statute thereby, overpowering State law. This unprecedented one sided mal-law protection allows drug companies to know there will be no reprisal for their hand in causing the Autism epidemic. It is unbelievable, Big-Pharma now thinks they can put whatever chemicals they want in vaccines and they are protected by this mal-law liability shield. In fact, the Autism epidemic will only make them even more profits from selling drugs that will supposedly combat those stricken with Autism. This allows those who are accused of creating the Autism epidemic to profit from their negligence; a self-created market that will fill their bottomless profiteering bag. One can conclude since, they are certainly, aware of the chemicals they put in vaccines that they have purposely causing health demise, created health problems and have intent to profit from their created Autism epidemic. They have no economic reason to end chemicalization Autism or stop using harmful chemicals in vaccines; they will continue distribution of chemical vaccines as long as it is profitable and

there is no recourse. Parents must be free to seek to prove that the AUTISM PLAGUE upon children IS MAINLY CAUSED BY VACCINE CHEMICALIZATION.

Those who seek to not only continue to profit from the inequitable fact that vaccination is mandated but now also by the restrictions of the mal-law of the Vaccine Compensation Bill unjustly, makes vaccine producers impervious to any economic loss from injury directly related to vaccination. This has taken the major weapon of litigation or negligence law from parents whose children suffer vaccine induced injury; leaving children naked with no parental recourse against being victimized and/or injured by vaccine chemicalization. Yes, parents should be allowed to prove in a valid civil court of law that their children were injured by vaccine injections. If all pointers are pointing in the same direction of fault and/or culpability, if vaccines are shown to be the cause in fact, of Autism; then it can be proven in a court of law that Vaccines Producers created the Autism epidemic. Loss of freedom to litigate is loss of ability to stop the autism epidemic!

In addition, since the Autism epidemic is well underway it opens an entirely new market era of drug profiting, a new built–in market to sell drugs for an autism epidemic that was mainly caused by Big-Pharma's chemicalization of tiny babies, little infants and small children. Autism increasing to epidemic levels is only a positive for the profiteering vaccine/drug cartel. Mandated vaccine drug sales are the main etiology of Autism and now it has created the need for new types of drugs and its usage which, surge because of the epidemic. Mandated vaccination that causes Autism and the new market of drugs to treat autism is a win-win situation for Vaccine/Drug Producers. Drug syndicate profit by the law mandating vaccinations as it enforces the public to be vaccine chemicalized and they are rewarded for this negligence; they have spawned a built-in market, a win-fall of profit from the new generation of drugs sold to treat Autism. They profit from the epidemic it created!

Parents whose children have become Autistic after vaccination must be allowed to try to prove in a valid Civil court of law that the cause in fact of the Autism was the chemical vaccine injection or that the Vaccine/drug syndicate knew and/or know that the chemicals in their vaccines are injurious. Vaccine Producers and/or drug/vaccine makers will have major additional profits obtained from the treatment of vaccine induced Autism sufferers. They have spawned the need for a new drug market. Billions will be made in additional profits obtained from the treatment of vaccine induced Autism sufferers. The vaccine industry considers it bad business to make the Autism epidemic go away; if the Autism epidemic thrives they can treat the Autism masses with their new breed of profit making drugs which, will generate billions. They have the opposite of strong stimuli to end the Autism epidemic; distributing unclean vaccines perpetuates AUTISM and profiteering. Lobbyists have achieved the unconscionable inclusion of the Vaccine Compensation Bill stealthily in the body of the Homeland Security Act in order, to self-serve Drug Makers. The American people are tired of a rigged system; one that places money before safety. Children will continue to be chemically experimented upon and chemically compromised; the autism epidemic will continue until CORRUPTION is ended and vaccines come CLEAN!

Just as the Vaccine Producers lobbied for mandated vaccinations and for their liability protection the Vaccine Producers will also attempt to have their new Autism drugs sales

guaranteed. There antics will not stop; Vaccine Producers will soon lobby to have government pay for their new generation of Autism palliative drugs to assure prices will be high and that their self-generated need for Autism drugs are distributed and/or definitely paid for. The merry go round of vaccine/drug taking and its harmful chemical doping of children's brain cells will escalate. More and more drug dependence will occur and spiral further and further out of control unless, parents take command of the situation and their children's healthcare destiny. Ending the Autism epidemic requires abolishing vaccination slavery chemicalization. The way to end the Autism epidemic is the implementation of the TWO STEPS OF CORRECTION. Children are being chemicalized; safeguard them from it!

One might think **Frist is bent on stopping parents' ability to seek justice from the actual source of their child's injuries** and/or **not** make Vaccine Producers pay for their negligent act of causing injury and/or Autism. While Bill Frist was running for office the National Republican Senatorial Campaign Committee received $226,000 from you know who. In addition, Eli Lilly was strangely compelled to buy **five thousand copies** of an illiterate book of Frist's. Full price was paid for these costly books; there was no normal bulk discount given and they probably were not even read. You might conclude all this as an inducement or an unjust reward or some might say a **pay-off for the inclusion of the voted down Vaccine Producers protection Bill** sneaked into the Homeland Security Bill. One can begin to paint the real picture of why and how this failed Children's Anti-Safety Rider became mal-law under the cloak of Homeland security.

Vaccine chemicals distort the natural chemical homeostasis; unnatural to the body or alien to the body or foreign to the body and/or **TOXIC to the body chemicals must not be in vaccines.** Furthermore, the CEO of Eli Lilly was sitting on the Homeland Security Advisory Committee and although, the existence of this obvious conflict of interest Eli-Lilly was perfectly positioned to **influence the inclusion** and enactment of the ill-Rider and thereby, self-served in protecting Eli Lilly. This in combination with the Frist agenda and folly sealed the fate of parent's attempt to protect their children and prevent parents from justly seeking justice for their children's vaccine induced injuries. Safety of our children and/or vaccine safety were dealt a lethal blow when the **Rider was snuck in** under major conflict of interest.

This sick folly does not secure our children from harm; quite the opposite, it places our children in grave danger. It promotes vaccine chemicals for profit instead, of children's safety. It allows injection source injury (chemicalization) to continue unchecked and leaves parents without legal recourse when their children are injured from vaccines and/or from Vaccine Producers negligence. **How in justice's name can the People be expected to just sit back or be complacent with vaccine injection SLAVERY or under any enforced healthcare? Parents need to demand the TWO STEPS OF COREECTION in order, to best protect their children. The spoils of political contribution and/or lobby tactics promote improper law making; it must be forbidden or stamped out for America's best interest and survival.** Drug Companies have been intimately involved with major GOP fund-raisers to assure Children are enslaved to suffer its profitable vaccine chemical injections. **All medical intervention should be at the discretion of the People. Stop enforced chemicalization and you prevent autism. Right what is so very wrong. Stop chemical experimentation and chemicalization autism!**

How pervasive and/or high up are the chains of connections that keep children enslaved to be vaccinated and unfairly protect producers of vaccines from rightful lawsuits? President Bush and Eli Lilly, the developer of Thimerosal the mercury-based preservative used in vaccines, have very close ties; Bush sat on the Lilly board. Lilly's former chairman and chief executive, Sidney Taurel was appointed by President Bush to serve on a presidential council. Eli Lilly's former executive, Mitchell Daniels, Jr., was the White House budget director. Close ties to drug heads perpetuate the wrongful protection of Vaccine Producers, in the form of a shortsighted and ungrounded anti-liability for Vaccine Producers. From the top of the hill and on down there is links to protect Vaccine Producers and not our children and these connections reek of impropriety. Parents need to protect their children from chemicalization and attack those that chemicalized!

It is in the best interest of children for parents to be free to prevent or delay chemicalization. The particulates of vaccines destroy the perfected chemistry of health. The intestines have a certain flora of bacteria; this sensitive bacteria flora is susceptible to the chemical propensities of vaccines. Beneficial intestinal flora can keep disease producing microorganisms under restraint whereas; a bacterium that suffers chemical exposure poisoning does not. Chemical poisons can promote unnatural bacteria strains to grow. **Health and disease prevention is all about chemistry.** The anti-health chemicals must be removed from vaccines. In a November 2012, Congressional Autism Hearing, CDC officials failed to site even one study backing up vaccine safety claims. Most health conditions are from chemical exposure; most **women who have breast cancer have foreign chemicals in their breast fluids**. The infiltration of chemical promotes disease. **The best guarantee for health is to steer clear of chemicals.** Autism is a chemical manifestation; vaccine chemicalization is the primary cause of the epidemic.

The mandated vaccination law is at odds with parenting, morals and natural health standards of excellence. It is a violation of personal space and body; it enforces unnatural chemicalization. We must have liberty to protect and control our children's healthcare. Unvaccinated, healthy children are forbidden from entering school on mere speculation that they will fall ill. This exclusion is quarantining, ear-marks people as different and results in prejudicial treatment of the unvaccinated; it produces inequality and is discriminatory. Such a mistaken law violates human Rights and does not allow for equal citizenship. This unsound law blatantly violates the Right to education and equality of education opportunity. **It is justifiable civil disobedience not to succumb to submitting your children for unwanted vaccine chemicalization or to refuse to take part in a chemical injection experiment.** Mandated vaccination is not what the People want; it is what the Drug Company's want and is self-serving.

Freedom to govern our very own health and/or healthcare is liberty to control what will or will not be injected into our blood or body. **We must be free to decide what is in our children's best health interest; free to protect our children from unwanted chemical exposure and/or enabled to legally refuse unwanted vaccine chemical injections.** Health is dependent upon having the proper chemistry. There is a chemical and magnetic signature of optimum health. Autism has a chemical component; vaccination induces chemically compromised children! Vaccine anti-health chemicals produce a less health resilient state; inducing an Autism reactive state. Recognize that the **laws of chemistry apply to the human body** when chemicals are injected. **Autism is not idiopathic as they would have you believe; it is chemically induced**.

The chemicals of health do not include the chemicals found in vaccines. Children's internal chemistries are bastardized by vaccines. We must prompt cleaner, chemically free vaccines. Children are being used as human guinea pigs in a chemical mixing experiment; free Americans must be free not to submit to experimentation. Vaccines denature the health generating chemistry. Do not disengage from parenting; your children need your protection and you, need to protect your children from the vices of unnatural vaccine chemicalization. BEST PROTECT YOUR CHILD'S VITAL CHEMISTRY WITH LIBERTY TO PROTECT YOUR OFFSPRING! Vaccine Producers must be sufficiently punished for its use of chemicals that injure in its vaccines and the people must be free to refuse unwanted healthcare, NOT ENSLAVED to vaccinate; this will GET THE CHEMICALS OUT of vaccines and best serve our children's best health interest.

Let a jury determine if vaccine producers are negligent and their vaccines cause Autism! To be precluded from having your day in court because of some special treatment of vaccine producers is inequitable and is grossly un-American. The American system of justice and jurisprudence has it that the fact finders are a jury made up of ordinary citizens and that the jury will decide the facts. They have hijacked government by making it impossible for parents to even attempt to prove in a traditional civil court of law that vaccination destroyed their children's excellent health and spawned autism. A competent jury of your peers would easily find that the injection of vaccine chemicals which, has unnatural to body chemicals is at minimum inducing the vaccination recipient to be a human guinea pig used in a chemical experiment and that the injection of these alien chemicals is injuries to the natural perfected chemistry required to be optimally healthy. In addition, the fact finders would readily find that autism is in fact, caused by exposure to chemicals that disrupt, distort and make abnormal the internal chemistry of those that suffer an injection of such, chemicals. The American tradition of negligence law must be steadfastly applied to vaccine manufacturers and the American legal system that we have come to rely and depend upon for consumer safety for anyone injured seeking justice must be fully restored. TWO STEPS OF CORRECTION will end these abuses and violations. Be chemically safer; consider only chemically SAFER vaccines. Unnatural to human biology chemicalization is not harmonious with health. Parents do not be misled or misinformed; protect your children's vital chemistries!

Unnatural to the body chemicalization causes harm especially, if injected. It is a strict case of vaccine producers' profit from its chemicals for profit in vaccines that is children's health loss! The health problem from vaccine and/or medicine chemicalization is very real and extremely disconcerting; the cause of death from opioids more than doubled in 2016. If we do not act to do something about the opioid epidemic and the autism epidemic or the unnatural to human biology chemicalization epidemic now our future will continue to spiral downward. There is no legitimate reason to inject unsafe vaccines into children when SAFER vaccines are available or can be made available. Parents must do what is in their children's best interest by seeing to it that children are not exposed or injected with unnatural to human biology chemicalizations; be FREE to protect your children!

CHAPTER 7

LAW MUST BENEFIT THE PEOPLE AND BE WHAT THE PEOPLE WANT

Our government has been hijacked by special interest groups that only serve their agenda. Among these governmental hijackers are the 13,000 Big-Pharms lobbyists that represent vaccine producers' self-serving agenda. The laws that they often write word for word find its way into enactment not by chance. Mandated vaccination regulation that has overstepped its time for being mandated and now is antiquated law has been erroneously expanded upon and holds our children enslaved to endure and suffer multiple unnatural to the body chemicalizations. These mal-laws that keep us shackled or chained to non-consented to vaccination slavery are not at all what the PEOPLE want! Vaccination benefit has been overshadowed by its negative chemicalization health effects. To be enforced to inject a tiny baby, little infant or small child with unnatural to the body chemicals is objectionable to free Americans. No one wants their offspring exposed to chemicals that do not benefit the body or be commanded by mal-law to suffer it!

The clear majority of people do not want vaccine chemical injections to be mandated by law! Almost 100% of parents asked thought it **best that Parents be permitted to refuse any vaccination** that they determine too dangerous to inject or not in their children's best interest, it is practically unanimous that the People want and require to have this **basic freedom**. So why is it not so? Vaccinations are predominantly mandated because those whom profit from them make sure it is so. Vaccinations are a big business and the big money machine dictates its mandate. Children are **ENSLAVED** to be vaccinated to assure Vaccine Producers profiteering. Mandated vaccination laws are primarily not for the public's benefit but rather, are a direct product of the Drug industry's lobbyist efforts and for their self-serving profiteering agenda. In addition, the mandate eliminates the cost of important quality control measures for safety. The People want more vaccine quality control not less; they want vaccine producers to be accountable and liable.

Mandating vaccine **CHEMICALIZATION** transgresses one's internal chemistry and is an egregious Constitutional violation. People are subdued by the oppression of vaccination slavery and are made to witness children's chemicalization. Parents are feeling guilty for not stopping the vaccine chemical insult of their children however, they are not to blame; they are **VICTIMS OF VACCINATION SLAVERY**. Mandated vaccinations are not in the best interest of children; **they are in the best interest of big Drug Corps. If there was no profit to be made by mandated vaccinations, there would be no vaccination mandate**. Liberty to refuse vaccines is essential for vaccine quality or safety and for our basic freedom. To carry on a **FREE** civilization there can be no mandated or enforced chemicalizations or inability to deny unwanted vaccines. Mandated or enforced vaccination is not of benefit or what the People want; it cannot remain law!

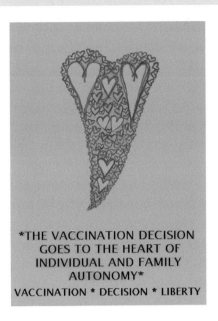

*THE VACCINATION DECISION
GOES TO THE HEART OF
INDIVIDUAL AND FAMILY
AUTONOMY*
VACCINATION * DECISION * LIBERTY

Unnatural to the body chemicals in vaccines once injected into babies, infants and children of all ages are of tremendous burden to their forming bodies and are extremely destructive to health. No rational parent, no fair-minded citizen wants to be exposed to such chemicals; the People never want their children to be injected with vaccines containing such chemicals. People do not agree with being enslaved to vaccinate; they want the freedom of healthcare decision! The puppet government of vaccine producers must not micro or macro manage our health decisions or master over our vaccination decisions. Making us enslaved to vaccinate is the epitome of being ruled over instead, of properly governed. The scale of public opinion demands that we are not enforced to vaccinate.

The introduction of alien to the body chemistry into the highly vulnerable systems or cells of our offspring is the cause of autism and vaccine chemical injection is the main cause of the autism epidemic. The People's understanding that unnatural, vaccine chemicalization is the main cause of the autism epidemic is based upon documented observation of vaccinated children's health demise and is supported by the science and laws of chemistry and/or chemical reactions. The People do not want to be forced by law or regulation to compromise their offspring's chemical integrity or be induced to sacrifice their children's perfected chemistry! Mandated vaccination has opened the door to chemicalization and/or use of chemicals for profit not safety; it must end! It is most reasonable for parents to keep children healthy by not allowing vaccine chemicalization.

You are not secure in your person if you are enforced to inject vaccine chemicals against your will. It is seizure of your healthcare decision and actual health to be enforced to vaccinate. The Fourth Amendment of the Constitution grants to the People the supreme, preeminent Right to be secure in their persons and/or against unreasonable seizures. Mandated vaccinations are an unreasonable seizure of a person's health, healthcare and/or body. Article Six, second paragraph, states that the Constitution is the supreme law of the land; therefore, no State can enact a law that violates the Fourth Amendment. **Reason to mandate vaccination is negligible and inconsequential as compared to reasons not to mandate. It is an unlawful seizure that violates the Fourth Amendment, people are not secure in their person; it seizes control of People's healthcare and/or bodies. It seizes vaccination decision control and/or one's self-control. People long**

to be free to self-regulate their health! Parents must submit their children to be injected and/ or exposed to vaccine chemicals; a seizure of healthcare decision and parental protection. Mandated vaccinations DO NOT BENFIT THE PEOPLE OR ARE WHAT THE PEOPLE WANT; it mainly serves those who profit from it and perpetuates unsafe vaccines that have chemicals for profit, not safety. These unnatural to the body vaccine chemicals pose an unnecessary imminent threat to our children's health; people do not want vaccines with such, chemicals.

Not only are mandated vaccinations against the natural order of things, they violate individual's natural Right to be left alone or not violated by unwanted injections of vaccine chemicals. People want to self-control their children's healthcare and prevent unwanted chemical injections. People want volitional; **SAFER** vaccines. Drug Companies strong political persuasions is much too pervasive; a wrongful protection of Vaccine Producers from liability and mandatory medical intervention has spawned as a result. Vaccine production irresponsibility and/or unnatural to the body chemicals in vaccines is now rampant. Rights and health choices must never take a back seat to profiteering from vaccination. Above all parents must be free to zealously protect children the way they think best and that includes, refusing vaccination and/or chemicalization!

A sure way to prevent lobbyists from pushing through laws that are ill-conceived or not in the public's best interest is to allow the public itself to vote on each law; cell phone or computer voting will soon be an option to allow for this. In the very near future one will be enabled to vote from home or from any convenient location by fingerprint recognition on your cell or computer; a truer democracy without law making corruption will emerge. Millennium generation are not as willing to expend their precious time and energy to go vote at an archaic voting booth and are leery that the voting machines could count votes inaccurately. Soon, people can use their online or cellular devices to vote. Image being enabled to vote on every issue; a true democracy! There is no room for lobbyist pushing law through in a true democracy; only the will of the People. The will of the People is not to be enslaved to vaccinate or be enforced to over parental objection! The will of the People is to hold vaccine producers accountable and liable if its' vaccines injure!

Money making agenda must not overshadow liberty; freedom and children's safety are essential, a must. Children's welfare is placed at risk by vaccination being mandated and due to the unethical and highly inappropriate liability shield that Big-Pharma has manipulated into existence. Mandating means you legally cannot refuse vaccination and that means even if the vaccine is bad it is has the legal fiction of being good; it also, means that vaccine producers do not have to properly worry or concern themselves about making vaccines that only have safe contents and/or satisfying parental safety demands. A liability shield means they can have chemicals that are hazardous to health in vaccines and the vaccine makers' have nothing to worry about if it causes injury; unjustly, they cannot be legally touched or hurt financially for any vaccine induced injury. The public, becoming aware of the injustice and lack of essential quality control by vaccine makers recognize what a danger mandated vaccination is to their offspring; they want the mal-law of mandated vaccination to be voided and for Big-Pharma to no longer have an unjust liability shield. The public seeks to assure their children's safety by making forcing vaccine producers to make vaccines that do not have unnatural to human biology or physiology chemicals. The public want children protected to the max and for parents to be free to protect!

The American system that is supposed to protect and benefit us is broken. The truth of the matter is that if the energy making discovery cannot be metered and/or profited from it will be suppressed and if a health generating discovery cannot be patented and thereby, profited from that discovery will be suppressed. We must be vigilant to assure discoveries can benefit us whether they make tons of money or make established or conventional uses or companies make a lot less money. Law must be for the publics benefit and be what the public wants; it must not only protect the profiteering of the well-established, it must protect our present and future well-being. Discoveries need to be available and you to decide what is best for you!

Natural healthcare discoveries compete with Big-Pharma and very often totally prevent the need for drug or vaccines thereby, decrease profiteering by Drug/chemical companies. Because natural substances decrease profiteering from drugs/vaccines there is self-serving agenda to suppress or eliminate the competition; this is a strike against the public good and/or welfare. Their droves of lobbyists see to it that law is enacted, which assure their profiteering and growing monopoly; **even though the law they manipulate into enactment is not of benefit to the People and that most of the People do not want such wrongful law. Money corrupts absolutely, if unconscionable profits were not made from mandated vaccinations, there would be no mandate of vaccination and the enslavement to be vaccinated would end!** They are attempting to make vitamins and minerals virtually inaccessible by making it required to be prescribed and thereby, price vitamins out of the market by regulation; making it so difficult and expensive it eliminates or controls the competition. Having to get a prescription for natural remedies makes it a lot more difficult get them and the price of a vitamin prescription makes it cost prohibitive. It is an attempt by Big-Pharma to corner the market, take over the natural remedy market or eliminate competition. Making it a requirement to first obtain a prescription to obtain vitamins or minerals is economic waste, limits access to natural remedies, is not in the best interest of the public and is, not what the public wants. It is not in the best interest of the public that vaccination is mandated or that vaccine producers are deregulated, unaccountable or made not liable for the chemicals they use in vaccines. The free market of natural cures must not be taken from us by special interest group mal-regulation.

They also have design to make us dependent upon certain few food types and manufacturers by putting into regulation that the seeds that grow into plants are patentable and therefore, private property. This is unprecedented and unnatural that seeds, food and/or life can be patented or OWNED. Food should be for all and not owned! They even dare to hide the truth by not labeling it GMO; taking our freedom of decision or choice away. If it is not natural or if is man-made it should be labeled so! To patent food ownership or pass GMO's off as unlabeled food is not regulation for the People and it is not what the People want. Mandated vaccinations, in perpetuity, are not for the benefit of the People and are not what the People want. Unjust law enactment has perpetuated the egregious oppression of our Right to self-determined healthcare and choose what we feed our family; it has caused the runaway negligent infiltration of our children's vaccine supply with unwanted harmful chemicals and forced us to eat what we may not want to eat. Assuring profiteering from vaccine sales must no longer take precedence over the common good and/or what is in the best interest of children. The food we are choosing at the supermarket must not be cloaked or hide anything about it; there must be full labeling to assure total transparency. Truth will set you free and can keep you healthy; know what you eat and know what is in the vaccines that might be injected into your offspring's delicate systems!

Chemically laced vaccines are cause for growing distrust in vaccine safety and/or in the vaccination program; it has caused an erosion of credibility. Immediately after the passing of the Homeland Security Bill, which cloaked the passing of the Vaccine Producer liability shield, federal court was motioned to **permanently seal the records** on all thimerosal (mercury) related information and/or material handed over by the government. Wow talk about cover-ups, now pertinent information relating to the health of our children and/or the harm caused from vaccines was sealed, not allowed to be viewed; **a cover-up**. Permanently, sealing records or temporarily sealing records in such an important issue serves only to protect those that can be injured by those records; vaccine makers'. The protection of Vaccine Producers and the cover-up **does violence to the protection of children and of human and parental Rights**. Politicians, more than appear to be in collusion with Big-Pharma; the campaign contribution afford special treatment, bias and protection. The bias stands out when you compare it to how someone's unvaccinated health status is not sealed or rendered private; and yet they seal records of Autism cases. The record suppression is slated and stops further inquire into the true cause of the autism epidemic; vaccines. Prompting the removal of anti-health chemicals from vaccines and attainment of much better vaccine safety for our children is the number one priority, it must take precedence!

Big-Pharma's influence to give it special treatment and money-making bias is rampant. One example is called upon here to illuminate the pro-bias treatment and/or corruption. In 2016 the CDC after a year of purposeful doing nothing to alert the public, allowed the public and government to spend in access of 200 million dollars on a FluMist finally stated it did not work; after a year transpired of knowing it did not work. The CDC had not one but three studies showing the FluMist was a dud; it did not work, was a waste of time and money. The CDC inaction allowed Big-Pharma to rip-off 200 million and caused the public to be infiltrated with unnatural to the body chemicals via the chemical mist being inhaled. CDC is in collusion with Big-Pharma. We need to prompt the CDC to do what is in the public's interest not what is in Big-Pharma's money interest.

An outrageous example of how far their factions will go to suppress new discoveries or avenues of different means of treatment that interfere with the already established mega money-making monopoly, is the total elimination of Dr. Wilhelm Reich's books, manuscripts and potential healing inventions. The FDA not only decreed that Reich's books be withheld from distribution but outrageously, FDA agents orchestrated the destruction of his books; Reich's books were actually burnt, incinerated. Confiscation of learned information, scientific research or proposed patient treatments and/or book burning should not take place in a FREE America. The decree and/or injunction for the destruction of Reich's invented benefit for humanity (Reich's Orgone Accumulator) were drawn up by the FDA and the U.S. Attorney; it called for its destruction and the destruction of all of Reich's published research bulletins.

I am in no way advocating Reich's work or stating that his inventions had any merit however, we will never know if they were a source of health benefit since, it was snuffed out. In the land of the FREE, to allow an individual's proposed benefit for humanity to be snuffed out or totally suppressed is outrageous. For your information, Reich's background indicates that he was an extremely intelligent person and a highly respected professional. Sigmund Freud used to send him patients for psychoanalysis and he was a well-known neuro-psychiatrist he certainly, did not have the earmarking of a quack. It is highly likely, that his work did have some degree of merit or that another genius innovator could have stood upon his shoulders and seen further to improve upon his initial work for humanity to benefit however, because of corrupt powers we will never know its possible benefits and humanity will likely, suffer for it. There were claims and patient studies that gave every indication his therapy was beneficial in the treatment of cancer. Suppression of potential new health benefits and scientific books being burned are crimes against humanity! Inequitably, the Vaccine Companies that have a sorted past, can put whatever, they want in children's vaccines and government does little about it and parents are supposed to do nothing about it and are unjustly legally blocked to refuse their injection. **Law must be for the People and what the People want; not for corpocracy or for what corpocracy wants!**

Vaccines have chemicals that cause all kinds of health problems because it manipulates the chemical consistency within. Take for example, Fluzone High-Dose, it was somehow approved by FDA but was finally taken off the market long after it was reported to cause low platelet counts, enlarged lymph nodes, life-threatening allergic reactions, extreme shoulder pain and paralysis and Guillain-Barre syndrome and convulsions. You never know what you are releasing with the chemicals of any vaccines being injected or breathed in; signs and symptoms are just indicators that the vaccine has altered your internal perfected chemistry of health and it is destroying your chance at optimum health and increasing your chances of health problems including, autism! To allow vaccines to have unnatural to the human biology chemicals is the reckless endangerment of the public and to allow vaccine makers to skirt any liability is the reckless endangerment of the public and is ludicrous, insane and grossly negligent. To enforce vaccine injection by mandate is off the chart insanity and is the main cause of chemicalization autism. No one wants to be enforced by mal-law to inject one's child with unwanted chemicals!

The atrocity of allowing Vaccine Producers to skirt liability allows them to place anti-health poisons in vaccines; parents' must not be enslaved to chemicalize. In a time when it was cautioned that low level mercury exposure by eating fish was unhealthy; Vaccine Producers put mercury poison in vaccines and we were induced by mal-law to inject it into our children. **Between 1990 and 2000 vaccinated children were exposed to mercury levels more than the FEDERAL SAFETY LIMITS for adults**. There was a possibility of obtaining a vaccine that did not have mercury however, parents were unaware of it because informed consent and/or **informed DENIAL** wrongfully did not apply to vaccinations, no one really knew about the opportunity or the choice of an alternative. What the public was not informed about vaccines without mercury or that single doses did not need mercury and/or have mercury and that there were other preservatives instead of the extremely toxic mercury preservative to be had. **Informed DENIAL/consent** of vaccine injections is crucial to adequately inform patients and protect children. Let us prompt **SAFER** vaccines and fill the gap between parents and children, with **informed DENIAL or consent of vaccinations**. Let us not have law that cause runway negligence or that enslaves!

The consensus among those who have thoroughly investigated the apparent relationship between Vaccine Producers and the law makers is that there certainly is major conflict of interest because of their close ties and arrangements. In fact, Rep. Dan Burton during his chair position of the Subcommittee on Human Rights and Wellness raised the question on May 3, 2003, "**Is there collusion** between the pharmaceutical companies and our health agencies?" Burton's answered his own question, "the appearance in many cases is that **there is**." Burton's conclusion came after an extensive three-year investigation into vaccines and Autism in which his staff and himself reviewed all the relative documents, literally thousands of pages that involved the CDC, FDA and political committees. **Parents must not surrender their children to the vices of conflicts of interest. Parents must protect children from vaccine chemical doping by injection. Parents must be free to refuse what they consider unsafe vaccine injection CHEMICALIZATION.**

Recognize that this corrupted system perpetuates violence to our children's health and to our Rights. The introduction of anti-health vaccine chemicals into the blood chemistry of children sets the stage for the abnormal. Injected vaccine chemicals alter the natural chemical configuration within the bloodstream, placing the gears in motion for Autism. The rendered abnormal blood chemistry, from vaccine injected chemicals, rapidly penetrates the cells of the brain, chemically doping these critical cells. Once a tipping point is reached, a chemical critical mass syndrome ensues, spawning Autism. Knowing that the FDA, CDC, FTC and/or Government allows People to be exposed to more and more and more chemicals/toxins in the food we eat, the drugs we consume and the vaccines that are enforced; makes one realize that we must be in self-control to no longer be exposed to chemicals. People need to retake the healthcare decision of whether to vaccinate. Demand to be free to refuse vaccines and that vaccines have no anti-health chemicals. **Liberty of healthcare decision is having the freedom of healthcare choice! Healthcare slavery must end; VACCINATION ENSLAVEMENT MUST BE ABOLISHED!**

People are sick and tired of government telling them how to plan their life particularly, vaccination healthcare. Giving people no choice in the matter is incredulous, ill-conceived, a violation of the law and should be a crime! People know better than government as to what is best for their very own health or for that of the health of their very own children! It is outrageous for government to intrude upon the all-important health decision of vaccination. Government serves the People and not the other way around; government must not make people subjects of government and take control over their health decisions by mandating vaccinations especially, permanently. Most of the People agree that they must be **FREE** to control their own healthcare and that parent's control their children's health decisions therefore, government is not serving the People by mandating vaccine chemical injections; the mandate merely serves the Vaccine Producers interests. **There must always be measures in place that force producers of vaccines to first act to make vaccines safe and not place anti-health chemicals in vaccines; informed DENIAL/consent of unwanted vaccinations and being free to litigate against Vaccine Producers are those needed and essential measures!**

Can anything be stronger than the child parent bond; it is true parents have the most proximate relationship with child and have cellular, blood or genetic relationship; this makes parents the supreme decision makers for their child. Essentially, it is a natural Right to self-determine healthcare; it is not a government sanctioned Right, it is GOD given. Refusing vaccinations is a supreme natural freedom which should never be interfered with by government! Government must not take control of our health decisions. Parents' not government rule the decision of whether the child will or will not be administered vaccines except, if the parents have been found guilty in a court of law by a jury of one's peers of childcare negligence or child abuse. Make no mistake, mandated injection of unnatural to the body chemicals into tiny babies, little infants or small children is child abuse on a mass scale; autism is one of its negative results!

Many parents are naturally logic stricken about preventing chemicalization! Parents, have put one and one together, connecting the dots, that the causation of autism is the injection of unnatural to the body, vaccine chemicals. The mindless herd mentality of the vaccination program along with the threat of consequences for breaking the vaccination mandate/law keep us shackled or enslaved to submit children for vaccination; despite any logic to the contrary or rational fear of injury. Vaccine Producers have carved out a puppet government protection for profiting and an enslaved population that assures vaccine chemical sales. Lobbyists buffer or vaccine producers from being directly connected with all this pro-vaccination government bias. Government or rather, lobbyists need not, should not and must not supersede parents in deciding what is best for the health of children. Why is that parents freely decide what their child eats, drinks or everything and anything else that has to do with the securing of the welfare children but not what chemicals if any are **TO BE OR NOT TO BE** injected? Parents are certainly, the ones that are supposed to make all of their offspring's' life protective decisions; why not vaccinations! Money making is the root of vaccination slavery! Parents' not government, are meant to make their immature offspring's health decisions. Parents' are empowered by natural law to decide what is best for their children; the natural order and/or the highest authority, our GOD, makes it so. Preventative vaccination decisions or what chemicals if any, to accept, is for parents to make!

Mandated vaccinations violate the Constitution and our fundamental freedoms. Our Right to Privacy and/or the protections afforded by HIPPA compliance are violated. Our Right to Self-Govern our own internal being and Self-Preservation are violated. Our Right to be left alone or not have our bodies violated with unwanted medical intervention is violated. Our Constitutional freedom to freely travel between states is violated due to the heavy burden of having to become vaccination compliant when we attempt to travel into a State that has more severe vaccination requirements as compared to the State one might originate travel from.

The Constitutional requirement that our Government must not favor one religion over another and/or establish one religion over another is violated by mandated vaccination State requirements; by favoring those with religious vaccination with school entrance and at the same time deny entrance to those who's religion does not require a religious exemption. Those that do not have the required religious exemption and remain unvaccinated are prejudiced for not having the right religion by not allowing school entrance or rather, government by its act of allowing school entrance of unvaccinated children with the right religious belief is the act of establishing one religion over another. The act of different treatment based upon religious belief is the establishment of one religion over another. The act of basing school admittance based upon religion establishes one religion over another. The act of treating unvaccinated children being treated differently based upon one's religious belief or religion is the government establishing a religion over another religion. The act of allowing school entrance for unvaccinated based upon religious exemption is establishing that religion as superior, favored or as required. By virtue of their religious belief one can enter school, or one cannot. Those who do not have the special favored religion must be vaccinated; **they favor those not vaccinated who have the religion not to be vaccinated with school entrance and prejudice the non-favored religions that are not vaccinated with enforced vaccinations or forbid school entrance; this is government wrongfully establishing one religion or another.**

The religious exemption analysis is fraught with illegality. Through arbitrary and capricious methodology, they miraculously, determine if one's religious belief is sincere and if the religious exemption is valid; this **religion witch hunt** is against the law. They actually can ask the question is one's religious conviction not to be vaccinated sincere and check the validity of sincerity based upon how long one has had one's belief. One might have a long held religious belief or one that was formed that day; either way people must be taken for their word after all, it is their belief. Separation of Church and State forbids this line of questioning at any level! No free practicing religious American should be required to confess their private religious beliefs and moreover, no one should be questioned if their belief is sincere. What is controlling whether it is legal or not legal is the fact that one's body is one's temple therefore, government's mandate to vaccinate is a violation of Separation of Church and State and thereby, unconstitutional.

It is very important that we stop our children from being violated by unnatural chemical exposure and save them from becoming autistic; parents must be free to stop what they think might or will cause autism and prevent their offspring from encountering it. The fact, that vaccines have been found to harbor chemicals that violate one's natural chemistry with unnatural to the body chemicals is proof that parents must protect their children. It is well within the preview of parenting to not subject their offspring to such, chemicalization and/or vaccine chemical infiltration; and it so happens to be very, very, very smart parenting. People are programmed, their senses dulled into being vaccination compliant slaves. Awaken your spirit of freedom to do what is best for your family's health as you determine it; no longer be enslaved to vaccinate!

The requirement that law be equitably applied to all citizens or that law not single out a certain select group or not be discriminatory in its application or in its effect is violated by the erroneous vaccination mandate. Perfectly healthy school worthy children, who are not vaccinated, are singled out and prejudiced with a fiction that they are not school worthy. Children are entitled to attend school; the healthy, unvaccinated, are not. Schools are given incentives to monitor that children are vaccinated. Child Services can be called in to take these children away from their parents to enforce vaccinations. Our Right to our day in court and/or to litigate directly against the party that caused the injury is violated because we are legally forbidden to litigate directly against Vaccine Producers when their vaccines cause an injury. Our Right as parents to protect children from harm and/or potential harm is violated and our childrearing freedom and/or family autonomy are all violated because the **VACCINATION ENSLAVEMENT LAW does allow refusal**.

The mandated vaccination law is arbitrary and capricious in that it singles out only childhood vaccinations for mandate while not mandating the more dangerous Flu or any other healthcare. No other healthcare is mandated making the vaccination mandate arbitrary and capricious. The Flu can be fatal or devastate health much more than childhood disease. Influenza starts to be transmitted the day before you become sick whereas, childhood diseases become transmitted upon sickness and sometimes days after the tell tail signs and symptoms of sickness occur; this allows for the precaution of quarantining childhood diseases. Therefore, is not only arbitrary and capricious to mandate childhood vaccinations, but rather, there is less reason to mandate childhood vaccinations and more reason to mandate Flu shots. Each drop of vaccine that has mal-chemicals, is a desecration of blood that can catalyze and effectuate **AUTISM. GET THE CHEMICALS OUT** and stop mandating vaccination!

Mandated/enforced vaccinations are draconian in nature. During these modern healthcare times of respecting the patient's decisions in healthcare and/or respecting informed consent/ DENIAL requirement, to be forced by law and coercion to receive a vaccine injection is

repugnant and an enigma in the healthcare delivery system. **It is much too severe, too iron fisted to deny an individual and/or parent for their child, their Right to refuse an invasive medical intervention such as, vaccine chemicalization injection.** The limited Police Power of the State, which allowed for mandated vaccination during an epidemic period has long passed; the People no longer need or want to be under the burden of becoming vaccination compliant particularly, when vaccine is laced with unnatural to the body chemicals. It is now an abuse of power to maintain the continual onslaught of more and more vaccinations. Mandated vaccinations have been enforced upon the People for too long; for an inordinate, improper and impermissible length of time. Vaccination has turned into a big business, a profiteering machine that impermissibly expanded the limits of the Police Power. Perhaps, vaccination can be mandated during a crisis or exigent circumstances or an epidemic but absent the emergent circumstance there should be extraordinary measure of mandated vaccination. **The People do not want to be under the oppression of perpetual mandated vaccination or be made to violate their religion.**

Religious Exemption from Vaccinations.

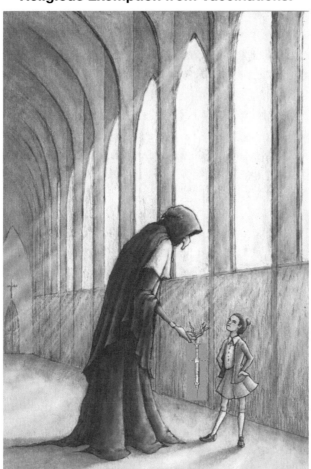

The Constitutional Right of FREEDOM OF RELIGION protects you from suffering an unwanted, unnatural to human biology vaccine chemicalization, if it violates your religious belief or prevents the FREE exercise of your religion. Stand strong against what violates one's religion!

Benjamin Franklin said, "If you give up your freedom for safety, you don't deserve either one." Freedom must never be sacrificed! Mandated vaccination is a loss of liberty. It is weak argument to enforce vaccinations for safety especially, vaccines with unnatural to the body chemicals; this loss of liberty is what Franklin warned about. It is absurd to argue that the mandate is safe when it enforces chemicalization! All the lame excuses for mandating vaccinations and the idiotic contentions that injecting chemicals is safe or not harmful or is not a cause of AUTISM is absurdity piled on top of absurdity. This does not even rise to the level of giving up freedom for safety because the vaccines are not safe. We need SAFER vaccines; we need to GET THE CHEMICALS OUT! One should take into consideration in analyzing the need to GET THE CHEMICALS OUT of vaccines or if the present state of vaccination is worthy of injection that the chemicals combine in our bodies. Moreover, vaccinations are not tested for its cumulative effects; multiple exposures pose obvious adverse chemical interactions and many unknown health risks!

There are multitudes of humans that are resilient to disease or are practically health perfect; do these individuals have Rights that endow the person to not be injected with the chemical chaos of the multiple vaccinations? Do those that choose to rely upon pure natural means of healthcare have to bow down to the pressure of vaccination fanaticism and hysteria? What about all the people that have done their homework and have come to recognize that there are chemicals in vaccines that do not serve any benefit and in fact, are completely alien or unnatural to human biology and/or physiology and/or for many rational controlling reasons do not want vaccine chemicalization to be circulated into their highly vulnerable systems; are they not to be free to protect themselves and their offspring from the threat of such, chemical destabilization? NO FREE AMERICAN should be enforced to distort or manipulate one's natural chemistry; NO FREE AMERICAN should be made to stand down as responsible parents in their protection or prevention of their children from unwanted chemical exposure! ABOLISH VACCINATION SLAVERY!

Police Power of the State has its power limitations; it must not enforce vaccinations for long periods of time or mandate vaccines that cause injury and it must not supersede the power of parents in keeping their perfectly healthy children safe. The vaccine industry lobby use this Police Power for its own self-serving gain; creating a bottomless pit, a Grand Canyon of continuous, ever increasing, mandated vaccinations that dominates us to endlessly vaccinate in perpetuity. In perpetuity mandated vaccination is the improper use of the Police Power; the vaccination mandate was never meant to be prolonged or in perpetuity. Mandating injections of anti-health chemicals is a wrong exercise of the Police Power of the State. Adding vaccine after vaccine to the mandate or continuing the mandate when there is no epidemic or imminent threat of an epidemic violates the proper use of the Police Power. Having no end in sight for the finalization of the mandated vaccination program is wrong; it oversteps the proper use of the Police Power of the State. **There certainly, should be and needs to be, reasonable restraints or limitations on how many or how long vaccinations are mandated. Police Power, enforcing vaccination mandates with no end in sight, is intolerable and is a severe oppression of our Right to self-determine health. The vaccine industry wants us enslaved to be vaccinated forever to assure profits; they have manipulated the continual mandate.**

Out of the multitudes of people asked, it was almost unanimous that vaccines need to be free of unnatural to the body chemicals and that parents must be legally able to refuse an unwanted, vaccine CHEMICALIZATION injection. People think that the decision regarding children's vaccination, to either accept or deny a vaccination, should be and needs to be

in the hands of the children's caring parents; this is the tradition and/or golden rule for basically all healthcare for children. It is best to entrust healthcare decisions and overall welfare with none other than the children's parents. Children must have **perfect security** in their parent's liberty to protect them! Parents require freedom to refuse unwanted medical intervention, such as an unwanted vaccination. **Parents are their children's great pillars of strength and protection.** Parents must be entitled to control children's healthcare!

Coinciding with the good standard in healthcare, doctors are free to properly council their patients, to direct patients and lightly remonstrate with patients. However, doctors must not command or unduly influence patients to vaccinate. The ultimate decision to accept or deny care must always rest with the patient and/or the parents, for the child patient. Parents may be interested in what authorities have to say on the subject however, parents legally must never be made to adhere to another's thoughts or conclusions. Perfectly, healthy children must be secure in their parent's protection from an unwanted suspect vaccination. Parents must be secure in their own basic protection responsibilities, enabled to protect their perfectly healthy children from all unwanted medical intervention, such as, an unwanted preventative vaccination. There must be parental freedom to protect children the way the parents' think best; without undue influence or enslavement to another's thoughts or conclusions. **There must be no vaccination SLAVERY!**

A child's vaccination destiny must be freely decided by the child's parents and law that controverts this must be deemed mal-law! The puppet governmental infraction of enslaving children to be injected with vaccine chemicals must be remedied through the **TWO STEPS OF CORRECTION**. The infraction against our freedom of healthcare choice and/or self-determined healthcare can no longer be masked by puppet government which only pretends to care for our children's welfare but, primarily cares about securing Vaccine Producer's profiteering on the grandest scale. **If there were no profits from vaccinations, you would see mandated vaccinations disappear in the blink of an eye**. Penetrate the façade of why vaccinations are mandated and protect your children from unwanted vaccine **CHEMICALIZATION AUTISM**! The **mandated vaccination enslavement law** is an unprincipled law. The public by self-preservation Right must be free to be both cautious and flexible when it comes to vaccinations, being free to refuse an unwanted chemical injection or postpone vaccinations or pick and choose vaccinations. There is an unacceptable lack of coherency for children's best interest if vaccination is decided by puppet government and/or profiteering Vaccine Producers. Parents hold children's welfare as their primary life directive and must be in control of the vaccination decision! Parents must demand informed **DENIAL** of injections and Vaccine Producers must be held liable for vaccine induced injuries! Injecting vaccine chemicals that parents conclude are too dangerous to inject is not in the best interest of children. **Be free to reject injections; freedom to refuse is essential!**

INFORMED DENIAL OF VACCINATIONS secures healthcare freedom and vaccine safety. Determining the vaccination decision is a priority decision for parents. **Vaccinations are a quintessential health decision that is for parents not government to make**! The knowledge that vaccines do contain anti-health or unnatural to the body chemicals, makes it an extremely important decision, **a paramount PARENTAL protective decision**. To be enabled to refuse a vaccine chemical injection is a must to fulfill one's parental child protective obligations. Individuals must be free to choose; not merely be a statistic but rather, be a statistic breaker! People must have healthcare options and not be boxed into the same approach as everyone else or be handcuffed to an approach that does not suite them. People must be free to think outside the box and demand a personalized approach! **Freedom to decide when or if vaccinations take place is essential to assure vaccine quality/safety, child protection and individuality!**

To place anti-health chemicals in vaccines and state that vaccines are safe or advocate that they are safe to inject violates the very precept that the vaccination program was founded upon. To cover-up the horrific facts that vaccine chemical injections do cause health problems or is the main etiology of the Autism epidemic is a disservice to the American People. There are vaccination advocates who purposefully turn the blind eye to the dangerous propensities of unnatural to the body chemicals, stating unequivocally that the chemicals of vaccines pose no threat to health and that vaccinations have nothing to do with Autism. Who are you going to believe your own eyes and ears that see, hear and/or observe as your children's health degenerate proximate in time to receiving a vaccine **CHEMICALIZATION** injection or are you to believe those which, are profiteering off the sales of vaccines? Just understanding the laws of chemistry is all one needs to access the danger of injecting unnatural chemicals or to fathom the harm from such, an occurrence and that chemicalization autism is spawned from doing so!

Learn the very denaturing character of the chemicals in vaccines; recognize its anti-health property or propensities. Do not be blinded by all the hype of vaccine advocates rhetoric, do not be so gullible or taken by cover-up stories; injections of vaccines are the main etiology of chemicalization Autism, they are perpetrating chemistry experiments on your children. Principles of chemistry control the reactions in the body; you do not want unnatural to the body chemicals to penetrate and dope your tiny baby's brain cells! Rely upon what is logical and the laws of chemistry; believe in what your own heart tells you. Injected vaccines chemicals upset the natural chemistry of the blood and brain cells. Do not allow self-proclaimed Vaccine Producers to act as demigods bent on making you submit children to suffer vaccine chemicalization; do not let the monopolized profiteering of vaccine chemical sales make your child an autism statistic. **If there were no profits to be obtained from vaccinations the mandated vaccination law would be non-existent; the lobbyist would simply concentrate on another adventure to bring the pharmaceutical industry profits**. Mandated vaccination and its enforcement is much too harsh; **it is draconian!** No **FREE** minded parent wants their offspring to suffer an unwanted vaccination!

Prompt increased quality control and safety that is brought about by having a free market competition applied to vaccination by ending the mandate of vaccination. Inexcusably, there is no need for vaccine producers to assure vaccine safety; they have a monopoly on childhood disease prevention, a most unintelligent, anti-safety for children vaccination mandate makes it so. A reason why vaccines have fallen into doses of chemical destabilization is because there is no competition when it comes to vaccines; they have a government sanctioned monopoly. Vaccine producers wallow in the fact, its vaccines are mandated therefore, people have no realistic choice in the matter. There will be full utilization of their vaccines no matter what chemicals are vaccines. Having no free market permeating throughout the vaccination market place has given vaccine producers the green light to put whatever, chemicals they please into vaccines and harmful and/or unnatural to the body chemicals are found in vaccines as a result. There are chemicals in vaccines that generate the most profit; they have no requisite concern about safety. The free market instills consumer protectionism that requires SAFER vaccines; it prompts vaccine producers to be extremely concerned about vaccine chemical content and/or safety. It is health wise that the producers of vaccines be held accountable and liable if its vaccines are found to be laced with unnatural to the body chemicals. The public wants a free market place to be applied!

Moreover, to mandate vaccination is counterproductive to the obtainment of SAFER vaccines; it places our very young children safety in grave jeopardy, it ignorantly, makes all parents to have to rely upon only the untrustworthy vaccine producers, leaving it up to their whim or greedy minded self-serving agenda! The mandate places vaccine chemical dice in the hands of parents and enforces parents to throw the chemical dice and gamble with the chemicalization outcome; parents are forced to live with the chemicalization results. Chemicalization autism is a direct result of the mandate! There may be fleeting moments of keeping vaccines clear of unnatural to the body chemicals, but the mandate's tendency promotes less quality control for safety not more and thereby, renders vaccines unsafe. The unwise mandated vaccination created monopoly must be curtailed by allowing childhood disease prevention diversity, competition, free market and accountability. If Big-Pharma did not want a guaranteed way to profit from vaccines, there would be no mandated vaccination and if Big-Pharma was held accountable and liable for vaccine induced injury, there would no longer be the strong tendency to use chemicals that derive the most profit and not the most safety! For the sake of vaccine quality control for vaccine safety and/or children's welfare, vaccination must be volitional; **NO VACCINATION MANDATE! Liberty to reject injection will set you free from being injected with unwanted chemical infiltration!**

What the People want is the basic dignity and freedom to decide what is best for their young offspring. Parents want to be free to steer clear of vaccines that they determine has contents that are questionable or that the parents realize as harmful. When parents realize the vaccines have unnatural to the body chemicals or have chemicals that are not inherent or natural to their children's delicate systems and/or bodies; parents must be free to protect and save their children from what parents determine is unnatural to their children's natural chemistry or stop an unnatural chemicalization. People want to freely refuse what they think might cause health problems especially, chemicalization autism. There must be liberty to prevent autism the way you as concerned parents think best; to stop vaccine chemicalization is a most rational parental want or need and basic liberty!

It is innately intelligent or perfectly natural and/or instinctive for children to depend upon their parents FOR IMPORTANT LIFE DECISIONS especially, for health-related decisions. There is no such, intelligent design to have State-government make children's vaccination decision. No other entity is so perfectly suited and situated to make life decisions or holds the child's best interest in as, high regard and/or no one wants what is best for the child's welfare or strives to keep the child out of harm's way than the child's parents. As far as doing what is best for children, parents', as compared, to government and its lobbied for regulation, have incorruptible integrity, consummate wisdom and insight instinct in deciding what is best for children. **Parents must call the shots** by being fully empowered to refuse vaccine chemical injections for children. Enslavement to vaccinations must be abolished, we must re–establish family autonomy and wisely put an end to the spiraling out of control Autism epidemic. **THE PUBLIC DOES NOT WANT TO BE ENSLAVED TO INJECT DOSES OF VACCINE CHEMICAL DISTABILIZATION!**

Liberation from vaccination slavery is essential to truly live free, to render vaccines reasonably safe and/or to secure the well-being of all vaccinated. Being free to refuse vaccine chemical injection is fundamental to parenting. **The vaccination mandate laws are mal-laws with no regard to parental protection right of children and causes less not more vaccine quality control. Law must not command injections of vaccine chemicals especially, against the will of the individual or parent. The mandated vaccination law place children in harm's way, separates children from their parent's protection and/or impedes parental protection. No law should so generally forbid parents from protecting their children from chemical exposures and no law should allow Vaccine Producers the unprecedented government sanctioned quasi-legal escape from negligence liability or be impervious to pay compensation when their vaccines cause injury and/or Autism. There must be no poisons in vaccines; the liberty to refuse unwanted vaccines and the unfettered freedom litigate against vaccine producers for allowing vaccines to be laced with any unnatural to the body chemical poison will achieve this most rational desire and goal of vaccine purification. GET THE CHEMICALS OUT; vaccines are too dangerous!**

The argument that unvaccinated children somehow pose a threat is based upon mere and false conjecture that ASSume perfectly healthy children's unvaccinated immune systems are inherently weak and will not only encounter childhood disease but will fall victim to it and upon extended mere conjecture that those vaccinated are going to become ill from those who are unvaccinated and fallen ill because the vaccination will not protect them. If the vaccination supposedly works then it should be justified that we can rely upon the fact, that the vaccinated are not at risk from those unvaccinated that are ASSumed will become ill. Perfectly healthy unvaccinated children pose no real threat it is just a fiction. If the purpose of the vaccination holds any promise, then those vaccinated should be protected even if the fiction comes to fruition that an unvaccinated perfectly healthy child falls sick with a childhood disease. Speculation or fiction piled on top of speculation or fiction is not rational reasoning to mandate vaccination. Mandating vaccinations based upon speculation after speculation should be impermissible law. The perfectly healthy unvaccinated cannot be rationally ASSumed to become ill and in fact, those that are unvaccinated who have not been dosed with vaccine chemical destabilization or chemically compromised stand a greater chance of remaining optimally healthy; the laws of chemistry applied to human biology and/or physiology dictate it so. Law must not be based on mere fiction!

This above reasoning for vaccination mandate pales compared to the reasoning and/or arguments that parents have for not mandating injections of chemical destabilization! 99.99999999% of parents think children's vaccination decisions is best determined by parents and that there are chemicals in vaccines that must not be injected; for all intents and purposes it is unanimous that the public does not want vaccinations to be mandated. The dangers inherent with enslaving the populace to be vaccinated far outweigh any one-sided pro-mandated vaccination enslavement argument. Consumers' choice and freedom dictate that if vaccinations were SAFER vaccines, worthy of having they would not have to be freely utilized and not be forced upon us by mandate; they need to be based upon consumerism and freedom of healthcare decision! People know what is good for their children they should be highly suspicious of any government command to inject chemicals for profit or insistence to do so especially, if it is against what a parent thinks is best for their child! The power of healthcare decision for children must generally always remain in parents; there must be no vaccination mandate in perpetuity!

If vaccinations work they grant immunity therefore, the unvaccinated pose no major threat to all those protected by vaccinations. Vaccinations do cause injury, so it is wise to correct what is in the vaccines that is causing injury; the chemicals of vaccines need to be analyzed to determine what chemicals are unnatural to the body. We now know that cancer and most if not all degeneration of health is related to chemical exposures and/or altering the normal body chemistry. Vaccine chemicals must not destabilize one's perfectly formulated internal chemistry; **GET THE CHEMICALS OUT** of the vaccines that are unnatural to the body. Parents' are becoming logic stricken and are concluding that vaccine chemicals are too dangerous to inject. Parents' have the Right to live freely without being enslaved to submit their children for vaccination enslavement. Your body is your temple; it must be entirely up to you to accept or deny vaccine chemical infiltrations! The People want **vaccination decision freedom**; not slavery!

The Autism epidemic will begin to subside only when **ALL** of the foreign, unnatural, alien to the body chemicals are out of vaccines; making vaccination a matter of freedom of choice, basing vaccination strictly upon informed consent/DENIAL and properly holding vaccine makers' accountable and liable will **GET THE CHEMICALS OUT**. Litigation liberty, to bring vaccine producers to justice and/or to be free to seek damages against producers of harmful vaccines is the proper application of negligence law to vaccines; instilling a reasonable degree of safety. The People want **SAFER vaccines** and to not let vaccine manufacturers off the hook when it is found that they put chemicals for profit, not safety, in vaccines and vaccine induced injury results. People want their children to have the greatest degree of safety and not continue to allow what promotes unsafe vaccines. **TWO STEPS OF CORRECTION** are needed!

Wake up America, in order, to secure the chemical integrity and/or safety of our children we must assure that they are not exposed, infiltrated, injected or administered unnatural to the body chemicals! Make no mistake, vaccine producers will have to forcibly be induced to **GET THE CHEMICALS OUT** and the **TWO STEPS OF CORRECTION** is the sure way of doing so! Vaccine industry autonomy and vaccine producers' priority to make money above all, must no longer stand in the way of serving children's best interest! The welfare of children is under chemical attack; we desperately need to correct what is so terribly wrong by assuring children's chemical integrity! Basing vaccinations on informed consent/**DENIAL**, on a totally **voluntary basis is key to securing safety; it will vastly improve vaccine quality control.** Vaccinations must be restricted to a voluntary system; vaccinations should only be administered if **true informed consent** is first obtained from the potential vaccination recipient. In addition, there needs to be an **equitable holding of vaccine companies liable for vaccine induced injuries; the vaccine injured must be enabled to pose lawsuits directly against the maker of the vaccine that caused the injury**. Children are best protected if the protection of their parents is not restricted by a vaccination mandate. Parents' properly empowered or enabled to refuse unwanted vaccines and enabled to freely litigate if injury occurs best protects children.

In addition, there is **no imminent crisis calling for a governmental intrusion of the magnitude of enforced multiple chemical injections; there is only the crisis created by Vaccine Producers and their puppet government enforcing children to be injected with vaccine chemicals. Fundamental freedom requires that parents be empowered to protect their children from unwanted injections and/or be left alone, undisturbed to enjoy their family autonomy with personal healthcare decisions. Refusal of unwanted chemical injections is consistent with**

being a free American and being autonomous. Vaccines will no longer have the anti-health chemicals once parents are enabled to refuse unwanted vaccines. Parents empowered to deny an unwanted suspect vaccine injection will directly stimulate Vaccine Producers to produce vaccines that are not laden with chemicals in order, to satisfy parent's health concerns. Make no mistake; Vaccine Producers need to be prodded to **GET THE CHEMICALS OUT** of vaccines. Children deserve safe vaccines and a safe vaccination schedule.

Together, these positive actions will **prompt** the needed degree of vaccine quality control to get the chemicals out of our children's vaccines, rendering vaccines much safer. Strangers should not decide how much, if any, chemical exposure your child will be exposed to; parents' must way out the risks of vaccination and decide if it is too dangerous to inject. Therefore, the control of whether a vaccination shall or shall not be given wisely and rightly is only vested in the hands of the children's parents. We need to assure that vaccine companies are brought to justice when their vaccines negligently cause injury. We need to institute these corrective measures to **GET THE CHEMICALS OUT of vaccines; to produce much, much, much safer vaccines. We do not begin to understand even one percent of the negative to health consequences, which result from injecting children's blood with CHEMICALS of vaccines. Mandated vaccination, by its definition is a violation of the Right to decide what is best for one's offspring and violates one's children with vaccine chemicalization by injection; it must not be tolerated, for it is enslavement to healthcare that can be very unhealthy!**

It is known that unnatural to the body chemicals take no part in the normal reactions of the body, it serves no benefit instead, it burdens the body and causes abnormality. It is just insane to have these chemicals in vaccines which, can be injected or inhaled or by any other means, enter the body. To purposely administer such chemicals into developing tiny babies, little infants or small children is an act of gross negligence, is child abuse by chemicalization and should be considered criminal if the one administering the tainted vaccine has knowledge of the toxic fact. Chemicals for profit not safety in vaccines have made vaccination too dangerous to inject. Certainly, parents' must be informed prior to the vaccination of the presence of any degree of unnatural to the body chemicals and be absolutely, free to save and/or prevent their offspring from being exposed to vaccine chemicalization! We desperately need vaccine producers to GET THE CHEMICALS OUT! The vaccination option must be as safe as possible and have a vaccination option that is most beneficial and, not detrimental. It is ludicrous to enforce parents by vaccination mandate to stand down and allow the injection of their children with vaccines of any kind and it is preposterous and an act of child abuse to enforce the injection of vaccines that have any degree of unnatural to the body chemicals! Parents' need to stop the sheer madness of the epidemic of unnatural chemicalization! There is no imminent threat of a childhood disease epidemic however, the epidemic of injections of vaccine unnatural to the body chemicals is real; so, let's stop the epidemic! People want SAFER vaccines that do not chemically compromise their children.

Parents' must be free to sit back in their chair of Rights and be afforded their freedom to protect offspring the way they think best and to rely upon proper law or government to secure them in this all-important Right and fundamental parenting responsibility! The real reason why government is too often lead to take actions is not because it is in the

common good or what the People want or is approved by the People rather, it is the lobbyist influence upon law-makers so that some special interest group can readily obtain unfair and non-consented to monetary gain. Do not let lobbyist manipulated mal-law enactments destroy your Right to decide what is best for children; parents need to decide what is best not wayward government. The law must be just, not cause injury and be what the People want! Fluoridation of water, restriction upon vitamins and minerals so that it requires a prescription and a wasted doctors' visit to obtain them, mandatory antibiotic drops put in newborns' eyes without the permission or knowledge of the parents, GMO so called food being unlabeled to replace our non-GMO natural and/or organic food choices at the supermarket and mandated multiple vaccination are to name some of the choices taken from the public and we are being made subject to. The choices that have been ripped from us is not what the People want or in the Peoples' best interest! Just how important is it to free Americans to have the capacity to protect their very young children from what parents conceive or recognize as an imminent threat or danger is off the scale of importance. Without question, parents' want the freedom to deter any harm that a parent thinks and/or determines is placing their child in jeopardy. PARENTS' REQUIRE THE LIBERTY TO PROTECT THEIR OFFSPRING FROM ANY CHEMICALIZATION!

The influx or injection of unnatural to the body chemicals is no small violation to one's health; it is a grave offence. Unnatural to biology chemicalization act to destabilize the normal reactions of the body and unleashes a gamut of renegade abnormal reactions. The laws of chemistry apply to the chemical reactive propensity from vaccine chemicals. To purposely inject such, chemicals in the name of the common good is a concept that is flawed; there is a misconception that these harmful chemicals will not take its unhealthy toll or spawn autism. Drugs are chemicals and we know that chemicals impact the central nervous system causing it to abnormally calm down or hype up. Unnatural to the body chemicals induce abnormal reactions; the autistic child demonstrates being neurologically compromised, unable to relax when one normally would or could. Chemicals are drugs and drugs are chemicals; you would not take a drug unless you had a problem. Chemicals all have effects and it is not health wise to be exposed to unnatural to the body chemicals when you are perfectly healthy, and it is sheer madness to inject unnatural to the body chemicals in perfectly healthy and/or in quickly developing tiny babies, little infants or small children. Free, normal, responsible parents do not want to be mandated to inject!

At what risk do we dare put our children under must not be up to wayward government or the puppet government of vaccine producers who are bent on profiteering from vaccination; PARENTS MUST BE SECURE IN SECURING THEIR CHILDREN'S WELFARE! If there is a benefit from vaccination it must be carefully weighed against any actual or unknown negative to health consequence of vaccination. CHEMICALIZATION AUTISM is something that parents must be free to guard against and that must include refusing vaccine chemicalization. There is growing oppression upon our liberty to be self-sufficient or self-regulating individuals; lobbied for regulation is destroying fundamental liberty. The clear majority want to know what they are eating thus, want GMO's labeled and yet, they keep us in the dark; uninformed that the it is GMO. The public wants freedom of consumer choice and do not want most of the food they eat to be GMO. Because GMO's are patented, can be owned and meg-profited from, it is pushed upon us. It is lobbyists securing a way to make unconscionable profiteering from GMO's that make it permeate the market place as undetected; with no consent or approval of the People and it is not in the best interest of the People. GMO's are taking over; the corn and soy products in supermarkets are now 90% GMO. Freedom of choice and/or decision as to what is best to eat is being severely limited. Vaccination mandates is what has seeded or lead to this anti-freedom way of life; it has spawned the pathway to further enslaving. Big-Pharma, chemical industry, Monsanto's and/or lobbyists dictate, mastering over us; liberty and the American way of life is all but lost. Proper law is what the People want and is for the best interest of the People! Securing America, with the TWO STEPS OF CORRECTION will make order out of chemical chaos and stop the escalating chemicalization autism epidemic.

We must be extremely diligent and careful not to have our tiny babies or very young exposed to chemicals that have magnetic signatures or chemical propensity that is disruptive to the homeostasis and/or biology of their quickly developing bodies and systems. **Autism results from chemicalization of the body with chemicals that are unnatural to the body. Vaccines are laced with alien, unnatural to the body chemicals that seed/spawn Autism.** Vaccine chemicals are injected according to the recommended high frequency vaccination schedule. These multiple frequent vaccine chemicals are directly injected into our children; unwisely, brain cells are being doped with all these chemicals. A type of allergic response first occurs but rather, the attractive, repulsive and other molecular chemical properties of the vaccine chemicals results in chaos and abnormal manifestations within the blood and brain cells. Be free to reject injection!

Health requires a natural to the body chemistry; a developing child's nervous system is reliant upon chemical homeostasis. The nervous system malfunctions with improper chemistry; neuronal synapses cannot produce required impulses because of abnormal chemistry. Parents' not government, have the Right to determine if the risk from vaccine chemicalization is too great! Parents must be free to make the vaccination decision and if necessary agonize over the pros and cons of vaccinating or not vaccinating. Parents need to be **informed** about the pros and cons in order to either give their **informed** consent or **informed DENIAL**. Parents should look beneath the surface of things; access the truth about vaccine chemicals and/or know the chemicalization negatives and **be free to refuse** vaccinations. Know unnatural to the body **chemicals are the enemy** and injected ones are the worst! The number one way to prevent autism is maintaining one's internal chemical homeostasis and/or purity; parents must not be enforced to compromise their young offspring's chemical makeup! The People do not want mandated vaccination slavery!

We need to first be convinced that a vaccine is safe to consider it; we need to have an improved understanding of all vaccine particles and their deleterious propensities. Its properties and what transpire must be properly traced, mapped and/or its behavior captured; otherwise, we are blindly injecting these chemical laden vaccines. All the known signs and symptoms of a post vaccination negative reaction must be given to parents, so they can make an educated/informed decision and be on the alert for negative reactions. The signs and symptoms, post vaccination, are only the tip of the iceberg of health degeneration related to vaccine's toxic chemicalization. A fuller and much deeper analysis and examination is required! Once parents are properly informed they must be **FREE** to deny or accept all vaccinations. Chemicalization of healthy children is unwarranted and too dangerous! The normal chemical reactions within children are abnormally altered or mutated by unnatural vaccine chemicalization. Those who fall victim to **VACCINE CHEMICALIZATION**

AUTISM are not the exception; it has become common place and is the cause of the autism epidemic! Know what is in every vaccine!

What have they done to vaccine's that make parents so upset? What chemicals have they used in the vaccine's production? What have they exposed our children's developing and susceptible brain cells to? What can parents do to protect their children from unwanted, chemically laced vaccine injections? The answers to all but the last question will be quite upsetting to rational caring parents however, the answer to the last question will be a sure road to relieve parents from the untenable position in which parents have been placed. **Parents have been placed in an untenable position by the erroneous vaccination mandate law, which improperly gives Vaccine Producers and enforcement of vaccination much too much power over us; rendering parents devoid and/or divested of their natural Right to protect children from unwanted, invasive medical intervention and/or vaccine CHEMICALIZATION. While it is true that not all unnatural to the body chemicals are equal; it is certain the presence of such chemicals in human cells is a recipe for health disaster. If you question how unnatural body chemicals impact health can negatively just look at how invasive Chemotherapy not only causes healthy cells to dysfunction; it can cause cellular death. Parents do not want vaccines to have unnatural to biology or body chemicals for profit.**

My long-ago prognostication, about the harm caused from vaccine's unnatural to the body chemicals that are injected into the homeostatic or natural chemical contents of the blood, will be proven absolute, as detection ability improves. Indicting what chemicals are in vaccines that are unnatural to the body and what negative to health reactions are caused by these chemicals will be slowly but surely be recognized for what is. Currently vaccines are unfit for injection and vaccine producers are woefully unprepared or have the capacity to secure children's chemical stability and/or safety. The **TWO STEPS OF CORRECTION**; will accomplish the end to such, chemical Russian roulette before this total understanding of how and/or why injecting unnatural to the body chemicals is so, so bad! It is a no brainer; injecting vaccine concoctions of who knows what of unnatural to human biology chemicals will be considered one of medical history's worst blunders. The blunder is the gross violation to the vaccine recipients' right to be healthy and parents' right to self-protect their young children! The health decay and/or negative health transformations that have been witnessed, time and time again, by observant parents and by the children's observant doctors, must be adequately researched and parents must be **ADEQUATELY WARNED** before the vaccination decision is to be determined. **Without liberty to refuse vaccinations; vaccines will not be safe, and our children remain at grave risk!**

Healing chemicalization Autism and/or chemically induced autism needs parents to assist in assuring their children's chemistries are purified having only chemicals that are natural to the body, utilized by the body and needed to be maximally healthy and once a near normal chemistry is achieved and the consequences of being injured by such chemicals are corrected then health may be restored to an improved degree and perhaps possibly to a normal degree of health. Within only 2 or 3 months if it is done accordingly these positive changes will begin to have normalizing affects such as, but not limited to the start of increased focus or improved attention and demonstrating an improved capacity. Recognize that assuring a proper natural structure and/or having a spine that is optimally positioned will allow for normal function and assuring the proper natural chemistry will allow for

normal function; both spinal proper position and chemical excellence equals a normal healthy condition and that the pursuit of excellence for both will best achieve optimum health and prevent or recover from chemicalization autism and/or induced chemically spawned autism. For the sake of children's health, know this! The infinite biological paths are blocked or interfered with when unnatural to the body chemicals are present. We must stop the relentless industrial machine of mandated vaccine chemicalization. Unnatural to the body chemicals degrade function; there comes a tipping point, a chemical tipping point that spawns' autism! Once chemicalization is stopped there is an enormous capacity to self-heal and recover rapidly!

It is very sad that our legal system has been hijacked by lobbyists who push for law enactment that one-sidedly benefit certain corporations but not the public; mal-law results such as, the mega-money generating vaccination mandate that causes unsafe vaccines and consequential, children's health demise. Mal-law enactment is enslaving parents to surrender their children for unwanted harmful chemical infiltrations which are injections of unnatural to the body or biology chemicals. One's chemistry dictates health or autism. The right chemicals are needed to make molecules that are required to remain healthy and the wrong chemicals spawn abnormality and/or autism. Needed for health molecules depend upon building block chemicals; effecting the nervous system, endocrine system, metabolism and on and on and on. The cells of the body all have receptors for molecules that command cellular function therefore, the chemicals within impact molecule formulation character and thereby, effect cellular function. Unnatural to the body vaccine chemicals have adverse effect on required for health molecular formulation and causes formulation of abnormal to the body molecules that should not be. Be aware that we need chemicals which, are the building blocks of molecules, health or life and steer clear of chemicals that are unnatural to the body which, are the chemical stumbling blocks of health. GET THE CHEMICALS OUT; by having vaccination based upon the TWO STEPS OF CORRECTION! Mandated vaccination has unhealthy results!

One cannot trust in a money-based vaccination system, it will not do the right thing to protect us in fact; one is accurate in trusting that the system is geared to make the most money and not protect us. They have breached our trust by allowing unnatural to the body chemicals in vaccines; a destabilizing chemicalization of our babies, infants and very young children. Because of profiteering from sales of chemicals or increased profiting by putting these unnatural to the body chemicals in products; the products and/or food we eat and vaccines we inject are all tainted with these chemicals that maximize profit. The unnatural to the body chemical exposure problem is saturating the market and unless you become aware of it and do something about it; your children will fall victim to it! Subway' food chain and many others put chemicals in bread to keep bread soft when it naturally would get hard; this chemical is the same chemical that they put in yoga matts to make them rubbery and we are eating this chemical garbage. There is regulation that baby's blankets must have fire retardant in them and it has been found that these chemicals have found its way into the blood of our children. They put fluoridation in the drinking water of many communities in a mere effort to prevent cavities and this chemical is suspected of causing cancer; the money machine of the chemical/Drug industry lobby for it. The farm industry uses a vast array of chemicals to make fruit appear perfect and they use way too many chemicals that manipulate growth such as, to thin the number of fruit grown so that the fruit grows larger. Among the long list of farm chemicals, we are exposed to common names are Ethephon, Carbaryl, DNOC, NAA, NAAm, Alsol, Oxamyl, Cytokinin, Gibberellin and Silvex. However, it is the multiple injected vaccine chemicals that by far is greatest chemical insult to children's health; chemicals for profit, not safety is in most if not all vaccines. Chemicalization warfare is being posed upon us; be acutely aware of it; avoid it!

Taking antioxidants are the rave for assuring health. Vaccines test as oxidizing, which is the opposite of an antioxidant. Oxidation is the process of rusting, or the browning of an apple; the effect of oxidants injected into the body is that they lead to the breakdown of cells. OXIDATION has been shown to be the cause of accelerated DEGENERATIVE DISEASE. The chemicals of vaccines trigger abnormal reactions, magnetically alter their surroundings and change the environment that the cell's genes are commanded from. People need the basic dignity to be left alone and not have to inject substances that oxidize. FREEDOM TO REFUSE INJECTIONS THAT OXIDIZE IS ESSENTIAL. Injected chemicals are the most dangerous of chemical insults; steer clear! Parents do not want to take any part in abusing children with injections of unnatural to the body and biology chemicals. Do not dope your offspring's blood and brain cells with chemicals that have no beneficial presence or that cause cell dysfunction or destruction! Do not stand by an allow your children to be violated; the injection of unnatural to the body and biology chemicals is unhealthy, a direct strike against one's welfare. People do not want to be mandated to be vaccinated and want SAFER vaccines.

The People want vaccination, perhaps, one of man's greatest gifts to man, to be a rational, safe option. Being vaccinated must not compromise one's chemical integrity or poison one to any degree in the process. There is absolutely, no health benefit to having chemicals for profit and not safety in vaccines. Yes, parents want this option to protect their offspring from childhood diseases however, they do not want to be enforced by mandate to do so! The enforcing of vaccination is a main reason why vaccines are not chemically pure as possible and therefore, not as safe as they should or could be. The People want vaccines to be as safe as possible and want every implementation applied to vaccines in order, to assure our children's vaccines are optimally safe. Prompting vaccine producers to not use chemicals for profit and not safety in vaccines, is crucial; not having unnatural to the biology or body chemicals in vaccines must be instilled in those that produce vaccines. The TWO STEPS OF CORRECTION assure children's optimum safety!

Individuals must be masters of their own domain and/or personage; parents must hold their offspring's welfare without undue influence by outside forces and not be commanded to have their perfectly healthy children be subjected to unwanted vaccine chemicalization. What is injected into oneself or into one's children must be up to the individual or the parents of the potential child recipient. Injecting vaccines impact health and thus, is more egregious to not have liberty to self-regulate one's internal chemistry. Vaccines are not as alkaline, efficient or effective or as safe as parents' might want for it to be injected into children's delicate and susceptible bloodstreams. The People want the basic freedom to decide what is best for their health and not be forced to do otherwise! If one wants to safeguard their natural chemistry and/or assure one's alkalinity by not bastardizing one's chemistry with unnatural to the body vaccine chemicals that individual must be free to do so. CANCER has been shown to thrive in ACIDIC environments therefore, in pursuit of keeping blood and/or body as alkaline as possible you must assure alkalinity and/or be free to refuse acidic vaccines. Many rationally conclude that vaccines cause cancer and is the main cause of the autism epidemic since; they are acidic and have anti-health chemicals with degenerative propensities and cause unnatural electro-magnetic upheaval. FREEDOM TO REFUSE INJECTIONS IS ESSENTIAL. The People want to be free to protect their children by preventing unwanted chemicalization injections!

The inherent danger of chemically doping children is what parents need to be free to prevent. Parents require the basic liberty to say yes or no to any preventative healthcare. Unnatural to the body vaccine chemicals increase the risk of a critical mass chemical syndrome; the individual's blood chemistry becomes saturated with vaccine chemicals (a chemical tipping point is reached) spawning abnormality and/or autism. The chemical doping of brain tissue alters the normal environment of the cells causing a corresponding dysfunction of the brain cells. Once the critical mass is reached an unstoppable unleashing of negative to health reactions ensues; nervous system malfunction is inevitable, and Autism is spawned. Chemical toxicity creates inescapable negative to health results. Autism is the direct result of the reaching of a critical mass chemical syndrome chain reaction and/or chemical doping of the brain. Vaccine chemicals that are unnatural to the body are contaminants, toxins; poison. FREEDOM TO REFUSE VACCINE INJECTION IS ESSENTIAL FOR HEALTH AND IS A FUNDAMENTAL LIBERTY!

Do not be foolish by leaving the fate and/or health of your children strictly in the hands of those who profit first above all or Corporate America or be subjects of the whim of Vaccine Producers. Do not let them enslave you to chemicalize your children! It is far better that parents be legally enabled to perform their natural parental responsibilities; allowing parents to determine just what is best for their perfectly healthy children especially, in a non-emergency need of care situation. Truly, parent's freedom to protect their children from corporate greed, happenstance and/or chemical exposure is essential. Parents' controlling whether a vaccination will or will not be delivered best serves to promote safer vaccines and is in the best interest of children. Parents need to be free to not expose their children to chemicals or unwanted chemical injections. It is much too harsh, too draconian, to enforce unwanted CHEMICALIZATIONS.

What parents reasonably require is the Self – Preservation Right of INFORMED CONSENT/ DENIAL prior to any vaccination and the informing aspect must be thoroughly realistic and/ or legitimate. The infusion of foreign to the body vaccine chemicals into children's delicate and susceptible bloodstreams is a critical recipe for breaking apart good health that leads to health abnormality including but not limited to Autism. The mandated vaccination law with its resultant coerced/forced takeover of the natural control of our bloodstream puts us at undue risk; this will go down in the annals of medical history as one of its darkest moments as it is, tyrannical medical intervention. We need to be totally released from onerous mandated vaccinations to live in a state of freedom. FREEDOM TO REFUSE INJECTIONS and/or to control your and children's healthcare destiny is self-preservation and parental protection of children. This freedom is crucial whereas, mandating vaccination is comparatively, trifling and yet; very dangerous.

You never know when your child may be placed in some unexpected danger but as a parent you want to be sure you are free to spring into action to protect your child if it is at all possible to do so. When parents know in advance that a danger is imminent or estimate that something will cause a health problem in their child; parents absolutely want to be free to stop or prevent any imminent threat targeting their child or prevent any possibility of harm to their beloved child. Ongoing vaccine chemicalization regimentation is this threat on steroids. Mass quantities of parents are now recognizing mandated vaccination as a strong possibility of harm. The People want to be free to be parents, in fact, free to be the very best parents that they aspire to be! When parents decide that any vaccine chemical concoction is too dangerous to inject or will subject their child to any degree of harm or that the vaccination is not in the child's best interest then without question, without doubt; parents must be completely free to protect their child by refusing the vaccination! No parent who determines that a vaccine is too dangerous to inject should be coerced, enforced or be enslaved by vaccination mandate to subject their precious child to any unwanted vaccination and/or perceived of danger! Parents are the natural guardians of their children; they must be empowered to protect! No law shall disenfranchise, diminish, lessen or disembowel parental protection of children! Parental freedom to protect children from unwanted vaccines must control all vaccination!

Our children are all normal in that, they are all naturally sensitive to unnatural to the body chemicals and will have an allergic type reaction if the chemicals are toxic enough and/or the chemical quantity is significant enough. Unfortunately, the chemicals that have been found in vaccines would most probably insight negative to health consequences and/or the possibility of allergic reaction. Allergic response shows observable signs of a problem; indicating that an ongoing gamut of harm is occurring. In addition, how these chemicals enter the body has to do with the level of harm or abnormality caused. Vaccine chemicals are directly injected to quickly find its way into the blood and circulate into brain cells; the natural chemical balance is thrown off. It can shock the system; its injection gives these chemicals an overpowering bad effect. Vaccine chemicals upset the intricate chemical world within the blood. There is a spontaneous breaking down of the vaccination recipient's homeostasis; optimum health is rendered less possible. This break down initially registers as signs and symptoms, (side-effects from the vaccination) that is proximate in time to the vaccine injection. As this alien, foreign to the body, vaccine chemicals fester within the vaccinated child; their mid-term and long-term presence have deleterious impact; causing Autism. Vaccine **CHEMICALS** are injected directly; it quickly enters the blood; thus, the chemicals have greater negative to health impact. Parents' protect your children's delicate health!

An example, of how vaccine chemicals cause major life-threatening health problems is Intussusception from the Rotavirus vaccination. The Rotavirus vaccination given to children was taken off the market, after it was finally recognized that it caused a life-threatening problem known as Intussusceptions. Intussusceptions, a condition in which part of the intestine slides into another part of the intestine, called telescoping, can be life-threatening. Science cannot explain the mechanism behind how the **UNNATURAL to the body** Rotavirus vaccine **CHEMICALS** cause intestines to be so unnaturally commanded or caused to do such an abnormal, life threatening thing; it is like an alien has taken over one's intestinal track and it can kill you. Vaccine chemicals have properties that dictate and/or cause abnormality. The fact is that all alien, foreign to the body chemicals are transgressors of health; injecting such, chemicals is a **chemical ticking time bomb. Fact is, that the chemical toxins of vaccines take their unhealthy toll on everyone; just more so in individuals who are already chemically compromised.** Imagine, if the chemicals constituents of just one vaccine can cause such a horrid, life threatening intestinal telescoping; certainly, the array of chemicals from all the other multiple vaccine chemicalizations must be avoided. **STOP CHEMICALIZATION AUTISM!**

Unnatural to the body vaccine chemicals do cause horrific problems. Proximate to the time of injection problems are not often that detectable. In addition, vaccine chemicals from the multiple vaccination exposures interact over time to cause degenerative health. Many related health problems are insidious; showing themselves slowly over a long period, eventually, there are abnormal changes with mental, physical and/or visual manifestation. Logically, there are many undetected harms that mandated vaccinations do cause. Know that harm comes from the entire list of unnatural to the body, vaccine chemicals such as, but not limited to glutamate and aluminum; that is being infiltrated into our children by injection slavery! The health uncertainty principle from undergoing unnatural to the body chemicalization is enough reason to be free to refuse. We must free ourselves of being subjects of vaccine chemicalizations by **ABOLISHING VACCINATION SLAVERY. Be in control of your children's blood chemistries'; make sure you remain connected to your children and not be distracted by mal-law monopolization!**

Parents must be completely free to decide if the benefits of the vaccine outweigh the risks and/or when a vaccine is too dangerous to inject be free to decide that it is best to refuse it. Proper parenting does not allow for children's well-being to be contingent on anything external to themselves - not the will of others, not the wayward regulation of vaccination mandate and/or what vaccine producers dictate, and certainly not anyone else's decision to have your children suffer a vaccine chemicalization that you the parents' think is unwise, unhealthy, too dangerous and/or not in your offspring's best interest. Is it safe, is it safe, is it safe; should keep repeating in the minds of parents as they contemplate the vaccination debacle. What perfect strangers to your children think is safe or what those who are bent on mega-profiting from vaccination determine is safe is probably not what those who truly care about children think is safe and is not at the proper level of safety of parents. So why on earth or in heavens name are we enslaved to submit to what strangers think best! The People want vaccination decision freedom; the People want to abolish vaccination slavery. Are vaccines safe to inject or in the best interest of your children; decide for yourself and never submit to vaccination SLAVERY!

Parents are adept at taking care of their children, they dominate in knowing what is best for their offspring whereas, for government to do so or command vaccination or intervene, control or supersede is a wayward concept and fraught with conflict. The general rule is that parents control their children's health decisions and so must be true for the vaccination decision! Enforcement by mal-law to have children punctured by unwanted needle and injected with unwanted chemicalization must stop! Power over one's blood chemistry must be self-directed and not commanded over by government or private industry; this ruling is pure law, natural, and/or divine law. Harm is being perpetrated upon our children due to the mal-mandate. It is not for government to decide if vaccines are safe to inject; it is for properly concerned parents!

The pure chemistry of health is being adulterated; this atrocity is taking place despite parents not giving their true informed consent and without parents being free to litigate against vaccine companies for negligently produced vaccines that cause injury. Vaccines destroy the individual's purely natural biological chemistry. The **CHEMICALS INSULT** of vaccines causes abnormal reactions, which continue to react over months and years. Chemically, induced transmutations take place and optimum health is rendered impossible. It is understood that **the life of the flesh is in the blood**; any unnatural to the body chemicals introduced by injection into the blood pollutes the blood and thereby, the flesh is polluted. **The cells of the brain are directly negatively impacted by vaccine chemicals injected into the blood; malfunction results. Mandated unnatural to the body vaccine chemicalization is cause of internal chemical turbulence and overpowering someone by enforcing it causes mental internal turbulence. People must not be molested or battered by unwanted vaccine chemicals; be free to control oneself! Every chemical has intent and/or an energy; it is extremely important to health to remain chemically natural or pure and not be poisoned by alien chemicals which, are unnatural to one's biology, physiology and/or is not part of the homeostatic chemistry.**

According to an October 2005 article in "JAMA Pediatrics", approximately, 28% of pediatricians might dismiss you for refusing any single vaccine, and 39% of pediatricians dismiss patients who refuse all vaccines. What these doctors are forgetting or are breaching is that informed consent/ DENIAL law affirms the patient's right to control their healthcare destiny and protects the patient freedom to refuse unwanted healthcare such as, vaccines. Doctors are acting unethical when they dismiss a patient or are coercing or enforcing a vaccination mandate with the threat of dismissal or rather, patient abandonment. When parents' fear vaccination or think the chemicals in the vaccines are not in their child's best interest; they must be free to refuse it! **Transmutation of the normal chemical reactions of the body is caused by the infusion of vaccine chemical toxins. Transmuted end products follow; releasing who knows what upon our children's internal homeostasis. Chemicalization, distorts the once pure health generating atmosphere. The initial shock of the chemicals injected, and their interplay can in itself cause a critical chemical mass syndrome that leads to autism. The once healthy environment is turned into a polluted environment that commands our genes, alters internal chemical reactions and leads to the destruction of health; Autism is spawned. Science confirms this understanding of renegade chemical reaction and/or alteration; it is indisputable that chemicals dictate the reactions and the end results of reactions. We must prompt the end of enforced CHEMICALIZATION; abolish vaccination SLAVERY!**

The FDA and/or the vaccine industry refuse to recognize that **CHILDREN ALL HAVE A NATURALLY SENSITIVE CHEMISTRY and that vaccine chemical exposure is a problem**. They would lead us to believe that only certain children are uniquely sensitive but in reality; all children's health are put in jeopardy by vaccine chemicalization and that is why there is an autism epidemic. **The chemistry of children that have already been manipulated or rendered unnatural will be more sensitive to vaccine CHEMICALIZATION but make no mistake; vaccine chemicals are the real problem. Injection of vaccine chemicals is an unnatural chemicalization that upsets the chemical homeostasis required for optimum health. Chemical toxins of vaccines take their unhealthy toll on everyone, reactions from vaccination are not because your children have some freakish, "unique sensitivity"; it is the vaccines that are to blame and not your healthy children that all react negatively to it!**

The FDA has been hijacked by Big-Pharma, it has become a master of distortion, deception and manipulation of the truth instead, of properly, being a master of securing our children's well-being; they refuse to acknowledge that vaccines have bad chemicals and that **it is vaccines that are the real problem.** FDA's deceptive contention that is only certain children who have a "unique sensitivity" to vaccines is hogwash. The FDA has shut its eyes to the harm caused from vaccine chemicals and is too slow to recognize related insidious neurological and endocrine developmental problems. In order, to have prevented the Autism epidemic we needed proper leadership with no conflict of interest. It was very foreseeable that injecting such, unnatural to the body chemicals would cause health problems. FDA has too long been on constructive and actual notice of the dangers of injecting unnatural to the body chemical toxins (poisons). The FDA operates under conflict of interest; **it receives 40% of its funding from the pharmaceutical industry** that they are supposed to be policing. The FDA does not analyze drugs at an arms-length investigation either, for approval or to be removed from the market. Many FDA employees have benefited financially from the pharmaceutical industry further evidencing a major conflict of interest. FDA commissioner, Margaret Hamburg is said to have received 2 million dollars from the pharmaceutical industry. Do you think that the highest-ranking officer of the FDA has a conflict of interest? Do you think money can induce one to turn a blind eye in the drug/vaccine approval process? **Parents' must be children's ultimate protectors and not the FDA or government!**

The FDA certainly, appears to be doing the pharmaceutical industry's bidding by protecting them and/or their drugs. The FDA inexplicably and inequitably allows drugs that cause injury and even death to stay on the market and yet it attacks natural cures vehemently thereby, eliminating competition for their best financial friend. The FDA looks after the Drug Company's best interest by attacking natural cures and wrongfully banning natural cures. The FDA is very quick to act to shut down natural remedies and/or call them ineffective and dangerous even though they have no credible evidence for it whereas; it strongly supports and bolster drugs and/or their use even though there is strong proof that a drug causes major injury. This bias behavior is repetitive, shows a pattern of preferential treatment; acting to benefit Big-Pharma. In addition, the FDA appears to be helping Big-Pharma by eliminating natural cures or competition.

The FDA wrongfully, inequitably and **QUICKLY** banned the use ma-hung, a natural source of Ephedra, merely citing that ma-hung only appeared to be linked to 153 deaths and yet the FDA wrongfully allows big money-making drugs such as Vioxx stay too long on the market; it was confirmed that 100,000 have died consuming it. David Graham, the FDA's Deputy Director of the office of Drug Safety said that the "FDA is currently incapable of protecting the public against another Vioxx, we are virtually defenseless.", and "The FDA is incapable of protecting America from unsafe drugs or another Vioxx." He repeatedly stated that there is **undue influence** going on at the FDA and that "there is **INCENTIVE** to review the drugs as quickly as possible, approve the drugs a quickly as possible and **don't stand in the way of making profit." The approval process for drugs and vaccines is now CORRUPT; there no longer is a reliable legitimate investigatory approval process. Parents must never place children's health decisions in the hands of conflict of interest or FDA incompetence or be enforced to suffer a mandate.**

Yet another example of FDA one sidedness is how it completely ignores the fact or turns away from the fact that Aspirin kills over 2000 people a year. The pattern is crystal clear; the FDA purposefully chooses to be blind when it comes to big profiting drugs and/or vaccines and is over reaching when it comes to natural remedies that may diminish Big-Pharma profiteering. The constant attack on natural health remedies and its continued irresponsible allowing of harmful drugs to stay on the market is dangerous and not in the best interest of the public. There are many claims that Drug Companies produce ads which, make purposeful falsehoods and misleading statements about their drugs and that the FDA is aware of it and does nothing. To the rational or observant person, the FDA is not the one to entrust your children's health to; it will not assure children's health by assuring vaccines are safe. Parents' controlling children's healthcare decisions (vaccinations) can be trusted. I will state more than once in this book that vaccines have unnatural to the body, anti-health chemicals that cause Autism and that the **TWO STEPS OF CORRECTION are needed to GET THE CHEMICALS OUT and end the autism epidemic. Mandated vaccination is the mandate of chemicalization child abuse on a mass scale!**

Expose a person to unnatural to the body chemicals and optimum health becomes impossible until those chemicals are eliminated. We are exposing our children to more unnatural to the human biology chemicals than ever before. Spraying or exposing your underarms to chemically laden deodorants leads to breast cancer; note underarm lymph nodes are usually removed when the breasts are. Eating foods that have pesticide chemicals leads to tumors. If the cells of the diseased tissue are analyzed, it is likely to show chemical anomalies because of the chemical infiltration exposure. Injection of a vaccine that is tainted with chemicals leads to Autism. Injection of chemicals bypasses our natural defense against a negative to health chemicalization; making its injection that much more devastating to health. It is insane to have such, chemicals in vaccines; chemicals for profit, not safety, in vaccines must end, this utter madness must stop!

Protect children from chemical exposure and you protect them from suffering CHEMICALIZATION AUTISM! Do not let them become drunk on vaccine chemicals; If you object there must be no injection! **It is the laws of chemistry and physics applied to how unnatural to the body chemicals impact biology and/or physiology that make it clear not to denature one's internal chemical make-up or configuration**. Tumors often have pesticides in them and under the arm lymph nodes malfunction do to antiperspirant chemicals; a major cause of breast cancer. **Where do the chemicals of vaccines go after injection? Too many vaccine chemicals are injected over the young years of children; children's brains are doped by vaccine chemicals and it is up to you as the children's parents to prevent it. The next time you are faced with vaccination be sure you want the vaccine chemicalization and are not programmed or coerced into it. Make sure there are no chemicals for profit and not safety in the vaccine. The decision is yours to make; protect your child to the best of your ability!**

If the FDA deters from banning drugs or **vaccines** because of the negative financial impact on Drug Companies, then it becomes obvious that we must never let anything, or anyone interfere with parents protecting their children from what they understand as an unnatural to the body chemicalization or a vaccine that is just too dangerous to inject. The FDA may give a drug company time to supposedly, voluntarily reformulate their product without being ostracized or severely impacted with an immediate recall or ban; this is at our health expense. Parents' cannot afford to allow their children's welfares to be dependent upon such, fragile or subjective ground. The FDA's slow semi-removal of mercury from vaccines and the mercury still in FLU shots is the reckless endangerment of children and must be considered gross negligence. The FDA is very aware of health problems from all the anti-health chemicals and/or unnatural to the body chemicals in vaccines but, it does not act to protect us; meanwhile, our children's health is rapidly being lost and the Autism epidemic rages on. Another example that shows many drug chemicals are placed into the market and called; "safe" when they are not and stay on the market for years and are not banned but rather, merely given a (health advisory warning and/or removal mere suggestion) is the health advisory about drugs that contain Phenylpropanolamine. History strongly indicates that parents need to protect their children; it is much wiser to demand your Informed consent/**DENIAL in order, to best protect your children**!

Phenylpropanolamine (PPA) in products increases the risk of hemorrhagic stroke (bleeding into the brain or tissue surrounding the brain). This was a conclusion of a study that finally called the FDA into somewhat action to remove the chemical from the market. However, the FDA issued a mere warning in November 2000 and sat on its hands allowing Drug makers to take their time to voluntarily remove it from their products thereby, reformulating their products. In 2005 the FDA finally issued public warnings about PPA chemicals and listed products containing PPA; by that time too many unneeded injuries occurred, and products were already reformulated. This apparent ineptness or reckless endangerment is at the publics detriment and at Big-Pharma's financial benefit. The surfacing of this mal-behavior is only the tip of the iceberg; we dare not blindly trust Big-Pharma mega-maniac money makers to replace parents as supreme protectors of children. By natural law and the natural order; parents must be free to refuse unwanted healthcare and that includes drugs or vaccine chemical concoctions!

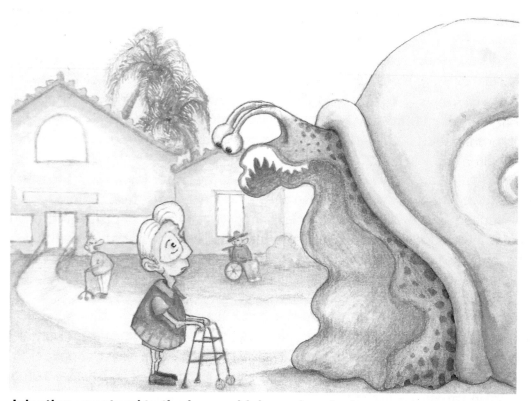

Injecting unnatural to the human biology chemicals can cause monstrous to health consequences. BE AWARE: Most flu shots still contain the forbidden mercury. Demand a flu shot without mercury!

On December 22, 2005, after all the bad and/or injury were done the FDA finally issued a notice reclassifying PPA as nonmonograph (Category II); not generally recognized as effective and safe.

It took 5 years too long to reach this life saving conclusion and there was never really a complete banning. It certainly appears, the FDA is doing damage control for the drug companies and/or trying to make them look good by making it appear as if the Drug industry voluntarily did the right thing. Countless injuries could have been prevented by quick and decisive action on the part of the FDA; we certainly cannot and must not rely on the bias FDA for our safety. Children can be saved from a life time of chemicalization autism if vaccines are prompted to become clean and adults can be prevented from succumbing to Alzheimer's disease by alerting the public that FLU shots still have mercury. Let us prompt the end of injected chemical exposures and/or **GET THE CHEMICALS OUT OF VACCINES; with the TWO STEPS of CORRECTION**. Individual's Right to Self-Determine Healthcare must control and there must be liability for negligent vaccine production to induce vaccine purification and safety. I must mention that lobbyists are ruining this country; they finance and actually draft law making. There are over 13,000 lobbyists to do drug business. Legislators' have term limits, they are here today, gone tomorrow, **which makes career lobbyists that much more powerful in influencing law**.

Think of your most prized possession or your most valuable item being taken from you and now times that by infinity and you still do not come close to grasping the importance of what the money mongrel, ill-conceived, vaccination mandate has taken from you. What has been taken from parents is the most precious right to decide what is best for their offspring in that by a mal-law, one's children must be vaccinated despite the fact, that the parents' do not think the vaccine is safe or the vaccination is not in their offspring's best interest or even if you as parents' think the vaccine will cause irrevocable harm and/or chemicalization autism to one's children. The level of personal and/or privacy violation is so off the charts that it is an absurdity. The People want and desperately need to be free to protect their children the way they specifically think is best! The corruptible or insensitive or bias FDA, CDC or puppet political hacks of Big-Pharma must not dictate or supersede parental decision as to what is best for their offspring; parents must rule! The FDA or any other non-parental entity do not have to be found guilty, by a court of law or by public opinion to have it that parents can properly protect their children; for it is the natural order, that parents be empowered to protect children and it is a perversion to have it otherwise.

The FDA and the CDC maybe being awarded for extreme pro vaccination actions or inactions and have been accused of receiving major monetary assistance or perks or **golden jobs** from Vaccine Companies or their lobbyists. The former **HEAD** of the CDC, Julie Gerberding soon after leaving the CDC became the president, of Merck & Company Inc's **VACCINE DIVISION**; you cannot have a more blatant conflict of interest. Despite the horrific optics or obvious conflict of interest and all the controversy that would follow her new found golden paying job the job was given anyway; perhaps her past performance required such a blatant disregard for appearances. This smells so bad or reeks of impropriety that one could not reconcile such a move unless they think they are above the law or could do anything they want. This attitude of doing anything they want is readily understood when one investigates how they allowed unnatural to the body chemicals for profit and not safety in vaccines. This is a gross disregard for doing what is right for the public and an in the face disrespect for public safety. Lucrative job offers from the vaccine giant during or after an individual's CDC rein is so wrong that it cannot be considered right. It is clear and convincing evidence that the CDC and Big-Pharma have strong financial ties or that performance at the CDC is tainted and/or not purely in the public's and/or our children's best interest. Yes, there are individuals that are pure at heart and incorruptible however, the possibility of making money and/or landing a lucrative job is a temptation that is over influential.

Jobs mean money and prestige, both are strong stimulus to unconsciously and/or consciously treat your real boss (Merck) with kid gloves and/or with reciprocating favor. **Power over what or how many vaccines are mandated or how vaccines are scrutinized for injury causation must never have ties to bags of money that the drug industry lobbyist carry or to the mind-bending incentive of a top paying job at the company that they are supposed to be policing; it is a horrendous conflict of interest. Parents have no conflict of interest when it comes to children; parents must have absolute control of the vaccination decision. Parents preventative health decisions must not be overpowered; we must reestablish the proper balance of power by allowing parents the dignity and liberty of self-governing their offspring's health especially, the preventative healthcare of vaccination! The grave injustice of parents' freedom to protect children being limited needs to be resolved!**

There is a code of omerta (silence) to not recognize when vaccination is the cause of injury or when Vaccine/Drug Producers do not act in the publics' best interest. Adverse events after vaccination are not being documented and are being suppressed. When parents complain of injuries from vaccination they are too often dismissed or snubbed as unrelated. To even suggest the chemicals of vaccines are injurious is an uphill battle on an icy slope. Adverse side-effects or health problems that are unwontedly recognized are minimized or put in extremely small, unreadable print or rattled off at hyper speed to make it seemingly, unimportant, unrecognizable, incomprehensible and/ or purposefully illegible. A code of omerta exists among Vaccine Producers, the CDC and FDA; **POWERS THAT ARE SUPPOSED TO PROTECT US ARE NOT**. The CDC and FDA grant unjust favor and bias protection for Vaccine Producers as they allowed **thimerosal for profit in vaccines** in the first place and later by purposely not recognizing its obvious dangerous propensity; even in the wake of countless scholarly warnings and parent's post vaccination complaints. In addition, no one recalled **all the heavy mercury laden vaccines** that were stock piled on doctors' shelves, even after it was declared that vaccines could no longer be produced with thimerosal; thereby, stopping the need for recall and consequential loss of profits. **Vaccine Producers were saved major cost for vaccine returns (CDC and FDC protecting the pocketbook of Drug/Vaccine companies) however, countless unneeded injuries from the stock piled mercury laden vaccines that were not recalled occurred. There are many other chemicals remaining in vaccines; we must stop this chemicalization. Do not be dominated or regulated by those who side with profiteering and not child safety!**

The conflict of interest that the higher ups of the CDC and the FDC have has festered into the obvious creation of danger for our children; allowing unsafe vaccines to be injected and enforced upon our children. Perhaps an extremely lucrative job with Merck & Company is for a job well done or rather, better recognized as a job not done. An elementary school student can readily discern that what has been found in vaccines is too dangerous; entrusted professionals, who are charged with securing the safety of children, to not recognize the obvious danger from injecting vaccine chemicals; is just unforgivable. Perhaps clear, valid judgment was clouded by vaccine money or made it so they would not see the apparent danger. **The 1976, Swine Flu debacle or hoax gives a perspective on how the CDC pushes unsafe or untested vaccines.** Flu shot X53A was not even tested and the CDC falsely stated celebrities' got FLU shots to convince and push the public into it. Wake up America; children are at risk without parental rule!

The mission is supposed to be to make vaccines safe and prevent harm. To sit on their regulatory hands or to fall asleep at the helm of protection or to purposely not act to protect children from further exposure to mercury in vaccines is the reckless disregard for children's welfare. Mandatory flu shots for 150,000 NYC children **still contain lots of mercury places children at further risk of Autism. Flu shots and many drugs still contain mercury; this is extremely negligent. Children and adults must not be shot-up with unwanted chemicals; there must be freedom to refuse chemicalization. People do not want to be enforced to submit their children for chemical injections and made to take the risk. People want the liberty of decision. Free people are not made to submit to injections; they do not bow to others ignorance or are thrown into a sea of chemical exposure without recourse! Free people do not have to face health uncertainty or health degeneration probability or autism because they are told they must by some renegade mal-vaccination enslavement!**

Mandated vaccination law is a modern-day enslavement law; enslaving parents to surrender their offspring to subject them to whatever vaccine chemical concoction that Big-Pharma want to profit from. This most egregious violation of parental rights and self-determined healthcare has been perpetuated upon the People with the falsehood that it was temporary and needed as an extraordinary measure during the extraordinary circumstance of an epidemic. Absent the extraordinary circumstance of an epidemic there must be no extraordinary measure of vaccination mandate! The epidemic no longer exists and there are now many healthcare options even if there was an epidemic. The emergency no longer is present and the so called need to supersede parents' protective right of their children has long ago come to an end. Vaccination was never meant to be permanent or in perpetuity! If there were no profit to be made by mandating vaccination they would not be mandated; it is all about the money and not about what is in children's best interest. Generally, parents', not puppet government are best at knowing what is best for children. Parents' decisions for the health of their children must not be blocked or superseded by mal-law vaccine chemicalization mandates. The People do not want to be enslaved to vaccinate; they demand the freedom to decide what is best for themselves and their children without undue government interference or coercion! The time to ABOLISH vaccination SLAVERY is here and now! Be free to protect your babies, infants and small children to the best of your ability; live free to reject unwanted chemicalization injections! Do you want to be dictated to inject your children with multiple vaccines even if the vaccines are laced with unnatural to human biology chemicals? Law must be for the people and what the people want; most people do not want to be forced to be injected.

CHAPTER 8

WHY CHILDREN MUST NOT BE INJECTED WITH TOXIC VACCINE CHEMICALS

VACCINES ARE NOT AS SAFE AS THEY SHOULD, OR CAN BE

The dangerous propensities of chemicals found in vaccines speak for themselves. It is understood that chemicals can cause cancer; it needs to be understood that chemicals can cause Autism. Every chemical you internalize has a physical property propensity and an energy that will either strengthen or weaken you. It's obviously a good idea and essential to health to eliminate the chemicals that weaken you, since these chemicals or energy signatures are obstacles to creating health and are building blocks of autism or not being optimally healthy. Parents should have an abundance of caution when it comes to vaccine chemicalization; have your wits about you and dig in to do the best you can to prevent unwanted unnatural chemicalization. It would be ill-advised to touch or contact certain vaccine chemicals; to inject them is so counterintuitive, so counterproductive to health that to knowingly inject it is CHILD ABUSE. Vaccine Producers do not want informed consent/ DENIAL of vaccinations because parents once informed; will wisely refuse vaccination. To inject certain chemicals of vaccines into the blood of infants must be considered an act of gross negligence and will be considered one the greatest atrocities of the practice of medicine. The lack of informed consent/DENIAL is a strike against safety. Not elaborating on the dangerous propensities of chemicals in vaccines is a malicious act against children and parent's obligation to protect them. No one should be demanded to place their child's chemistry in jeopardy or by law be enforced to expose their children to multiple vaccine CHEMICALIZATIONS.

Your body is like a chemical laboratory. The body requires a normal chemistry to function optimally and be free of abnormal health conditions such as, Autism. Parents must be free to safeguard their children's chemistry, to avoid an interfacing or formulating infant's pure chemistry with that of the chemicals in vaccines. Here is a partial list of injurious poisons, that has been found in vaccines: Aluminum, known to be associated with Alzheimer's disease and seizures and cancer producing in lab mice, aluminum phosphate, aluminum hydroxide, formaldehyde (a known cancer causing agent), polysorbate 80, polymyxin B, Neomycin, Streptomycin, 2-phenoxyethanol, Monkey Kidney Cells, Newborn Calf Serum, Ethylene glycol (antifreeze), Phenol also known as carbolic acid (this is used as a disinfectant, dye), human diploid cells (the dissected organs of aborted fetuses), chicken embryo, Formalin, gelatin, Amino Acid, Soy Peptone, Yeast extract, embryonic guinea pig cells and glutamate. We must be free to deny any chemicalization, free to self-preserve and free to protect children to the best of our ability.

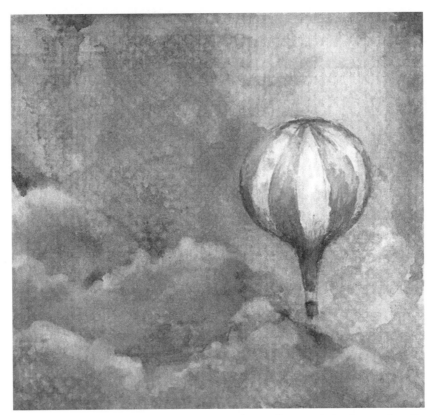

Be FREE and rise above the oppression of mandated vaccinations.

Vaccines are cultured in animal cells and that is problematic without adding all the chemicals to vaccines; open your eyes to what might be injected into your babies. In the vaccine process they infect African Green Monkey kidney cells with viruses. Viruses need live cells to replicate; so, vaccines actually come from diseased animal tissue. The separation process of vaccine from animal cell structure is far from perfect and too often contaminations of vaccines occur. Informed parents do not want their infants injected with this spew. Most people make sure the food they eat is safe; make sure vaccines are safe! Parents should be a million times more concerned about what is being injected into their children's blood than what they eat. The Autism epidemic is man-made, from injecting all the chemicals found in vaccines into babies' bloodstreams. Be aware, stealth and/or cancer-causing viruses have been found in vaccines. The vaccination industry is an uncaring business and what can be found in vaccines is definitive proof that our children are not safe. You would be astounded to learn what is in vaccines; demand to be informed.

There are many chemicals in vaccines that must be removed to render vaccines much SAFER; we must act to GET THE CHEMICALS OUT. There are a lot of smart parents out there that know vaccine chemical exposure causes Autism. Parents have become aware that the vaccine industry is more concerned with profits than their children's safety; they put chemicals for profit, not for safety, in vaccines. Children's health is dependent upon safe vaccines and it is up to parents to make sure that the vaccines are safe. Refuse unsafe vaccinations! Parents should know that vaccines have anti-health chemicals. You owe it to your children to refuse unwanted chemically laced vaccines. Vaccinations must not be mandated and parent's Right to refuse trampled upon, out of vague and remote fear that perfectly healthy children will become ill; this is especially, true when childhood diseases are not prevalent, or no emergency healthcare intervention is required. Parents must have the Right to weigh-out the risks of vaccinations and decide what is best. The impact of injecting chemicals can be staggering. Vaccine Producers and their puppet government do not recognize parent's all important need to protect their children from chemical exposure and/or unwanted medical injections. The present state of vaccine chemicals and its delivery system and/or mandate is the reckless endangerment of our children. We must be FREE TO DENY chemical injections, FREE TO POLICE one's very own bloodstream, FREE TO DECIDE what healthcare will be accepted or denied for our children and FREE TO PARENT our children.

It is outrageously unjust and dangerous that Vaccine Producers are free to put whatever chemicals that they want in vaccines and not be litigated against or punished in the event their chemical concoctions cause harm. Vaccine Producers do not have a legal care; they never will face or suffer a monetary loss when their vaccines are negligently produced with anti-health chemicals and injury is caused. **The CHEMICAL DOPING of children, via chemically laced vaccine injections, can be corrected via the TWO STEPS.** Non-parents, to the children being vaccinated all have their price, which makes vaccine safety become questionable therefore, parents legally must be free, as **GOD** intended, to protect their children from unwanted vaccine injections. Vaccine Producers and/or their vaccines wrong doings are not that rigorously investigated as they should be. Parents are left to fend for themselves; they must be the ones that protect their very own children. The good of vaccinations from shocking the system with injected antigens to induce immune response is now overshadowed and superseded by the bad from chemical harm of vaccination. Vaccination is superfluous due to the mandating of vaccinations and consequential chemicals for profit in vaccines. Parents must be free to protect their children from chemical harm. Mandated vaccination is **SLAVERY OF A DIFFERENT NAME**.

There have been no adequate double-blind studies and/or any accurate studies that prove that even a singular dosage of vaccine does not cause harm, let alone multiple vaccines harmful tendency. There have been absolutely, no studies of the cumulative consequences of exposing children to the multiple dosages of vaccines over time. Wisdom necessitates that parents have abundant precaution and not submit their children for unchecked vaccines. Exposure to the chemicals from one vaccine is a major cause for alarm and even more disconcerting are the chemical interactions from multiple vaccine chemicalizations and their long-term negative to health consequences. Vaccination being a one size fits all can be devastating to health; size counts. The fact that the rate of Autism is higher in boys signifies how different, different body chemistries are; we really do not know what we are doing when we introduce vaccine chemicals. Accumulation of the chemicals in children from multiple vaccine chemical injections is a major cause for alarm; it is a meltdown of health, a critical mass chemical syndrome, which spawns Autism.

Chemistry titration experiments indicate just how sensitive chemical reactions are; there is a finite range of chemicals to achieve the reaction you are looking for or expect. GOOD HEALTH OR RATHER, AUTISM PREVENTION IS COMPLETELY RELIANT UPON A FINITE NORMAL RANGE OF CHEMICALS INTERNALLY. The introduction of foreign to the body chemicals such as, the present state of chemicals in vaccines send the normal health generating chemistry into a degenerating health chemistry or rather, an Autism generating chemistry. Once the normal chemistry is distorted or disrupted by vaccine chemicalization there is no knowing just how harmful the results will be however, your children's optimum chemistry has been compromised and the odds are now in favor of Autism. The diagnosis after vaccine chemical exposure can range from allergic reaction, Autism and/or brain injury. Be wise; do not expose your children to chemicals not indigenous to the normal body chemistry or normal chemical reactions of the body.

Mandating chemical injections is destructive to children's health, not constructive;it sets in motion less quality control. Knowing that all children are naturally sensitive to abnormal changes to their blood chemistry and that vaccines cause internal abnormal chemistry; it comes as no surprise when vaccinations induce intussusceptions, convulsions, seizures, inflammation of the brain, fever, which may end in AUTISM. These signs and symptoms are testament to how dangerous vaccine chemicalization is and/or if disruption of the normal chemistry occurs. Unnatural to the body vaccine chemicals cause systemic and neurologic problems and are indeed the major cause of Autism and other health ailments. More indications of the onset of Autism are: no babbling or pointing by 12 months, no single words by 16 months and lack of brief phrases by 24 months and loss of language or social skills. The unleashing of injected chemicals creates a raging reaction WAR within. Every unnatural chemical plays a role to cause health degeneration and establish Autism. The war between normal reactions of health and negative reactions of Autism wages on with each vaccine chemicalization. Chemicals in vaccines for profit and not for health and the mandating of their injection, destroys the perfected chemistry of normal health. CHEMICALIZATION is the ENEMY of HEALTH and the SEED of AUTISM.

The erroneous mandated vaccination law is a VACCINATION ENSLAVEMENT LAW that enforces the exposure of children to chemicals; it is literally an act of chemical warfare upon the recipient's chemistry. Enslavement to be injected with vaccines and the unwise liability shield granted Vaccine Producers are why vaccine quality control has faltered and has resulted in children's brains being systematically chemically doped. Children's brains are bombarded with vaccine chemicals, which race through their bloodstreams after injection. We must endeavor to see to it that vaccines are produced with safety first and/or produced without unnatural to the body, anti-health chemicals. Chemical doping the brains of children must end to stop the prevalence of Autism and parents must not be plagued with the monumental impasse of a vaccination mandate.

The highest degree of quality control to assure safe vaccines must be instilled. Each chemical exposure may lead to abnormality. The least exposure to chemicals the better off our children will be. Injected chemicals pose a truly ominous threat to health. Injected chemicals do not go through the bodies filtering system such as, the selective digestion absorption or elimination process. Injected chemicals are extremely harmful because they enter the bloodstream quickly and reach the brain cells in undiminished concentration. Once the cells are infiltrated with the chemicals of vaccines the normal chemical processes of the cell are compromised. The normal transformation of one set of chemical substances to another is bastardized; chemical reactions become unstable. The vaccine chemicals in the blood enter your cells as reagents or reactants of the metabolism of the cells. Expected or optimal chemical reactions do not occur; the yield of products is altered. The precise reactions and products that are necessary to sustain optimum health are altered or lost and anti-health reaction begin; all resulting in the spawning of Autism.

The chemical equilibrium of the vaccination recipient is thrown off by the introduction of the alien to the body vaccine chemicals. Metabolic pathways are manipulated and/or interfered with because of the presence of these vaccine chemicals that should not be there. The spontaneous chemical reactions of homeostasis can no longer normally take place; reaction rates are changed, and chemical synthesis is altered. The chemicals that are present dictate what reactions take place and the reactions, which can or cannot take place, rule one's health outcome. So, called elementary chemical reactions of the body are manipulated by the presence of the alien to the body vaccine chemicals. Abnormal reaction after abnormal reaction occur because of the multiple chemicalizations of vaccinations. A critical mass chemical episode of abnormal reactions will lead to Autism. The presence of vaccine chemicals will cause renegade chemical synthesis and interfere with the normal cellular activity. The nature of chemistry is that if foreign to the reaction chemicals are present during the reaction those chemicals can interact in the chemical reaction. Electrons move when there is a chemical reaction leading to the formation and breaking of chemical bonds. There are abnormal electron movements when the chemicals of vaccines react with the chemicals of the body; abnormal formations and breaking of chemical bonds. Parents should not risk altering their children's normal biochemistry, to do so jeopardizes well-being and will likely cause abnormal bioreactions that will lead to abnormality.

Parents must not remain powerless to prevent their children from such chemical exposure in the face of what is already acknowledged about the harms that vaccine injection can and have caused. Parents' must not wait until the entire world or for those who negligently put unnatural to the body chemicals in vaccines, to wise up or have an epiphany that chemicalization causes health problems and/or Autism. Together, we must go on an anti-chemical doping of our children campaign. We need to instill protection of our children by demanding **PARENTAL SAFETY SATISFACTION**. To prevent the chemical doping of children the **TWO STEPS OF CORRECTION are required,** which requires **INFORMED REFUSAL of a parentally unsatisfactory vaccines** and holds Vaccine Producers traditionally **LIABLE** for vaccine induced injuries. The **TWO STEPS** are crucial to obtain safer vaccines and to end the Autism epidemic.

Parents should not be put in the untenable position of placing their children at risk of vaccine chemical exposure but rather, vaccinations must conform to parent's rational safety concerns. In the face of the multitude of scientific papers and the laws of chemistry that support such rational parental concern; parents must not be induced to vaccinate against their will and better judgment. **Parents must demand that no unnatural to the body chemicals be in vaccines and refuse vaccinations until they are offered clean vaccinations.** We want the purest vaccines for our children, the quintessential form of vaccines; we want safer vaccines.

Parents must not be forced by vaccination mandate to gamble with their children's lives and/or health. Parents must be free to avoid having their children exposed to vaccine chemicals. Signs and symptoms proximate in time to vaccinations confirm that exposure to vaccine chemicals is an etiology of Autism and other related health problems. The laws of Nature and/or of chemistry applied to vaccine recipients confirm that all children are sensitive to even the slightest changes to their natural chemical environment. To be enforced by law to inject a chemical vaccine is tyrannical medical intervention and is nothing less than **enslavement; it is slavery of a different name and/ or kind. Vaccinations must be an exercise of free will.**

Chemically laced vaccines abnormally alter the body's natural chemical environment. Altering the natural chemistry of the blood alters the natural chemistry in the cell and effectuates an altering of the chemical environment of the genes. An abnormal chemistry surrounding the genes causes the genes to dictate abnormal messages, a genetic abnormal expression; a type of genotoxicity. Cellular biological chemistry impacts cellular function and can allow bugs and/or pathogens within the body to multiply out of control thus, illhealth or disease. Children should not be made to endure unwanted chemical manipulations by an enslaving vaccination mandate. We must be masters of our own health and not tolerate government control of it. Parents need to free their children from the oppression of vaccination enslavement; liberate them from chemicalizations.

The cutting edge, new sciences of SIGNAL TRANSDUCTION and that of EPIGENETICS, support the understanding that if the chemistry within the body is changed, we simultaneously, change a lot more than chemistry. A change to the microenvironment will lead to a macroenvironmental change. A change in chemistry makes a world of health difference. The injections of alien, unnatural to the body vaccine chemicals, into our children's ultra-sensitive chemical/environment have significant life changing and/or negative to health consequences. Unfortunately, the present sorry state of chemically laced vaccines being injected will damage our children's genes and effectuate problems not only in them but in our children's children. Injecting anti-health chemicals is of course unhealthy but there are also genetic complications. Your genes master health and/or sickness however, chemicals master the genes; the chemicals dictate genetic expression. Stems cells placed in a Petri dish will differentiate into fat, muscle bone or whatever, depending upon, not their genetic make-up (stem cells are all the same) but rather, the environment of the Petri dish; the chemicals turn on the genetic differentiation. Autism is more a chemical problem than a genetic problem. Chemicals induce genetic expression and over time cause genetic mutation and/or weakness. Vaccine chemicals alter metabolic reactions of the body and can negatively mutate genes over time. BY RIGHT, CHILDREN'S INTERNAL CHEMICAL MATRIX is for parents to determine and have ultimate control over!

A host of abnormal changes will incur as the chemicals that have been injected are circulated throughout the bloodstream. **The transgressions from these chemicals can and will impact the individual in negative health degenerating ways; optimum health is rendered impossible.** Cytological specialization and/or cellular differentiation can be interfered with in the presence of toxins. The individual cells that are assigned to specialized tasks cannot optimally perform do to chemical toxins in the biological matrix. The pattern of cell differentiation loses efficiency thereby; the child's ability to be optimum is diminished in the presence of a chemical toxic environment. Parents must be **FREE** to protect their children from all unwanted chemicals. Big Pharma sells vaccines and vaccine recipients are the buyers of vaccines. Buyers' require the fundamental consumerism liberty to decide if the vaccine is worthy of buying and/or not too dangerous to inject into their precious and susceptible children. Vaccination must be based upon consumerism and not be enforced upon the public in order, to stop unsafe vaccine production. In addition, vaccine producers need to be held liable, made to pay when vaccines cause injury. The priority is assuring **SAFER** vaccines in the best interest of children and not the profiteering from vaccine sales; our children's welfare must be secured by the **TWO STEPS OF CORRECTION**.

Before you hand your child over to the powers that be for injection of a vaccine, do be a responsible parent; demand to know every chemical that is in the vaccine! Parents' should immediately recognize that certain vaccine chemicals that can be found in vaccines are toxic. Many of the chemicals that have been found in vaccines have a propensity to cause health problems and are extremely unwise to be injected into the blood. It is a 'no brainer' that certain chemicals used in vaccine production are health degenerating, having no business being used for our children's vaccines. A vaccine that has mercury is hazardous waste if you were to dispose of it, it should be put in toxic dump therefore, it is insane to inject it and is considered an act of child abuse to do so. In fact, if this vaccine vial broke and spilled on the floor it would be considered a toxic spill and/or hazardous waste. There is no excuse for vaccine producers' omission and/or commission of allowing foreign to the body chemicals in our children's vaccines or for the takeover of our government or regulatory agencies to allow such, chemicals in vaccines. They have destroyed the trust, which parents blindly placed in them. The FDA and the vaccine industry surely should have concluded long ago that having certain chemicals in vaccines is counterproductive to health and downright dangerous. **Parents' need to stop being so blind; parents' must take back their children to best protect them!**

How dare they not urgently, tell us or strongly warn us, about the dangerous chemical content of vaccines or not give us choice or chance to refuse such, chemicalization! It is nonsensical, or rather; it is tragic that parents' sit back, handcuffed to a mal-law that commands us to jeopardize to any degree, the optimum health of our children! They forget that these are our children not theirs and parents' have the SUPREME RIGHT TO PROTECT children from chemicalizations and/or the unwanted medical intervention of vaccine chemicalization by injection. Parents' do not want children to be in contact with dirty water and they are reverent about keeping their children's blood clean and/or free of chemicals; not exposing them to chemical folly. Chemicals are in vaccines because Vaccine Producers cannot be touched when their vaccines cause injury and do to the fact, that informed consent/DENIAL does not rule vaccinations; no matter what they place in vaccines they can get away with it. They only concentrate on putting chemicals for profit in vaccines; they do not have to concentrate on children's safety. There is a much HIGHER DANGER OF AUTISM because of mandated, anti-health chemical vaccine injections; there is loss of optimum health ability when anti-health vaccine chemicals are pumped into you. VACCINES, HARBOR DANGEROUS CHEMICALS AND CHILDREN ARE BEING STRUCK DOWN WITH AUTISM BECAUSE OF IT.

Without question, the injection of unnatural to the body chemicals into rapidly, developing children is a destabilizing force upon health, is destructive to resistance against disease, causes health problems and/or promotes abnormality. Does the placing of such chemicals in vaccines rise to a level of gross negligence or criminal activity, is a question that may need to be answered by a Jury of our Peers? The advent of vaccination was surely one of scientist's great accomplishments however; its greatness is now overshadowed by human weakness to make money. This has led to tainting vaccines with alien to the body, harmful chemicals and a wrongful continual enforcing of vaccinations upon the public in order, to mega-profit. We need **SAFER** vaccines in order, to secure our children's well-being. There are now chemicals in vaccines for profiteering reasons that have nothing to do with health. **Vaccination slavery and a consequential health epidemic have resulted from a profit first and health second attitude which, is bent on continually forcing impure vaccine injections that are too often against the will of parents and not in the best interest of children. The quasi-legal blanket immunity that was unfairly and unwisely, granted vaccine producers in 1989 allows for runaway unnatural to the body vaccine chemicalization without proper accountability and liability. The time to correct this vastly inappropriate and extreme wrong is long overdue; the TWO STEPS of CORRECTION will be our salvation!**

As science, moves forever forward it must be carefully monitored; not allowing money making to dictate or slate it. If it was not so unconscionably, profitable to keep vaccination mandated, then there would be no vaccination mandate! There is no valid reason why the vaccination decision is not allowed to be a matter of freedom of choice or for parents to decide when a vaccine is or is not to be administered or is or is not in the best interest of their children. There are so many things that parents should take into consideration before making the vaccination decision; become educated about the vaccine. It has recently been discovered that 8% of the human genome comes from viruses. The fact that viruses have infiltrated or become part of the human genome gives a clear warning that purposely, injecting vaccines with attenuated viral material could cause accelerated or additional viral takeover of our genome and/or cause a genetic disruption of the normal genetic human code. This is yet another reason why parents must weigh out the pros and cons of vaccines or genome manipulation, along with all of vaccines inherent problems from unnatural to the body vaccine chemicalization to make a decision that is in the best interest of children. Certainly, parents need to be FREE to decide what is best and not be commanded by a TYRANNICAL VACCINATION MANDATE to be made to suffer one's children with! Protecting one's child, as parents see fit, may be our greatest liberty!

Merely because there are vestiges or proven vaccination success, it does not mean that parents should not do their due diligence or safety checking and parents must always be free to refuse a vaccination. No one should be forbidden from protecting their children from vaccine chemicalization or harm. No parent should blindly accept vaccine injections or ignorantly trust that vaccinations have no major health risks. Discern if the vaccine has unnatural to the body chemicals to discover if they are dangerous. Simply **FIND OUT** whether the chemicals of vaccines that are injected into the bloodstream are considered natural or not natural to the bloodstream. Generally, if the chemicals are natural to the bloodstream; **NATURAL CHEMICALS OR MOLECULES ARE THE BUILDING BLOCKS OF LIFE and/or HEALTH** however, if the chemicals are not natural but rather, **UNNATURAL** to the bloodstream, these **CHEMICALS OR MOLECULES ARE LIFE'S and/or HEALTH'S STUMBLING BLOCKS** if they are injected. Allow your children to be chemically safer; consider only chemically **SAFER** vaccines!

Injecting vaccines or flooding a baby's blood and/or body with unnatural to the body chemicals will cause aberrant or abnormal reactions and will be a stumbling block to the needed creation of necessary proteins and enzymes. A vaccine (CHEMICALIZATION) alters, upsets, disrupts and makes impure the perfected chemistry of the body. This consequential

chemical upheaval from pumping a baby with alien to the body chemicals is what SAFER vaccines' the tax-deductible charity is determined to prevent by rendering vaccines devoid of such chemicals which, are utilized in vaccines to either maximize profits (CHEMICALS FOR PROFIT) or are in vaccines because of stupidity, ignorance or lack of taking children's best interest into account or as, first and foremost. There are some promising results with enzyme therapy in the gut to prevent Autism however, this is a mere band-aid on the problem; what needs to be addressed is the cause of why the gut therapy is needed and/or why the gut lacks needed enzymes. The abnormal or unnatural to the body chemicalization is the cause in fact, of one's inability to produce required for health enzymes. Vaccine chemicalization is the primary cause because it's chemicals are injected, circulate in the blood and penetrate brain cells, unimpeded; doping brain cells (a much more direct hit). Whereas, ingesting chemicals you have somewhat of an efficient and effective way to rid your body of the harmful chemicals; it selectively, defecates and urinates the bad chemicals out of your body. Safer vaccines' the charity works to assure your baby will not be bombarded with anti-health, unnatural to human biology and/or physiology chemicals. Let us act together to save children from unnatural to the body chemicalization! It is imperative you assure that your quickly, growing baby has a normal chemistry thereby, promoting health. A compromised chemistry will not produce normal proteins or enzymes; spawning Autism. Promoting SAFER vaccines that do not harbor unnatural to human biology or physiology chemicals is the goal and proper issue.

Everyone seems to be on the same page about the danger of ingesting or breathing in abnormal to the body chemicals such as, arsenic, mercury or aluminum or any other alien to human physiology chemical; parents are all considered right on target when they act to prevent such exposure upon children. Why is it that when parents strive to avoid abnormal chemicalization by injection, it is so often condemned? It is likely, that people are so programmed to trust in vaccines are only good and that it has no unnatural to the body chemicals. Many vaccines have chemicals which, if in food, the parents would readily refuse or protect their children from. Take control of your children's welfare, protect them from health demise by chemicalization! Do not sleep on your parental rights, do not acquiesce into unwanted, too dangerous to inject vaccines! Most parents if not all parents, become extremely, upset when strangers take control of their children especially, if that control can have negative consequences or negatively impact their children's health and especially, when what is being done to their children is not what the parents agree with. "Whose child is it anyway" is core to who should be in control. Basic liberty requires that parents be in control of their perfectly healthy children! Before your children enter a DEGENERATIVE HEALTH SPIRAL, take it upon yourself as, responsible and reasonable parents; assure YOUR CHILDREN have SAFER vaccines.

The vaccination decision for children is only for parents to make; there must be no enforced vaccination! Government has a limited power to enact laws that supposedly, protect us however, this power must remain limited and not supersede or over power parents' health decisions for their children. Corporations do have rights however, they must not supersede the rights of parents. Big Pharma' puts whatever chemicals in our children's vaccines that it so chooses however, parents must always be FREE to refuse any vaccine chemicalization that parents think as, unsafe. If the slightest amount of arsenic were put into someone's food that would be criminal and of course you are **FREE** to refuse it. Big Pharma puts poison to the body, toxic to the body, unnatural to human biology/physiology chemicals, in its vaccines such as, but not limited to. aluminum and mercury. Arsenic, aluminum or mercury or any other chemical that is not health promoting should not be in vaccines and should outrage any potential vaccine recipient. There is no health reason for these chemicals to be in vaccines; these chemicals can only cause health detriment! Just as, it is an outrageous concept that we be enforced to accept doses of arsenic; it is equally, outrageous that people especially, tiny babies, little infants and small children are enforced to accept doses of mercury or any other unnatural to the body chemical. **BE FREE, TO REJECT INJECTIONS OF UNWANTED, CHEMICALIZATION!**

Chemicalization of the brain with unnatural to the brain tissue is the cause in fact, of autism in our young population and Alzheimer's in our adult or senior population. It makes perfect sense that if you distort the needed natural chemical balance necessary for normal functionality that dysfunction will inevitably occur. Although, the laws of chemistry make it clear that distorting brain cell chemistry with unnatural to the body chemicals some foolish skeptics wanted to see proof that the natural chemical makeup of the brain cells is actually occurring. In examining the levels of aluminum in the brain, it has been discovered that the level of aluminum in the brain of those diagnosed with Alzheimer's is higher than the general population who do not suffer from Alzheimer's. Even higher levels of aluminum are found in those exposed to unusual high amounts of aluminum in the workplace or in the environment. Aluminum just as mercury, are accepted as, known neurotoxins. As we age our brains begin to accumulate aluminum in the brain as life exposes us to it however, the amount of aluminum is higher in those stricken with Alzheimer's. Professor Chris Exley, from Keele University, says "his latest research confirms aluminum plays a role in cognitive decline." The injection of vaccines that contain aluminum, mercury or any other unnatural to human brain functionality is something the public needs to be warned about (such injections are a direct hit upon brain cells with no abatement of its toxic load. Many adults after they receive a Flu shot which, contains aluminum, mercury or other unnatural to human physiology chemicals show signs of dementia and are soon diagnosed with Alzheimer's. On the side of our very young; many parents report that their children cognitively degenerate after vaccine chemicalization and then are eventually, diagnosed with Autism. The key to health and prevention of Alzheimer's and Autism is not to be chemically exposed to such, chemicals! **SAFER** vaccines, the charity, is dedicated to making vaccines with no such, chemicals.

It is absolute mad science to inject unnatural to the human biology chemicals in tiny babies, small infants and little children; only health degeneration can result! **SAFER** vaccines' the charity, quest is to end this madness by perfecting vaccines. **SAFER** vaccines strive to induce producers of vaccines to be held accountable and liable for vaccine induced injuries and grant parents there most essential protective right of children and thereby, assure the chemicals for profit are taken out of vaccines. There is a moral obligation to save lives when you can, to improve life when you can and/or make **SAFER** vaccines when you can; we must implement the **TWO STEPS OF CORRECTION**. There must be a fiduciary duty placed upon vaccine producers to achieve only **SAFER** vaccines. Parents holding their children close state what madness is this, that mandated vaccination mal-law commands parents to surrender their children for vaccine chemicalization especially, when parents know the fact, that a vaccine can contain unnatural to human biology, unnatural to human physiology and/or unnatural to the body chemicals. The fact is, there are chemicals put in vaccines for profit and not safety that are unnatural to the body chemicals; take every measure to avoid such, **CHEMICALIZATION.** Mandated vaccination is an attempt at absolute power ruling over us, allowing man's great gift to man (vaccination) to be corrupted by profit. Assure your children's SAFETY by assuring SAFER vaccines through your dominant control of the vaccination decision!

Chemical exposure is the main etiology/cause of Autism and Alzheimer's. The very first suspect and/or what doctors ask when a patient present with memory problems is, "what list of drug/medicines the patient is on"; doctors know the number one cause of mental problems is the chemicals the patient is exposed to. AUTISM and/or mental or neurological problems in children also, are primarily caused by abnormal chemicalizations and the primary source of abnormal chemicalization is vaccinations! Unnatural to the body chemicals opens the door to disease. Healthy chemicals are natural to the body and are required in order, to function properly and/or are needed to stay healthy and generate optimum life. Infiltrating the body with anti-health, **unnatural to the body chemicals** degenerates' health and can generate Autism and Alzheimer's especially, chemical or compounds like aluminum or mercury (known neurotoxins). Exposure to such, vaccine chemicals young in life can lead to Autism and exposure to such, vaccine chemicals found in the Flu shot later in life can cause Alzheimer's. **Flu shots and many drugs still contain mercury; that is crazy negligent.**

How can parents keep their children SAFE? Parents' need an unabridged ability to protect or decide what is best for children; SAFER vaccines' the charity recognizes this parental right and instinct as essential to the production of SAFER vaccines which, are not laden with unnatural to the body chemicals. It is most logical that unnatural to biology chemicalization is the cause in fact, of Autism in children and Alzheimer's in adults; 100%, optimally functioning brain cells are rendered impossible! Parents want their freedom to do what they think will assure optimal function! The brain and nervous system is like a fine-tuned chemical/electric grid and obviously, aluminum is a conductor of electricity therefore, it should not be in injected into babies! It is common knowledge that aluminum is highly, conductive thus it must be considered mad science or gross negligence or criminal to inject a vaccine with any degree of it. As far as mercury is concerned, it is off the scale of insanity to suffer our children with any degree of it. Know what is in the vaccine you are contemplating; use SAFER vaccines Org. to learn what is in the vaccine. Your baby needs you to assure that the vaccine will not chemically compromise and/or cause injury.

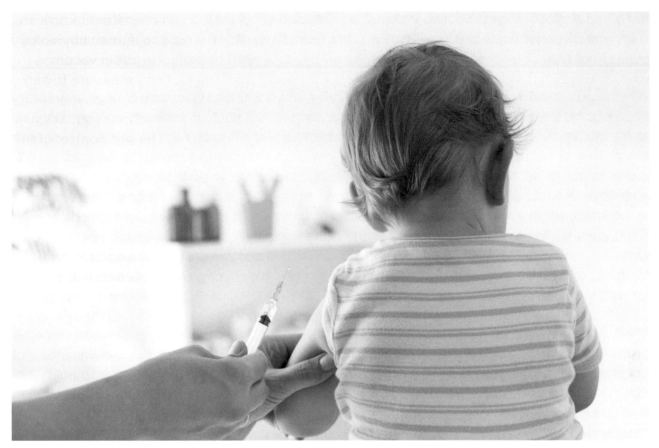

As responsible parents, before allowing a vaccine CHEMICALIZATION, determine if there are anti-health agents or unnatural to your child's biochemistry particulates in the vaccine.

Concentrating on thimerosal, the **mercury**-based preservative, it is alerting to note that although, thimerosal was banned from usage in childhood vaccines it remains the most frequently used preservative **in Flu shots**; **this is crazy and negligent**. The highly renowned biologist and immunogeneticist, Dr. Hugh Fundenberg, MD, with approximately 850 published in peer review journals, has linked Alzheimer's with the Flu shot. According to Dr. Fundenberg, individuals who received, "Five consecutive Flu shots between 1970 and 1980 (the years studied), his/her chances of getting **Alzheimer's disease is 10 times higher** than if they had zero, one or two shots." Please, understand that if you inject unnatural to the body chemicals into the blood that all kinds of abnormal processes will ensue, and health will not be preserved. The above study indicates that **chemical infiltrations are the enemy** and vaccines need to be cleaned-up. Furthermore, the unnatural to the body chemicals in vaccines is the main cause of **AUTISM**. Do not undergo unwanted chemicalization; protect your children from the same! Demand that your child's vaccines are **SAFER** vaccines; vaccines you rationally, can approve of! Flu shots for preschool children especially, if it has mercury must never be mandated as was done in NY city.

Health Alert: Flu shots are available **that do not have thimerosal,** but they are hard to come by and you must ask for them or beg for them. Grandma and Grandpa keep every IQ point you can, stay on top of your game, do not chemicalize; if you inject the Flu shot at least inject the one that has the least harmful chemicals. **People have a Right to know what chemicals lay in wait in vaccines.** People must be warned/informed about what chemicals in vaccines are not natural to the body. It must be acutely brought to attention; so that people can make an educated decision to accept or decline the proposed vaccination. Demand vaccines with no chemicals of concern; **if anti-health chemicals are in a vaccine it is controlling, rational reason, to refuse. History will reflect that countless people were injured by unneeded chemicals in vaccines.**

Why would a parent choose a vaccine that is laced with unnatural to children's biology, physiology and/or body; they, would not! Vaccines can be made without such, chemicals; making choosing to be vaccinated a much more rational choice, being a **SAFER** vaccine. The purity of children's blood, free of pollutants and/or chemical infiltrations should be monumental to parents; as it is monumental to health. To not be free to stop chemicalization is earthshaking. The anti-health chemicals of vaccines once injected will rapidly enter the bloodstream and infiltrate the brain; this is extremely unwise and detrimental to health. Let us see to it that vaccines are produced with the understanding that alien, unnatural to the body chemicals and/or anti-health chemicals are extremely unhealthy to inject. We must protect our children and seniors from the vices of medicine for profit and/or being injected with harmful chemicals. We must prompt the removal of such, unhealthy chemicals in vaccines through the **TWO STEPS OF CORRECTION**!

There are chemicals in vaccines not natural to the blood, they have alien to the body reactive properties, having propensity to create abnormality; making it a stumbling block of life and/or of optimum health. These chemicals induce renegade reactions and abnormal biological functioning; making the vaccine unsafe. Children should not be subjected to enforced injections or be infiltrated with unwanted vaccine chemicals. Protecting children's delicate and naturally sensitive chemistry must be the highest priority; allowing **informed parental denial** of vaccine injections will do just that by prompting vaccines to be produced cleanly. **Vaccines will have to pass the Sanity Test before they can be considered for injection** (to be explained later).

Why on earth or in heavens name are parents forced to blindly rely upon anyone else but themselves to discern the vaccination healthcare question or forfeit their parental control. Live by your own opinion, intelligence and convictions when it comes to the safety of your very own children. Let parents decide if a vaccine is safe enough for their children! Children's healthcare decisions must not be controlled by anyone other than the children's parents. Parent's authority or control over their children's healthcare must not be disempowered or undermined by lobbied for government rules, regulations or mal-law. Be FREE to keep YOUR child's bloodstream devoid of unwanted chemicals and/or vaccine chemicalization! What has and still is occurring to parents who refuse unwanted, conceived of as too dangerous to inject vaccination, in their honest effort to best protect their children from chemicalization impurity verges upon thogoracy. Vaccine companies and its puppet mal-government has manipulated and hijacked our legal system in an illegal attempt to void parents of their right to protect their children. Parents are being wrongfully accused of child abuse for protecting children from what parents deem too dangerous to inject vaccine chemicalization. Those responsible for the mandate of vaccination especially, when it is against parents will need to be accused of child abuse. Mandated vaccination of unnatural to the body chemicalization is child abuse on a mass scale in that, it suffers multitudes of children with such, unnatural chemicalization!

It is absurd for parents to be coerced or forced to inject their child and it definitely, should not be up to the FDA or government or anyone else except, the parents of the child, to

determine if a vaccine is worth the risks of injection. Personal healthcare decisions must be up to the individual otherwise, they are not private and/or personal! Vaccination decisions are personal and private, just like all other healthcare decisions; vaccinations must be **a matter of personal decision/choice and a matter of privacy. The bottom drops out of parenting when parents cannot protect their children from unwanted chemicalization. Decisions, about vaccination or injections of unnatural to the body substances are monumental; they are major life decisions that only parents should make! Even if the fantasy came true, that the drug, surgery or vaccine were perfect and totally safe; the patient still must have control over oneself and over one's own children; you must have the final say, being positively, FREE to accept or deny all proposed healthcare. This freedom is supreme especially, in preventative healthcare such as, vaccination.**

People must remain in control of their healthcare destiny unless, they volitionally, allow otherwise. The individual must be totally **FREE** to decide if popping a pill every time she or he is mentally or physically not feeling perfect is or **is NOT** the answer or if the individual will permit or not permit all healthcare. Even in an emergency, if, the individual is conscious and of sound mind; that individual can accept or not accept the care or accept going or not going to a hospital. There is absolutely, no valid reason, for an individual and for parents for their children, to not to be in control over themselves or for parents to be control of their children's healthcare. Basic liberty and dignity require that citizens, (**FREE AMERICANS**) have absolute control over their own bodies and that of their young children and in that freedom, decide to accept or deny of vaccination, under what is commonly understood as, **INFORMED** consent/**DENIAL**! Moreover, without exception, questions of preventative healthcare especially, surrounding perfectly, healthy children such as, is the usual case of vaccination, need to be under the supreme power and/or self-control of the individual or parent for their child. Drugs, surgery and vaccines are powerful tools when they are not forced upon us or overused. **Vaccination can be a great gift to mankind or a curse, depending on whether vaccinations are volitional or are forced upon us or overused or contain unnatural to the body chemical contents. There must be no medical intervention mandates in a FREE America. Be FREE to reject injection! Be FREE to decide the path you desire; determine what is best for you and your children! People often have rational and compelling reasons to decide against medical intervention.**

People have come to recognize that every time a drug is introduced into the body in an attempt to remedy condition A or correct function A, the drug creates a different condition and/or inevitably throws off function B, C, D or Z. We are now savvier about how to achieve health, more optimum health intelligent; we now know better; do not allow your children to have even the slightest exposure to chemicals that are not life's building blocks and/or are chemical stumbling blocks to optimum health. **People should not be enforced to inject vaccine chemicals just like people should not have unwanted pills jammed down their throats. Consumer's freedom to decline proposed healthcare is basic to our liberty and is paramount to health care quality control.** Parents must be completely **FREE** to deny vaccination and/or be entitled to refuse a vaccination that the parents are not convinced is in their child's best interest.

Even if they falsely **ASS**ume there is no risk from the medical intervention and/or vaccination the **Patient's Self – Preservation Right** must take supreme control and/or Informed consent/ **DENIAL** of care must rule. **If there is no proven risk or any risk however, minor or remote from** being vaccinated, the patient/individual must be in control of their own healthcare destiny and have supreme jurisdiction over their very own body, internal being and/or healthcare decision. DECISIONS, DECISIONS, DECISIONS, parents make all the important decisions regarding their children certainly, their decision to refuse unwanted chemically laced vaccine exposure must be honored and not subjugated or deterred!

Parents should not be pushed into doing something for their children that they do not think is in their children's best interest; parents must not acquiesce or stand idle instead, they must take matters into their own capable hands. If you think vaccines are not in your child's best interest; take control of your child's welfare! **We need not continue to suffer the consequences of vaccination industry's mass lack of intuitiveness and/or its agenda to keep us enslaved to unwanted vaccination. The FDA, Drug Companies and their puppet politicians have partnered in governance to dictate, command and enslave us to be subjected to unhealthy vaccination. They have robbed parents of their supreme Right of Protection of Children. How many of chemicalization injections and/or how many chemical concoctions must be commanded to assault and battery your children with before you scream "STOP"; I need to protect my child from chemicalization? Parents' must fend off this assault and battery upon their children and violation against parent's Right in order, to protect their children.**

Vaccination slavery is modern day slavery and interestingly, the mock vaccination Court's authority that resides over matters and renders a decision is not called a Judge but rather, appropriately, is called a **"MASTER".** In addition, those who command us to undergo unwanted chemicalization and/or do not recognize our plight and/or that we require the most basic freedom of control over what will or will not enter our bodies or bloodstreams must be considered our **"MASTERS".** Perhaps their short sightedness is because they are not personally impacted by the problem or that they all have a conflict of interest or they want to stay in control, having domination over us and thereby, assure the meg-profit vaccine machine continues without interruption or parental input. **Regardless, if parents grasp the gravity or danger of the vaccine chemicalization situation they absolutely, unequivocally, must be FREE to protect what is theirs to protect, (their children) and thereby, disallow suspect vaccines that harbor these alien/foreign chemicals from being injected or pumped into their children.**

Parents' who have done their due diligence or think it obvious that unnatural to the body chemicals create chemical imbalance or disharmony when injected into children's delicately balanced blood chemistry must be endowed to perform their inborn parental responsibility of protecting their children from this very real danger! It is incredulous that the powers that be have transgressed our trust in them by allowing such, chemicals in vaccines. It has been many a parent's worst nightmare when their children are injured by the chemicals in vaccines or upon discovering the disruption to children's natural chemical make-up or natural chemistry. Keep your internal chemistry as pure as possible and you will be as healthy as possible! Parents must be **FREE** to keep their children's internal chemistry pure and/or seek chemical excellence. Parents deciding **"NO"** to vaccination must always mean, **NO** vaccination!

The public and politicians were repetitively, given a major falsehood when we were first all duped to be shackled under a vaccination mandate that "vaccines are absolutely. safe". It is appalling how vaccine producers in the past and still today are almost deified as, all knowing, and how we acquiesce to this obstinate position that alien or unnatural to the body chemical vaccines are good ("absolutely, safe") and/or have no negative impact upon health. We **ass**ume them correct, we blindly trust that vaccines do no harm; and we have been programmed to not even question if vaccines are safe or unsafe and/or have unnatural to the body chemicals. It is established that vaccine safety or efficiency and effectiveness cannot be questioned even, in the face of differing credible reports, viewpoints, pure logic and **VALID LAWS OF CHEMISTRY. Thin ice pillars hold these deities above all contrary logic, intellectual opinion and parent observations that vaccines are not safe; rational and accurate evidence is crumbling the thin ice pillars. Science and technology should not be worshiped; it must be questioned!**

Just as, individuals are **FREE** to follow their technological gods or never question the efficiency, effectiveness and safety of vaccines; there also, must be **LIBERTY TO NOT. Individuals must be FREE to NOT be obedient to vaccination ideology or extremism** but rather, **LIVE A NATURAL LIFE and/or only be an advocate of natural healthcare;** not being shackled to invasive medical intervention or made to endure or suffer unwanted vaccine chemicalization. What is best for oneself or one's children or if a vaccine is safe enough to be injected, must be under the **individuals' self-control and determination**. It is the individual's bloodstream which, we are talking about; not the vaccine producers'. **WE MUST NOT LIVE UNDER THE CAPTIVE SYSTEM OF MANDATED VACCINATION ENSLAVEMENT!**

Healthcare decisions can be considered a matter of one's personal religious belief **as, all major questions in life are often decided upon by one's religious belief. The vaccination decision is understood by many as, a religious decision and this decision must be allowed to be lived by as it part of the blessings of religious freedom! For the sake of your children's safety, know that you are FREE TO REJECT VACCINE INJECTION; particularly, if you are religious about it! Philosophical objection or intelligent, well thought about decision not to allow your children to undergo vaccination are too often not under the freedoms that are vehemently, protected whereas, religious liberty to care for your temple (body) is a supreme Right that is protected under the highest law of the land (THE CONSTITUTION). The parental right to protect one's children from a vaccine that is conceived of as, too dangerous to inject is just as important of a right. To not grant parents this most fundamental right, is very wrong, and needs to be corrected. Parental protection of their children should be a supreme law; parental vaccination decision needs to rule over vaccination. There is such, a thin line between one's religious belief and parental decision about vaccination that it is the same. Parents deciding what is best for their children and parents' intelligent determination of whether a vaccine is safe to inject or is not in their children's best interest can be considered a religious decision. What you decide for your body or welfare or for your children's healthcare is a matter of outmost privacy, a personal decision and/or a matter of religious conviction; a freedom of religion!**

There now is an immense number of scientists, doctors, chemists and a growing rational population of trusted, intelligent individuals who warn us about the dangers of a long term, mass vaccination program and/or the harms from vaccine's chemical injections and/or that suspect vaccines are just too dangerous in their present state to inject. The sheer magnitude of parents that have steadily been reporting adverse reactions from vaccinations is cause for alarm and for the need of improved, **SAFER vaccines**. Parents crying out, swearing that children were caused Autism due to vaccinations should instill research into why its occurring and a change in safety and/or how vaccines are produced. **Presently, a vaccine injection is an influx of anti-health chemicals. SAFER vaccines, the charity, is aware of the problems parents observe after injection and is determined to render vaccines SAFER with less or NO harmful chemicals!**

With the long list of unnatural to the body chemicals that have been found in vaccines it is obvious that what vaccine producers think is safe for our children does not meet the reasonable parental standard or of the good manufacturing standard for consumer. Vaccines are laced with alien, foreign to the body chemicals such as, formaldehyde, aluminum and mercury, to name just a few and this is intolerable to most if not parents. Parents should be cautious in deciding if a vaccine injection is in their children's best interest; be in control of whether a vaccine will or will not be injected into your children's bloodstream. **BE FREE TO REJECT VACCINE INJECTIONS and vaccines will be prompted cleaner; it is in children's best interest and it will help END THE AUTISM EPIDEMIC.**

I applaud parents who demand to protect their children to the best of one's ability. Parents are recognizing that to being enforced to submit children for unwanted, conceived of as, too dangerous to inject vaccine chemicals is the **WAGING OF CHEMICAL WARFARE** upon the precious and delicate health of children; causing destruction of children's normal chemical integrity. Health is dependent upon maintaining the normal chemistry of the body; injected vaccine chemicals alter this sensitive chemical make-up. **SAFER** vaccines, the charity, recognizes that fewer unnatural to the body chemicals in vaccines the better children will be off. Parents must have a choice not to vaccinate in order, to prompt vaccine purity. Recommending vaccines with anti-health chemicals as, preventative healthcare, is counter intuitive and will cause health degeneration rather than, health resiliency. Vaccinate with only SAFER vaccines that are approved by SAFER vaccines charity.

It is a blow to one's mental health to be enforced to submit children for vaccinations and even more mentally destructive when you are convinced that the chemicals are unhealthy to inject, and one is devastated when your child suffers **VACCINE CHEMICALIZATION AUTISM.** People are steeped in their belief systems and it is mentally and physically injurious to be forced to go against one's deep rooted healthcare belief which, is too often the case with mandated vaccination. **When parents determine that an unnatural to human biology and/or physiology chemicalization will occur if the vaccine chemicalization takes place then there is no telling the severity of mental trauma perpetrated to parents and family when enforced against their will or parental decision not to inject!** Parents who concluding a vaccine has chemicals that are not safe to inject and if their children understand that their parents think vaccines are unsafe are all being injured mentally when enforced to vaccinate. Much has been written about the mind and body connection; there is a psychosomatic component to enforcing injections against parents' will and/or fears. When you are being injured mentally it has its negative to health physical ramifications. Not only is the Autism epidemic caused by enforcing unwanted, unnatural to the body vaccine chemicalization but also, an epidemic of mental trauma if done against one's will and/or if one recognizes that they are being **ENSLAVED to vaccinate!**

Today, the number of vaccine doses have increased to a point that it is considered an overburden and give great reason to be extremely alarmed over this burden of vaccine chemicalization. The adage, "the straw that broke the camel's back" can be applied to the

onslaught of overly burdensome multiple vaccinations. One mandated injection against one's will is slavery; multiple mandated injections are an enslavement that is torturous. There has never been more reason to clean-up vaccines, **MAKING SAFER** vaccines by enabling parents to be **FREE TO REFUSE** unwanted vaccine chemicalization will, help achieve cleaner, **SAFER** vaccines. If parents think vaccination is not safe or not in their child's best interest, they must refuse the vaccination. **TO GET THE CHEMICALS OUT OF VACCINES**; vaccination must be voluntary and vaccine producers must be held liable for vaccine induced injuries. Chemicals in vaccines is the **MAIN AUTISM CAUSATION!**

Vaccines are laced with anti-health chemicals making them utterly unclean and not healthy to inject. We must endeavor to make **SAFER** vaccines in fact, we need to induce or see to it that vaccine producers produce much cleaner vaccines, rendering vaccines devoid of unnatural to the body chemicals in order, for the vaccine to be rationally, considered by parents, for injection! Vaccines that are laced with unnatural to human biology and/or physiology chemicals are extremely, objectionable and not fit for injection! All vaccines must never be coerced and/or enforced however, coercion and/or enforcing of chemically tainted, unclean vaccines, is unethical, negligence gone wild and should be considered criminal and/or **ILLEGAL**. No one, should be held in a no-freedom situation when it comes to the welfare of one's children, giving parents no realistic choice but to submit children for unwanted chemicalization especially, unclean vaccines! Injecting vaccines which, are unclean; rendering children's bloodstreams unclean is a form of child abuse. Vaccine producers must be made to pay for its injurious negligence and/or when it jeopardizes our children by putting unnatural to the body chemicals in vaccines. The **TWO STEPS OF CORRECTION** will render **SAFER** vaccines and end the Autism epidemic!

All manufacturers of goods are traditionally, held accountable and liable for its products; it is an enigma that vaccine producers are not; this renders children unsafe! The power of the purse and/or its lobbying agenda has left our children less safe because this unconscionable liability shield gives less reason for vaccine quality control instead, of more. Unconscionably, Big Pharma, carved out an unheard-of total liability shield for vaccine producers to escape the rule of law (negligence law). Children desperately, need more safety measures not less; we need to hold vaccine producer's feet to the fire when its vaccines' content cause injury. Holding vaccine companies accountable and liable for vaccine induced injuries will achieve cleaner vaccines and consequently, a lot less vaccine induced injury will occur. In addition, the vaccination flood gate has been opened wide because of vaccination enforcement slavery; it has led to a breeding ground of too numerous, enforced vaccine chemical injections and there are a lot more in the planning. Vaccination frenzy extremism has occurred with vaccination domination over us. Refusal of unwanted vaccine chemicalization is a parenting obligation and an essential freedom that induces more vaccine quality control and/or **SAFER** vaccines; it protects children!

Profiteering vaccine producers are bent on jamming more and more vaccines into our children without affording parents the common decency and respect of **TRUE INFORMED** consent/**DENIAL**. They have design to vaccinate our very young children in Elementary school, **WITHOUT EVEN PARENT'S KNOWLEDGE** of this major impacting to health event. There is an inordinate amount of vaccines being enforced upon our very young, perfectly healthy children. Each vaccine has its known and unknown risks and there are the risks from the combination and accumulation of all the vaccines over time. Chemistry rules outcome and/or function and it is imperative to keep your quickly, developing baby's' chemistry pure and not injected with unnatural to human biology and/or physiology chemicals. If, these unnatural to the body vaccine chemicals are within your quickly, developing child optimum health is impossible and degeneration of health likely. The chemicals within us dictate whether we are formulating health or Autism/ADHD. Injecting these vaccine CHEMICALS is a recipe for health disaster/AUTISM.

There are risks from vaccinations that may occur over the long duration of time. The various vaccines' chemicals accumulate overtime within the body and in combination can cause problems that are unique to their combination presence. The presence of these chemicals over the lifetime of the individual can cause one to be more susceptible to health problems and/or poor health and sickness in one's later years of life. Vaccine's chemicals can remain within the vaccine recipient's body and eventually take their unhealthy toll when the overall internal body chemistry dictates it. Chemicals rule over one's reactions, metabolic production and command function; keep your chemistry pure!

Vaccine chemicals are opportunistic deleterious entities that become part of one's internal environment; they can take their toll immediately or interact when the molecular ratio allows for renegade reactions or when the chemical environment or geometric chemical proportions initiate abnormal sequences of destructive to health compounds and/or bio-hazardous formulations. Anti-health vaccine chemicals are the building blocks of Autism and the stumbling blocks of optimum health, causing health disaster; they must not be injected. Like any threat, by innate, natural and/or God given Right parents must be enabled to stand in the way of the threat and protect their children. Preventing vaccine chemicalization harm is a liberty that parents need to best protect their children. Working in partnership with the National Home Education Research Institute (NHERI) Dr. Anthony Mawson led a research team that found a relationship between vaccination exposures and acute or chronic illnesses in home-schooled children. THE VACCINATED CHILDREN HAD A MUCH HIGHER RATE OF AUTISM AND ADHD, AT A RATE OF 470% THAN THOSE THAT RECEIVED NO VACCINATIONS. The vaccinated were also, more vulnerable to ALLERGIES, ECZEMA and more frequently, suffered PNEUMONIA and EAR INFECTIONS. This study reveals what occurs after unnatural to the body chemicalization!

Parents possess the basic instinct to protect their children and protecting children is fundamental to parenting, it is parents number one priority whereas, government officials claiming that they know what is best for children and that it is in children's best interest to be vaccinated with vaccines containing unnatural to the body chemicals, do not have this requisite caring and nurturing priority to oversee the vaccination decision. Children must always have the benefit of their parents' supreme protection authority. Parents have what Big Pharma does not and Big Pharma has what parents do not which, eliminates vaccine producers and its lobbied for government vaccination mandates from the vaccination decision equation! What vaccine producers have that parents do not, is the burning desire and number one priority to make money above all and the enforcement of vaccination serves to assure its profits. Profit dictates its decisions; it is the most important priority not

our children's welfare. Parents must be **FREE** to protect children from unwanted, **PERCEIVED OF AS, TOO DANGEROUS TO INJECT, VACCINE CHEMICALIZATION**. Parents must always be secure in their basic instinct of protecting children. Parental protection of children needs to be supported by law, so parents are **FREE to protect children from** medical tyranny and stop **unwanted vaccine chemicalization!**

The mandated vaccination law undermines parents care and protection of children. Parents find themselves at odds with the onerous vaccination mandate especially, when parents become logic stricken about the unnatural to the body chemicals in vaccines. Following the erroneous vaccination mandate becomes secondary to parents when parents deem vaccines too dangerous to inject. Parents need to be **FREE** to do what they think is in the best interest of their children and/or what will secure their children's safety and well-being. **No law should disenfranchise parent's protection of their children or infringe upon their ability to do exactly what only parents do best, that is, protect the flesh and blood of their children. Protecting children from unwanted vaccinations is within the purview of this supreme parental authority. Parental decisions in healthcare must never be GOVERNMENTIZED; medical intervention must not be decided for parents or be commanded or enforced!**

As healthy, **FREE Americans, we must never be enslaved to accept any medical intervention or be commanded or held in bondage to have children vaccinated against parental will. Freedom of healthcare choice and/or informed consent/DENIAL protects us from this medical tyranny. There is a mass of documented cases that are in the public domain and have been published on the United States Court of Claims website from the decisions of Special Masters who preside in the National Vaccine Injury Compensation Program, often referred to as the "Vaccine Court" which, is absolute proof that vaccines are not only causing injuries, but that the injuries are horrific in nature and occur at an alarming rate. To enforce the masses of our children to suffer injections of unnatural to the human biology and/or physiology is truly, an act of child abuse on a mass scale. We need SAFER vaccines in order, to protect our children! We need SAFER vaccines in order, to make vaccination a rational choice! Protect your children by protecting their chemistry! SAFE vaccines and refusal of what you deem as, unsafe vaccines, is YOUR RIGHT!**These cases are in the public domain and have been published on the United States Court of Claims website from the decisions of Special Masters who preside in the National Vaccine Injury Compensation Program, often referred to as the "Vaccine Court."These cases are in the public domain and have been published on the United States Court of Claims website from the decisions of Special Masters who preside in the National Vaccine Injury Compensation Program, often referred to as the "Vaccine Court."These cases are in the public domain and have been published on the United States Court of Claims website from the decisions of Special Masters who preside in the National Vaccine Injury Compensation Program, often referred to as the "Vaccine Court."

The mal-act of government enforcing vaccination which, parents determine are too dangerous to inject, goes far beyond proper Police Power of Government; it is by far, an extreme overreaching by government and a wrongful paternalistic structuring by government that violates our Right to be left alone and/or in control of oneself. It commands parents to submit their children for vaccine chemicalization that distorts the perfected natural blood chemistry required for optimum health. **Parents duty to care and protect children to the best of their ability is not only subverted**

169

by the mandate to vaccinate; it completely disembowels the parental responsibility and authority about this most important to health and/or life vaccination decision. Mandated vaccinations violate and enslave people! People must be secure in their person; individuals' have a right to be left alone, unvaccinated; not violated with unwanted chemicalization injections. People require their most basic freedom to life, health and/or being in self-control of their healthcare, as individuals and family. Vaccination that is enforced by law, is freedom depreciation! **You are enslaved to vaccinate**; there is no realistic choice in the matter!

When it comes to perfectly healthy children there should be no regulation or mandate that overshadows or replaces parental authority about healthcare decisions. Government goes too far in its improper exercise of power to mandate vaccination especially, in perpetuity. The inappropriate vaccination mandate prompt the production of unsafe vaccines because consumerism is not being applied to vaccination. We need vaccination to be part of the arsenal that parents consider for their children's welfare and in order, for vaccination to be a viable, rational choice, we must GET THE CHEMICALS OUT. There must be no chemicals that are not indigenous to the body, not normally utilized for biological and/or physiological development or functioning in vaccines. We need to stimulate more safety control or quality control; the application of consumerism and/or INFORMED consent/DENIAL to vaccination and being FREE to litigate against vaccine producers for injuries caused by vaccine CHEMICALIZATION are necessary to induce vaccine producers to do the right thing and/or produce SAFER vaccines. To not allow refusal of unwanted vaccination that is perceived as, too dangerous to inject and to not hold vaccine producers accountable and liable for vaccine induced injuries is to place our children in jeopardy. To end the erosion of confidence in vaccines, vaccines must be made clean, be made a matter of freedom of personal choice! SAFER vaccines demand we instill what is needed to achieve optimum safety!

The mandated vaccination law wrongfully and immorally acts to make parents surrender their Right to decide what is best for their children and/or dismisses parents' ability to protect children from a conceived of and/or actual vaccination danger; it basically, eliminating parental freedom of healthcare decision for children. Mandated vaccination mal-law infringe upon parenting and at the same time, assure mega-profiteering by vaccine producers. This callous and most egregious law, grants parents no realistic choice, they must submit children for unwanted chemical injections, against parent's better judgment and/or effort to only, do what is in the best interest of their children. **Mandated vaccination regulation subtracts from parents' Right and obligation to assure the best health for their children. Parents who dare protect their children from the dangers of vaccination are often wrongfully, labeled as, child abusers; this is a prejudice and false labeling. It is not parents who refuse to allow children to suffer vaccination who are the child abusers or that violated their sacred obligation of properly caring for their children but rather, it is those that enforce unnatural to human biology vaccine chemicalization that are the ones that should stand accused of child abuse; it is child abuse on a mass scale! ABUSERS OF CHILDREN' expose children to unnatural to human biology chemicalization by injection or other means. All this inequity and injustice is occurring while vaccine producers crookedly smile since, they are impervious to legitimate legal action; in that it cannot be litigated against from parents who claim their children's injuries were caused by** vaccines. All this subversion of parenting is meant to ASSure MEGA-UNCONSCIONABLE PROFITEERING by vaccine producers.

The aforementioned, is a prejudice and mislabeling of parents who in reality, are acting as responsible, caring parents when they reject injection of their children with unnatural to the body vaccine chemicalization. Thoughts or words like, "The nerve of parents thinking they have the Right to not vaccinate children" adds to the stress that parents are under when they come to their children's rescue or aide. Generally, parents know better than the puppet government of Big Pharma that sees to it that vaccines are mandated and that children are enslaved to undergo vaccine chemicalization as often as it wants. Parents' are putting one and one together to come to realize that it is Drug and/or VACCINE lobbyists who are actually the ones that command us to spend money on vaccines and/or see to it that vaccinations are mandated; enslaving us to endure vaccine chemicalization and keep us forever under the vaccination enslavement law. Parents are concluding that injecting vaccine after vaccine or rather, dose after dose of unnatural to human biology chemicals into babies, infants and children will THROW OFF THE INTRICATE CHEMICAL BALANCE OF HEALTH. This chemicalization will cause health problems such as, cancer, asthma, allergies, early organ malfunction and/or diabetes, loss of mental optimum capability and a runaway epidemic of AUTISM. The above prejudices, deceit, violation and its command over us are why the TWO STEPS OF CORRECTION are needed to secure SAFER vaccines and/or children's NATURAL CHEMISTRY OF HEALTH!

When it comes to children's vaccination parents need their full voice and maximum power of decision. Without question, the vaccination decision is an important life decision and therefore, children's vaccinations must be decided by parents. A child's chemistry safety calls for the child's parents to decide what is best or if a vaccine chemicalization is beneficial or harmful. Vaccination advocates dare to be in control of all children's blood chemistry's, with ambition and direction to inject whatever, chemicals that are in vaccines; even if vaccines have chemicals that are unnatural to the body and/or cause injury. Fever and convulsions are just some of the injuries caused by vaccination and an AUTISM epidemic has been spawned and is spiraling out of control. Parents' need to regain control of their children's welfare to assure no more multiple infiltration of such, chemicals. We can achieve SAFER vaccines without the unnatural to the body chemicals.

Mandated vaccination' delivers a market that is handcuffed to vaccination which, induces easy money making for Drug/VACCINE companies and allows it to only be bent on making money and not health. If you cannot refuse vaccination that means it makes no difference what chemicals are in the vaccine or if it is objectionable because any objection is a moot point since, you cannot refuse it. MANDATED VACCINATION SLAVERY MUST BE ABOLISHED! Loss of control over one's own internal chemistry is a loss of essential liberty! This loss of self-control over one's very own blood and/or blood chemistry causes pandemonium; injuring people mentally and physically. Most parents submit children to be vaccinated not because they have weighed out the pros and cons of vaccination but rather, because it is the law and they have no choice but to submit; this is VACCINATION SLAVERY. Children are reduced to the status of slaves because they are enforced to endure vaccine chemicalization injections against their parent's will and/or judgment that the VACCINE

CHEMICALIZATION is not in the best interest of the children; it is a most egregious slavery, a gross loss of personal liberty and healthcare freedom. We must ABOLISH VACCINATION SLAVERY with the TWO STEPS OF CORRECTION!

In the interest of self-preservation do you think you ought to prevent the injection of unnatural to human biology and/or physiology chemicals? Do you know what chemicals are in vaccines or do you want your children injected with any abnormalizing chemicals? **Is it important to the well-being of children that parents demand SAFER vaccines that are devoid of chemicals for profit and/or chemicals that have no health benefit!** Vaccines can be made without such, chemicals. The magnitude of the chemicalization problem is exacerbated by the fact, children are expected to receive 48 doses of 10 vaccines covering 14 diseases, compared with just 3 vaccines for 7 diseases in the 1970's. **As vaccine doses skyrocketed so did Autism; an epidemic was spawned!** Now that children have become pincushions for more and more vaccines it is now of monumental health importance that we minimize the unnatural to the body chemicals within vaccines and thereby, achieve **SAFER** vaccines. The consensus, the most popular understanding and the comprehensive, all inclusive, sweeping viewpoint, about who should determine whether a vaccine is safe enough to inject; is that it is best determined by the general population of parents. The masters of vaccine production or its lobbied for puppet government cronies must not control. Parents must not be told what is safe but rather, the parent population needs to decide for themselves and as mass consumers always do, decide what the good standard is and/or what is considered safe enough to inject. **Demand SAFER vaccines!**

The fact, that vaccines carry unnatural to biology chemicals is sufficient that it can cause Autism. Brain cells functionality are completely dependent upon maintaining a perfected natural chemistry. The laws of chemistry apply to our children's delicate and sensitive biological reactions and the injection of unnatural to human biology/physiology chemicals from vaccines promotes adverse, abnormal and renegade reactions. The normal reactions within the brain cells cannot be 100% in the presence of such, chemicals. Brain cells cannot function optimally, in the presence of unnatural to human biology chemicals. We need to **GET THE CHEMICALS OUT! Vaccination needs a quality control that is instilled by consumerism. Vaccine producers will strive to satisfy parent's safety concerns in order, to sell vaccines; parents will do not submit their children for unwanted, unnatural to the body chemicalization. Individual after individual's insistence for safer vaccines is the key. Parent after parent refusal of chemically tainted vaccines and their demand and acceptance of only safer, chemically free vaccines, will CALL THE SHOTS; prompting vaccine purity and safety and will GET THE BAD CHEMICALS OUT of vaccines.**

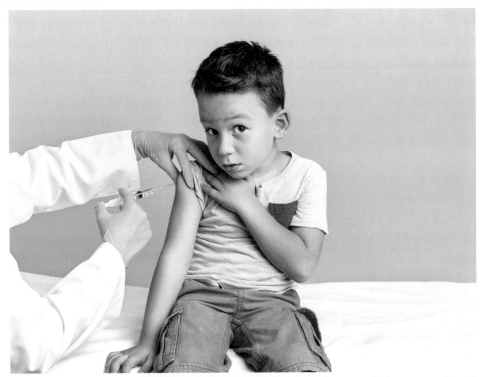

When a vaccine CHEMICALIZATION is injected, containing unnatural to human biology chemicals, it is massively disruptive to required for health biochemical reactions. Inject only SAFER vaccines!

Pertinent to children's optimum health is to minimize exposure by injection to unnatural to the body chemicals and the surest way to do that is to apply consumerism to vaccination and thereby, allow parents the Right to decide if a vaccine is or is not in their children's best interest and/or empower parents to refuse vaccines that they determine are chemically, too dangerous to inject. The general population of individuals or society's ideas on what contents cannot be in a vaccine is much more effective and efficient and American than merely relying upon the too few too powerful vaccine producers, or its puppet government. Being enforced to accept just any vaccine or a vaccine that you think has chemicals that are unhealthy is counterproductive to safety or quality control. Strictly, making vaccination acceptance or denial a parental decision or a consumer determination will help guarantee **SAFER** vaccines which, are in the best interest of children. **Vaccine producers have conflicts of interest that cloud their judgment and their numbers are far too small to DICTATE what chemicals are safe to inject. Your children must always be yours to protect; parents pure at heart health decisions, must rule!**

The collective determinations of every parent contemplating the vaccination decision will impact vaccine sales and vaccines' contents. Parents policing vaccines chemical content and determining if vaccines can or cannot be injected is consumerism properly, applied to vaccination. Parents" deciding if the contents are safe or what contents are permissible or not permissible in a vaccine will command vaccine producers to make SAFER vaccines; the way rational parents deem fit for injection. This vaccination delivery system is much more just and equitable. **The vast number of the population disagrees with what vaccine producers think is okay to put in its vaccines.** All parents giving their individual assessment, input, needs and/or requirements will trickle down to activating any needed safety changes in vaccines, rendering **SAFER** vaccines in accordance with the People's demands and expectations. **This is truly the American freedom minded way**

173

to secure SAFER vaccines. Vaccines must stand on their own merit and not be enforced upon us; safety depends on it! Safety is best achieved by refusal of unwanted, conceived of as, too dangerous to inject vaccines! In one's devout effort to not denature your offspring's perfected chemistry with an unnatural to biology, vaccine chemicalization; leave no stone unturned, make sure you know every chemical in the vaccine that is being considered for injection! This parental scrutiny and freedom will bolster and assure SAFER vaccines; making vaccination a much more rational choice.

We need a vaccination delivery system that does not coerce parents to give up their parental protective Rights or enforces unwanted chemicalization under the guise of a trumped-up Government Police Power protection. **We require that our children's vaccine supply not be tainted with chemicals for profit, chemicals that preserve the vaccine but does not preserve the optimum health of children and/or have no unnatural to the body chemicals. We need to make vaccine producers much more vigilant and caring to produce vaccines without such, chemicals. The very word parent and essence of parenting are defined by caring for one's children and/or protecting children the way parents determine is best. There is nothing more important to a parent as their children's welfare. There is nothing more important than making money to a Vaccine Company. Vaccination slavery grossly interferes with the fundamentals of parenting and what defines being a parent. Parenting authority must reign supreme when it comes to accepting or denying vaccines. Parents refusing unwanted suspect vaccine injections for their children are in children's best interest. Health is built on mere sand when children are injected with unnatural to the human biology and/or human physiology chemicals; we must see to it such chemicals are not in vaccines. We desperately, need to implement the TWO STEPS OF COTRRECTION!**

If parents detect or determine that there is something wrong with vaccine quality and/or safety, there must be LIBERTY to say "NO"; the basic intelligent design to REFUSE or STOP the vaccination. Placing the brakes on vaccinations is a freedom that must exist! Parents' being enabled to refuse unwanted vaccine chemical injections is fundamental to protecting children from harm; not being enabled to refuse or "put the brakes on vaccination" is not in children's best interest. Having vaccination mandated, with no realistic legal ability to be refused or put the brakes on the vaccination delivery, is like driving a car down a very steep decline without brakes; disaster will inevitably occur. Just as you would never place your children's safety in jeopardy by driving with no ability to brake if you detect a danger; parents should not be enforced to be careless parents by being made to place their children's vaccination destiny in the hands of strangers; with no legal ability to apply the safety brakes to vaccination or slow down the vaccination timing. Parents must be completely, FREE TO PROTECT CHILDREN! There must be parental legal brakes for vaccination in order, to prevent children from being placed in harm's way or prevent injury from chemicalization. You should not drive a car without brakes or consider vaccination if you cannot stop it! Stopping the injection of chemicals is a basic liberty.

Parents' require the Right of Legal Protection of Children; being FREE to REFUSE unwanted vaccine CHEMICALIZATION in order, to best protect their children! It must be required that parents first give their true informed consent and/or clear permission for a vaccination to take place. It is medical quackery and law enactment quackery to demand vaccination over parental objection. Parental liberty to refuse vaccination is essential in order, for parents to protect their children from a conceived of or actual danger. The decency and self-preservation of informed consent/DENIAL must rule over vaccination! Vaccines often are undesirable and chemically dangerous. All the signs and symptoms after vaccinations are testament to the fact, that vaccines are chemically dangerous and/or harmful. The special so called "Vaccine Court" has overseen damage awards from vaccine induced injuries that amount to about a billion dollars and that is with unfair caps being placed on the award amounts; this is testament to how dangerous vaccines are, and that vaccine do cause injury. Chemicalization from vaccines must never be enforced upon us!

Do you want to be FREE to REFUSE chemical injection exposure? PARENTS' YOUR CHILDREN ARE A PART OF YOU AND IT IS YOU WHO ARE ULTIMATELY, RESPONSIBLE TO ASSURE THEIR WELFARE; DO NOT BE SUPINE WHEN IT COMES TO VACCINATIONS OR RENDERED INCOMPETENT PARENTS BY A BARGAINED FOR MAL-LAW MANDATE THAT IS IN REALLY FOR THE BENEFIT OF BIG PHARMA AND NOT YOUR BELOVED CHILDREN! You and parents for their offspring have a Right to live undisturbed in body and health! Control the vaccination decision; do not be under the control of others for your children's vaccination destiny! Healthcare freedom assures vaccine purity and/or vaccine quality control. Be acutely, aware not to expose your children to unnatural to the body chemicals; it is the enemy. Autism is the result of chemical exposures and tainted vaccine chemicals is a main source of this chemical exposure. BE FREE TO PROTECT YOUR CHILDREN FROM VACCINE CHEMICALIZATION! The energy of unnatural to the body chemicals is destructive to the normal energy and health of brain cells; as these chemicals dope the brain cells its destructive alien energy is unreleased. Mercury, aluminum and other chemicals in vaccines are unnatural to the body negative energy.

Government vaccination delivery mandate positions itself superior to parents as, children's protective guardians and its insistence that children must be vaccinated despite parental objection is beyond unreasonable. This unnatural positioning enforces and/or enslaves children to be vaccinated in perpetuity despite parents' determination that the vaccine chemicalization comes with too much risk of injury. It is an actual taking of one's children, to be made to suffer an unwanted piercing of the skin by needling and injection of vaccine contents that have unnatural to human biology and/or physiology chemicals. Parents unbridled commitment for their offspring's' safety and health is compromised by this callous positioning. The money-making agenda of vaccine producers or its lobbied for vaccination mandates put a wall up between parents and their children that at times is impregnable. Vaccine safety is lost, and our children's welfare is jeopardized because of these erroneous vaccination mandates. The **TWO STEPS OF CORRECTION** are essential to remedy this intolerable situation!

Exposure to unnatural to the body vaccine chemicalization will never end if it is up to the profiteering vaccine industry. The **TWO STEPS** will stop this perversion! We need to regain our legal system and reestablish the natural order. State Police Power has wrongfully been used to mandate vaccination in perpetuity. Justice and general health are not served by permanently enforcing vaccination that violate parental Rights and dismembers parental authority. There is no extraordinary situation of an epidemic that may require urgent/crisis action or expanded Police Power of the State however, there is the present emergency and/or urgent need is to correct the man-made, chemically induced

Autism epidemic! The emergency calls for the prevention of unnatural to the body chemicalization! Perfectly, healthy children are falling victim to unhealthy chemicalization. Children must always be under parent's protective care in order, to prevent unwanted chemicalization. Vaccination is preventative care and must not be forced upon children! For the healthy, healthcare liberty must be at its highest level; especially, when the medical intervention is preventative healthcare or under a non-emergency situation. **People need to take a sober look at what chemicals are in injections of vaccines. There is no health reason why unnatural to the body chemicals are in vaccines; we must initiate the TWO STEPS OF CORRECTION in order, to GET THE CHEMICALS OUT and protect our children!**

The level of intrusion from enforcement of the vaccination mandate is off the scale when it comes to family privacy, your Right to live undisturbed or unmolested and your authority to be in parental self-control over the health and welfare of one's children. Of all the things that are proper for government to ask citizens to endure; the injection of children without the true informed consent of parents and/or without giving parents any legal room to refuse invasive chemical vaccine injections is certainly, not one. No parent should be made to go against their instinct or judgment that the chemicals within vaccines pose too great of a risk. Parents having the liberty to decide what is best for the health of their children or what is in their children's best interest is paramount to parenting and in the best interest of children. The essence of freedom itself is lost if, We the People, have no choice but to vaccinate. Parents' protecting their own children the way parents individually think best is in the best interest of children and is a fundamental liberty.

Children's vaccinations must not be mastered by government; it is too often dictated to by self-serving special interest groups or the very strong lobbying of Big Pharma. Permanent regulation that enforces vaccination is unconstitutional; it is a modern form of SLAVERY that hits at the heart of our most basic freedom of what we do with our own bodies and/or what will or will not be injected into us. In addition, emergency or crisis condition measures must never be in perpetuity. Once, the crisis is no longer a crisis, the law enforcing health measures must sunset and come to definite end; for we must not live under a permanent state of emergency especially, when the emergency no longer exists.

Vaccination slavery eliminates our most precious of FREEDOMS; the caring for our very own children, the way parents personally think is best and/or children's FREEDOM to remain unmolested; not violated by unwanted medical intervention. Parent's LIBERTY to decide what preventative vaccination healthcare choice will or will not be accepted or denied and/or parent's fundamental responsibility, privilege and/or FREEDOM to determine whether or not a vaccine injection is or is not in their child's best interest is violated. Vaccine injections must not be mastered over us; it must be a matter of FREDOM of choice. Parents' must be legally enabled to refuse an unwanted injection. The parental obligation of protecting and/or caring for children is controlling and must reign supreme. ENFORCED VACCINATIONS DESTROY OUR ESSENTIAL FREEDOMS. Parents' should not have to have a first-class defense attorney at speed dial for merely, deciding against allowing vaccine chemicalization injection when the good intentioned parents determine a vaccine is too dangerous to inject and is therefore, not in their children's best interest! Mandated vaccination is much worse

than the forbidden "taxation without representation", it is Vaccination without parental representation and/or ability to protect one's children!

When it comes to the health of your children why muddy up the waters with legalisms and/or mandates; parents need their control of their children's welfare. **Do not be compelled or handcuffed to paid for and/or lobbied for mandates that call for unnatural to human biology chemical infiltrations (CHEMICALIZATIONS). Do not just blindly, trust in vaccine safety, question medical intervention and question is your child going to risk a critical mass syndrome or suffer a chemical mass syndrome from the proposed vaccine chemicalization.** Only, parents are the **primal natural protectors** of children. When it comes to perfectly healthy, school worthy children; government must not infringe upon or sever this primal natural protection or violate the **Parental Child Protection Right**. Healthy, unvaccinated, school children must be allowed in school and without punishment or prejudice. Children not injected must be considered school worthy and not singled out or be prejudiced for following their parents' personal healthcare choice/decision or religious belief not to vaccinate. **There is no actual threat from children who are unvaccinated.** Freedom to Self-Determine vaccinations or being unvaccinated by virtue of **FREEDOM of HEALTHCARE or FREE exercise of RELIGION; permits one to enter school to receive a basic education and not be molested for doing so.**

If we are not free to care, protect and decide what will or will not be allowed to be injected into our very own children; America the land of the FREE needs a major overhaul! There is nothing more important to parents than the health or welfare of their children. It is beyond uncivil, beyond obnoxious and a travesty of justice to be enforced to inject your perfectly healthy children with a vaccine that you disagree with or recognize as, unsafe or that harbor's unnatural to human biology chemicals. The atrocity of mandated vaccination and its unnatural to the body chemical pay load must come to an end; it no longer should be allowed to violate our rights and children's bodies and/or brain cells. Some argue that the possibility of harm from vaccination is too remote for there to be concern, some think the harm is far too great, either way; if it is your body or your child it must be entirely, up to you whether you vaccinate. Be FREE to be the very best parent that you can be! The level of intrusion is off the charts; enforcing unwanted, perceived as, too dangerous to inject vaccine chemicalization is an intrusion of the worst magnitude. Many parents agree that they would rather suffer their house broken into and precious valuables taken or stolen, than to have their children taken or made to suffer unwanted chemicalization!

Parents' must be unmolested when they decide to refuse an unwanted, perceived of as, too dangerous to inject, vaccination for the sake of their children. When children are perfectly, healthy and their parents in good faith, think the vaccine is not in their children's best interest or the parents conclude a vaccine is too dangerous to inject or the parents are not convinced of the vaccines' safety; the parents must be completely, FREE to protect their children by rejecting the vaccine chemicalization.** Government's continual selective mandate of vaccination is a farce at taking care of children and should not be permitted to overshadow parent's decision about vaccination. The vaccination mandates keep our children shackled to suffer multiple vaccine chemicalizations for the benefit of Big Pharma. There is an ongoing and ever-growing ring of deceit about why vaccination is mandated; in reality, it keeps the vaccine industry in the money, allowing it undeserving, unconscionable mega-profits. Vaccine producers has hijacked government with its droves of big money lobbyists so that the real beneficiaries of vaccination mandates are vaccine producers and not children. It has manipulated an improperly, government sanctioned monopoly which, guarantees vaccine sales by mandate with an endless supply of children to inject its vaccines into. Politicians' who support this welfare illusion often gain financial political/monetary support for doing so. This self-serving agenda must come to an end; it has allowed chemicals in vaccines that must not be in vaccines!

It is apparent that mandated vaccination is mal-law, is the epitome of government overreach and best serves Big Pharma, not children's best interest. There must be no unnatural to the body chemicals for sheer profit in vaccines; safety needs be made to always, come first. Parental informed consent/**DENIAL and the holding of vaccine producers accountable and liable for vaccine induced injury are the TWO STEPS OF CORRECTION that will GET THE CHEMICALS OUT of our children's vaccine supply. The presence of unnatural to the body chemicals makes optimum health impossible; it breaks down our natural defenses, is destructive to normal biology and function. It also, can make an environment for dormant viruses and cancer cells to spawn and proliferate. Infiltration of unnatural chemicals cause dementia (Autism in children) and (Alzheimer's in adults).**

Without question, parents are pillars of reliability and credibility when it comes to making decisions which, are in line with children's best interest whereas, Big Pharma/vaccine producers not only have major conflicts of interest with doing what is in children's best interest in that it too often makes decisions based upon what obtains the most profit which, too often does not coincide with the best interest of children. Make no mistake; the history of the drug industry clearly, indicates that parents should not and must not be rendered inferior when it comes to vaccination decisions. Remember, Big Pharma was made to pay the all-time biggest fine for wrong doing and this makes it that much more obvious who can be trusted to have our children's vaccination fate in its hands; parents are the perfected decision makers. Lobbyists or more precisely VACCINE/Drug Companies have induced government to set up a monopoly, so that vaccinations are mandated, and the producers of vaccines are unchecked **PRICE FIXERS** that put **whatever chemicals they want in vaccines**. Vaccination being mandated assures that vaccines find their mark (children's bloodstreams), is far out of the realm of proper and into the realm of improper. Drug industry has set the agenda and have practically, total marketing freedom and government paid assistance to market their vaccine chemical products. There puppet government assures vaccines find their mark into the bloodstreams of children even if the children's parents are against the injection influx of chemicals. Children must suffer the chemicalization despite parent's objections because it's the law. **YOU LOSE** vital quality control and safety whenever you mandate healthcare; vaccination must not be mandated.

Certainly, everyone recognizes that there are calculated risks and uncalculated risks with being vaccinated or not being vaccinated however, when unnatural to the body chemicals are being injected the risk of altering your normal chemistry is definite. No one other than the potential vaccine chemicalization recipient and parents for their children must be in charge of whether or not a vaccination will or will not occur. The common signs and symptoms after vaccination are considered a degree of injury and severer injury is also caused by vaccination. No one should be enforced to suffer any injury, no matter how insignificant the injury. The People have the Right to remain unvaccinated and to live by their **FREEDOM** of decision not to be vaccinated. **People**

must be free to refuse a vaccination in order, to best protect the children and/or improve vaccines. When parents are not convinced that injecting a vaccine is safe or in their child's best health interest; it is excellent reason to refuse the vaccination. **Harassment or coercion upon parents to submit to vaccinations must end! Vaccination based upon mere speculation of childhood disease must not be enforced.** Children need perfected parental protection! Informed consent, better named "**INFORMED DENIAL**" should control the vaccination question; parents' quest or decision to protect children must be respected!

The mandated vaccination mal-law is a theft, a taking of parental protection of their children; it robs parents of their quite essential vaccination decision. Parents must regain their full empowerment, having 100% parental authority capacity and thereby, enable parents to protect their children to the best of their ability. It is high minded lunacy that commands parents to lay down their parental authority and responsibility of protecting their children. There must be no law commanding parents to submit perfectly, healthy children for vaccine chemicalization; no one should be enforced to expose their children's bloodstreams and BRAIN CELLS to unnatural to the body chemicals. There must be unfettered freedom to refuse unwanted vaccines and we need to initiate the TWO STEPS OF CORRECTION in order, to be secure in this liberty. Vaccines will become much safer once these TWO STEPS are in place. We must not be commanded to adhere to a certain regimentation of healthcare. There must be liberty to discern your own healthcare destiny! Authority of control over children's healthcare must rest with parents; not government!

Autism signs usually appear around the age of 2 to 4, if a parent thinks it wise or best to delay vaccination past these most frequent Autism onset ages it must be their prerogative to do so. Certainly, as the children's parents, the decision to post pone a vaccination or completely deny it, should be for parents to decide or to know what is in their offspring's best interest. Moreover, if a parent has determined that vaccines are suspect because unnatural to the body chemicals are in vaccines or because vaccine companies are impervious to traditional litigation against any vaccine induced injuries; then parents are properly, concerned and must be **FREE** to not allow vaccination. Generally, a parent's ability to protect their children, as they see fit, must be adhered to. **Opting out of injecting a suspect vaccine and/or flatly saying "no" is a freedom parents require and that children rely upon in order, to be adequately protected.**

Vaccines will no longer be suspect, once the **TWO STEPS**, which are continually stressed in this book, are delivered. Each **CORRECTIVE STEP** will be a **champion of SAFER vaccine excellence and a higher level of voluntary vaccination compliance will result**. Excellence in vaccines is not be accidental; it will be the direct result of the implementation of these needed **TWO STEPS**. Prompt, the high intension, the sincere effort and skillful execution needed to produce **SAFER vaccines. Vaccines must earn parental approval** in order, to be considered for injection. **Freedom to refuse** vaccination will stamp out vaccination **SLAVERY. Do not volunteer to chemicalize your children and never give up your liberty of decision! Surely, you would choose to give your child as much brain power or the highest intelligence; certainly, good health and/or optimum intelligence is dependent upon perfecting one's chemistry.**

Presently, vaccines are a health disruptive chemical source. Vaccinations upset the normal chemical balance of the body and when it penetrates the brain the cells of the brain are

caused dysfunction. Vaccinations interfere with homeostatic chemical reactions of the body. The presence of these foreign to the body chemicals, prevents the normal optimum chemical reactions of the body and/or brain from taking place and induces abnormal reactions; both of which, result in abnormality and negative health effects. There becomes a danger of a critical mass chemical toxic episode. **A naturally, pure chemical composition of the bloodstream plays a critical role in health optimization.** The introduction of unnatural to the body, biology and/or physiology chemicals from vaccines into tiny babies, small infants and developing children is disruptive to the chemical composition of optimum health Signs and symptoms associated with vaccination indicate a health problem has ensued. Subtle, abnormal changes that are much more difficult to detect, over time also, occur. **Be warned; be aware!**

Anytime you engage in anything that is fundamentally unnatural, expect unnatural results. A good layperson visualization of what negative consequences occur from injecting foreign to the body chemicals into one's bloodstream is the comparison of a great chef in his preparation of an exotic meal; the chef relies upon the quantity and purity of the ingredients used and/or the chemicals he mixes together in order, to achieve the magnificent result otherwise, the exquisite meal will not result. This is analogous to your body, blood and brain dependence upon a consistent proper level of naturally utilized chemicals; with no alien chemicals to foul up the precise formula of optimal health. Just as, the chef would end up with a disaster of a meal if foreign ingredients and/or chemicals were injected into his broth or mixing bowl; so, it is, that your body will end up with a health disaster when unnatural to the body chemicals are injected into your children's very susceptible and delicate systems. **Do not mix unnatural to one's biology chemicals in vaccines, into the broth of your children's vital blood chemistry instead, be wise and be safe by refusing such, chemicalization; demand much SAFER vaccines! The charity, SAFER vaccines, is dedicated to achieving SAFER vaccines and informing you!**

The injections of vaccine chemicals cause the destruction of the natural biological chemical formula which, is required for optimum health and needed to safeguard against Autism. Your best defense against Autism is to maintain your natural perfected chemistry! The altering of the chemical composition and reactions within the bloodstream have unhealthy end results. Alien to the body, unnatural to the biology and foreign to one's physiology chemicals that have been found in vaccines, are a negative presence when injected into one's bloodstream; a wave of abnormal reactions or abnormality result. We try to assure that our children do not eat unnatural to the body chemicals and yet, many do not hold the same vigilance against like vaccine chemicals. How wildly, wrong is it that such, chemicals are being injected into our babies? We must all be on guard to avoid injections of vaccines that have any degree of unnatural to the body chemicals. Children need and deserve SAFER vaccines! SAFER vaccines, the charity, is where you can find out the chemical facts about vaccines and secure the welfare of your children. You take all kinds of measures to assure health; take what is perhaps the most health measure by only considering SAFER vaccines that have passed the "SANITY TEST", have been made SAFER by the TWO STEPS OF CORRECTION that has GOT THE CHEMICALS OUT!

It is apparent that the introduction of chemicals into our biological make-up is extremely unhealthy. Why are products allowed to enter the market, which have anti-health chemicals? For example, hand sanitizers that contain triclosan or triclosan containing products, can destroy health by disrupting the endocrine system and causing injury to your immune system. In addition, when bacteria are exposed to the chemical concoction of triclosan it can stimulate antibiotic resistance. There is a natural chemical balance that if not maintained degenerates' health. Swing the chemical pendulum too far or upset the natural selection by introducing anti-health chemicals or anti-health agents it causes health degeneration. **We must be careful not to expose the outside of bodies to non-natural biological chemicals. We must be much more careful not to expose the inside of our bodies to such, chemicals; in fact, it is wise to be fanatical about safeguarding the internal purity. Injections of vaccine chemicals are the gross upset of the fine-tuned, highly sensitive, chemistry of human bio-physiology.**

The goals are to grant the potential vaccination recipient a Self-Preservation Right which, is secured by informed consent/DENIAL and to equitably and most wisely, hold vaccine manufacturer's liable for vaccine induced injuries; both goals once achieved will prompt SAFER vaccines that are produced with no unnatural to the body chemicals. A reduction in **CHEMICALIZATION AUTISM** frequency will occur due an achieved lack of unnatural to human biology chemicals in vaccines and/or a decreased risk of a **chemical critical mass syndrome.** Protecting and maintaining the health promoting natural chemical homeostasis of the body will be secured through the prompting of the quintessential form of **SAFER vaccines. The TWO STEPS OF CORRECTION require liberty to deny vaccination, no constraint to self-determine healthcare, no depriving parents from deciding what is best for their children and holding vaccine producers accountable and liable for any vaccine induced injuries.**

Let the application of our Rights and a properly applied negligence legal tort system set us **FREE** from the oppression of unwanted mandated vaccination and thereby, **GET THE CHEMICALS OUT** of vaccines; chemicals that are too dangerous to inject because it is unnatural to human biology and/or physiology. If there is no rational or plausible ability to refuse vaccination or avoid punishment for not vaccinating, then **we are not free**! Withholding of entitlements or benefits or fundamental education for not being vaccination compliant, are the whips that keep enslaved to be vaccinated. By no means can vaccination compliance be considered voluntary under the threat of no school entrance or that child services will be called in to take your child away from you to be vaccinated against your will and you will may be deemed a child abuser for standing in the way of vaccination. Is there no armor that can protect us from the arrows of unwanted vaccination? The doctrine of informed consent/**DENIAL** is the armor you need that can protect you against such, violations. Liberty to litigate directly against vaccine producers for the atrocity of chemicalization negligence is not just armor, it is a like a knight in shining armor with a sword of justice. Both armor and sword are aspects of the **TWO STEPS OF CORRECTION** that will bring about **GETTING THE CHEMICALS OUT** of vaccines and procure SAFER vaccines!

Be extremely careful not to expose your developing baby to unnatural to the body chemicals and do NOT be so foolish to inject such, chemicalization! Be acutely aware that injected chemicals quickly circulate to the brain and can dope the brain with whatever chemical pay load is in the injected vaccine. A chemical is a like a tiny package of dictating information, energy and reactive propensity. In addition, the new discovery or confirming science of epigenetics makes it clear that chemicals influence our genetic expression; triggering a genetic expression that is characteristic of the chemical environment that surrounds the genes. The crazy concept of injecting alien or unnatural to human biology chemicals

that are found in vaccines into quickly, developing babies is the epitome of mad science. We now know that chemicals have its influence and that the wrong chemicals will cause one to be unhealthy therefore, safeguard your children from unwanted chemicalization. The science of epigenetics confirms the fact that unnatural to the body chemicals can transmute genetic expression. Know that many of the unnatural to the body chemicals in vaccines are wreaking havoc with human homeostasis. Chemicals have reactive character or propensity, have magnetic fields and/or its energy signature. The presence of unnatural to human biology chemicals in the blood and/or brain cells of quickly, developing babies, will have negative impact upon development and/or function. Such, chemical presence manipulates the natural perfected environment of brain cells and can trigger abnormality and/or abnormal genetic expression. Do not inject unnatural to human biology chemicals; it can have devastating results; demand SAFER vaccines! Vaccines need to be SAFER, more intelligently designed and in order, to do so, parents must be FREE to make an informed decision for their children's vaccination healthcare.

Mandated vaccination and its enforcement of unwanted vaccination is an intolerable invasion of THE PARENTAL RIGHT to decide what is best for one's children. It is a gross interference of parents Right to protect children from what parents determine is a wrong or what parents deem is a too dangerous to inject, vaccine chemicalization. To overpower parental protection of their children is governmental overreaching. To inject unnatural to the body chemicalization under the guise of doing something for the welfare of children is fraudulent and is medical intervention extremism. Let us, establish that no individual shall be compelled by law to enter a doctor's office or healthcare facility to undergo unwanted or enforced treatment, whatsoever! No individual shall be restrained, molested or burdened with unwanted medical intervention; that means, no one should be made to endure unwanted vaccine chemicalization! No one shall, because of their health choice, opinion or belief, be singled out and treated different or prejudiced for it. Parents must be FREE to be parents for their children! Without question, the fact, that vaccine producers put unnatural to the body chemicals such as, but not limited to mercury and aluminum, is an absolute betrayal of the trust that the public has blindly placed in vaccine producers and in the governmental enactors of mandated vaccinations. Whenever, you penetrate all our children's bodies with chemicals that are fundamentally unnatural to the body expect there to be unnatural results; abnormality like the Autism epidemic!

Children in perfect health, with no emergency need for healthcare, do not need medical intervention mandated; parents can and should decide what preventative healthcare is or is not in their children's best interest! There must be liberty of vaccination decision especially, during non-epidemic situations, when no imminent threat or emergency is at hand. Mandated vaccination in perpetuity must be declared unconstitutional and recognized as, medical intervention enslavement! Healthy children should not be enforced to have unwanted medical intervention and parents must never be accused of child neglect when children are perfectly healthy or when parents refuse vaccination for their children. When parents decide, what is best for children it must be respected. When parents decide, not to vaccinate it is more than likely, for a very good reason such as, parents deeming a vaccine not safe enough for injection. Free Americans must have liberty to deny unwanted healthcare including, any vaccine chemicalization! There must be liberty to live by one's opinion in matters of personal healthcare and in doing so, in no way diminish or negatively, effect civil capacities and/or education privilege! Government intervention in the area of personal healthcare choice must be denounced! **There must be total Separation of an Individual's Health Autonomy and State. The same excellent reason behind the Constitutional requirement of Separation of Church and State is also, excellent reason for Separation of Personal HealthCare Decisions and State**.

Just as government must not establish a religion and/or enact law that favors, coerces or enforces individuals to submit to a specific religion analogously, it must not establish a particular mode of healthcare preference and/or enact law that coerces or enforces individuals to submit to a specific medical intervention, such as, vaccination injections. There are many people who if they had the liberty to decide how to combat childhood disease would rather, choose to establish health by all-natural means and not be dependent upon vaccination. There are many ways to secure health or be resilient and strong against childhood disease and/or its aftermath risks; being vaccinated it just one way to bolster resistance to childhood disease. Individuals and individual families must be able to enjoy freedom of healthcare choice, determine what is in their best interest and be **FREE to deny unwanted medical intervention**. Government must not choose the mode of healthcare or command it! Government must not put undue pressure or coercion upon individuals or upon parents concerning their children, which deters free thinking or freedom of personal choice in healthcare. Children require the blessing and comfort of their parents' protection; without government intrusion! Children need their parents to protect them from unwanted vaccine chemical injections, without government dictating otherwise! Parents must be secure that their children will not suffer unwanted injections or be coerced into it! **There must be no vaccination without parental representation, confirmation and/or consent!**

Crawling all by itself, on unsound legal ground; vaccinations are the only healthcare that is mandated. It is unjustly and immorally the single exception to the legitimate and well - established **safety rule and requirement** of informed consent/**DENIAL** which, controls if the treatment is or is not delivered. We the People, have been unjustly, stripped of our dignity and individual Right to Self-Determine the vaccination question and consequently, are devoid of our Right to Self-Govern our body and/or what is allowed to be injected or flow in our very own blood. Unconstitutionally, and unethically, we are enforced to submit ourselves and our children for vaccinations. Oppressively, vaccinations are coerced and enforced upon us, despite the fact, that the parents are against having their child injected and never give their true informed consent.

Vaccinations are administered despite the fact, that **no true legal permission to have the child vaccinated is granted**. Informed consent must be required in order, to administer a vaccination! The adage, "a dollar short and a day late" is not strong enough to depict vaccine producers finally acting to remove mercury from childhood vaccines. Too much damage has been done. Understandably, the public's confidence and trust, blind as it may be, in vaccines and/or the vaccine industry has fallen sharply and because of the vaccine industry's reckless, uncaring unintelligent and callous utilization of unnatural to the body chemicals in vaccines it has caused a turning point in what can be allowed in vaccines and who decides if a vaccine will or will not be delivered. It is now beyond the point of no return, there must be a change in the rules governing vaccination; people must no longer be mandated to suffer unwanted vaccine chemicalizations. No longer should parents and/or the public tolerate or stand idle under the oppression of unwanted chemicalization injections or for not being **FREE TO REFUSE** vaccine chemicalization. **The TWO STEPS OF CORRECTION** must set things right; parents must be **FREE TO PROTECT their children with refusal** of unwanted vaccination and vaccine producers must be held responsible, accountable and liable for vaccine induced injuries in order, to **GET THE CHEMICALS OUT**!

The golden rule in healthcare is for doctors to always first obtain informed consent in order, to render any proposed care. Rendering care that is not consented to is considered a violation and is actionable**; unconsented to care is considered an assault and battery**. Administering vaccination with no true volitional consent because of coercion is a violation. Mandated vaccination equates to no real freedom of choice to decide for or against vaccination, no realistic ability to decide not to consent and/or deny vaccination; it is unethical and violates the Rights of those who do not really want to be vaccinated. People are submitting for reasons other than a good health decision and this must be considered illegal and it makes the delivery of a vaccination unethical, an act of medical malpractice and a violation of the doctrine of informed consent. Parents too often collapse under the pressure of the vaccination mandate, submitting their children to suffer an unwanted vaccination; not because parents think the vaccination is in their children's best interest. The vaccination delivery system must be corrected with the **TWO STEPS OF CORRECTION**. Parents' decision must rule; parents' need the decisive control of whether the vaccination is in the best interest of their child's welfare. The enforced vaccination system is an enigma to the strongest custom and safety requirement of informed consent. Informed consent/DENIAL needs to rule over vaccination; as it is the golden rule of healthcare. **YOU MUST BE FREE TO DENY OR ACCEPT HEALTHCARE and that includes vaccination**!

This is not a case of needy sick children that are in desperate need of medical intervention. Not only are these perfectly healthy children not in need of medical intervention their parents are all mentally competent, having full capacity to decide all their children's healthcare and/or health choices; they are legally competent. This clearly indicates that there is no cause to mandate vaccination; children are healthy, and parents are competent. Moreover, this is a case of mere preventative health measures, there is no crisis condition that may call for governmental intervening and/or a reason for a mandate. **People must be FREE to serve and protect their children; to keep children out of harm's way.** If a parent refuses a vaccination because they have determined the vaccine injection not safe; it must be **legally understood as, an act to keep children out of harm's way, an act of protection! Parents need to assure their babies develop cognitively proper, so their children develop executive functioning with ability to control impulses and in order, to do so it is imperative that one's offspring are not injected with unnatural to human biology or developmental chemicals. Choose and demand SAFER vaccines without such, UNSAFE chemicalization! Obtain SAFER vaccines by the TWO STEPS PF CORRECTION; choose vaccines wisely!**

Whether vaccines are a cause of Autism or **THE MAIN CAUSE OF AUTISM,** is not the primary issue; it is who should have control of the vaccination decision or be in charge of whether or not it shall or shall not be delivered. **The general rule must always be that PARENTS' BE IN CHARGE and IN CONTROL over all of their children's important life decisions and vaccination is an important life decision! Make no mistake, chemical infiltration is the leading cause of all abnormality. The main cause of the Autism epidemic is the unwise injection of chemicals into children. As the number of vaccine dosages went viral or exponential so did the spawning of the Autism epidemic. THE LAWS OF CHEMISTRY APPLY TO WHEN A CHEMICALIZATION OF OUR BABIES OCCURS AND REVEALS HOW UNNATURAL TO THE BODY VACCINE**

CHEMICALS CAUSE ABNORMALITY AND/OR REACTION UPHEAVAL. Chemicalization of children has caused an epidemic of Autism. Unvaccinated children remain normal; are comparatively healthier, robust and have vitality. Chemically compromised, vaccinated children too often are plagued with health issues. Corporate greed and vaccine chemicals for profit have plunged children into an Autism epidemic.

Parents are the ones who decide what care to accept or deny even in the direst circumstances or when the condition of their child is perplexing or complicated; parents are vested with control over decisions on cancer or heart treatment for children. There is absolutely no valid reason why parents are not free to decide upon vaccination. Certainly, parents possess the capacity to decide the comparatively simple vaccination medical intervention question. The main reason why parents have been disempowered in their vaccination decision capacity is to assure profiteering to Big Pharma from vaccination; it is all about the money. Parents are considered having the capacity to decide much more complex healthcare questions than the vaccination question and are certainly more than capable to decide any preventative healthcare question such as, vaccination medical intervention. There is no controlling reason to supersede parents by governmentalizing the vaccination decision or enforcing vaccination upon our perfectly healthy children. **In general, parents know what is best for their children! Parents have unbridled commitment to only do what is in children's best interest**. Parental vaccination control requirement needs to become the law of the land; it needs to be consistent with all other healthcare. The tradition is the decision power rests with parents for all of children's proposed healthcare, without exception. **Parents are sophisticated, their level of knowledge is far too great, to allow for the injection of vaccine chemicals (chemicalization) by mandate! To place bargained for government vaccination mandate above parental decision power foolheartedly leaves children vulnerable to unscrupulous profiteering by enforced vaccine chemicalization! Chemicals for profit, not safety, have found its way into our vaccines! We require SAFER vaccines that are not laced with unnatural to human biology chemicals!**

Perhaps, long ago the extraordinary circumstance of a real numbers epidemic gave rise to the extraordinary invasive measure of mandated vaccinations. However, this extraordinary measure was only supposed to obfuscate or usurp parent's Right to decide what is best for children during only the temporary period of the epidemic crisis; absent the crisis of an ongoing epidemic there must be no further loss of parental Right to decide if a vaccine is safe enough to inject otherwise, it is an unwarranted violation of our Rights! However, even during a proven epidemic, no parent should be mandated to suffer their children with vaccines that contain any degree of unnatural to human biology chemicals! Parents should always be completely FREE to do what they think best for their children!

At the time of the spawning of vaccination mandates it was falsely **ASS**umed that vaccines were "absolutely safe"; it is now known that vaccinations, do cause harm and/or **now harbor anti-health, unnatural to human biology chemicals**. The fact, that vaccines are an unnatural chemicalization is controlling reason not to mandate vaccination and supersedes any reason to mandate vaccination. In addition, there is now greater understanding of what keeps one healthy or have resiliency against childhood disease and how to prevent any severe harm if a childhood disease does take place. There is also, now understanding that if a child does have a natural occurring childhood disease that the child may be better off because it will give the child lifetime immunity whereas, when a child is vaccinated the immunity obtained is not lifetime, it wanes over time and thereby, leaves a person susceptible later in life when the impact can be more devastating. People must be **FREE** to weigh out the pros and cons of vaccination and/or decide when it is best to vaccinate or not vaccinate at all. **Our goal is to prompt SAFER vaccines so that choosing to be vaccinated becomes a rational choice.**

There no crisis of a childhood disease epidemic however, there is the crisis of a horrific Autism epidemic and that is where most of our effort needs to be concentrated. There are now, multiple known precautions to prevent a childhood disease epidemic whereas, there is not enough action being taken to decrease or eliminate the unnatural to the body chemicals in our children's vaccine supply. Proper nutrition, keeping one's, immune system strong, adequate cleanliness and the use of newly developed super antibiotics are to name just a few of the ways, in these modern more intelligent days, to control childhood disease. When all else fails, quarantine is yet another option to curtail the quick spreading of childhood disease. **This all marks the end of the extraordinary measure of enforcing vaccination! The alerting fact, that unhealthy chemicals are in vaccines is controlling reason to FREE THE PEOPLE from the oppression of being enslaved to vaccinate.** Enforcing vaccine **chemicalization** against the better judgment of parents is counter intuitive and the **ruthless disregard of human life and dignity. BE FREE TO REJECT INJECTION! Be FREE to decide what is best to secure your children's optimum health! The main way to curtail the Autism epidemic is to make sure that your offspring are not infiltrated with unnatural to the body chemicals. The primary exposure or worst kind of chemicalization exposure is the injected kind. Be safe, make sure you only consider SAFER vaccines; demand they GET THE CHEMICALS OUT!**

Government should not dictate healthcare or take dominating control over children's internal welfare or overpower parent's Right to protect their children from any unwanted medical intervention. To mandate increasing numbers of chemically laced vaccinations, with no scheduled end in sight or sunset of the mandate is a gross infraction against our personage and Right to be left alone. Government is not meant to rule over us and certainly, it must rule over what we will inject into our bodies or what must be injected into our babies and/or children! The vaccination mandate and its enforcement tactics coerce parents to allow the injection of vaccine chemicals into their children even when the parents truly do not agree with it or the parents deem the vaccine too dangerous to inject. It results in parents being obedient to the vaccination mandate and disobedient to their instinctive and superior obligation of taking care of children to the very best of their ability. It induces parents to abandon their parental responsibility of protecting their children the way they think is best; it places parents under duress to go against doing what they have determined is in their children's best health interest. It induces parents to be negligent parents because it coerces parents to disregard what they know is best for their children. The mal-law forbids or disallows parents from acting and/or living by their parental protective conclusion that a chemically laced vaccine is too controversial or too dangerous to risk injecting into their children. There is an unprecedented urgency to GET THE CHEMICALS OUT of vaccines; the chemicals that are in vaccines for profit and not health, must be removed. Mandated chemicalization is an enslavement act, a mal-law, is immoral, unprecedented, unjust, unconstitutional and un-American; IT IS LAWLESSNESS!

No one should have a monopoly on healthcare; we must be FREE to decide for oneself and for one's children what healthcare to accept or deny. It is extremely offensive to be enforced to vaccinate or be made to trust that vaccines are just good or not harmful. It is a disgusting, grotesque attack on our children that vaccine producers put unnatural to human biology chemicals such as, the chemical formulations of mercury and of aluminum in vaccines which, they knew would be injected into our tiny babies, little infants and small children's fragile, developing bodies. No offense or blow to freedom is greater than being enforced by mal-law vaccination mandate to suffer one's children with unnatural to human biology chemicalization. Human dignity and parental nurturing protection of children from unwanted vaccine chemicalization means no more to the people that enforce vaccination for profit than pebbles on the beach. Pro-vaccination authorities would overthrow our Right to care and protect our children and destroy our self-preservation liberty and/or usurp our self-governing of ourselves and our children. The very liberty that we so highly prize is undermined unless, we stand dedicated to the preservation of the principles that our country and all healthcare is founded upon. In order, to **live FREE,** parents' must be **FREE to protect** their own flesh and blood from unwanted medical intervention; **FREE to decide** if a vaccination will be given and **FREE to deny** an unwanted or perceived of as, too dangerous to inject vaccination. **These are not scant freedoms; they are dynamic freedoms that we zealously need to protect and are inseparable from being a FREE AMERICAN and AUTONOMOUS individual and/or family**!

There is no greater satisfaction for parents in life than to feel and know that they have done the best job possible in the caring and protection of their children. The People must not be deterred from their primary mission in life; caring and doing what is best for their children. If parents determine that vaccines are not in their child's best interest or are not trustworthy or are too dangerous for injection; then by Natural or God given Right parents must be FREE to reject the injection and/or refuse the unwanted vaccination. The vaccination compliance rule jolts parents and their children from their seat of control over healthcare. If parents are not obedient to the compulsory vaccination requirement they risk being attacked for it. Children and their parents are abused by the vaccination law; children are abused by enforced chemicalization and parents are abused by coercion to submit children for unwanted vaccination. Parents must not be made or abused to inject their children! Tis abuse renders its victims enslaved to vaccinate! We must clean-up vaccines and free-up the control to self-govern. Liberation of protection of children is essential to end vaccination enslavement and/or medical intervention tyranny.

Now that you are aware that there are unnatural to the body chemicals in vaccines would it be negligent to not safeguard your children from such, chemicalization or to not stop vaccine producers from doing so? We all were duped or negligent to have trusted that vaccines do not contain such, chemicals or that the pharmaceutical industry would not put your children in harm's way. In a MSNBC broadcast, November 2, 2006 entitled "Bayer Exposed (HIV Contaminated Vaccine)" it was exposed that the Drug Company new that it's Factor 8 vaccine was tainted with HIV and yet the company shipped the tainted drug overseas in order, to make a profit. You need to determine if the Drug Company's actions or inactions were proper and decide what character it truly has. Now do you think it is worthy of your blind trust or its vaccines are safe or that it does not put unnatural to the body chemicals in vaccines or will not put people in harm's way in order, to make a buck?

In addition, the FDA did nothing to stop them from shipping its tainted vaccine; allowing injuring of innocent children with this harmful drug and to the best of my research no one has ever been penalized or punished for doing so. For vaccine producers' money rules over safety but for parents; safety rules! Let this revealing scenario teach parents that PARENTS MUST BE IN CONTROL OF WHETHER A VACCINE IS SAFE OR WILL OR WILL NOT BE INJECTED! Do not blindly trust that vaccines have no anti-health chemicals; do not ASSume vaccines safe. Vaccine safety is not trustworthy; keep your children out of vaccine's harm's way. Many chemicals in vaccines should not be injected! If a vaccine is harmful they may sell it anyway to obtain what is most important to them, money, caring first about profit; not safety. Children need their PARENTS to protect them from vaccine chemicalization harm by being FREE to do so; FREE to reject injection!

Think about it, literally everything has its unique chemical formulation that makes it what it is and if that chemical formulation is altered it can have major impact. It is of extreme, monumental importance that A DEVELOPING BABY HAS A NORMAL/HEALTHY CHEMISTRY. Injection of unnatural to human biology and/or physiology chemicals DISRUPTS THE NEEDED CHEMISTRY FOR NORMAL DEVELOPMENT! If you were a child would you want your parents blocked by mal-law unable to refuse vaccine chemical injections or not be free to protest or forbid the chemicalization of your body, blood and/or brain cells? Brain cells cannot even come close to functioning optimally if they have been infiltrated with non-indigenous to the brain cells' chemicals. The facts show that the Drug/VACCINE industry for profit has tendencies to falsify research, falsify documents, mislead the public, give false data, and perpetuate false or misleading information about their products. For government to disembowel parents, taking away their parental Right of protection and/or their control over whether a vaccine will or will not be injected is a violation of mega-importance that is beyond unreasonable and is against humanity and/or parenthood that is so unjust that it is un-American. The mandated vaccination mal-law strips parents of their Right to protect their children; disemboweling or destroying their natural and fundamental liberty of protecting their very own children from unwanted chemicalization. These violations have led to chemical chaos and/or unsafe vaccines. Parents must not trust profit-based organizations that have history of producing falsified, misleading or doctored product information. INFORMED CONSENT/DENIAL must control vaccination delivery! Parents' do hold children's best interest and are more than able to discern the vaccination pros and CONS. Liberty to control health or life must be yours!

Parents are FREE to safeguard their children from all kinds of unwanted chemicalization, there is no valid reason why vaccine chemicalization is the exception; in fact, it is a much higher priority for parents to protect their children from injected chemicalization. Harmful results from the smoke/chemicals are why parents do not want their children to smoke. Harmful results from vaccine/chemicals is a valid reason why parents do not want their children to be injected. Just as it is proper or correct for parents to not allow their children to be exposed to the chemicals from smoking; it is just as proper or correct that parents forbid and protect their children from being exposed to unwanted, deemed as, too dangerous to inject vaccine chemicalization. Exposure to anti-health chemicals should strike a deep fear in any rational parent. Government must not make mal-law that enforces chemicalization or that enforces smoking or the vices of vaccine chemical injection. Parents must be FREE to

protect their children from all unwanted chemicalization. Parents require the same liberty to safeguard their children from vaccine chemicals as they do from smoke chemicals. Parents must be FREE to refuse; say "NO" to unwanted chemicals; no matter what the source. Vaccination delivery must only occur with TRUE parental permission. When parents do not give permission, it means that no injection of vaccine chemicals can be given; no unwanted chemicalization!

We all want our kids to be as safe as possible therefore, we need someone to watch the vaccine companies carefully to make sure they are doing everything in its power to make vaccines safer and you can rely upon **SAFER** vaccines, the charity, to assure this; it is a primary mission of the charity. In fact, **SAFER** vaccines, the tax-deductible charity, pledge is to investigate and report back to the world what is being done and who is not doing what they should chemically. In the end, with public awareness, the vaccine manufactures will make the vaccines it produces even safer. Only with your tax-deductible donations can this happen. **SAFER** vaccines have monitored a problem with vaccines in that they contain unnatural to human biology chemicals and that means very probable health problem for vaccine recipients. What good is monitoring what vaccines contain without doing something about it! **SAFER** vaccines, the charity, intend to do something about it by implementing the **TWO STEPS OF CORRECTION** which, have been elucidated throughout this book. The mandated vaccination law is in direct conflict with the long history of **informed consent/ DENIAL requirement, which rules over healthcare delivery and supersedes outside of the family vaccination decisions**. The informed consent/**DENIAL** healthcare safeguard protection has become **COMMON LAW and is now considered a fundamental Right and/or a natural Right. It secures your autonomy and self-preservation; it assures that the individual is free to self-govern their own healthcare and/or body.** It is considered a **FUNDAMENTAL RIGHT** to be physically left alone undisturbed; not being molested or injected and/or have your body violated. **One must be FREE to live by one's own healthcare convictions and not be violated by unwanted medical intervention.**

As far as, being enabled to make the needed change in order, to go from less safe vaccines that are laced with unnatural to the body chemicals to **SAFER** vaccines we must set upon it by first admitting to the truth about vaccine contents; it is far better to tell the truth than to continue to ignore it. The whole truth and nothing but the truth is that vaccine producers purposefully put unnatural to the body chemicals in vaccines such as, mercury and the **EPA** (Environmental Protection Agency) **classifies it as a toxin**. Let this truth set you **FREE**; allowing you to protect your children from chemicalization disaster. Our children are far better off without such caustic to health chemicals in vaccines. **SAFER** vaccines, the charity, will not stand idle, it will always work feverishly to rid our children's vaccines of chemicals that their bodies are insulted or compromised by. Parents **FREE** access to being informed about what chemicals are in vaccines and being **FREE TO REFUSE** unwanted chemically tainted vaccines is required in order, to achieve **SAFER** vaccines. Holding vaccine producers accountable and liable for utilizing such, unnatural to human biology chemicals in vaccines is also, a step to achieve **SAFER** vaccines. The aforementioned are the major aspects of the **TWO STEPS OF CORRECTION** that will most certainly, **GET THE CHEMICALS OUT and is in the best interest of our children**.

There is something more important than following bargained for government mandates in this world, something much deeper and more real. **At all cost, at all avenues, parents need to be FREE to**

protect children to best of their ability and know how. It is not that I do not respect and love our government; it is that I love our freedom and children's wellbeing more. **We are FREE to disagree with enacted laws however, we must not break the law merely because we disagree with it rather, we should vigilantly work to correct what is wrong with the mal-laws. There are times when one law is inconsistent with another law and in this rare instance we should do our best to not break either law however, it might be necessary to be civil disobedient to a mal-law that is inconsistent with a more supreme law and/or a Constitutional law. Mandated vaccination is mal-law that is wholly inconsistent with one's supreme Right of parents to secure the welfare of their children. If parents determine that a vaccine has a poison in it or a neurotoxin or is not in their child's best interest even though the dictate that parents must allow the injection of a poison; parents have a higher obligation of protecting their child from harm. For the common good of all, we are set on this one battle to make SAFER vaccines. We must ABOLISH BEING ENSLAVED TO BE VACCINATED;** it so drastically impacts our lives and fundamental liberties. Parents alone must have the final say; parents must have vaccination determination power. Parents empowerment to protect children must no longer be extinguished by mal-law vaccination mandates; parents' decision about what is best for their children or determination as to when a vaccine will or will not be given must not be broken. Parents are the gatekeepers for all non-emergency healthcare; vaccine injections should not be the exception! **WE MUST BE FREE TO REJECT INJECTIONS**!

Just as, the power of a plant or tree is in the roots, the power that nurtures the health and the safety of children is in parents indeed, children's roots are their parents. The mandated vaccination law uproots parental empowerment of and for their children. Law must not weaken this power and children must be secure in their parent's protection. The mandated vaccination law separates children from their parent's protection by calling for the enforcement of vaccination even, in the instance when parents determine that the vaccine chemicalization is not in their children's best health interest. When parents object to vaccination the law must not violate their parental decision not to vaccinate! Children must not be cut-off, uprooted, from their parent's protection! Parents must not be stripped of their natural obligation and/or God given Right of protecting their children. The **vaccination enslavement law** renders children barren of parent's protective decision; leaving children totally susceptible to vaccine injected chemical harm.

Children need to be able to rely upon and be secure in their parent's innate, caring and intelligent judgment. Government oversteps its boundary of jurisdiction when it intrudes upon parents' rightful dominion over the welfare of their children; it is the jurisdiction of parents to make the vaccination decision. Parents need to stand firm in their decisions over what is best for their children and be enabled to do so without interference from an overreaching vaccination mandate mal-law. Parents must not have their will broke under the overpowering, undue pressure, of vaccination compulsion or its coercion antics. Perfectly healthy children that remain unvaccinated have a Right to go to school and not be treated as if they were lepers' or with discrimination for their unvaccinated status. Parents must BE FREE to protect children as they see fit; their decisions allowed to protect children! VACCINE CHEMICALIZATIONS DO CAUSE HARM!

It is wrong if there is even the slightest decrease in parent's freedom to take care of children's health concerns because it places children in danger. In general parents are forever committed to their children best interest and must not be hamstrung or diminished from doing so or doing what they think best for their children's welfare. Parents need to be **FREE** to trust in their reflexive caring judgement for their children in order, to best secure the general welfare of all children. This is particularly true when it comes to questions of preventative healthcare and especially true when their children are perfectly healthy with no immediate need of medical intervention. It has become common knowledge that very often prescribed medicine or surgery can cause all kinds of health problems in fact, the adverse reactions or complications are just too long to list. **WHEN YOU DO SOMETHING UNNATURAL EXPECT UNNATURAL RESULTS! The injection of unnatural to human biology chemicals into the body creates unnatural to the body results.** Even though there has been a mountain of damage control to not let it become more readily known that vaccine chemicalization is fraught with adverse reactions that even surpass the problems caused by other medical intervention make no mistake; unnatural chemicalization of quickly developing babies is disastrous to the achievement of optimum health!

Do not trust that a vaccine is safe; know what chemicals are in it! Injection of unnatural to human biology chemicals is devastating to our precious children. Parents do not stand for being sidelined for anything involving the welfare of their children. Parents are aghast when they learn what chemicals have been found in vaccines and become extremely concerned and even outraged that they are sidelined from the vaccination decision. Recognizing that they were made to suffer their children with unnatural to human biology vaccine chemicalization is a stab in the heart for parents who trusted that vaccines would not chemically compromise their children. Unnatural to human biology chemicals cause cancer, mental problems and cause Autism; such chemicals in vaccines cause abnormal reactions and that equals abnormality.

Getting a handle on the magnitude of the problem caused by injecting unnatural to the body chemicals is imperative. You grasp how dire the situation really is when you come to learn that Depression or Bipolar disorder is caused by chemical imbalance or abnormal chemistry of the brain; you begin to get an inclining of just how crazy or unhealthy it is to inject tiny babies, small infants and immature children with unnatural to human biology chemicals. It is no wonder that someone with Autism is having mental dysfunction. Abnormal chemistry is the cause in fact, of Autism and the multiple injections of unnatural to the body vaccine chemicalizations are the main causation of the Autism epidemic. **Vaccinations are given to perfectly healthy children; too many of these perfectly healthy children are no longer perfectly healthy after injection.** Vaccines have become vessels for unnatural to the body chemicalization. If you control whether a vaccination takes place; **you control its safety**. Parental freedom of the vaccination healthcare decision is essential to the prevention of unsafe vaccines. Understandably, parents are wanting to back away from having children vaccinated with tainted vaccines that are untrustworthy for safety. If you are going to vaccinate why vaccinate with a vaccine that has for profit chemicals in it which, are chemicals that are unnatural to human physiology and not of one's natural chemistry! **SAFER vaccines**, the charity, want to make choosing vaccination a much more rational choice by seeing to it that the vaccine industry **GET THE CHEMICALS OUT**; rid vaccines of chemicals that are not indigenous to the body or normal chemical homeostasis. The atrocity of taking our freedom of choice away and not holding vaccine producers' feet to the fire of negligence law have caused vaccine contents to become too dangerous to inject, **RESULTING IN VACCINES BECOMING AN INJECTION OF UNNATURAL TO HUMAN BIOLOGY CHEMICALIZATION**.

At minimum parents should view vaccine safety with a **HEALTHY DOSE OF SKEPTICISM** and make anyone who recommends a vaccine first prove to you through the unmasking of the vaccine's chemical content that the vaccine is indeed, among the vaccines that can be considered a **SAFER** vaccine. It is the golden rule in healthcare delivery that informed consent/**DENIAL** rule over it. Parents protect their children by deciding if the vaccine contents are too dangerous to inject! Another very important safety measure of how you best protect your children is to make sure you can litigate against the vaccine company and doctor if the vaccine that the doctor represented is safe does in fact, cause your children an injury. This liberty to litigate keeps manufacturers vigilant about safety! Unfortunately, vaccine producers have made it very hard for you to protect your child with the blessings of negligence law; unlike all other medical intervention you may not be enabled to litigate when it comes to vaccination. However, demand this freedom to protect and/or litigate, under the liberty of contract law. Your liberty to contract is a Constitutional right and supersedes such, lobbied for inferior law. If there is any hesitation on the doctors' part, you not only should walk out of the doctor's office; you should run! **PROTECT YOUR CHILDREN!** You absolutely, want your doctor and the vaccine company to be accountable and liable in case there is any vaccine induced injury! A clear indication that your child's welfare is at risk is if you are forbidden or will have increased difficulty in seeking damages in the more likely, event of an injury. Vaccine producers lobbied for liability shield places its welfare above that of our children!

Mandating vaccination has played a major role in instigating vaccines to become tainted with chemicals that are not harmonious with optimum health and is so counter intuitive to health safety that it verges on negligence. The result of not applying consumerism and/or not allowing parents their most important responsibility to refuse a vaccine that parents deem unsafe or unsuitable or too dangerous to inject has spawned the production of unsafe vaccines. We need **SAFER** vaccines; not vaccines that are laced with unnatural to the body chemicals that are considered unsafe vaccines! The questions that need to be asked are did vaccine producers know that its vaccines were being rendered unsafe or harmful or to any degree less safe by its utilization of certain chemicals especially, chemicals that assure higher profits that have no benefit to the vaccine recipient? Did it put vaccines for use without adequate warnings or did they assist in orchestrating that there be no freedom to refuse vaccine injections? Children desperately need to have the safest possible vaccines and **THE TWO STEPS** best assure **SAFER** vaccines. Healthy children come from pure blood as, health comes from the blood is a basic truth. Liberty to prevent vaccine chemicalization is a blood purity essential.

More times than not the public is not given the truth or are outright deceived about the safety of products. Diet soda was hailed as the "healthy alternative" to regular soda, too many drugs to mention were put on the market as "safe" and vaccines were sold to the public as, "absolutely safe"; all have turned out to the furthest from the truth. Even when there is an uproar over how unhealthy a product is the product usually stays on the market or is finally not allowed on the market and the manufacturer just changes the name of the product or keeps the forbidden content in other products. For example, Olestra (fat free) chemicals were found to interfere with needed absorption vitamins and yet virtually the same product with just a new name (Olean) is still on the market with the same chemicalization danger and supposedly toxic mercury was prompted to be removed from childhood vaccines and yet vaccine producers still have most of Flu shots laden with mercury and the flu shot is often recommended or mandated for children. This lunacy of chemicalization is what parents absolutely need to be FREE to reject, prevent or refuse! Children are properly dependent upon their parents for protection against harm and government must not supersede this parental protection or deny it or replace it! It is proper parental jurisdiction not wayward government jurisdiction to oversee healthcare or health management. The safety of children requires full 100% parental protection. Parents should be welcome to raise the level of safety for children and not be so deterred. SAFER vaccines, the charity is what is needed to achieve safety; SAFER vaccines are the trusted guardian of the children! Protect your children by only using SAFER vaccines!

Parents entrusted vaccine producers to not place their children in chemicalization harm's way and they were deceived for doing so. The deceit is that unnatural to the body chemicals are in vaccines and that children are being injured by vaccines despite reassurances otherwise. If we could only refuse vaccination or litigate against vaccine producers for vaccine induced injuries vaccine would quickly become SAFER vaccines. Unfortunately, vaccines have become unsafe because of the public not being legally enabled to refuse vaccination thereby, making informed consent/DENIAL a moot point. In furtherance of making vaccines unsafe what instigates the placement of children in chemicalization harm's way is an unconscionable liability shield for vaccine producers. Filthy rich, Big Pharma lobbied for and manipulated into procurement an anti-safety measure which, gives vaccine producers an unwise liability shield that has resulted in the production unsafe vaccines. This total liability shield measure renders vaccines which, are produced with less call for vaccine safety quality control. Children desperately need their vaccines to be much SAFER. The self-serving total liability shield allows producers of vaccines to not intensely care about what chemicals it uses. It can use whatever chemicals it pleases without accountability for doing so; it pays not a cent to the injured.

Where do we go from here? One must wonder what is the relevance of injecting unnatural too human biology chemicals into babies? The negative health affects of altering the normal biochemistry with injections of unnatural to human biology CHEMICALIZATION is measureless as the sands on the seashore. We must be forever vigilant not to bastardize our children's delicate chemical balance with such, alien chemicals. It is the mission of SAFER vaccines, the charity, that you can choose SAFER vaccines. We know that absolute power corrupts absolutely, so we must not to be under the absolute power of vaccination mandates. Vaccine producers must not utilize whatever chemicals it so chooses. Know all the chemicals in all vaccines and be FREE to refuse if it dangerous. We have the responsibility of our children for what seems a short time; let us be FREE to care for them to the best of our ability. It should not be such a titanic struggle for parents to prevent vaccination that they deem too dangerous and not be a titanic struggle to bring vaccine producers to justice when parents accuse them of negligently producing a vaccine that causes an injury. Vaccines can be made much SAFER FOR OUR CHILDREN! SAFER vaccines' the charity, TWO STEPS OF CORRECTION will make them much SAFER.

CHAPTER 9

PARENTAL JURISDICTION NOT GOVERNMENT JURISDICTION

Government making our vaccination decisions is much too intrusive. To make personal choices about significant aspects of life and/or healthcare is the highest valued Right. Whomever controls what will or will not be injected into children controls the children's health and/or welfare. In the healthcare environment, it is PARENTS' JURISDICTION TO DECIDE what will be allowed for their children and vaccination should be no exception! The basis of a full life expression is being FREE to decide what is best for your children. FREE will is a gift that no individual should be asked or coerced to give up or be made not to live by. Parents should not be made to sacrifice their children for unwanted vaccine chemicalization. The healthcare choices of an individual are strictly the purview, business and JURISDICTION of the individual; it is not a government jurisdiction and if one argues that it is it certainly, is not superior. CHILDREN'S HEALTHCARE IS THE PROPER JURISDICTION OF PARENTS! Preventative healthcare decisions of parents should not be overruled or superseded by government; parents must not be enforced to suffer or sacrifice their children to the vices of vaccine injections. Mandated vaccination is tyrannical child abuse by chemicalization! True freedom dictates that the People have the complete control over what preventative healthcare they accept or deny. Individual's choices in healthcare, to accept or deny medical intervention must be respected especially, in matters of prevention or when the individual's health is optimum. Government has no valid jurisdiction in commanding permanent chemicalization injection slavery. Parents are justified in securing control over their children and/or over their healthcare; parents have jurisdiction to protect their health. It is a fundamental liberty to decide what is best and/or protect children as parents are meant to do. To be shackled to medical intervention or to be enforced by a mandated vaccination law to bring your perfectly healthy children to suffer an unwanted vaccine CHEMICALIZATION injection and/or to be commanded to do so despite parents determining the vaccine unsafe or not in their children's best interest is to be ball and chained, imprisoned to vaccinate and not free to be parents.

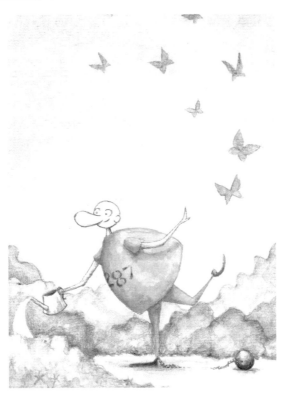

It is a fiction of freedom to live under the oppression of being handcuffed or ball and chained to suffer unwanted vaccine chemicalization under mandated vaccination.

Unfortunately, the standard for manufacturing vaccines has been compromised by greed, it is now flawed as it tends to put unnatural to human biology chemicals in to allow for higher profits without regard to its anti-health consequence. People can get a sense of the atmospherics of injecting their children with chemicals that are alien to the body or unnatural to human biology and rationally reach a conclusion about the consequences of such, chemicalization. SAFER vaccines, the charity will act to **GET THE CHEMICALS OUT** and thereby, bless children with **SAFER** vaccines. The vaccination decision surrounds preventative healthcare and children that have no apparent sickness or emergency need for government emergency measures or mandated medical intervention; there is no valid reason for a government vaccination mandate. Our destiny is to be in ultimate control over our very own internal welfare, for what insanity would there be if otherwise. A mandated enforcing of vaccinations annihilates individuality and free thinking. **The enforcement of vaccinations wrongly concentrates power to care for children in the hands of centralized government; encroaching upon and violating parents' jurisdiction of caring for and protecting children.** What the government says goes-or else, shackles the human spirit. Permanent mandated vaccination is an over extension of government power and is not the proper jurisdiction of government. Mandated vaccination has been bargained for by the vaccine industry! **It guarantees the vaccine industry profits at the expense of our liberty and safety of our children!** Freedom to refuse vaccination is required to assure **SAFER** vaccines and liberty to litigate against vaccine producers will prompt proper quality control to achieve **SAFER** vaccines.

In order, to secure **DOMESTIC TRANQUILITY and FREEDOM** the People must be endowed with the fundamental Right to determine their healthcare and/or health destiny and that of their children. **You see it is incumbent upon parents to give their children the very best chance at optimum**

health therefore, parents must not be made into zombie parents by a mal-vaccination mandate which, forbids parents from refusing vaccination particularly, when parents deem a vaccine chemicalization as, too unsafe or too dangerous to inject. Governmental domination over our healthcare decisions disrupts the domestic tranquility and enslaves our bodies and minds; it forces conformity to government commanded medical intervention. Government should not be so dominating that it intrudes upon the private vaccination decisions of individuals. Government overreaching into personal vaccination health- care decisions is a prime example of government getting too big and is essentially the destructive and wasteful business of minding another person's business. For the sake of quality control in healthcare and freedom of health decisions, medical intervention must never be enforced upon the public; it should not be dictated by government. The jurisdiction of government is not in the internal space of the human body. Government has no permanent realm of jurisdiction in the People's preventative healthcare decisions and no superior jurisdiction that can overrule the decisions of parents for their healthy children. During non-emergency situations government must not dictate preventative healthcare. In a free society healthcare is not controlled by government!

WHO IS A BETTER STEWARD of children's welfare and/or blood chemistry; parents are! The People do not need or want invasive nanny government that singles out certain medical interventions for mandating such as, mandated vaccinations, or for that matter, any form of healthcare nanny government. The People want a government that serves the People and has reasonable restraints of power, allowing parents to protect their children from unwanted chemicalization injections. We must not serve government through the unlawful takeover of children's healthcare or health destiny and/or parent's vaccination decision authority. Government must not obfuscate parents nurturing, caring or decisions in healthcare for their children. Law must not infringe upon fundamental parenting or shackle parent's protection of their children or anguish the spirit of parenting. We must be free to decline unwanted vaccinations for the sake of vaccine quality and in the best interest of children. Liberty to control health is the freedom to boycott unwanted vaccines. For example, why accept a vaccine that has a preservative that in unnatural to the body. Salt is a natural to the body preservative that the public should have it as a choice as a preservative or no preservative whatsoever. Injecting vaccines with mercury as a preservative is unwise, unhealthy and are acts of child abuse by chemicalization. Those who support mandated vaccination especially, of vaccines that have unnatural to human biology chemicals are complicit with child abuse by chemicalization.

In order, for parents to be on purpose as parents, on point or focused on what is primary to parenting (the protection of their children); parents must be enabled to refuse a vaccine chemicalization injection if parents deem the vaccine too dangerous or not in their children's best interest! Whomever controls the vaccination decision shall win the war as to what chemicals are in vaccines. Parents need to be FREE to access what chemicals are in vaccines and once informed decide if the vaccine will or will not be injected. No manmade law can be allowed to supersede parents in this crucial, natural parental realm. Children need and deserve the blessings of their parents' protection; children's well-being depend on parent's full spectrum of protection and this includes the rejection of unwanted vaccine chemical injections. Law must not sever children from the protection of their parents; it is the natural order. Parents must not be limited in making healthcare decisions especially,

preventative vaccination health decisions. Parents must have dominion over what is right or wrong for their children and/or whether a vaccine is in their children's best interest. The parental Right of deciding what is best for children comes from GOD!

Wise men say "government is best, which governs least"; this is especially, true when it comes to health choices and/or vaccinations. Government is best if the government governs least for decisions in health. Parents do not need government intruding upon their private healthcare decisions and do not want to be commanded to submit their children to be vaccinated. The premises that the mandated vaccination law is proper law because it is for the common good of the masses or a price we must pay for living in society or that vaccinations supposedly do more good than bad are all flawed. **We the People' must live FREE** and not merely have the illusion of freedom. We must act to prompt the removal of harmful unwanted chemicals in vaccines by granting The People' their basic freedom to self-protect themselves and their children in health and in sickness. The public good is best served and people are truly **FREE** if the individual can control their very own bloodstream. **FREE** will is a gift and no parent should be asked or coerced to not live by their **FREE** will. **True freedom requires that people have the unmitigated control over their personal health affairs and/or the vaccination decisions.** One's individual choice in deciding what healthcare to accept or deny must be respected especially, in matters of mere prevention and/or when an individual's health is optimum. Our destiny is to be in ultimate control over our very own internal welfare, for what insanity would there be if otherwise. A mandated enforcing of vaccinations holds down individuality and **FREE** thinking. **The mandated enforced vaccination law wrongly concentrates power to care for our children in the hands of centralized government instead, of with children's parents.** What the government says goes-or else, shackles the human spirit. Mandated vaccination is government over-powering liberty! **Liberty to refuse vaccine chemicalization is freedom not to be mastered over in healthcare**.

I do not mean to denigrate Government officials or legislators however; they should not make promises to self-serving, pro-mandated vaccination lobbyists; at the loss of our liberty and expense of children's health. It is common sense to want to keep your offspring's blood **FREE** of unnatural to human biology chemicals and it illustrates that vaccine producers either have no common sense for lacing its vaccines with such, chemicals or it has agenda is to put profiteering ahead of our children's welfare. **If it can be proven that vaccine producers had knowledge that a chemical or chemicals it put in vaccines caused health problems or even health risk and/or they knew that it could produce the vaccine without such, a chemical or chemicals then that can be considered a prima fascia case for culpable negligence.** Harsh chemical preservatives in vaccines may give vaccines longer shelf life which, means increased profits however, it gives children unneeded, unhealthy chemicalization. There are other much more natural preservatives like salt, which, are not near as unhealthy for vaccine recipients and there is also, the option to at least offer potential vaccine recipients a vaccine that has absolutely, no preservatives whatsoever. Big Pharma has played the dominate role in assuring that vaccines are mandated despite the fact, that doing so destroy parents Right of protection of children and/or ignores children's need to be protected by their parents when parents determine a vaccine is too dangerous to inject. The general welfare is not served by mandating vaccinations or having vaccines produced with alien, foreign to the body chemicals. The general welfare is best served by giving people the Right to determine if a vaccine will or will not be injected into their bloodstreams, enabling parents to protect their children and thereby, stimulating higher safety standards for vaccines. **Furthermore, granting**

informed consent/DENIAL best protects children. In addition, holding vaccine companies liable for vaccine induced injuries is indispensable to secure SAFER vaccines and thereby, put an end to the Autism epidemic.

When the vaccine companies were under siege for all of the justified lawsuits brought against it, due to vaccines being manufactured with chemical negligence causing injuries, the action taken by vaccine producers was reprehensible in that it did not properly seek to stop its negligence, and/or the reason vaccines caused children injuries instead, it unconscionably decided to make itself impervious to lawsuits stemming from its vaccines. It used government as its puppet and with bias and baseless reasoning gave vaccine producers an unwarranted, impregnable protection from litigation (a total liability shield). This assured vaccine mega profiteering could not be affected by lawsuits but, allowed for continued runaway negligence thereby putting business protection ahead of children's safety! Vaccine company's lobbyists and big money donations assured there would be no punishment for negligent vaccine production; an anti-safety negligence liability shield was perpetrated. Not too many people know about this total liability shield. **SAFER vaccines charity' wants to turn this around and make children's safety the priority and end this unconscionable and unwise anti-safety liability shield that vaccine producers manipulated into existence!**

Instead, of government hitting the vaccine companies squarely right between the eyes with punitive fines, treble damages and supporting honest and justified lawsuits; government was lobbied to unduly protect vaccine producers by enacting regulation that government/tax payers' money would pay the compensation to those injured by vaccines instead, of vaccine producers. Vaccine producers rightfully should pay, not our tax dollars for its negligence; this inequity was done under the mal-enactment of the National Childhood Vaccination Injury Act of 1986. Tax payer's dollars used to pay for vaccine production negligence is insane, unjust and at our children's health detriment because there is no negligence deterrent, no punishment for harmful vaccine production. It makes vaccine companies impervious to lawsuits when our children are injured by vaccines and only assures that the vaccine supply will continue to be produced negligently and/or with unwanted chemicals. Vaccine companies cannot be hurt financially when vaccines cause injury, so it will continue to put chemicals for profit and not safety in vaccines. Children need to be protected by negligence law and parental freedom. Children's welfare; demands **SAFER** vaccines!

Big Pharma too often puts a drug or vaccine on the market that causes major injuries and it is accused of pushing doctors to prescribe a drug and higher doses of it even though the drug causes harm or the patient does not need the higher more expensive dosage. The drug industry is often being accused of unethically influencing doctors to write more and more prescriptions of a new drug and/or for higher doses even if the patient is happy taking a drug that does the same thing and cost less money; too often the new drug or upped dosage can expose the patient to far greater health problems. The brand name drug Subsys is one drug held in such, controversy. In a wrongful death lawsuit, it was plead that Insys, the pharmaceutical company that makes Subsys, "infiltrated the medical community with lies, misinformation, kickbacks and financial awards and that its reps routinely spoke directly to patients." Subsys (fentanyl) a sublingual spray, is known to cause life-threatening respiratory depression. Hundreds of deaths are being linked to Subsys and over dosing by prescription is one of the causes of death. It is plead that doctors over prescribe or jack up the patients' dosage because everyone makes more money. Apparently, this drug company looks at its bottom line or how much money it can illicit rather, than patient need or protection. It is said that doctors are rewarded and/or that one doctor was paid $35,000 by the drug producer of Subsys for writing Subsys prescriptions or increasing its dosages however, the pitiful doctor ridiculously claims it did not influence his reason for prescribing the drug. People could be dying and yet doctors overprescribe, and Big Pharma continues its business as usual, selling its drugs. The FDA is not adequately protecting us, and its inaction is shameful. This is just one glaring example of why we must be **FREE** to protect ourselves and why parents always need to be completely **FREE** to decide what is best for their children and protect them accordingly. The FDA or any governmental branch or vaccination mandate has no business or jurisdiction to overrule parents' protective decision about healthcare for their perfectly healthy children! **Parents' have the real true caring and JURISDICTION over children's welfare and the DELIVERY OF VACCINATIONS MUST BE RULED BY THIS SUPREME UNDERSTANDING!**

There is a litany of chemicals that need to be removed from vaccines! Obviously, there are unnatural to the body chemicals in vaccines that may have to remain in order, for a vaccine to be a vaccine. However, are unnatural to biology chemicals that desperately need to be removed that do not even have to be in vaccines. Toxic chemicals that are mainly in vaccines to increase profit (chemicals for profit) must be removed. The potential vaccine recipient or parents of the potential child vaccine recipient must be the ones that decide whether to allow the vaccination otherwise, it will spawn chemicals for mere profit in vaccines. Please, notice that the mission statement of **SAFER vaccines**, the charity is to **GET THE CHEMICALS OUT** but not necessarily, all the chemicals. A primary goal is to remove those chemicals most concerning like mercury and aluminum or other known harsh or toxic chemicals. If we do not implement the **TWO STEPS OF CORRECTION** vaccine producers will continue to put **CHEMICALS FOR PROFIT and not safety in vaccines, chemicals that do not have to be and should not be in vaccines.** In order, to achieve much **SAFER** vaccines, **SAFER VACCINES THE CHARITY,** strives to make the public aware of the pertinent fact, that unnatural to human biology chemicals are in vaccines and that it is very unhealthy to inject such, chemicalizations. Certainly, chemicals are in vaccines not for our children's welfare but rather, to generate or assure maximum profits and parents and the public need to become aware if this and be proactive to have these chemicals removed. **THE TWO STEPS OF CORRECTION WILL GET THE CHEMICALS OUT!** Our precious freedom to decide what will or will not be injected into our children is essential to secure **SAFER** vaccines. Holding vaccine producers properly accountable and liable for vaccine induced injury is another vital **STEP OF CORRECTION** in the securing of **SAFER** vaccines and our children's welfare.

The National Childhood Vaccination Injury Act has it all wrong in that it renders children less safe by not deterring negligence; it holds that vaccine producers are not accountable or liable for when its vaccines cause injury, they pay nothing. This leaves the vaccine industry's negligence unchecked, promoting runaway negligence, placing our children's welfare at severe risk. It renders Big Pharma above the law and/or not subject to negligence law and that is just the wrong thing to do. The application of negligence law keeps companies concentrating upon safety when producing its products; to not apply the law to our children's vaccine makers' is a disaster in the making, our children's welfare is placed at great risk. This has given the vaccine producers way too much leeway and promotes irresponsibility and is much too much power over children's welfare. It prompts more negligent content, not less and/

or the production of vaccines that are **TOO DANGEROUS TO INJECT**. Anything of power left unchecked will become villainous over time. The vaccine industry has been left unwisely unchecked by the lobbied for enactment of the National Childhood Vaccination Injury Act of 1986 which, resulted in the vaccine industry only having to concentrate on maximizing profits instead, of our children's utmost safety. This mal- Act and no informed consent/**DENIAL** protection are counter to vaccine safety and children's best interest. The vaccine industry must be stopped from putting certain unnatural to the body chemicals in vaccines. **Such, chemicals injected into tiny babies makes optimum health impossible or at the very least implausible.**

If you sprinkled aluminum onto a circuit board it would interfere with its functionality since, aluminum is a conductor of electricity. The brain is electrical in nature, it is like an electric circuit board; it is logical and probable that when you inject a vaccine with aluminum and that aluminum infiltrates the brain to dopes the brain cells, it will be extremely destructive to the brain functionality (a short circuiting). Knowing the dysfunctional propensity of aluminum makes it presence in vaccines an act of gross negligence and/or culpable negligence. Autism in our young and Alzheimer's in our adults are mainly caused by injecting chemicals like aluminum or mercury and other unnatural to human biology chemicals. Vaccine producers have breached our trust and destroyed our confidence that vaccinations are safe for putting such, chemicals in vaccines. It is only, safe to say that vaccines are unsafe and whichever side of the vaccination debate you are on the statistic of onset of both Autism and Alzheimer's have spiked while more vaccinations came on line - WHY - is the question? All indications are that the unnatural to human biology chemicals in vaccines is the cause of these raging epidemics. Many doctors', chemists' scientists' have concluded that such, chemical content is extremely unhealthy to inject. Many parents have become logic stricken about the correlation and are rightfully concerned about injecting their children with vaccines that have unnatural to the body chemicals. Not all unnatural to the body chemicals are equal; some chemicals found in vaccines or used in vaccines should not be injected. While the Big Pharma Industry says there is no correlation to these alignments and its vaccines which, is a page right out of the playbook of the tobacco industry; there must be a reason for such, epidemics and we are now asking a very logical question based on a logical analogy between the electrical function of the brain and a circuit board and that the laws of chemistry apply when this alien to the body chemicalization invades a baby's blood or brain cells. Parents want answers and no longer submissive to unwanted chemicalization injections. **People must be FREE to decide for oneself what chemical will or will not be injected!**

Do not play **CHEMICAL RUSSIAN ROULETTE** with your offspring's' chemistry! Put abnormal to the body chemicals into rapidly developing babies expect abnormal results. There should be an abundance of caution when it comes to what chemicals children are exposed to! The vaccine industry has crossed the line with its utilization of unnatural to human biology chemicals in vaccines. It is not wrong to desire the best for your child or want to protect your child from being infiltrated with chemicals which, are not indigenous to normal biology. Those who have seen to it that vaccines contain unnatural to human biology chemical have taken it upon themselves to distort the normal chemistry of our children without regard to its negative to health results. Mandated vaccination has spawned an abnormal chemicalization upon our quickly developing children that is disruptive to the obtainment of optimum health. Children's perfected chemistry is bastardized by this unwarranted vaccine chemical infiltration. The mandate makes quality control a moot point and renders vaccines chemically intolerable and/or dangerous. We want to support the generation of **SAFER** vaccines that do not make vaccine recipients risk the consequences of abnormal to the body or unnatural to human biology **CHEMICALIZATION**. Parents must be totally **FREE** to protect their children from unwanted **CHEMICALIZATION**! The first manufacturer of vaccines that successfully produces a vaccine that does not violate the vaccine recipient with chemicals for profit and/or chemicals that are not harmonious with health will corner the market and the public will flock to reap the benefits of vaccines without the unneeded risks of unnatural to human biology chemicalization. We must secure our children have the chemical building blocks of optimum health and assure that they are not compromised with chemical stumbling blocks to health and/or not violated with unwanted **CHEMICALIZATIONS.** Do not throw the chemicalization dice.

Be **FREE** to not let your children risk being short circuited by heavy metal chemicalization by injection. The fact, that vaccines have been found to harbor heavy metals such as, mercury and aluminum is horrendous and gives any parent pause to allow their children to be inoculated. The charity **SAFER** vaccines is dedicated to giving people a choice not to be injected with such, chemically laden vaccines and to the procuring of **SAFER** vaccines that make vaccination a much more rational choice. Mercury is a heavy metal and a **SUPER CONDUCTOR** that should not be in vaccines; it is classified by the **EPA** as **TOXIC WASTE** and is a known neurotoxin. Despite the profiteering fact that mercury is a preservative, it is health insanity to have in vaccines; **SAFER** vaccines, the charity is working to have it removed. Aluminum is a metal that is extremely conductive, as is mercury; the brain is like an electric grid and this makes the concept of injecting such, chemicalization as faulty, unhealthy and even life threatening. **SAFER vaccines charity is determined to protect your children, working tirelessly to GET THE CHEMICALS OUT**! Your children deserve the best chance to be healthy please, help by donating to **SAFER** today. The main reasoning why vaccines have devolved to become vessels of unnatural to the body chemicals is because people cannot legally refuse vaccination, it is mandated and in addition, vaccine producers are impervious to litigation, not having to pay a single cent in damages when injury occurs because of vaccine chemicalization since Big Pharma lobbied for and carved out an unethical, unprecedented and unconscionable total liability shield. **SAFER vaccines**, the tax-deductible charity has a plan is to help orchestrate the **TWO STEPS OF CORRECTION that will protect your children's welfare BY PROMPTING SAFER vaccines**.

What lunatic put chemicals that are good conductors or super conductors in your children's vaccines? Why on earth or in heavens name would parents want these toxic, life-force interfering chemicals to be injected into their tiny, quickly developing babies? No one really knows the true negative to health consequences of such, chemicalization. One thing is completely known that these chemicals are totally alien to human biology and/or physiology and the presence of these unnatural to the body chemicals cause abnormal chemical reactions to take place in the body. Chemicals have reactive propensities and heavy metals, or chemical configurations of aluminum and mercury have reactive propensities and electromagnetic signatures that are very disruptive which, must create ABNORMALITY. SAFER vaccines, the charity, is working to GET THE CHEMICALS OUT to secure your children's safety. Make no mistake, protect your children's vital chemistry!

If parents took it upon themselves to inject some of these unnatural to the body chemicals which, have been found in vaccines they would more than likely be brought up on charges for reckless endangerment and/or child abuse even if they did it in the name of good or

had these chemicals mixed in with something that is determined beneficial. **Should not vaccine producers be held to the same good standard of care and be brought up on the same charges for purposefully putting unnatural to human biology chemicals in its vaccines?** There are chemicals in vaccines that are in vaccines which, are considered more for profit and less for safety. Parents become outraged to learn that vaccine producers have put such, chemicals in its vaccines and that vaccine companies have manipulated into existence a total liability shield for when its vaccines are proven to cause injury. **Too many people are losing confidence in vaccine safety because of the chemicals that have been found in vaccines and due to this unprecedented and unwise liability shield. SAFER vaccines, the charity is well aware of these concerns and inequities and will act to correct what is so wrong by being a strong advocate of the TWO STEPS OF CORRECTION.** The People need to be empowered with the freedom to control their own healthcare destiny and not be dictated to in this private area! Vaccine companies must be held accountable and liable! **SAFER** vaccines will be the voice of the voiceless; those not wanting to be forced into injections will be heard! **WE ARE ENDOWED BY THE CREATOR WITH CERTAIN INALIABLE RIGHTS SUCH AS, THE LIBERTY FOR PARENTS TO PROTECT THEIR PERFECTLY HEALTHY CHILDREN FROM UNWANTED MEDICAL INTERVENTION AND DECIDE IF A VACCINE CHEMICALIZATION IS OR IS NOT IN THEIR CHILDREN'S BEST HEALTH INTEREST!**

FREE PEOPLE are not enforced to undergo vaccine chemicalization by injection or be made to rely upon vaccine producers or its puppet government that does its bidding. Vaccine content safety is placed in major jeopardy if we are enslaved to vaccinate; we must be **FREE** to protect our children by deciding for ourselves if vaccine content is or is not safe to inject. **As soon as, CONSUMERISM is applied to vaccination there** will be **PRESSURE placed upon vaccine producers TO REMOVE ITS CHEMICALS FOR PROFIT and thereby, rid vaccines of its chemical contents that parents are rightfully concerned about.** The fundamental liberty of parents deciding what is best for their children is part of normal parenting, the natural order of things and is basic to the very premise of **FREE** will. This liberty promotes **SAFER** vaccines because of consumer choice and/or freedom to refuse an unwanted vaccine. We must get off the crazy train of enforcing injections of vaccine chemicalizations. Instead, let us set upon a sure path, with laser sharp focus, to promote a vaccine production that respects the natural integrity of our children's pure bloodstreams and passes the rational safety concerns of parents. **Restore the natural order so parents can once again do what is instinctive; protect their children from a conceived of harm as an unwanted medical intervention of vaccine chemicalization.**

Mandated vaccination is an enormous system of injustice. What can enter a person's bloodstream is their own private affair; no one or mal-law should command you to inject vaccine chemicals into it. The liberty of healthcare decisions goes to the very heart and essence of freedom. No one can be considered free if they are forced, enslaved to have their own or their children's precious skin pierced by an unwanted needling and injected with unwanted vaccines. The fact that people must vaccinate despite the fact they fear needles or are apprehensive the vaccinations will cause harm or know it will cause harm and/or signs and symptoms indicates the high degree of oppression that people suffer under mandated or enforced vaccinations. The enlightening fact that vaccines have alien, foreign to the body contents and that vaccinations do cause harm; makes it that much more egregious that vaccinations are mandated and the act of vaccination enslavement that much more outrageous. **The FREE exercise of healthcare decision and/or health choice is the most** primary of freedoms; enforced vaccination is a form of medical intervention slavery and considered a most terrible violation and crime. The fact, that no living cell can function normally or survive in the presence of mercury tells us or strongly indicates that vaccine producers put chemicals or molecular chemical compounds in vaccines that parents should be FREE to object to and/or refuse injection!

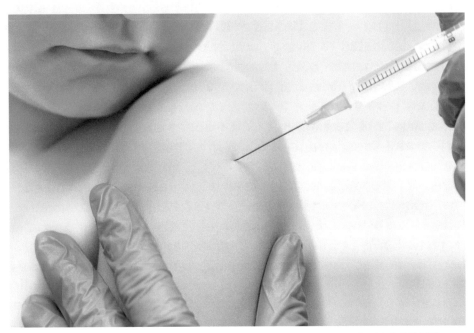

DO YOU KNOW WHAT CHEMICALS ARE IN THE VACCINE?

Picture a needle being pointed at your tiny baby, taking aim to pierce her skin, in an attempt to inject a vaccine that has chemicals which, are unnatural to human biology. You have become somewhat educated about the harm or logical risk that can come from injecting such, vaccine chemicals and do not want to upset, distort or manipulate your healthy daughter's perfected natural chemistry. You personally know too many parents who claim their children were injured by such vaccine chemicalizations and many say that the injections caused their children to become Autistic. In addition, you have learned that millions of dollars have been paid out to compensate victims of those proven injured by vaccination and you are aghast to learn that negligence law really does not apply to the producers of vaccines in that they have an unconscionable total liability shield. You want and need to protect your children to the best of your ability! You really do not agree to inject vaccines that have chemicals that obviously cause harm however, because your children are blocked from entering school if they are not vaccination compliant; you feel you have no real choice in the matter and are coerced, whipped into submission so you are forced to submit your children for unwanted vaccine chemicalization. Inexplicably, the law dictates that you must submit your child to be vaccinated even if you conclude the vaccine is much too dangerous to inject. So, Child Services do not take your child from you and to assure your child can easily gain entrance into school, you hesitantly and begrudgingly submit your child to be shot up with vaccine chemicalization. You never do give your true informed consent, you crumble under the undue pressure, you are coerced to allow your child to succumb to chemical injection, your will is broken; you are reduced to a VACCINATION SLAVE and suffer your enslaved child with unwanted chemicalization.

Instinctively you may have felt chemical vaccine injections were not good for your child, but you were coerced and forced to submit. Perhaps, your intelligence smacked you in the face that the vaccination is an abnormal chemicalization of the blood. You want to afford your children the benefit of vaccination but without such, unnatural to human biology chemicalization. You do want to vaccinate however, you do not want to regret that you did not protect your child from chemical doom. You demand a clean shot, one without anti-health chemicals; you want a SAFER SHOT BUT, IT DOES NOT YET EXIST. SAFER vaccines' charity is dedicated to giving parents better vaccine choices; vaccines which, are less an unnatural to human body chemicalization and more of a rational choice to become vaccinated. SAFER, strives to prompt vaccine producers to rid vaccines of the chemicals that many parents object to and that have become known not to be so wise to inject. Parents must not be robbed of their ability to protect children, parents must be FREE to nurture and safeguard their children's health. Of all things, sacred and most important to parents is the well-being of their children; for government to intrude in this highly private area of parental jurisdiction is unwarranted, unprecedented and the highest level of personal invasion. Preventative healthcare for the perfectly healthy is strictly the purview and jurisdiction of the individual and/or parents for their children. Government has no jurisdiction, no authority or business, in intervening or commanding parents to submit children for any preventative healthcare especially, unwanted chemical invasions!

Even the most sensitive of persons could not imagine the remorse, sorrow or uncompressible anger and the incomprehensible devastation caused to parents from having to submit their child for a vaccine chemicalization against the parent's will. Times this anguish by an exponential number and you begin to understand the life changing grief that occurs to parents and their children when an unwanted vaccine induced injury takes place such as, AUTISM. Having to do something against your will is always unpleasant however, having to do something to your children that you think not in their best interest can be devastating especially, when your child is injured because of it. Parents are coerced to submit their children; they are enforced to allow an UNWANTED vaccine chemicalization. Parents' are left devastated, having to live with the quilt and health deterioration if their children suffer a vaccination induced injury. It should be a heinous crime to enforce parents to put their children in harm's way with unwanted, denaturing chemicalization. There is a growing population of people that are so distraught over this enforced vaccination system that they are taking a stand against it; standing united against tyrannical medical intervention and the oppression of VACCINATION SLAVERY. A JUSTIFIED CIVIL DISOBEDIENCE is at hand! SAFER vaccines' the charity has TWO STEPS OF CORRECTION that will save your children from being abnormally chemicalized and this will prevent the growing civil unrest!

The chemicals that have been found in vaccines strongly indicate that vaccine producers are unstrained from putting whatever chemicals it wants in our children's vaccine supply and do so with impunity from lawsuits. SAFER vaccines' want to put normal and rational restraints on vaccine producers with the TWO STEPS OF CORRECTION. Parents are rightfully concerned about what chemicals are being injected into their children. Perhaps one of the greatest, if not the most important aspect of life is procreation and the fulfilling of all the pleasures and pains of parenting. Protecting your children is understood as a primal instinct and/or natural Right; a biological imperative. No man-made, mal-law should stand in the way of this longing, need or primal function of protecting one's own flesh and blood. **If a parent deems something as detrimental to the well-being of their children, they are endowed by natural law to safeguard their children from this perceived of or actual danger.** Parents commonly make the healthcare final decisions for their children! In combination of these universal laws and understandings, parents' that perceive a vaccine to be controversial or too dangerous or not in their children's best health interest must be **FREE** or entitled and/or empowered to prevent the unwanted vaccination danger and thereby, **stop the assault and battering of their children!**

Controlling or overpowering someone in their vaccination decision or to ignore parents' protective decision to not inject their children with vaccine chemicals or disempowering parents are links in the chains of bondage of enforced, VACCINATION SALVERY. Intellectual and spiritual wisdom tells us that without liberty to protect one's children or decide what is best for one's very own children and/or not be FREE to determine if a vaccine injection is our children's best interest; then WE ARE ENSLAVED to vaccinate our children. Wisdom and/or liberty is the ability to monitor oneself and one's children; to be in control, to self-direct, to decide just what is best and to possess the self-preservation authority to accept or deny any chemicalization by vaccine injection.

Injection must not be given without parent's true informed consent, there must be valid permission! Parents must always remain FREE to protect their children. A law that impinges upon parent's freedom of childrearing protection must automatically be held as suspect and assumed to be mal-law or warped attempt at law and/or a perversion of the natural order. **Vaccination mandates enslave parents** to immorally shriek their parental responsibility of deciding what is best for their children; forbidding parents from protecting their children from unwanted, conceived of as too dangerous to inject vaccine chemicalization. It violates the parents most fundamental Right to care for their children to the best of their ability. This mal-law makes any parent who does not vaccinate their child a dissident and/or a law breaker and improperly can call for Child Protective Services to act against these good intentioned **parents who validly act to protect their children from harm.** The mandated vaccination law violates children through the assault and battery of unwanted, perceived of as, too dangerous to inject, vaccines. If parents determine or are convinced that the vaccine should be given in the best interest of their children then by all means, with parental unadulterated permission the vaccination can and should be administered. **Vaccination must be voluntary** and not mastered or enforced upon us!

People are calling for an end of the enforcement of unwanted vaccine chemicalization, to put an end to enforced unnatural to the body chemicalization; the time has come to **ABOLISH VACCINATION SLAVERY**! There has been talk of protests to end the aggressions improperly placed upon us and/or to straighten out all the destructive mess that self-serving lobbyists and the callous political machinery have created. I sympathize with the oppressed and might someday have to stand shoulder to shoulder with them in their freedom fight; however, I prefer the viable peaceful solution to this untenable situation; **THE TWO STEPS OF CORRECTION SOLUTION**! Positive change and justice must come; parents must be **FREE** to protect their children from unwanted chemicalization by vaccination. To **ABOLISH VACCINATION SLAVERY** and to send a justice message to the political machinery; we must implement the **TWO STEPS.**

In order, to best safeguard children if I must choose between the righteousness of parents being FREE to protect their children from unwanted, conceived of as, too dangerous to inject vaccine chemicalization and peace, I choose righteousness! We can act civilly to **FREE** ourselves from these overburdens by having the proper awareness and commitment to make the needed changes and thereby, quell the need for drastic measures. To rid ourselves of these oppressions we must take strategic **FREEDOM STEPS OF CORRECTION. Abolish vaccination slavery,** restore freedom and the natural order of things with these **CORRECTIVE TWO STEPS**. Vaccine companies need to be slammed with a strong dose of **freedom reality**. Empowering parents to have the decision control in the care of their children is the perfect and natural right thing to do and best protects all our children. **It is as natural as breathing for parents to be responsible for their children's well-being; parents must have ultimate protective power and control over if a vaccine will or will not be injected. Vaccine producers must not have unchecked absolute authority over what is in vaccines and must be held accountable and liable for its vaccines that cause our children injury. Parents need liberty to bring vaccine makers to court to seek justice and COMPENSATION for their children's vaccine induced injuries. We must self-rule over our very own blood and body!**

Vaccinations are a contradiction, a union of opposites. On the one hand, vaccines have antigens that hopefully elicit somewhat of a lasting immune response however, in opposite union to health, vaccines have alien, foreign and/or unnatural to the body chemical content that destroy the brain cells' normal chemical homeostasis; disrupting one's optimum health and/or promoting a gamut of health problems including, Autism. The **uncertainty** of vaccine safety and the **certainty** of ill-effects on health make for an **uncertainty and certainty principle**, which affirms and demands that parents be empowered to call the shots; being endowed to decide if a vaccine will or will not be given and protect their children from unwanted vaccine chemicalization. **Importantly, one of the reasons why vaccination induces an immune response is because vaccines contain alien, foreign and/or unnatural to the body chemicals that your body recognizes as such and jumps into defensive action in an immune response to the alien chemicalization. The immune response from vaccination is not so much from the antigens inside the vaccine but rather, the unnatural to human biology chemicals in the vaccines. The immune response stresses and injures the immature developing immune system and the majority of the immune response does not give lasting immunity from the childhood disease in fact, the immune response produced from chemicalization is quickly fleeting.**

Moreover, because foreign to the body chemicals presently exist in vaccines health problems will result and/or a great deal of health uncertainty. The health problems or uncertainty is very problematic, and parents need to take it into consideration in protecting their children. **Experts have varying opinions about the safety of vaccines, at best, vaccines are found to be consistently, inconsistent; safe by some experts and not safe by others. It is my strongest opinion that many of the chemicals in vaccines have no benefit to health; only health detriment. Vaccines CAUSE HEALTH PROBLEMS; if they have unnatural to the body chemicals and not based upon informed consent/DENIAL and if vaccine producers cannot be litigated against for vaccine induced injuries.** Vaccinations can and do **Vaccine chemicalization must be a matter of freedom of choice; with liberty to refuse!**

Parents have a venerable position in deciding healthcare for their children. The vaccinations delivery system must respect this venerable, supreme authoritative position; parents traditionally decide if any healthcare will be accepted or denied for their children. There is no logical reason to treat the vaccination question differently. Mandated vaccinations are an enigma, like a rogue shark doing damage; enforcing injections make it rogue. **The uncertainty principle of vaccines and certainty of being chemically compromised by vaccination are controlling reasons for parents to dominate in a venerable protectorate position; to have the ultimate authority of protection for children and be the ones to decide what is in their children's best health interest. Parents' must be in control by having the conclusive authority over vaccination, deciding "YES" or "NO" to vaccinations. In deciding the vaccination debacle realize that the bill always comes due when you break the law of nature by injecting unnatural to the body chemicals into babies; all babies are chemically sensitive. You should be and need to be FREE to not denature or distort your offspring's chemistry! Support the charity, SAFER vaccines as, SAFER works tirelessly to bolster safety by striving to achieve SAFER vaccines for the sake of your children's well-being.**

There are too many parents' swearing up and down or claiming that soon after their children received a vaccination that their children's health quickly degenerated and/or that autism was eventually diagnosed. While there may be a few parents that may merely wrongfully determine that a vaccination was the cause of autism the sheer magnitude of reports cannot be wrong especially, when vaccines do indeed contain unnatural to human biology and/or physiology chemicals. SAFER vaccine, the charity wants to GET THE CHEMICALS OUT, the unnatural to human biology chemicals in order, to render SAFER vaccines. One parent told me that they were shot while serving in the armed services defending this great nation and lost a leg as a result however, they would rather, have lost both legs than to have watched their child health demise after a vaccination. The injuries are prevalent and the unnatural to the human biology chemicals in vaccines are the culprit. The CDC list of signs and symptoms that occur after injection is enough to make one recognize the very real danger of vaccine chemicalization however, it is just the tip of the iceberg of problems that can stem from unnatural chemicalization. Parents by supreme Right should be enabled to decide if a vaccine is or is not too dangerous to inject instead, of being coerced or forced or enforced by law to vaccinate! Children's welfare is much more the jurisdiction of parents than wayward mal-mandates!

It is my strongest understanding that we need to have the chemicals that take part in building our bodies and health thus, this type or kind of chemicals are designated the CHEMICAL BUILDING BLOCKS OF GOOD HEALTH and perhaps more important to being healthy, is that we are not exposed to and/or do not need the chemicals which, have nothing to do with health but all to do with being unhealthy and these chemicals are designated the CHEMICAL STUMBLING BLOCKS OF GOOD HEALTH. Unnatural to the body chemicals are synonymous with CHEMICAL STUMBLING BLOCKS OF GOOD HEALTH and absolutely, must be avoided. Our children are placed in jeopardy when such, anti-health chemicals are allowed in vaccines or put in vaccines to merely bolster profits. These STUMBLING BLOCK CHEMICALS are an ANTI-HEALTH CHEMICALIZATION that can only serve to cause abnormality and never good health. Such, chemicals do not take part in the normal, everyday needed reactions of the body for health and alien to the body, anti-health chemicals are

not even part of human biology or physiology. Know that these stumbling block chemicals stress the body, cause abnormal reactions and/or cause abnormal reactive results that adds up to abnormality. These unnatural to the body chemicals do nothing that the body needs or requires to be healthy in fact, it is toxic to the body only having abnormal to the body chemical reactive propensity. These chemicals are considered foreign, alien and/or unnatural to the body and is like a waste product that the body has no use for. Save children from such, chemicalization and you preserve health!

When anti-health chemicals in vaccines are injected into your child's body a defense mechanism reaction ensues and this should ALARM YOU THAT WHAT WAS INJECTED IS INJURIOUS. Headache, redness at the injection sight, fever, vomiting, loss of normal consciousness or behavior, inconsolable shrill crying, loss of eye contact, starring and convulsion are some of the signs or symptoms and/or ALARMS that indicate an injury is occurring from the abnormal chemicalization. What is commonly seen, witnessed or experienced are these signs and symptoms indicate a problem has ensued. The body is no fool it recognizes an abnormal CHEMICALIZATION for what it is and reacts to it as the body attempts to deal with being chemically compromised. Unnatural chemicalization will cause abnormality and the early on reactiveness shown by signs and symptoms indicate that problems are just beginning from the unnatural to the body chemical infiltration. These reactions of the body alert the conscious person to the problem. Vaccine abnormal chemicalization and its negative reactions cause less than 100% optimum health thus, these chemicals are not building blocks but rather, stumbling blocks of good health. SAFER vaccines, the charity wants to research what unnatural to the body chemicals are in vaccines, alert the public to it and instill the removal of chemical stumbling block from vaccines. SAFER vaccines, the charity wants to assure your children are offered SAFER vaccines which, do not chemically compromise those who become vaccination recipients!

The vaccination mandate disregards parents as if they are not capable of making the vaccination decision, ignoring parents' right of decision in fact, the mal legal mandate totally obfuscates parental authority and/or what parents think best for their children. Parents are FREE to decide what is best in all healthcare regarding their children and vaccination should be no exception. Once again, if vaccines were not so unconscionably profitable to be mandated, it would not be mandated. We are not feeble minded or machines or robots that need to be commanded or directed by someone; we are independent free-thinking Americans that decide for ourselves what is right or wrong or good or bad or is or is not in our best health interest. FREE people are not commanded to eat what they do not want or inject an unwanted vaccine chemicalization. People want the command over themselves and want SAFER vaccines that do not have such, unnatural to the body chemical content in order, for vaccination to be a much more rational choice. Parents hold a truly caring consideration for their children. Who do you think should have the ultimate power of decision for the sake of your children's welfare; YOU or someone else? Who should decide if an unnatural to the body chemical will or will not be injected into your chemically sensitive baby? It is YOU, YOU and YOU again that needs to have this rightful control and/or self-determination! In general, parents are most trustworthy and have the proper close relationship to do what is right and have unbiased judgement!

To be held hostage until your child becomes vaccination compliant, to not be given the dignity and respect of vaccination self–determination, to have to submit your child for an unwanted vaccination just because a mal-law commands it or because your child's schooling will be withheld places both parent and child in an untenable position; dominates and enslaves one to be vaccinated. The threat of being considered a law-breaker if you do not submit your children for vaccination gives one no realistic ability to refuse; it is strong coercion to submit to vaccine injection. **It violates health privacy and one's sacrosanct health autonomy and/or freedom of healthcare decision. This loss of basic freedom results in an enslavement to vaccinate.** In addition, the threat that if you save your child from what you deem is a too dangerous to inject vaccine chemicalization, Child Protection Services will be called, to take your child from you; this torture of your mind breaks one's parental protective resistance toward vaccination; making you to submit to **VACCINATION SLAVERY.** Torture will make even the strongest submit, even in the face of possible Autism. Parents are disarmed in their protection of children because of the vaccination mandate. **VACCINATION SLAVERY has no informed consent/DENIAL and has vaccine producers not held liable and/or punished for vaccine induced injuries; resulting in vaccines being less safe. We need SAFER vaccines!**

Vaccination slavery is a most egregious **enslavement**, an unlawful taking of body and mind; an unnatural taking control of our children's health and/or healthcare. Obtrusive mandated vaccinations offensively, take charge of our children's bodies, obliterating our parental vaccination self–decision. Freedom of healthcare decision is of primary importance and privacy. Moreover, being endowed with the power to decide your and your children's healthcare vaccinations is basic to be an autonomous free-thinking individual and/or parent. The vaccination delivery system must be corrected to be consistent with **freedom of healthcare decision**. In a freedom minded society, it must be considered extremely unconscionable to force parents to have their children vaccinated especially, when parents deem the vaccine as, too dangerous. Coerced and/or forced vaccination is totally one-sided, a domination over us and caused vaccines to become unsafe!

When the vaccination mandate was enacted it was during the extraordinary time of an epidemic and under the falsehood or misconception that vaccinations were "absolutely safe". **If vaccines were once "absolutely safe" it no longer is true because of the chemicals now in vaccines and/or due to the fact, that there has been vast amount of proven cases of children being injured by vaccination**. Since, the vaccination mandate, vaccines have been infiltrated with chemicals for profit instead, of safety; now making vaccines too unsafe. Carrying agents and preservatives in vaccines are to name just a few of the chemicals that have rendered vaccines too dangerous to inject. Indeed, the blind trust that the public has placed in vaccination has been breached by such, chemicalization. The extraordinary continued obligation of mandated vaccination is now unrealistic, too extreme for the times and too draconian. No one contemplated that vaccines would become so injurious or that the number of vaccine dosages would grow exponentially or that lobbyists would see to it that vaccine injuries would be swept under the rug and/or that vaccine producers would manipulate an unconscionable total liability shield. Unconscionably, vaccine producers have manipulated that they are above the law in that negligence law is no longer applied to them; it does not impact them, and this means children are less safe and/or vaccines will be produced negligently without any deterrent. When a vaccine causes injury vaccine producers cannot be touched or legally concerned and that is just crazy!

No one anticipated or contemplated, nor wanted vaccination to be a permanent fixture and/or be enforced upon children in perpetuity. Mandated vaccination was not meant to last for any major length of time and, not in perpetuity; it was to be in place until the epidemic was over and the infringement or violation upon parental rights would cease and desist. Vaccination was not meant to be mandated during **NON-EPIDEMIC TIMES** as is, the situation of today. **Absent the extraordinary situation of an epidemic there must be no extraordinary measure of vaccination mandate. Freedom can be suppressed for only so long; the need for vaccination mandate has long ended and the time for liberating parental Rights is now too long overdue! Long-term oppression of freedom of health decision promotes lack of quality control rendering vaccines unsafe. Perhaps, during an emergency parental authority can be set aside for that instance in time however, absent the emergency parental jurisdiction over their children's welfare and/or vaccinations must rule supreme!**

Modern healthcare is now armed with the knowledge that proper nutrition, sanitation and clean water play the major role in childhood disease prevention and recovery. In addition, there now are super-antibiotics if childhood disease gets out of control and/or if medical intervention is called for. Moreover, the implementation of less invasive chiropractic care, homeopathy, herbal remedies, vitamin and minerals and the conservative use of antibiotics place our children at very low risk of injury from childhood disease. **The greater risk is now from the unnatural to human biology chemicals in vaccines and not from the risk of childhood disease; making THE NEED FOR SAFER VACCINES IMPERATIVE! Under the present circumstances vaccines are unsafe and mandated vaccination is now very antiquated and too egregious.** To continue to trample our Rights during these very different set of circumstances is clearly inappropriate unjust and/or unjustified. It has become apparent that too many numbers of vaccines are now mandated and that vaccines are now big business; making forceful vaccination mandate that much more unjust and/or wrong. **Our Right to self-determine health for our healthy children must now rule supreme!** Today, it is understood that medical intervention is only permitted when the patient agrees to it, giving their informed consent therefore, mandated vaccination is now **antiquated mal-law**. In addition, the ill-conceived law was based upon the falsehood that vaccinations are "absolutely safe" therefore; it is **faulty law** that must be stricken! **SAFER vaccines, the charity, will achieve SAFER vaccines that make sense to inject!**

There is now basic understanding that health or abnormality are dependent upon one's chemical makeup. There are good chemicals and there are bad chemicals; chemicals that are needed to be healthy and chemicals that if present will disrupt the natural chemical reactions of the body and thereby, spawn abnormality. Chemicals not indigenous to the normal chemical homeostasis, that are alien or foreign or unnatural to normal human biology or physiology will cause abnormality. **Inject something abnormal to the normal metabolism of the body and expect an abnormal result! SAFER vaccines are vaccines without such, chemicalization!** This fundamental must be steadfastly applied to vaccine production, with it being a golden rule to never stress or insult a vaccination recipient with an unnatural to the body chemicalization. Vaccine producers are guilty of continually utilizing unnatural to the body chemicals that disrupt the vaccine recipient's delicate chemical homeostasis. **Many of these chemicals in vaccines are primarily used to achieve making more money and are not for children's safety. SAFER vaccines'** the charity calls these unneeded, unnatural to the body chemicals, **"chemicals for profit"**. Exposing babies, infants or developing children to such, abnormal to the body chemicals is considered by many as, child abuse. Parents must be completely **FREE** to protect their children from unwanted chemical infiltrations and/or unwanted vaccine **CHEMICALIZATION. Protect your children by making sure there are SAFER vaccines; a most reasonable requirement!**

A most important step in achieving **SAFER** vaccines is to strongly condemn the inequity that those injured by vaccination are blocked from seeking damages against the party that actually caused the damages. Customary negligence law or its obligations are drafted to avoid continued negligence. Negligence law must apply to vaccinations in order, to secure **SAFER** vaccines; it is anti-negligence, assures vaccine quality and/or a reasonable vaccine production quality control. Being able to have your day in court and be equitably enabled to seek damages against the actual party that caused the vaccination injury is fundamental to the relationship and most important to vaccine quality control. For something as important as our children's vaccine supply it is essential to hold vaccine producers accountable and liable for vaccine induced injury!

This is a call to end unsafe vaccines perpetuated by vaccination slavery and the unconscionable total liability shield that vaccine producers manipulated. Instead of the wrongful enslavement to be vaccinated, allow for fundamental freedom of informed consent/ DENIAL based acceptance or refusal of vaccinations to prevail. The mandated vaccination law takes control and overly intervenes' in people's lives, totally negating the choice-liberty in healthcare and this must cease and desist in order, to establish **SAFER** vaccines. If vaccination slavery exists people cannot refuse therefore, vaccine producers can put whatever chemicals it wants without objection or loss of business. Consumerism liberty must be applied to vaccination to assure vaccine safety. **We need to have the unmitigated autonomy to either accept or deny vaccination.** Vaccination compliance must only be achieved because the people think it best! **Citizens must not be enforced to inject! Even if a vaccine is considered safe by government or others; it must be up to the individual potential vaccination recipient to accept or deny the injection. Vaccination must not be enforced, and vaccination recipients must be free to seek justice against vaccine producers when accused of negligence!**

The collective trauma of being commanded to vaccinate an unwanted vaccination, to be made to endure an unnatural to the body vaccine chemical entanglement is so very wrong that it must be considered unjust and illegal. Wrongfully, there is immense prejudice posed upon those who dare to stand up for their Rights by refusing to inject their children when parent's in a good faith act to protect their children from vaccination harm. Most people fold and submit their children for the unwanted vaccination under the duress, coercion and stress posed. **Government has no jurisdiction, power or authority to over-rule parent's vaccination decision not to vaccinate. Parents must control their children's healthcare, they have decision making sovereignty over vaccinations, they have healthcare decision dominium, it is strictly parent's province, and it is only their turf; government must not trespass on parental territory or jurisdiction.**

To have to do something, anything, **AGAINST YOUR WILL** and/or **BETTER JUDGEMENT** is both painful and offensive and to have to bring your precious children to have an injection of unwanted unnatural to human biology and abnormal to one's metabolism chemical formulation is stratospherically painful, offensive and should be a violation of human rights and/or against the law. Jurisdiction of government must not trample into the personal health decisions of People. An individual's body or internal space is only for that individual to solely command over. The concept of governmental jurisdiction has no long arm reach into the private healthcare affairs of the People. A person's internal universe is not for government to command or rule over. Vaccinations are chemicalizations of the blood and body; it is an injection of chemicals into one's internal self-governed space and/or blood and body. Government was not formulated to dictate our health and/or control our healthcare decisions; government does not have the authority and/or jurisdiction to do so! Mandated vaccinations especially, during non-emergency times, are inappropriate and surely must be illegal. It is a fiction or mere conjecture that **perfect or healthy children** pose a threat to others if they are not vaccinated. It is sheer conjecture or mere **ASS**umption that perfectly healthy children will become sick if not vaccinated; law should not and must not **be based on mere conjecture or ASSumption.**

For the sake of our children's welfare it is of monumental importance that parents be at 100% capability and/or in control; in ultimate power to protect their children from all conceived of danger. Disintegration of a parent's control in caring for children due to the mandated vaccination law and the destruction of our Right to be left alone must end; we must not be violated by unwanted medical intervention. Government has no jurisdiction over preventative, personal healthcare when no emergency exists and cannot demand injection of vaccines that cause injury under any circumstance. These are all excellent reasons to end the madness of a vaccination mandate and clean-up vaccines to a satisfactory non - chemical level that parents can rationally approve of. **Parents need clean vaccines and LIBERTY to decide what is best!**

People require to be FREE and live their lives without being personally violated or have to surrender one's children for enforced injections of unknown consequences or potential harm. Parents are highly efficient and effective controllers of children's health needs and parents must not have their efficiency or effectiveness reduced or superseded by mandated vaccinations. Children are left vulnerable because the vaccination mandate eviscerates parent's ability to protect their children from unwanted chemical exposure. Enforced vaccinations eviscerate parental authority to care for and protect their children. The TWO STEPS OF CORRECTION will restore parents and thereby, allow parents to fulfill their parental obligation of parenthood. Parents need to be fully re-empowered to protect their children. Regaining capacity to protect their children will perfect parenting. Law-makers must always be conscious to not enact laws, which undermine parenting. Once parents are given back their rightful control of children and/or their children's healthcare, WE WILL SEE THE INSANITY OF CHEMICALS IN VACCINES END; no more dirty vaccines.

Someone commands you to put something in your mouth and swallow it but, you do not want to ingest it however, you are told "the government states it good for you and therefore, you are commanded to eat it"; what goes through your mind or what freedom is lost or what violation is being perpetuated upon you? Now, add the fact, that you have been warned by some helpful source that there are unnatural to human biology chemicals in what you have been commanded to eat and that if you eat it you often get signs and symptoms and an injury is possible; now what goes through your mind? You want to refuse but there is a law that requires it and weather you like it or not it will be jammed down your child's throat; what do you think, what do you scream and what action do you take? You find out that lobbyists have spawned this mal-law and that huge profits are being generated by it. What if the powers that be spawned a mal-law that made you suffer an injection or worse, made your children suffer multiple injections that have unnatural to the body chemicals in them; **what do you say or scream and what action do you take**?

States that sanction the trafficking of coerced or enforced vaccinations must cease and desist. The **TWO STEPS OF CORRECTION** are the armor against the arrows of enforced vaccine chemicalization. Chemical warfare by vaccine unnatural to the body chemicalization is attacking our children's brain cells. **Parents must become FREE to protect their children from unwanted, unnatural to human biology, CHEMICALIZATION**. In order, to establish justice and secure the blessings of liberty to ourselves and our posterity, we must establish that no vaccine should be given without the express permission of the individual who the vaccine is proposed for. Permission must be first obtained from the parent or rightful guardian of the children that the vaccination is proposed for prior to the delivery of any vaccination. The liberty and principle of self –determined healthcare must be equitably applied to vaccination, producing a balanced structure of power in which, justice, equality and liberty are in equilibrium; rendering vaccines **SAFER**.

The decision to accept or deny vaccination is for one's personal health benefit or detriment; it is not for government or doctor to decide or dictate. No State can be allowed to deprive a citizen of their basic self-caring health liberty or freedom to decide if a vaccine chemical injection shall or shall not be injected. An individual's healthcare must only be directed the way that individual thinks best. Your delicate blood chemistry must be for only you to protect; you must be **FREE** to refuse vaccination. One's very own bloodstream and/or what enters it must only have one master, yourself. **To have health mastered over you by a stranger ENSLAVES you; one who is dominated and oppressed instead, of being FREE and A MASTER OVER ONESELF. We must be completely FREE to live one's own life and protect the lives of our children! Parents must have this freedom capacity for their offspring until, they reach adulthood.**

You must be **FREE to control** and/or to decide upon your own vaccination destiny, **it impacts your and your children's lives;** to not be free in this capacity is a violation of the United States Constitution. How and all the many ways the Constitution is violated is made obvious in this book. For example, according to the United States Constitution, the supreme law of the land under the 13th amendment there can be no slavery. **As, is pointed out in this book, if we cannot be in self-control over our very own blood and/or body chemistry and/or are enforced to inject unnatural to human biology chemicals into our children against our will then the illegality of VACCINATION SLAVERY exists today, and MUST BE ABOLISHED to resurrect the Constitution. Mandated vaccination is slavery! It is in direct violation of the Constitution and therefore, must no longer be tolerated in that we must act to ABOLISH VACCINATION SLAVERY.** In addition, advocates of vaccination mandates wrongly argue that the People have no Constitutional Right to Self-govern their own healthcare or protect themselves from unwanted vaccination however; the Constitution does protect the **People's life and liberty**. Certainly, protecting one's internal chemistry is the protection of "life and liberty". Moreover, the Constitutional Amendment XIV [1868], "No State shall make or enforce any law which shall abridge the privileges or immunities of citizens of the United States; nor shall any State deprive any **person of life, liberty**, or property without the due process of law; nor deny to any person within its jurisdiction the equal protection of the laws." As you read this book you will become aware of the fact, that mandated vaccination laws are mal-laws which, can be proven unconstitutional. Parents by **GOD given law** have the supreme Right to protect their children.

Furthermore, parents are drawn to do what is best for their children, it is genetic, instinctive, it comes naturally and is parents' highest priority; law must not transgress what is a perfected natural nurturing or caring for children. The general rule of law must be that no one is more perfected than parents in deciding upon vaccination. The law must reflect the view that parents by a higher authority than man-made law must protect their children, and no one is better situated and suited in general to make the best vaccination decision for children. if parents have concluded that a vaccine chemicalization injection is too dangerous to inject or parents are not convinced of the vaccines safety then nothing should or can legally or illegally stand in the way of parents' decision not to vaccinate.

Some. wrongfully argue that the Constitution does not specifically have words that state there is freedom to decide what healthcare to accept or deny therefore, it is not a Constitutional protection. Merely, because the Rights that protect us from unwanted vaccinations were not enumerated word for word at the time of the writing of the Constitution it does not mean that this fundamental liberty is not protected by the Constitution; the Ninth Amendment allows for this future vital protection. The Ninth Amendment anticipated this in that, it allows for all basic Rights be protected and not deny People their **Rights vested in the future**, such as, the instant case of the denial of the **People's Right to refuse unwanted, vaccine chemicalization and/or medical intervention**. Rights that are obvious in the People such as, **the Right of an individual to govern what will or will not enter their own blood vessels are "RETAINED BY THE PEOPLE"**. The Constitutional Amendment IX [1791] states, "The enumeration in the Constitution, of certain rights, **shall not be construed to deny or disparage others retained by the people."**

We have all kinds of Rights that protect us however, if we are not vigilant our Rights can be weakened or destroyed, and we be violated for it; falling victim to oppression as is the case of being mandated by mal-law to suffer unwanted injection chemicalization. If we safeguard our Rights; our Rights will safeguard us and induce SAFER vaccines; we will be protected from being dictated to inject or commanded to be infiltrated with anti-health chemicals through a syringe needling and/or puncturing. Sticking needles into a perfectly healthy baby is gross enough to make any rational parent cringe and require the Right to not be so violated. Sticking needles and exposing your baby to unnatural to human biology chemicalization and/or emptying a vaccine vial that you have determined is too dangerous to inject is what our rights are supposed to protect us from. To not have the liberty to refuse needling and being injected with chemicals that are in vaccines which, you determine are too dangerous to inject is a horrid reality and must be declared an illegality. Children' normally have a high sensitivity to changes in their perfected natural chemistry; if you do not want your children to be injected with unnatural to the body chemicalization; it must be your Right not to do so. You must not be enforced to have your children suffer unwanted vaccine chemical injections; your Right to be left alone and/or liberty to life protects you from being so violated.

There are legal Rights (sometimes also called statuary Rights or civil Rights) that are Rights conveyed to us, codified into legal statutes by some act of legislation or implied enumerated Rights, and are contingent upon our beliefs, customs and laws. In great contrast, **NATURAL RIGHTS** (also known as **Unalienable Rights** or **Human Rights** or **Moral Rights**) these are Rights we are automatically vested with, we are born with; they are not contingent upon being put into a writing.

Natural Rights are thought of as **universal Rights which are understood that we are born with** or are **instinctive** or **God given. Natural law and Natural Rights** are closely related. It is understood that natural law and/or natural Rights are **supreme** as compared, to mere man-made laws and/or laws or Rights established through social contract, positive law and/or government enactments. **Natural protections such as, Self-determined healthcare and/or deciding what will or will not be injected into our body and/or blood is a so called, Natural Right or Unalienable Right or Human Right or GOD given law.**

Personal preference in healthcare and/or making the healthcare decisions that the individual thinks best for oneself and for one's children is basic to human existence and to natural law and/or to natural Rights as natural gets. We must correct the perversion of who has authority in caring for our children and/or who has supreme authority to decide our children's healthcare. The distorted idea that government can overrule a parent's protection of their perfectly healthy children is manifested in mandated vaccination mal-laws. Government paternalistically enforcing vaccinations upon us, ignoring parent's Right to protect their children is unjust. We must restore the natural order of things; return to the more civilized normal way of allowing parents to decide what is best for children. **Go back to what is highly proper, appropriate and natural where parents determine if healthcare will be accepted or denied for their children especially, the preventative health decisions for perfectly healthy children that are not in dire need of medical intervention such as, whether vaccine chemicalization is to be given or not given**.

The truth of the matter is that the media fire people if they allow anyone on television that is anti-Big Pharma and causes any loss of the giant advertiser's business. Most ads on television are from Big Pharma familiarizing and programming us to all take drugs and vaccinations without thinking or questioning it. They target our very young children by putting its commercials on during children's television time; children are very susceptible to its programing. We have become too complacent with this targeting! Vaccines are not adequately studied before being released for public use. Important studies of how the multiple vaccines react together over time has purposely never been done and there finally is a study that compared the unvaccinated with the vaccinated and it was very revealing. Dr. Anthony Mawson and his coauthors in a study, titled, 'Pilot comparative study on the health of vaccinated ad unvaccinated 6- to 12- year-old U.S. children'., showed that the unvaccinated compared to the vaccinated are healthier on many levels. **The vaccinated children were more often diagnosed with allergic rhinitis, other allergies, eczema/atopic dermatitis, a learning disability, AUTISM SPECTRUM DISORDER, neurodevelopmental disorders (NDD) such as, learning disability, ADHD or ASD and chronic illness. Instead, of this study being front page BIG news it has been censored as part of the vaccine industry's damage control.** Chemicals make or break health and the unnatural to the body chemicals in vaccines are causing many health problems.

Vaccine's chemical must react when injected into babies however, this is obviously not a primary concern to Big Pharma however, it is of monumental concern to parents who do not want to jeopardize their children's health. The widespread censorship must end and an honest conversation about vaccines and/or its safety begin to be presented to the public. The vaccine conglomerate surpasses all other lobbyists in this country; it by far spends more to assure vaccine sales, spending $2.6 billion a year which, is twice as much as what oil and gas spends. It also, gives $31 million to a year to federal political candidates and thereby, compromising all who receive Big Pharma's money. Instead, of all this wasted money going out the proverbial safety window most of it should go to research what **chemicals are in vaccines that are disruptive to health** and/or studies on vaccine chemical reactions once injected into children's child. Parents need to understand the ramifications of this and to be **FREE** to protect their children accordingly.

Your body is your temple and it is your NATURAL INNATE RIGHT, SELF- PRESERVATION RIGHT, and/or SELF- DETERMINED HEALTH RIGHT that protects you and your children from unwanted vaccination injection SLAVERY. You must not be precluded or repressed from keeping the blood of your children as pure as you personally want, free if you deem it so of unwanted injections of foreign to the body vaccine chemicals. **Parental informed consent/ DENIAL is your safety net that safeguards your FUNDAMENTAL RIGHT to live your life and control what is allowed or not allowed to flow through your blood vessels; allowing parents to protect children's health and/or blood purity to the best of their ability. There must be no legal or illegal choke hold on parents' ability to protect their children!**

People are amazing, magnificent, spiritual, beings and the law must treat people so. Government must serve the people and not the opposite. **Yes, it is of course good to have rules, but it is bad and impermissible to be ruled over. To be ruled over and/or commanded to submit your perfectly healthy children for unwanted medical intervention is this "impermissible to be ruled over" which, FREE people must not be subjects of. Mandated vaccination is the People serving the government, being ruled over and enslaved by government to vaccinate.** At the conception of this great country it was decided that the government is to serve the People. **Being enforced to have your children injected without parents true informed consent violates the essence of liberty.** The government laws should reflect the needs of the People and protect their children from unwanted, vaccine chemicalization. **Parents' by Natural Right must be able to deny an unwanted vaccination.** Vaccines conceived of as, too risky or too controversial to inject by parents must not be enforced. People want **SAFER** vaccines in that vaccine producers are held liable for vaccine induced injuries. **Vaccine chemicals have impact on health so, require your LIBERTY to reject injections! The holding of vaccine producers accountable and liable and the FREEDOM to reject injections are essential to achieve SAFER vaccines for the welfare of all children.**

Informed consent/**DENIAL** is your safety net for assuring the well-being of your children, a vital connector between you and your children and it is a safety instiller as it will prompt vaccines to be made **SAFER** and/or not have objectionable anti-health chemicals in vaccines. The blessings of Informed consent/**DENIAL** prevent one from being violated by unwanted medical intervention and prompts vigilance by vaccine producers for safety. It allows parents to prevent any unwanted, unnatural to the body chemicals from entering their children. To not have informed consent/**DENIAL** ruling over the vaccination delivery places children in jeopardy and promotes less safety or quality control for vaccines. **Children need this essential protection! There is no greater force of nature than a parents' longing and caring to protect children!**

If the chemicals that have been found in vaccines were to be put in quantity into a landfill that landfill would be designated a "toxic dump". Should we not safeguard our children's vital chemistry with even more zeal than we do our land. Parents need to protect children, so they are not treated as if they were a toxic dump and/or injected (pumped and dumped) with unnatural to human biology chemicals. **The biochemistry or molecular chemistry of babies dictates one to either be healthy or unhealthy. Quickly developing cells or systems of babies are dependent upon obtaining the needed chemical building blocks of health and avoiding its chemical stumbling blocks. Unnatural to human biology chemicals found in vaccines are health's stumbling blocks. When it comes to protecting children, parents would rather stand up for their Rights than sit down on their Rights; be in actual control of their children's healthcare and not be mere titular control figures. Parents have a need to fulfill one of life's primary purposes which, is the protection of children and this protection includes protecting children from conceived of and/or actual vaccine chemical harm! Liberty to reject chemicalization injections is required to adequately protect children!**

Vaccines are approved with mere theoretical safety; each vaccine that hits the market has **not been proven safe for children**. The FDA does not assure that only demonstrably safe and effective vaccines reach the market. Vaccines are not always tested on humans for their pharmacokinetic effects and there are **no long-term study** spanning a minimum period of ten years before a vaccine is released upon the public; **no vaccine is ever proven safe before released.** Since, the traditional study is not performed before a vaccine is released it can be considered potentially too dangerous to inject and/or illegal. We must not be subjected to vaccines that are not properly tested on humans; it is mere speculation or **ASS**umption that they are safe. Since vaccines are mainly aimed at healthy children and merely as a prophylaxis against diseases that they may never encounter it is totally unreasonable to rape parents of their Right to say "NO" to unwanted, vaccine chemicalization. **Presently, the only thing sure is that when a vaccination is given to a baby that baby is exposed to unnatural to the body chemicals. We can and must make it that SAFER vaccines become a reality!**

Government should not enforce citizens to walk the plank of vaccine chemical injection! The truth is vaccines are not that safe and that it is a fact, that vaccines harbor unnatural to human biology chemicals and have caused major injuries. The United States legal standard applied to vaccines defines them as, "Unavoidably unsafe products that are quite incapable of being made safe for their intended and ordinary use". As hard as it is to believe, certain chemicals that have been found in our children's vaccines are considered toxins. A sampling of the harmful chemicals that our children either are enforced to take orally or are injected are **formaldehyde (a strong carcinogen), aluminum phosphate and alum (a preservative) that are molecularly high on the scale of electromagnetic and is highly probable to cause interference or abnormality to the circuitry of the brain and nervous system, phenol (carbolic acid), acetone (a solvent used in fingernail polish remover) and believe or not, thimerosal which, is a derivative of mercury that is a highly toxic heavy metal.** Vaccine producers were prompted to stop using mercury in vaccines however, as crazy as it is, it remains in some vaccines. Parents' must be **free** to deny the injection of vaccine chemicalization of abnormal to the body chemicals; to hold otherwise, is inconsistent with liberty, parenting and health.

The understanding that unnatural to the body chemicals in vaccines pose an unnecessary risk and absolutely cause abnormal reaction results to vaccine recipients is the all-important revelation. The mission of SAFER vaccines charity is to rid vaccines of these burdensome and/or toxic to the body chemicals! Vaccines also, can contain poisonous foreign proteins such as, monkey kidney cells, rabbit brain tissue, and chick embryo and calf serum. These

harmful foreign proteins and the above toxic chemicals are destructive to our children's health. It is of no wonder that American children have such high rates of health problems that range from Allergies to Autism to Cancer since, children are enforced to assimilate multiple vaccinations laced with all these negative to health effectors. Freedom requires that we not be subjects of or subjected to toxic, chemical-buildup! Become a freedom fighter and/or protector of your children's chemical integrity, by donating today! Parents need to do what only parents do best and that is protect their children! Government must only support and protect this primal parental need. Parents' deciding what is best for children, is universally accepted and is the natural order.

It is very revealing that vaccine companies did not voluntarily remove mercury, a known neurotoxin and nephrotoxic from vaccines, it had to be induced to do so, strongly indicating why vaccines can and still do contain unhealthy chemicals. **Parents must not blindly inject; they need to be vigilant as to what is in vaccines!** Parents are understandably upset that vaccine producers did not timely act to render vaccines safer or immediately move to remove mercury. There are other chemicals in vaccines that vaccine producers know are unnatural to human biology and are lax or refusing to remove from its vaccines. The vaccine industry apparently, cares more for profit than children's safety and cares not to quell the rational health concerns of parents and health experts. **When a content correction has negative impact upon vaccine company's profit; the corrective measure or safety precaution will rarely occur, nor will they pay much attention to parent's outcries.** The removal of mercury only came after the proverbial "Chemicals hit the fan" and in response to the build-up of parent's long-term outcries and health experts' warnings. **This finally precipitated an Amendment to the Food and Drug Administration Modernization Act, which was signed into law on November 21, 1997. The amendment commanded that within 2 years the FDA compile a list of all the drugs and foods that contain INTENTIONALLY INTRODUCED MERCURY COMPOUNDS.**

Vaccine producers were callously aware that the FDA called for the mercury list and that its vaccines would surely be on this list; **yet the vaccine industry still did not act to remove the mercury from its vaccines, nor did it heed health experts' warnings or the mass appeal to remove the mercury; it reeks of negligence.** Make no mistake, this involves the chemical well-being and/or health of children so, it was totally improper for the FDA to allow 2 years to gather the **list of drugs and foods that contain INTENTIONALLY INTRODUCED MERCURY COMPOUNDS.** The FDA close ties to Big Pharma can explain why so much time was wrongfully afforded and at our children's health expense or why the FDA turns a blind eye to the unsafe, alien chemicals in vaccines. It is likely, that Big Pharma was given the excessive time because it allowed it to make as much money possible. For the future of our children we must never trust that Big Pharma will keep our children's vaccine supply optimally safe; **THE CHARITY, SAFER VACCINES' mission is to assure** vaccine safety through the **TWO STEPS OF CORRECTION!**

It is unwise to place your children's welfare in the untrustworthy and those who purposefully put such, chemicals in vaccines are untrustworthy! It is best to be in control of your children's welfare by knowing what chemicals are in vaccines and deciding for yourself if the vaccine is safe! Rational, parents should not even want their children to come in superficial or surface contact with some of the chemicals that have been found in vaccines and should become very concerned if such, chemicals are injected into their children. Remember, it was only after a time consuming and uphill battle that the removal of thimerosal from most childhood vaccines finally occurred by 2001. Injury caused by exposure to anti-health chemicals, still in vaccines is the main etiology of the ever-increasing **AUTISM and Alzheimer's epidemics. The most important Autism and Alzheimer's prevention is to remove the toxic, unnatural to human biology chemicals that are in vaccines. Make sure children are not injected with or exposed to unnatural to the body chemicals and children will be health resilient for it!**

Imagine how infuriated parents are after learning their child was injected with a vaccine, which still had mercury because vaccine producers **DID NOT RECALL** the tainted vaccines on the shelves in doctor's offices, even after they were told not to produce vaccines that contain mercury derivative. Imagine, being a parent of a child injected with mercury and your child is caused Autism. **PLACE TRUST IN YOURSELF BY PROTECTING YOUR CHILD WITH INFORMED CONSENT/DENIAL; KNOW WHAT CHEMICALS ARE IN VACCINES, MAKE SURE IT IS SAFE! HARMFUL CHEMICALS MUST NEVER BE INJECTED INTO BLOOD. INFORMED DENIAL AND/OR REFUSAL OF CHEMICALIZATION MUST RULE.**

THE SURE WAY TO REMOVE UNWANTED CHEMICALS FROM VACCINES IS THROUGH FREEDOM TO REFUSE A VACCINE AND/OR THE REFUSAL OF ANY VACCINE THAT CONTAINS UNWANTED CHEMICALS. If there is one thing that we can trust in is that the power of the purse will move vaccine producers into action to remove unnatural to human biology chemicals from its vaccines if they are causing its vaccines not to sell. Vaccine producers are experts in profit making and ultimately concerned about making as much profit from the sale of their vaccines as possible. We need to make unwanted chemically laced vaccines unsellable through the informed **DENIAL** or refusal of such vaccines. Vaccine Producers will then be prompted to produce vaccines without chemicals and with close attention to parental anti-chemical concern. Consumerism properly applied to vaccines will **GET THE CHEMICALS OUT. VACCINATION CHOICE, GRANT PARENTS THE VACCINATION DECISION; THIS LIBERTY ALLOWS ONE TO DENY UNWANTED VACCINES AND IS KEY TO SAFER VACCINES AND CHILDREN'S SAFETY!**

ALARMINGLY, the cumulative doses of mercury from vaccinations exceeded the protective guidelines set by the Environmental Protection Agency (EPA) at the time of the FDA Modernization Amendment and still the vaccine companies failed to act. Now, if this does not tell parents that they need to act to protect their children from such, horrific chemicalization perhaps, nothing will. For the love of our children and their welfare, how could we be so foolish and/or complacent to allow vaccine producers to do such, an unforgivable bad thing to our children; parent must protect their children! Law must not overrule parents' protective decisions or make parents give up their reins of parental protection; parents must be free to refuse vaccinations for the safe keeping of their children. Parent's ideas of what is in line with staying healthy or is health wise must be respected. Parents' must control preventative, non-emergency, healthcare decisions!

An abnormal sign that parents observe after vaccination is excessive secretion of saliva, (salivation) which happens to be a tell tail sign of mercury poisoning. Vaccine producers' put mercury in children's vaccines, this mal-action of placing this chemical in vaccines and omission of voluntary and timely removal gives a clear signal not to blindly trust them with your children's welfare and so, parents' must always demand an informed consent/DENIAL of vaccination to promote SAFER vaccines. Children's well-being, not profit is the motive for not using unnatural to the body chemicals in vaccines. THERE ARE STILL UNNATURAL TO THE BODY CHEMICALS IN VACCINES THAT GIVE PARENTS EXCELLENT REASON TO FORBID THESE UNSAFE INJECTIONS. DO NOT LET SUCH, CHEMICALS ENTER YOUR CHILDREN. DEMAND SAFER VACCINES! REJECT DIRTY VACCINES AND VACCINES WILL BE PRODUCED CLEANER; CHEMICALLY FREE!

Signs and symptoms from mercury poisoning are nearly the same signs and symptoms that Autism children and Alzheimer's adults display after suffering vaccine chemicalization of unnatural to the body chemicals. Where there is smoke there is fire and where signs and symptoms are the same, the causation is the same. Unnatural to the body chemicalization impact negatively upon neurological function and cause brain dysfunction and/or abnormality. Mercury exposure signs and symptoms are almost identical to that of Autism and Alzheimer's; they have a sign and symptom identical signature therefore, it is the same culprit!

Mercury exposure from food poisoning takes a vastly different course into the body than exposure from vaccination in that the mercury does not reach the brain as quickly or as much. Injected mercury by vaccine chemicalization and all the other chemicals of vaccines quickly gain access to the blood system and then this toxic blood hits the brain tissue, attacking brain cells with no buffering of the chemical exposure whereas, ingested mercury is somewhat eliminated by one's selective digestive process. Vaccine chemicalization is much more a direct hit upon the brain as compared to ingesting a toxin that can to some degree be eliminated by the selective digestive system. **Moreover, it is not the singular chemical insult of mercury that is the main etiology of Autism or Alzheimer's but rather, the entire spectrum of unnatural to the body, anti-health chemicals that are in all the vaccines being injected.**

It is not baffling that babies or quickly developing immature children develop health issues after being injected with toxins and/or unnatural to the human body chemicals! Put abnormal to the body chemicals into developing babies and abnormality will result. The finger pointing or the quilt over who is responsible for such, injected chemicalization chaos or anti-normalization is not what is so important; what is of extreme importance is that we learn and now stop being destructive to our babies' normal chemical homeostasis. Autism is not idiopathic; chemicalization is the main origin of Autism. Do not be mistaken or deceived, it is not just mercury; it is the entire array of injected anti-health vaccine chemicals that can spawn Autism. It is imperative that we make opting to be vaccinated a much more rational choice by achieving **SAFER vaccines; we must GET THE CHEMICALS OUT!**

It is obvious that babies who are not exposed to or suffer abnormal to the body chemicalization or unnatural to human development chemicals will be healthier than those that have and that the Autism epidemic has a chemicalization causation! If babies achieve and maintain the purest of natural or optimum to biologic chemical makeup they will be healthier for it and not be as susceptible to becoming an Autism statistic. These health principles steadfastly applied to vaccine production will END the AUTISM epidemic!

Parents who delay vaccine chemicalization of children until their children are older and of greater robust stature logically better withstand abnormal chemicalization; these parents report less Autism. Tiny babies are so highly susceptible to any upset to their natural chemistry which, is required to be healthy and/or resistant to Autism. Those who wisely spread shots out or break up the dosages and/or refuse multiple dosages are reporting less vaccine induced adverse reactions or Autism. This glaringly points to the fact, that vaccine chemical injections chemically dope brain cells of children! **By totally preventing or decreasing the chemical doping of children by only injecting SAFER vaccines will stop the raging Autism epidemic and the spreading out over a greater span of time of injecting any chemically unsafe vaccine will help deter the Autism epidemic. The goal is to prevent a critical chemical reactive tipping point and/or deter an unnatural to the body chemical mass syndrome. Anti-health, unnatural to human biology and physiology chemicals are enemy number one and primary cause of AUTISM!**

In a conversation with an Organic Farmer who was very proud of his plants and/or crops for being free of anti-health pesticides or other abnormal to the body chemicals I brought forth that the idea or concept of what assures that crops are healthy for you also, works for vaccines. Organic farming recognizes that in order, to get the end product the way you want it to be, being healthy as possible for the public to consume, it is ultimately important to see to it that the plants and/or crops obtain all the water and natural nutrients and/or minerals and to make absolute sure that no abnormal to human biology chemicals are in the soil or water that infiltrate the crops or plants. The farmer totally agreed with the aforementioned and when I said, "the same science or rule of achieving optimum health applies to babies; babies need their natural to the body chemical building blocks of health and need to avoid any anti-health, chemical stumbling blocks of health", the farmer's jaw dropped as he realized how true this is and why SAFER vaccines, the charity' mission to GET THE CHEMICALS OUT is so important to the health and/or welfare of all our children.

In the pursuit of SAFER vaccines, the force of consumerism (LIBERTY to decide what product to accept or deny and/or being enabled to refuse an unwanted vaccine injection) prompts needed quality control for vaccine safety and/or children's safety which, self-generates more confidence in vaccinations. Allowing for vaccine consumerism will generate SAFER vaccines and therefore, make choosing to be vaccinated much more rational choice and it gives vaccines a much-needed trustworthiness. To leave vaccines to the rank and self-indulgent production under the present enforced, no freedom of choice system continues to escalate distrust in the very concept of vaccination. To continue to callously not grant parents their basic parental authority and dignity to decide if a vaccine is or is not in their children's best interest and/or not allowing for SELF-DETERMINED VACCINATION CONSUMERISM; escalates distrust in the very concept of vaccination, inducing less vaccination compliance. Because vaccination is mandated and/or enforced, vaccine producers have not had the requisite level of safety for children consequently, it uses anti-health chemicals in vaccines. Parents want and need to be FREE to reject vaccines that have unnatural to the body chemicals. Vaccination compliance must become voluntary; based upon informed consent/DENIAL as is, all other healthcare. The facts that vaccines are not "absolutely safe" and/or are laced with unnatural to the body chemicals make vaccination mandates that much more immoral, intolerable and egregious.

Now isn't it crazy that our children are being mandated to be injected with such, chemicalization! The health of our children is at stake here and we must only trust our children's vital internal chemistry to those who are trustworthy. The fact, that certain chemicals are utilized in vaccines is not only disturbing or alarming, it is outright outrageous. How vaccine producers did not properly respond to parental concerns over vaccine's contents and just how Big Pharma did not jump into action or move at all to rectify the chemicalization reveals the Big Pharma to be what it truly is and that is, a big business that does not have the requisite caring safety attitude. The makers of clinical and laboratory thermometers at least showed that they care enough for public safety by stopping the use of mercury in their thermometers; out of the remote fear that a thermometer could break, and a contact absorption of mercury may occur. Moreover, they stopped using mercury in antiseptics (Mercurochrome and Methylate) to accommodate the growing rational health concerns over mercury exposure. Vaccine producers are ruthless money makers, they do not show caring or caution; they continued to expose your children to mercury and **to this day they continue to expose children to unnatural to human biology chemicals.**

Mega-profit minded vaccine producers did not rush to protect your children's health by removing mercury from its vaccines instead, they were prompted and/or forced to and its inaction speak louder than words. Vaccine producers need to be watched carefully, to assure it does not put profit in front of our children's safety and **SAFER vaccines charity'** is positioned to do exactly that. Vaccines also, need to be policed by parents and the way to do that is through the doctrine of informed consent or **DENIAL liberty. We have all learned a valuable lesson to never trust a profit-based company that has helped see to it that children are enslaved to be vaccinated; our children's safety will not come before profiteering. We must never again relinquish our healthcare safety Right of informed consent/DENIAL of vaccinations. Do not fall victim to unnatural to the body chemicalization; DO NOT INJECT anti-health chemicals! We must secure for our children SAFER vaccines to best benefit from vaccination with less risk!**

Without question the super, majority of parents would opt to not expose their children to the alien, foreign, unnatural to the body chemicals therefore, vaccine producers must be made to produce these achievable SAFER vaccines. Parent's most reasonable and animate desire to safeguard their children from chemical exposure is part of the natural expression of basic parenting. Nothing is more essential to parents than the protection of children from a perceived of harm and in the instant case a vaccination that parents have deemed not in their children's best health interest or too dangerous to inject. Therefore, let us work together to grant parent's their supreme power to deny unwanted vaccinations. Liberty to prevent this unwanted medical invasive procedure will stimulate the removal of alien, foreign, unnatural to the body chemicals from vaccines.

Mercury is just the tip of the iceberg, parents need to be assured for their children's welfare that all unnatural to the body chemicals which, are not absolutely necessary are no longer in vaccines and thereby, have the opportunity to allow their children to be injected with only a SAFER vaccine. Informed consent/DENIAL is the SWORD OF CHILD PROTECTION AND POSITIVE CHANGE to achieve SAFER vaccines. The holding of vaccine producers accountable and liable (no more liability shield) FOR VACCINE CONTENT AND/ OR VACCINE INDUCED INJURIES is the other needed STEP OF CORRECTION that will GET THE CHEMICALS OUT. The single most toxic fact about vaccines is that they contain alien,

foreign and/or unnatural to human biology chemicals. Abolish vaccination mandated slavery and this toxic fact will be no more. Freedom of decision and liberty to litigate are essential to our children's safety. Autism is an epidemic and numbers of chemical exposures has become so extreme that PARENTS and JUSTICE no longer can stand idle. Together, let us act to GET THE CHEMICALS OUT of vaccines by FREEING THE PEOPLE FROM VACCINE INJECTED CHEMICALIZATION SLAVERY!

Mercury is known to cause **thyroid conditions** because it disturbs the metabolism of cooper and zinc, the two minerals that are critical to thyroid function. Mercury also **disrupts immune function** therefore; children's resiliency against disease is more **HINDERED; NOT HELPED by such, vaccine chemicalization. Cells cannot survive in the presence of mercury**. Mercury is just one of the harmful chemical exposures from vaccinations that render our children Autistic (the tip of the **chemicalization iceberg**). **All THE CHEMICALS in vaccines lay a foundation for Autism. Until the clear majority of chemicals are removed from vaccines the Autism rate will either continue to rise or remain at unacceptable epidemic proportions.** Be not complacent with chemicalization; **GET THE CHEMICALS OUT, do it now**!

Vaccine proponents have had the audacity to belittle the fact that our children have been exposed to mercury from vaccines by insinuating that the kind of mercury that they are exposed to in vaccines merely has a biological half-life of approximately 7 days. Well who wants their children exposed to any form of mercury; no matter what the half-life. There are expert geniuses that tell us that the shorter the half-life the more dangerous it is and extremely health disruptive. They have a great deal of nerve to expose our children and then try to deceive or make light of the exposure. The "half-life" rhetoric is meant as a distracter from the truth. **THE FACT IS, the shorter the half-life, the more unstable the compound; destabilized mercury is likely, more dangerous for children than mercury that has longer half-life.** Moreover, mercury undergoing a rapid half-life (rapid abrupt instability) impacts the immediate area surrounding this abrupt decay, the molecular and magnetic concurrent changes can have greater negative to health consequences than if it had a more lingering, longer half-life. **The rapid decay of mercury can cause the rapid decay of our children's health**. The body of the child that has mercury, which is undergoing rapid mercury decay is subject to induced **abnormal changes in** vibration, temperature (heat transfer), metabolism, rate of chemical reactions, magnetic field; this results in electrostatic alteration and/or electromagnetic radiation. The burden of mercury and other anti-health vaccine chemicals make one susceptible to **CRITICAL MASS CHEMICAL SYNDROME. The array of injected anti-health, unnatural to the body chemicals is the primary etiology of AUTISM. All unnatural to the body vaccine chemicals have to be studied for its ill effects.**

Make no mistake; all forms of mercury are neurotoxic and nephrotoxic, it must never be injected into babies; to have it vaccines is crazy and those responsible for any degree of it in vaccines are madmen. To blindly place your children into the hands of such, madmen is ill-advised. To mandate vaccines that have unnatural to human biology chemicals is an act of chemical warfare upon the vaccine recipient and to mandate children be injected with such, chemicalization is mandated child abuse. **Vaccine producers' put a health destroying toxin in our children's vaccines, which means they have breached the blind trust that we put in them. Parents need always do their due diligence before considering the injection of any vaccine chemicalization**. Never place your children in chemicalization harm's way and choose to no longer be experimented on with chemicals or vaccines that are not proven safe. **Aluminum and many of the CHEMICALS IN VACCINES have NOT been proven safe or established as safe by experience. Remember, basic laws of chemistry apply to your children when they are exposed or infiltrated with unnatural to their body chemicals. Children must not be made to be vaccine chemically injected guinea pigs. Parental informed consent/DENIAL will protect your children from unwanted chemicalization and/or being experimented upon.**

Do not automatically ASSume that the chemicals in vaccines are safe to inject; because **many are not!** Parents need to be **FREE** to protect their children and not be enforced by mal-law to submit to unwanted preventative medical intervention and/or made to suffer unwanted vaccine injections of unnatural to human biology chemicalization. **FREE AMERICANS** are not held hostage to the insistence or vices of preventative medicine or made subjects of Drug Company's chemicalizations. Do not give up your children to whatever the mandated vaccination law says or even what the doctor recommends instead, do your own research on vaccination and exercise your parental Right to choose what is best for your offspring. Hospitals or doctors can and have taken it upon themselves to inject children with multiple doses and multiple shots that parents live to regret, as is the case of Crystal Downing of California who claims that her infant was caused to die after 8 simultaneous vaccinations. Doctors are certainly not all knowing, and many have very poor judgement and too many do not even know what chemicals are in the vaccines that they are injecting into your children. Some doctors stupidly give children vaccination that is not even recommended for children. When a vaccine induced death occurs it is often brushed off as a SID. SID, is Sudden Death Syndrome which, basically has no known cause of death. Please, for your children's welfare do look into what chemicals are in vaccines and do not allow a Chemicalization Russian Roulette to take its toll on your children! Only inject with approved of **SAFER** vaccines!

A stellar trust buster, against Drug Companies, is that on December 22, 2006, a US Court decided in Hoorman, et al. v. SmithKline Beecham Corp. that parents who purchased for their minor children Paxil(R) or Paxil CR(TM) (paroxetine) may be eligible for benefits under a $63.8 million proposed settlement. It was found that the Drug Company for prescriptions for children and adolescents withheld and concealed material information about the medications safety and effectiveness for minors. Most of the people involved in the litigation felt they were **not adequately warned in advance of the drug's side effects and addictive properties**. Analogously, Big Pharma does not adequately warn potential vaccine recipients of the fact, of the unnatural to the body chemicals. Slowly but surely, more and more studies will trickle in despite the callous effort to suppress honest, valid research which, clearly shows the chemicals in vaccines are causing major health problems. In Apoptosis, May 2012, Volume 17, Issue 5, pp 516-527, a study revealed that Hepatitis B vaccine induces apoptotic death in Hepa1-6 cells (liver cells). In addition, the researchers concluded that exposure of Hepa1-6 cells (liver cells) to a low dose of adjuvanted hepatitis B vaccine leads to loss of **MITOCHONDRIAL INTEGRITY, APOPTOSIS INDUCTION, AND CELL DEATH**, and other cells are negatively affected. This study points to the chemical additive aluminium hydroxide adjuvant as the cause of such, adverse side-effects. This information is being suppressed; you really must research to find it! The vaccine industry spends many millions to assure vaccines are sold and mandated and who knows how much it spends to suppress anything negative about vaccines or on damage control.

Trust in yourself, your intelligence, common sense and parental instincts to discern what is best for your children and DECIDE what chemicals you do or do not want your offspring to be injected with. **Do not stand for having your fundamental Right to self-determine healthcare taken from you or violated.** Your children are yours to protect and care for; the vaccination decision must be yours to make! Vaccination must be voluntary and based upon informed consent/**DENIAL**; it must not be enforced upon us. **Be a FREE thinking, FREE individual and not a VACCINATION SLAVE! Demand to protect your children to the best of your ability. Parents need to have design and control over children's healthcare; the acceptance or denial of vaccine chemicalization must be under the SUPREME POWER OF PARENTS!**

Remember, the old adage "an apple a day keeps the doctor away" well this life saving, or health philosophy has all but been put on the wayside as it is stifled, no longer being disseminated to the public on the regular basis it once was. The phrase an apple a day" does not mean that you all you need to be healthy is an apple; it is a symbolism for the proper health philosophy, "to let your food be your medicine and your medicine be your food". Eat right and/or consume what the body needs, and you can remain healthy or regain your health. Basic freedom requires that we not just hear these health philosophical words or health advisements but also, by Right; can live by them! No one should be forced to submit their perfectly healthy children for unnatural to the body chemicalization; there must be liberty to live by an apple a day principle and/or natural means to be healthy! Pretty soon if not already there will be a drug for every conceivable ailment, or symptom; we must not be blocked from choosing not to be drugged or vaccinated. Vaccination is an important option however, if it is forced upon us it becomes chemically corrupted. There must be liberty to take the drugs you want and refuse the ones you do not want.

It should not be up to wayward government or the omnipotent few who lobby government for vaccination mandates which, dictates who has the power of vaccination decision but rather, individuals need to be vested with the power to accept or deny vaccination preventative medical intervention! Freedom is bleeding by the infringing or violation of our liberty to decide as parents what is best for our children and the enforcement of unwanted vaccine chemicalization. Liberty, requires that we abolish mandated vaccination and thereby, end the oppression of enforcement of vaccination especially, those enforcements of the non-SAFER vaccines as is, determined by the charity overseer, SAFER vaccines. One loss of liberty leads to another, a slippery slope of loss of freedom; we must assure our freedoms are vehemently protected and not violated.

There are drugs for everything however, it must be up to the individual to accept or deny it! There is a very real danger of drugging for every single sign or symptom. One drug called Linzes claims to take care of and/or is prescribed for multiple health issues including, constipation. Today there seems to be a drug for every single function or aspect of life without taking care of the causation. There is no regard for doing what is right for yourself or adequately hydrating or eating properly so that you do not become afflicted with constipation. People are taking drugs to get rid of their symptoms without taking care of the cause of the problem or in the instance case what lead to the constipation affliction. Dehydration or diet can cause constipation; to just take an anti-constipation drug without taking care of the cause is very dangerous and is a disservice to the patient. To not be

hydrated properly or continue to have a diet without adequate or needed fiber can lead to chronic constipation and much more severe health problems. Also, remember, all drugs have chemicals and cause adverse side-effects. Drugs very often merely rid the symptom, masking the underlying cause; and not taking care of the cause of the condition is not the good practice of healthcare. Getting rid of the constipation by drug chemicalization or not recognizing that constipation is a sign or signal or alarm, alerting you to seek out the underlying causation, is unwise; it often leads to a problem becoming chronic or more severe or a more complex and dangerous to life problem. For instance, if you medicate to merely get rid of the constipation and do not rectify the dehydration, the dehydration will likely, continue and not being hydrated can lead to a more severe problem such as, but not limited to, Stroke. Take medication wisely and always address the underlying cause!

There is a long history of a wide range of health problems stemming from vaccinations. Way back in 1775 one of American history's greatest revolutionist Nathanael Greene reported a negative reaction from the Smallpox vaccination in that it left a cloudy spot in his right eye; I only bring this ancient negative reaction to vaccination case to the reader's attention to bring an eye-opening understanding that vaccine chemicalization is dangerous and is cause all kinds of injuries. Unnatural to human biology chemicals are very bad for your mind and body. Modern day reports of hundreds of lawsuits have been filed against a Drug Company by families that claim Paxil drove children to suicide. The brain's sensitive chemical balance and make-up is thrown into disarray by drug and vaccine chemicals. The anti-health chemicals of behavior disorder drugs cause male feminization (male boobies) and it is said to cause violent episodes and even, suicide. Children's chemical homeostasis is distorted by drugs or by the injection of vaccines. Purposefully injecting anti-health chemicals into children can be considered child abuse! Abnormality, results from such, chemicalization. Makers' of Paxil also, stand accused conspiring to hide its adverse effects in order, to obtain FDA approval. One is left to wonder is this mal-act business as usual for the vaccine industry when it seeks to obtain an FDA approval. **With all the unnatural to the body chemicals found in vaccines; the adverse effects from it may have been and still are being hidden or purposefully ignored.**

The use of unnatural to human biology chemicals in children's vaccines breaks the spirit of the mandated vaccination law and more importantly breaks the spirit of freedom and/ or parenting. Enforced vaccination proponents who do damage control to lessen the impact of vaccine induced injuries do the public a gross disservice. Without question; injecting such, chemicals distort, disrupt and is destructive to the vaccine recipients' normal chemical homeostasis. Liberty requires that individuals be in total self-control and have absolute decision power over what will or will not be injected into our vital body and/or blood chemistry. Deep pocketed lobbyists participate in a concerted regulatory arbitrage to get around our supreme freedom of self-determined healthcare and parental authority to decide what is best for our children's welfare. Only a voluntary vaccination system can be considered a valid law of the land. No rational minded person can say that the dumping or pumping of multiple vaccine chemicals into children will not cause severe health problems. Parents must be true to their mission of preserving their children's health; if you know a vaccine chemicalization will compromise your children's chemical integrity and/or likely cause health problems, do not allow it! Require freedom to decide what is best for your children! Many parents would rather their children risk naturally getting a childhood disease, which usually comes and goes, than face the long-term or permanent health problems or death from vaccine chemicalization. Law must not disconnect you from your essential parental responsibility or command you to be vaccine dependent. No one but you should control what enters your internal being!

There is an ongoing attempt to keep all citizens shackled in perpetuity to the vices of mandatory vaccination medicine, giving parents no choice but to submit their children for burdensome unwanted, chemically laced vaccine injections. There is improper undue influence to keep the vaccine market profitable via vaccination mandates and/or ongoing impositions placed upon parents, coercing parents to submit their children for unwanted vaccine injections. Mere monetary interests of Vaccine Companies and the oppression of parents' liberty to decide what is best for their children must not continue to keep children enslaved to be chemically injected. This oppression has led to vaccines becoming more chemically tainted and a lot less safe. Parental responsibility for children's welfare must have maximum effectiveness and our laws must support this most natural order of things!

How do you reconcile compromising the chemical integrity of children's health or children's general welfare; you don't! No one on the surface of this planet that is in their right state of mind would want their children unnecessarily exposed to unnatural to human biology chemicals, to any degree; and not from a vaccination. Furthermore, the fact that our precious children were and to this day can still be exposed to any degree of mercury, for whatever the half-life of the mercury is, is frightening. Parents have been kept in the dark about what chemicals are in vaccines; this is extremely troubling and of grave concern to the health and welfare of all our children. Parents cannot make an educated or intelligent decision about vaccines without being told the truth of what chemicals are in vaccines. To holdback chemical content information or to make slight of the chemical facts, is an injustice and places our children's welfare in major danger. To best protect children, parents need to be enabled to choose SAFER vaccines and not be blindsided by unwanted chemicalizations. Distractive nonsense and manipulation about what chemicals are in vaccines is being perpetrated upon consumers of vaccines.

In analyzing why people are healthy as compared to sick and/or remain healthy or live a long life compared to the opposite, I have concluded that it is due to not being traumatized mentally or physically but mainly, it is not being chemicalized by unnatural to human biology and/or physiology chemicals. Many of the old day story of those who lived long lives and had energy and vitality not only through their younger years but also, during their well-advanced senior years; ate smartly and ate from their own crops that were not chemically tainted. They managed to grow and harvest their nourishment themselves and what is, very revealing is that the exceptionally healthy either rarely took prescription chemicals drugs or never did at all and perhaps most importantly, were not injected multiple times very young in life with unnatural to human biology chemicals of todays' vaccines. It was only when they were very old that medication was taken. There is a lesson here and/or a way of life that is worthy being followed. WE MUST BE FREE TO FOLLOW THE LESSONS OF THOSE WHO HAD NO UNNATURAL TO HUMAN BIOLOGY CHEMICAL DEPENDENCE AND THROUGHOUT LIFE REMAINED OVERALL HEALTHY!

Those that may choose to withhold chemical content information know that no one in their right parental mind want to expose their children to toxic chemicals. The possibility of decreasing profits is sinister reason for not properly or adequately informing the innocent of the toxic fact, about the presence of unnatural to human biology chemicals in vaccines. Parents do not want to shoot their children up with chemicals and/or compounds such as, mercury, aluminum or formaldehyde that have been found in vaccines. Vaccine producers fail but, PARENTS' MUST NOT FAIL; parents must protect their children from any and all unwanted chemicalization and thereby, protect their children from chemicalization harm. Realize that injections of unnatural to human biology chemicals are catastrophic to children's health. It is commonsensical to not put such, chemicals in your body and/ or to inject it into children however, it is not commonsensical to vaccine producers. The producers of vaccines are not properly protecting your children from chemicalization harm so, YOU MUST! Demand SAFER vaccines for injection, approved by SAFER vaccines charity; protect your children!

Many have concluded that there is no lack of common sense on the part of vaccine producers but rather, is a profit based more sinister plan for such, chemicals in vaccines and explains why vaccine producers belligerently and unconscionably continue to use certain chemicals (chemicals for profit) in vaccines. To have purposefully utilize such, chemicals and/or have actual knowledge of the consequences of unnatural to human biology chemicalization sounds in gross negligence or actual criminal negligence. Either way we must confront this assault and battery upon our children, their chemical safety or natural homeostasis is being compromised; we need to establish that parents have the unfettered liberty to protect their children from conceived of or actual danger of vaccine unnatural to the body injections. Irrespective of whether vaccines producers remain belligerent; it is in the common good of all children that parents be completely FREE to protect children from all injected chemicalizations. Vaccine' content must fall in line with working with the body's design; for the safety of our children we must not permit unnatural to human biology chemicals in vaccines. Your children's welfare depends upon your LIBERTY TO PROTECT CHILDREN WITH POWER OF REFUSAL TO VACCINATE!

The threat of chemical exposure from vaccination is very real and very grave. We must have ABSOLUTE FREEDOM TO PROTECT OUR CHILDREN from this very real and grave threat. The CONSTITUTION and FUNDAMENTAL HUMAN RIGHTS dictates that we must be secure in ourselves and do not have to bow down to another's healthcare will. This is especially true when it comes to what is to be injected or not injected into our and our children's bloodstreams. Protect your Self-determined health and Parental Rights!

It is mindless to inject tiny babies, small infants and little children with chemicals that are not normally found in the body or that have no capacity in biology, physiology or participate in the functions in order, to be optimally healthy and/or have normal human existence. Furthermore, it is a dishonest operation to have these chemicals in vaccines and state that vaccines are good for you. Moreover, to knowingly inject such, unnatural to human biology chemicalization should be considered an act of child abuse. Vaccine producers and their support teams apparently are masters of deception as they attempt to make light of the fact, that they are exposing our children to unnatural to human biology chemicals from its vaccines.

They are bent upon reversing the blame and/or limiting their culpability for putting stressful unnatural to the body chemicals in vaccines by implying that "certain children have a unique sensitivity" instead, of admitting or concurring that vaccine chemicalizations are at fault and a major irritant. They wrongfully dismiss that its vaccine chemicalization is the main cause in fact of Autism and/or that innocent children have no freakish sensitivity but rather, that all children are all ultra-sensitive to unnatural to human biology chemicalization or generally negatively impacted by such, chemicals that are in vaccines. ALL CHILDREN have a severe sensitivity and/or susceptibility to such alien, foreign, unnatural to the body vaccine chemicals. Do not be sidetracked from the full realization of the dangers of injecting chemically laced vaccines. Vaccine producer's commissions and omissions indicate that they are not to be blindly trusted with our children's welfare. **Protect your children from unwanted vaccination harm! PARENTS MUST LEGALLY HOLD THE CONTROL AND LIBERTY TO DECIDE WHAT IS BEST FOR THEIR CHILDREN!**

It does not take a rocket scientist to discern that mercury or any unnatural to the body chemical should not be placed in vaccines; it only takes common sense. It takes money hungry uncaring individuals and/or those who are not worthy of **PARENTAL TRUST** to have put even a mere tincture of mercury or other unnatural to the body chemicals in vaccines. **Parents must be allowed to have a reasonable expectation of vaccine purity met and be entitled to refuse a vaccine, chemicalization or injection. One merely needs to understand that vaccines are injected into the body and blood of quickly developing babies and will take an unhealthy toll to discern that such, chemicals must not be in vaccines. It is beyond unreasonable and extremely dangerous to inject such, chemicals. Parents have an obligation, a need and a Right to protect children; informed DENIAL or REFUSAL allows you to protect!**

Unnatural to human biology chemicals are the seeds of health misfortune to those injected with them and is the main reason for the Autism and Alzheimer's epidemics. Many doctors, scientists, chemists and parents have rationally concluded that it can be or is catastrophic to the health of children and adults to inject the present chemically laced, unnatural to human biology chemicalization, state of vaccines. What is required for the achievement of SAFER vaccines are the liberty of decision (freedom to refuse vaccination) and holding vaccine producers' feet to the fire of consumer negligence law. THE PEOPLE MUST HAVE THE ABSOLUTE RIGHT TO REFUSE UNWANTED VACCINE INVASIVE INJECTIONS. Whose child is it anyway; YOUR CHILD EQUALS YOUR DECISION! The decision to inject or get the "jab", as they say in England, must be for parents to decide. Any level of alien, foreign, unnatural to the body chemical exposure can be considered an unsafe level. Parents' that want to safeguard their children's chemical homeostasis and thereby, protect their children from any and all levels of chemical exposure must have the unfettered liberty to do so. Mandated vaccination law is inconsistent with fundamental freedom of parental protection of children and one's Self-governing healthcare liberty.

Vaccine producers are not protecting children's safety as they should or could. The fact that even after a long peculation period and/or long after U.S. Congressman Dan Burton, Chairmen of the House Committee on Government Reform, requested an **immediate recall of all vaccines** that contain mercury; instead, producers of vaccines sat on its hands, it failed to immediately stop producing such, poor vaccines and it failed to recall the tainted vaccines that were in doctors' offices. This drastic uncaring and irresponsibly that allowed these vaccines to stay on doctor's shelves until injected is unforgivable and has likely caused children a bleak health future; causing unnecessary major injuries. **Apparently, money not safety dictate vaccine producers' actions and inactions.** In a Committee conducted hearing on July 18, 2000 appropriately titled, **"Mercury in Medicine: Are We Taking Unnecessary Risks?"** the FDA stated that **CHILDREN ARE BEING EXPOSED TO UNSAFE LEVELS OF MERCURY THROUGH VACCINES CONTAINING THIMEROSAL**. At this same Committee hearing it was determined that the **SYMPTOMS OF AUTISM AND THAT OF MERCURY POISONING MIMIC EACH OTHER. Parents' protect your children, no one else will; because money controls.**

Wow, the cat has really been let out of the proverbial bag; **vaccinations** laced with mercury **and Autism mimic each other**. A company that cares about children's welfare would act and act quickly and competently to safeguard children from such, vaccine danger; obviously Vaccine Producers do not care or care more for money. A huge monetary damage award is in order and criminal charges for the mal-act commission and/or the inaction omission. **Wrongly, Vaccine Producers' are practicality impervious to lawsuits regarding vaccine induced injuries; this is outrageous and makes no health safety sense. Hold Vaccine Producers accountable and liable; make them pay stiff penalties and/or the highest monetary awards permitted by law in order, to instill safer vaccines and assure better protection of children.**

We must never lose sight of the goodness of our cause, for it serves to best secure the well-being of our offspring. The charity, **SAFER vaccines**, mission is to cause vaccines to become reasonably **SAFE and thereby, secure the best interest of children**. Vaccines must not be laced with unnatural to human biology chemicals if we want to secure safety. **SAFER vaccines charity** salutes all efforts which, make vaccines safer and/or that might reveal the facts on how anti-health chemicalization causes health problems. As of, August 19, 2017 Rep. Bill Posey's bill, HR 3615 calls for the first federal study of the general health of vaccinated population and that of the unvaccinated population. Studies like this one are long overdue and must not be deterred in that it or ignorance allows continued vaccine abnormal to the body chemicalization negligence. The study will likely reveal obvious health problems caused to the vaccinated because they are being unnecessarily exposed to unnatural to the body chemicalization. When it comes to the health or welfare of your children one should not merely, think they are sure about the safety of vaccines but rather, be sure about it. Be sure your children are not being exposed to toxic chemical contents and/or unnatural to human biology chemicalization. Please, urge your Congressmen and Senators to support such needed studies such as, that of HR 3615! We are happy with any steps geared to make vaccines **SAFER and to improve the scientific integrity**. Please, be acutely aware that even when the vaccine industry is prompted to act to remove an unnatural to human biology chemical for example mercury that many vaccines still contain the poison. In 2007 128 million Flu vaccine doses were manufactured and that only 11 million were Thimerosal (mercury) free, a shameful percentage. The CDC recommended these mercury laden vaccines for children over 6 months and then every year of life. Children need parents to protect them from abnormal chemicalization!

It is absurd and repugnant that vaccines are not held to at least the traditional good standards of safety control. We need to assure that vaccines are required to go through the same rigorous approval process and safety testing that all drugs go through and that parents should not be satisfied with mere short-term testing. The consequences of injecting

230

unnatural to human biology chemicalization with chemicals such as, aluminum or mercury etc. must be studied over a more rational revealing period and not be so limited to such short periods because the chemicalization will more than likely, show its negative to health results over months and years of the chemicalization. These are our children's lives and good health that we are placing in harm's way if we do not put vaccines through the rigors of a traditional drug approval process. One can surmise that vaccine producer lobbyists have played a role in limiting or short-changing safety to get its vaccines approved and without revealing its real dangers. Parental informed consent/ DENIAL of vaccine invasive injections is required in order, to best control the chemical content in vaccines and to best protect our children. Big business, vaccine industry concentrations on profits; it has no business commanding what must be injected with parents' disabled to refuse. Parents are perfectly situated and are the best decision makers for children; parents must decide if vaccines are too dirty to inject and/or clean enough that they do not pose a threat to their children if injected. Mandated vaccination law not only violates and abridges Parent's Protective Right; it all but annihilates it.

One can very easily determine that vaccine companies are forever hellbent on the use of chemicals for profit in vaccines that make vaccines unsafe or not as safe as, they can and should be; this is causing potential and/or actual harm to those injected. WE NEED TO POLICE vaccine producers, TO ASSURE OUR CHILDREN HAVE MUCH SAFER vaccines. There must be a system of CHECKS AND BALANCES IN PLACE; applied to vaccinations and/or how vaccines are administered. Therefore, consumerism and its freedom to not be vaccinated must be steadfastly applied to vaccinations; rightfully parents must be FREE to refuse an unwanted vaccine and be completely FREE to disallow a vaccine that has unnatural to human biology chemicals. In addition, what is needed to achieve SAFER vaccines and level the playing field, the public must be FREE to hold vaccine producers' feet to the fire when its vaccines contain such, chemicals and/or cause injury. Moreover, hold vaccine producers accountable and liable for vaccine induced injuries; make Big Pharma pay damages to the victims of its faulty vaccine production and/or its negligence. Our freedoms will protect us; securing for us, SAFER vaccines!

Right now, there are vaccines that are not as safe as possible in fact, they are too dangerous to inject. The negative to health consequences from exposure to unnatural to human biology chemicalization is inevitable once exposed. The only thing in question is the degree of harm; not whether a harm occurs. The harm from willful exposure or unsuspecting innocent exposure to unnatural to human biology, vaccine chemicalization cannot be totally estimated. As, frustrating, baffling and crazy as it is, vaccines are being intoxicated with chemicals that cause biological interference and harm. There are chemicals in vaccines that have no normal presence in the normal, everyday reactions of the body and in fact, cause abnormality or foreign, alien and/or unnatural to the body anti-health reactions. Vaccines have been and still are vessels of unnatural to human biology chemicalization that intoxicate children with chemicals that are extremely abusive or are very disruptive to health; it should not be. Autism in the young and Alzheimer's in the older have a chemicalization causation component. For the sake of children's welfare vaccines need to be cleaned-up; allowing parents to be FREE to protect children from unwanted chemicalization and the holding of vaccine producers accountable and liable for vaccine induced injuries will achieve safety. The TWO STREPS OF CORRECTION achieves SAFER vaccines needed for child safety!

Know that 80% of the whopping global $24 billion vaccine market is under the one-sided control of Pfizer, Glaxo, Merck and Sanofi. They are in absolute control over what chemicals are in vaccines and do not want consumerism to ever be applied to its one-way monopoly market that does not grant parents the common decency of the vaccination decision. These masters of our internal chemistry act to prevent our freedom of vaccination decision and/ or make it impossible to refuse vaccine chemicalization and even act to stop Religious Liberty to deny vaccinations, a Constitutionally protected religious exemption. Be acutely aware, freedom of religion has already been destroyed as had occurred by the SB 277 mal-enactment in California. Italy and France now no longer have religious exemption for vaccinations. We must realize that our essential freedoms are under attack and that this loss of liberty has caused vaccines to be chemically unsafe. Please, help the charity, SAFER vaccines do something about it! If, The People, cannot refuse and unwanted vaccine chemical concoction and/or if we are not free to litigate against these vaccine makers then they can put any nasty, unhealthy or unnatural to the biology chemicals that it wants in our children's vital vaccine supply! On a positive note, as of July 2017 there are two bills that if passed will likely help end the above unconstitutionality, one bill in the Assembly, A8123a and one bill in the Senate, S8141c. Freedom of religious vaccination exemptions prompts vaccines to be produced with less or no unnatural to the body chemicals and thus, not as religiously objectionable! Government crosses over into impermissible governing when it seeks to investigate your religion or challenges your religious belief.

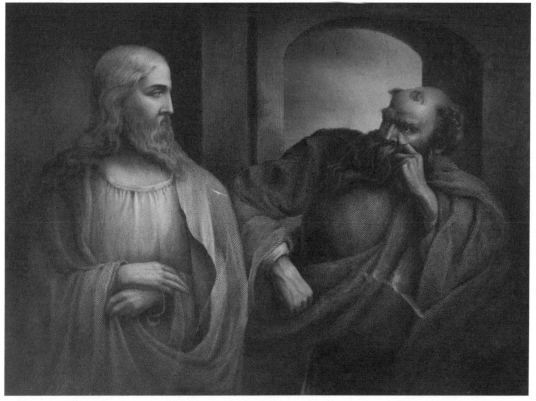

It is unconstitutional to be questioned or judged about your religion or religious belief.

Profiting above all is vaccine producers' top agenda. Despite knowing parent's safety concerns over chemicalization and a House Committee plea to remove mercury and scholarly warnings that the Autism epidemic is profoundly man-made, induced by vaccine chemicalization; vaccine producers kept pushing out vaccines tainted with mercury and never lifted a finger to remedy the situation until it had no choice to. By its purposeful mal-actions and woeful inactions, they are much too careless about what chemicals are in vaccines or could careless that vaccines are chemically unhealthy for our children. One thing is obvious from this debacle; parents' must be in control by being informed of all of the contents in vaccines and by being absolutely **FREE to deny** any and all vaccinations. It is in the best interest of all children that it be established for parents to control the vaccination decision and deem if vaccination is in their child's best health interest. There must be no injection when parents do not give their true informed consent and/or if parents give their **INFORMED DENIAL; parents** must rule over whether or not a vaccination is administered! Parents' being **FREE to refuse a vaccination** is in the very best interest of children and is absolutely needed to assure vaccine content safety!

It has been surmised that because of the FDA and vaccine company close ties and well paved road for golden jobs, along with the pressure placed from vaccine producer's lobbyists; the FDA has been overly influenced to not scrutinize vaccines for their content safety. It is said that the FDA now officially belongs to Big Pharma! The FDA may have saved vaccine companies millions of dollars by not issuing a recall of all mercury laced vaccines already stockpiled in doctor's offices and thereby, caused innocent children to be unnecessarily exposed to mercury. Irresponsibly, the FDA merely allowed pharmaceutical companies to phase out the use of mercury in vaccines over time (it as if the FDA works for Big Pharma and not for our safety). This FDA bias left our children's welfare in the self-serving hands and whim of the profit above all, vaccine producers to recall its mercury infested vaccines. Vaccine producers would never remove its vaccines from the market and cause itself losses; it did not do the right thing by recalling their mercury tainted vaccines and thereby, caused our children to suffer injections of mercury poison and/or unnatural to human biology chemicalization. This tells parents not to place blind faith in vaccine produces and/or Big Pharma's FDA, it was a real test of character and indicates we must not trust our children's safety with them. Do not trust that a vaccine is safe; make sure it is **SAFE! The charity, SAFER vaccines' works to assure that your children's vaccines are SAFE!**

Vaccine producers unconscionably did not recall their mercury tainted vaccines; in doing so they put money above children's safety. **This left untold numbers of children to be vaccinated with unfit vaccines; placing children in CHEMICALIZATION HARMS' WAY.** Innocent children and parents were kept in the dark, parents were not informed about the all-important fact, that there was mercury in the vaccines and were unconscionably injected into the delicate systems of these innocent children victims; all took place after the vaccine producers and doctors knew that the mercury had to be eliminated **This outrage could not have occurred if TRUE INFORMED CONSENT and/or INFORMED DENIAL OF VACCINATION existed. Logically, parents would refuse when they are informed that mercury is going to be injected. Informed DENIAL is the power which, can FREE us from this tyrannical medical intervention that enforces us to suffer CHEMICALIZATION CHILD ABUSE, ENSLAVEMENT! In reading, this book please, keep in mind that optimum health and the prevention of Autism in children and Alzheimer's in adults is mainly relies upon maintaining a near normal chemistry and/or homeostasis balance. Parents assuring their children's normal biochemistry and not distorting it with** injections of unnatural to human biology chemicalizations gives one the best chance at health and protects against Autism. We need to put the full court press on making vaccines SAFER by de-chemicalizing them!

In the year 2006 my book, Sting of the Medical Mosquito, linked Autism to vaccine chemicalization. It is my opinion that knowingly putting such, chemicals in vaccines like mercury or aluminum or other unnatural to human biology chemicals in vaccines distorts the normal chemical reactions of the body and that it is gross negligence to do so! In October 2006, National Institute of Environmental Health Sciences (NIEHS) released its report from its expert panel, "Thimerosal Exposure in Pediatric Vaccines", the findings revealed, "The researchers found statistically significant associations between thimerosal and two neurodevelopmental disorders: language delays and tics." These post vaccination language delays and tics are consistent with AUTISM signs and symptoms. The science or concept of vaccination has been hijacked, corrupted and bastardized by those who profit from it. There are chemicals put in vaccines that assure higher profits (chemicals for profit not safety) and these chemicals are ill advised to be injected into your chemically sensitive baby. Please open your eyes, your ears and mind to recognize that unnatural to human biology chemicals must not be injected into your baby if you want your baby to be optimally healthy and/or not become an Autism epidemic statistic. There is an ongoing misinformation agenda and/or a damage control campaign to prevent the realization of harm caused by vaccine chemicalization or subvert the truth of its mal-health consequences. Such, deceit undermines parents Right and ability to protect their children. Parents are properly concerned about what ingredients are in children's food, but they need to be a million times more concerned about what ingredients are in vaccines which, are injected to immediately flow unimpeded into children's biological systems and blood!

The vaccine industry is cloak and dagger and does not want the public to know how inefficient or ineffective its safety measures are; there is no transparency. Be aware, the CDC had to be sued, Civil action No. 11-Cv-01275 (ABJ), to have them somewhat respond to a freedom of information request about how it accesses vaccines and just how the CDC came to its forgone, absolute conclusion that vaccines do not cause Autism. It is troublesome that he CDC is not forthcoming with information which, concerns children's safety; when it comes to vaccines there is no transparency. The CDC's overt, absolute conclusion is wrong by their own research; apparently, the CDC is bias to vaccination promotion and its protection. Trust in vaccination is plummeting and the vaccination program is in a down spin crisis. It is troubling that parents are becoming resolved not to vaccinate however, you cannot blame parents for protecting their children from unwanted chemicalizations. Parents' are protecting their children by not blindly relying upon the superficial words of the CDC, FDA or the AMA. Vaccinations are a business; not a panacea. Did the CDC obstruct justice by redacting requested freedom of information material? The CDC knows that vaccines are causing injury! Is it not purposely revealing it or that a connection has been found between vaccines and Autism? If they have done the public a safety disservice perhaps criminal charges may need to be filed. The public should never relinquish its parental authority to refuse unwanted vaccine chemicalizations. Parents' must not blindly place their children's well-being with the CDC instead, come to your own logical conclusions! Control your child's healthcare destiny!

Something that the public should become aware of and warned about, is that lobbyists not elected officials very often draft the bills that legislator's put forward to be enacted into law. Often a bill can be word for word what lobbyists devised and not what politicians and/or what your Congressmen or Senators' contemplated. Too often these lobbyist laws are not in the publics' best interest but rather, more in the interest of the business that the lobbyists work for. It is my strongest opinion that only elected officials should have the authority to draft laws! Do not blindly trust that the laws enacted are devised by elected officials or that the law is enacted to serve the public. Moreover, do not blindly trust that vaccination mandates are enacted to best serve the public or think that vaccine producers cannot put whatever, unnatural to human biology chemicals in vaccines that serves it best; without having to worry about lawsuits or any negative to the business results. Money or donations or lobbyists have compromised our legal system; making laws that do not best serve the public and allowing vaccine producers to act with impunity and/or above the law. Children are too often mere pawns, in a chess game of profiteering. **BE FREE TO DECIDE WHAT IS BEST FOR YOUR CHILDREN; HAVE LIBERTY TO PROTECT THEM**! It is **PARENTAL JURISDICTION** to decide if a vaccine is safe or not and will or will not be injected!

Do not blindly trust that the AMA acts in the best interest of the patient; it has been shown that the AMA kept patients from access to alternative, safe healthcare. The AMA illegally tried to eliminate its Chiropractic competition, in a mal-effort to monopolize healthcare. AMA showed design to terminate technology that patients benefit from and are becoming reliant upon that is not medical intervention. On September 25, 1987, Judge Getzendanner issued her opinion that the AMA had violated Section 1, of the Sherman Act, and that it had engaged in an unlawful conspiracy in **restraint of trade "to contain and eliminate the chiropractic profession."** (*Wilk v. American Medical Ass'n*, 671 F. Supp. 1465, N.D. Ill. 1987). In addition, the "AMA had entered into a **long history of illegal behavior**". The AMA continued its destructive blockading of access to chiropractic, which does not rely upon chemical drugs and invasive surgery, during the long duration of litigation and trials. The above sited case indicates that the AMA's main concern is not the welfare of patients but rather, that it is in the business of wiping out competition in order, to secure its own welfare; not the welfare of the public. This case is just the tip of the iceberg when it comes to the AMA's lack of credibility and strategy to profit above-all.

MD's often urge patients into spinal surgery with the old sales pitch, "bad disc" when they know MRI's often indicate a false positive for a bad disc. Chiropractors can very often help true bad disc conditions without the use and side-effects of drugs or surgery and the AMA is acutely aware of it; but allow their patients to go down its one-way, dead-end, drug and surgery road. To this unlawful and unethical day, the probable reason why MD's or its organized AMA do not recommend their patients to see Chiropractors but instead, urge its patients to strictly rely upon its drugs and eventual spinal surgical procedures is because there would be a lot less unneeded surgery or drug taking and Chiropractors would become patients' nights in shining armor against back conditions of all kinds and become known as a great spinal surgery prevention. MD's push drugs and surgery for signs and symptoms and/or conditions that regularly can respond to Chiropractic treatment. These antics strongly indicate it unwise to blindly place trust in the self-serving hands of the AMA. **Parents' protect your children and protect yourselves from unneeded chemicalization and surgery!** Finally, in 2014, ethical MD's of the American Academy of Neurology took the position that doctors should be looking for other ways to help chronic pain patients, other than prescribing addictive and sometimes deadly opioid pain killers. Since, the 1990s, more than 100,000 people have died overdosing on opioid **chemicalization** and in 2009, there were more than twice as many deaths from prescription opioid overdoses than from cocaine and heroin put together. Think for yourself; know that drugs, vaccines or surgery may not be the answer and may in fact, be a tragic mistake and cause multiple health problems.

Chiropractic had started to become a major competitor that was impacting upon medical doctor's overly broad patient base and decreased the mega-profits of the AMA, (medical doctors). Chiropractic had become the biggest threat to their financial welfare and medical doctors thought it urgent to curb **chiropractic's growth**. Obviously, it is all about money to the defendant AMA and not what **is best for patients**. The patient's needs and/or benefits were blatantly ignored and/or injured; the AMA wanted an illegal monopoly and all the patient money. Moreover, the **United States Supreme Court on February 7, 1990 found the AMA QUILTY OF ILLEGAL PROPAGANDA against chiropractic. The AMA was ORDERED TO STOP its attack of the chiropractic profession.** This is proof of its design to control our healthcare and/or our healthcare choices. For the AMA, it is not about what is in the best interest of the patient; it is about securing the money. **Liberty of healthcare is crucial to secure against medical tyranny. All is lost if our healthcare choices are limited or we are mandated to accept a particular mode of healthcare. We must be FREE to choose what healthcare we think personally best and not have our choices limited or be enslaved to suffer vaccine chemicalizations! Follow the money and you gain why the AMA acts and why vaccines are mandated. If there was no unconscionable profiteering to be had from mandated vaccinations you can bet that they would not be mandated! There is a very real danger when healthcare is mandated or when the AMA is left unchecked in its actions that eliminate competition or patient liberty!**

The system is broken, and it is up to us to fix it. We must prevent potential healthcare monopolization from occurring and end any present monopolization! Mandated vaccination is a government backed and enforced, pharmaceutical and/or medical industry monopoly that assures unconscionable profiteering from a captured child-based market; holding the public shackled to unwanted and often at times unneeded vaccine chemicalizations. In addition, patenting anything to do with healthcare promotes its recommendation of the patented medical intervention for money instead, of actual patient need or being in the patient's best interest. Thus far, vitamins and minerals are not patentable and therefore, are not costing the public unconscionable amounts of money however, there is an attempt to make them only obtainable through prescription. If the powers that be make it that vitamins and minerals need to be prescribed its cost will skyrocket and then and only then you will see or witness a surge in medical doctors recommending vitamins and minerals; once again, the mighty profiting dollars will dictate what the AMA or its doctors recommend and not patient need. Greed or money should not rule patient healthcare! Absolute power over us corrupts absolutely and the vaccination mandate is absolute power over us, dictating what will be injected into our tiny babies' vital blood chemistries. Healthcare recommendations, healthcare coverage and healthcare mandates are being over influenced by lobbyists with deep pockets. The level of conflict of interest and/or corruption has become the rule and has rendered healthcare very often unsafe. The problem is pervasive; parents need to beware of it, and protect their children from unwanted, unnatural to human biology chemicalization.

The breast cancer prevention industry has been compromised by greed or what guarantees the most money and that is why the public has been locked into regular (yearly) cancer screenings that give an unhealthy dose of radiation (mammograms) and radiation is a main cause of cancer. Having year after year, (yearly) mammograms exposes the individual to crazy amounts of radiation; it is not wise and can actually cause what it meant to detect. Just put in perspective; the need to prevent cancer is greater the need to detect cancer, especially, when radiation is such, a cancer generator and when there are other non-cancer causing, cancer detection techniques or technologies. Many experts' opinion is that less invasive diagnostic techniques are available and far superior to the much more invasive radiation mammograms. It is not uncommon for an individual to palpate one's own breast tissue or for a competent doctor to efficiently palpate and detect an abnormality or miniscule lump in the breast tissue whereas, a mammogram completely failed to detect a precancerous or cancerous lesion and/or lump. Mammogram radiation is backed because it brings in mega-dollars and not because it is in the best interest of the public; it is way too much radiation! Breast cancer has become a mega-profiteering industry, bent on profit, not safety. Analogously, mandated vaccinations are for profit, not safety; run by corporations that are bent on profiting from children being enforced to be vaccinated. A brand-new market has been created for profit from all the vaccine induced AUTISTIC children. As harsh as these realizations are; you need to protect your children from vaccine CHEMICALIZATION with INFORMED DENIAL of vaccination. Parents become aware of what harmful, anti-health chemicals are in vaccines and then protect accordingly!

Women who are repetitively exposed to mammography RADIATION, year after year, are going to be more often diagnosed with cancer because of the exposure to the mammogram RADIATION. If you have too much of even good thing it can cause problems; to have too much of a bad thing is obviously, very unhealthy for you. Yes, you should consider a mammogram if you suspect something is wrong or on only rare instances however, recommending it for all and for each year is taking a diagnostic tool and turning it into an unhealthy habit and will cause the health problems that it is designed to diagnose. Overzealous medical intervention can cause iatrogenic disease; the degree of suffering caused by unneeded intervention or over prescribed mammograms, antibiotics and vaccine chemicalizations are dangers that we must be FREE TO REFUSE!

Children exposed to the full spectrum of multiple vaccine chemicalizations will be diagnosed with Autism more often than children not exposed, they have been chemically compromised by CHEMICALS FOR PROFIT in vaccines which, do not need to be in vaccines. These unnatural to the body chemicals render vaccines too dangerous to inject. We need vaccines to be as safe as, possible and not vials of unnatural to human biology chemicalization. Not exposing oneself to unnatural to human biology chemicals is most important to health preservation. So, make sure your babies are not suffering CHEMICALIZATION BY INJECTION! Lathering up your children with sun screen may protect them from extreme sun exposure but please, recognize that the chemicals in the sun screen will enter your children through their heated up expanded skin pores. The lesson here is to support the human biochemistry and not destroy it in order, to be healthy and prevent abnormality and/or Autism! To alter, distort or disrupt by injection the normal biochemistry with unneeded, unnatural to human biology chemicals in vaccines is the most unwise attempt at maintaining optimum health.

Underarm deodorants expose the breast tissue to aluminum and other TOXINS; via the lymph nodes in the armpits which, are part of the same lymph system of the breasts. Unnatural to the body deodorant chemicalization penetrate cells and eventuate cancer. The armpit pores are a major entrance and exit of the body; it is an entrance for underarm deodorant chemicals. For health, rinse your armpits with cold water after a hot shower to close these giant armpit pores, to prevent deodorant chemicals from easy entrance. Head hair is even porous; your hair will be and look a lot healthier if you rinse it with cold water to prevent applied hair product chemicals from entering the hair follicles. Injecting the chemicals of vaccines into muscle or blood vessels are a main chemicalization source that quickly reaches brain cells. The vaccination industry does not have children's best interest as its priority, as it uses harmful chemicals; if the chemical makes for bigger profit it is used. Drug Companies spend huge amounts of time, energy and money to see to it that vaccinations are mandated and that our children are ENSLAVED to be vaccinated.

You would hope that when it comes to our very own bodies and health's and of our dependent children that we are FREE to decide what is best and FREE to think for ourselves! Wrongfully, we are mandated, enforced and/or enslaved to accept, endure or and/or suffer medical intervention or we are programmed into it. The motivation behind this enforced or programmed healthcare tyranny is not so much, for our welfare but rather, it is for the profit it generates. There is hardly a message heard about vaccinations, drugs or mammography that is not profit motivated. What chemicals do you want your children or yourself to be exposed to; building block biochemicals or stumbling block synthetic chemicals? Parents are well advised to not allow their children to be exposed to unnatural to human biology chemicals especially; injected ones! Adults be aware of the chemical content in Flu shots it can cause Alzheimer's. Parents please, recognize that many sun screens have unnatural to the body chemicals and that these chemicals can enter your baby through your baby's skin especially when the skin is heated up by the sun, opening one's pores to the max. Deodorants applied under the arms especially fine spray deodorant chemicalization is a cancer causation source and should not be applied when one's underarm pores are wide open and/or immediately after a hot shower or shaving. Women' should be leery of yearly, mammogram radiation; it causes cancer! Constant psychological bombardment to "make sure your children are vaccinated or else…" or "be sure to have a mammography…" makes sure there are profits from droves of children to be vaccinated and mass indoctrinated women to incur yearly mammograms.

Using fear-based tactics or making inaccurate statements to induce parents to submit their children for vaccination such as, telling parents their children MUST be vaccinated or that the law requires it and that Child Services will take your child away from you to be injected or that your child will not be allowed in school or there is no way around being vaccinated, are all violating parental Rights and is the practice of tyrannical medicine. The breast industry induces women to have yearly, harmful mammograms by making them feel at great risk or negligent if you do not have it. The medical profession often will wrongfully tell a patient that the cancer patient will die early if you do not rush to undergo chemotherapy. Cardiologists too often tell every patient that they have 90% artery occlusion and that heart surgery will give great results and be as easy as a walk in the park. These scenarios rob people of their free will and coerce unwanted medical intervention. Stop exposing children's brain cells to unnatural to human biology vaccine chemicals and stop exposing breast tissue to harmful radiation and do not be wrongfully induced into any unwanted or unneeded healthcare! Be in control of your body and health!

Many vaccine chemicals are destructive and disruptive to health and are the main etiology of Autism. Injecting anti-health chemicals into the blood of all our children is the real epidemic that is the cause in fact, of the autism epidemic. Habitually taking drug chemicalization is another epidemic of iatrogenic disease. The U.S. and New Zealand are the only countries that mistakenly permit RX drug ads on television; these drug ads not only repetitively suggest taking drugs but rather, program our children that when they mature into adults to automatically reach for the drug bottles and/or be prescription drug dependent. The media is constantly filled with take drug advertisements. They spend tons of money to lobby Congress to assure we are bombarded with take drug ads; all in the name of profit. They see to it that natural remedies are always under attack. Natural living and/or natural remedies are suppressed, and freedom of healthcare is rapidly being eliminated. TEACH CHILDREN that health is dependent upon having the right chemistry and that injecting unnatural to body chemicalizations; is a sure recipe for health disaster!

Ask yourself this most pertinent question, are your children better off with enforced, mandated vaccinations which are lobbied for by the profit based Big Pharma or are your children better off having parents decide what vaccine is safe enough to inject or decide upon whether a vaccine chemicalization is or is not in your children's best health interest? Most parents agree that they need to always maintain control of their children's healthcare. The vaccine industry has manipulated a government sanctioned monopoly and an enforced child patient enslavement populace to assure their vaccines would find their mark and bring vaccine producers its mega-profits. We must defend our Right of Self-determined health and act to regain lost Rights, Privileges and Freedoms. The vaccine industry and its AMA collude together to assure profiteering from mandated vaccinations. Whatever chemicals that pass the cost/benefit test or makes the most profit will be found in vaccines; even if it is at the expense or health detriment of the public or it divests and/or deprives the People of LIFE (health) and LIBERTY. The mandated vaccination enslavement laws assure the pump and dump of vaccine chemicalization into children's blood and the chemicals penetrate vital brain cells; doping the cells which, sets the course for AUTISM.

Years ago, drugs were mainly used for only the very elderly or in critical or crisis care. Billions spent to program people to take drugs has exploded the drug market. The young have been induced to take all kinds of drugs; they have become drug robots, taking drugs for the slightest health issue. Many would not take unneeded and often dangerous drugs if they were in command of their own minds. They target children and constantly program us to submit our children for multiple vaccine chemicalization injections and we acquiesce to all their enforced chemicalizations. Regain rightful control of your children's health and vaccination decisions! Parents' are their children's natural and rightful guardians; be FREE to protect your child's chemistry! Health is all about having the proper chemistry, have the chemicals you need to be healthy but, not have too much excess of what you need and definitely, do not allow anti-health chemicals or animal cells or poisons from vaccines to be injected. Abnormal to the body chemicalizations from vaccines destroy chemical homeostasis, inducing chemical physiological and biological chaos! The result is that the body cannot be optimally healthy and cannot heal itself. The chemical building blocks of health are the natural to the body vitamins, minerals and/or chemicals whereas, the stumbling blocks of health are the unnatural to the body or to human biology anti-health chemicals that are not normally utilized by the body or take part in the normal biochemistry and thereby, are harmful and/or toxic. The impact of unnatural to the body, vaccine chemicals, is staggering; BE FREE, do not submit for unwanted chemicalizations!

Please be aware that we are being programmed, trained to take drugs and give up our nature to care for our children the way we personally think is best. The unending ads, the torrential flood of sensory information to take drugs and be vaccinated inundate and sweep us off our self-decision feet; inducing us to accept drugs or vaccines that we would otherwise, not. This barrage upon our senses makes involuntary healthcare appear as if it is a voluntary health decision; resulting in a fundamental distortion. This induced acquiescence or complacency renders one drug dependent and amenable SLAVES of vaccination. We have from early age, been indoctrinated by constant streams of advertisements to take this drug for this or that. We have been manipulated to give up our children for otherwise, unwanted drugs or vaccinations; despite the dangers of ingesting drugs or injecting vaccine chemicalizations. There is constant effort to induce us into an overwhelming feeling of helplessness and dependence upon drugs and/or vaccinations. They have succeeded in manipulating the public to the point that it is considered wrong or forbidden to speak bad of vaccinations or a cause of Autism or it not in the best interest of children. They have programmed us to form an automatic positive bias toward taking drugs and being vaccinated and have created an automatic negative reflex bias toward being unvaccinated. Just because it is considered unpopular speech or not mainstream choice does not mean it can be suppressed; people must be FREE to dissent, FREE to be independent without being condemned or coerced to do otherwise. People must be FREE to live by one's vaccination decision; not enslaved! BE FREE TO REJECT INJECTIONS!

There is above all agenda to prevent profit from vaccination decreasing, they know that vaccination mandate/SLAVERY assures profiteering; they jump to stamp out any anti-vaccination opinion or sentiment or any effort to end the erroneous vaccination mandate. They lobbied to allow drug or vaccination ads to be aired on television and with such frequency and/or programming skill that you are duped into vaccinations or automatically feel you must be vaccinated and this disrupts your free will; it induces one into dictated norms, actions, inactions, likes and dislikes. The design is to render you obedient and docile to what they want and they want to assure profiting through achieved obedient vaccination blind compliance; with no questions asked. We must no longer be induced to robotically vaccinate; we must be freed to learn to cherish our differences, specialness, individualism and enjoy the blessings of personal vaccination choice/decision!

You can be induced to go against what you naturally would not do, even extreme things; just look at the history of war. My father, a World War II hero, received multiple bronze stars for valor in battle. He told me horror stories of war and how he was trained/ programmed to hate the Germans, to shoot Germans and feel good about it through the watching of movies and propaganda. Dad' professed how astounded he was that he, a devout good, loving and religious person, could have been programmed or induced to kill another human being and feel good about it; like a good soldier, during war time. It took years after the war to realize how wrong it was to feel good about killing; for he had been programmed not to feel any remorse; to be a killing robot. You are programmed to not be your normal self; programmed to not protect your children from vaccine chemicalization harm and when harm occurs (Autism) not to blame the vaccine source for the harm.

You can be programmed to do anything including, having your children undergo dangerous vaccine chemicalizations and forgoing your parental protection of your children. Being programmed by repetitive conscious and subconscious messages produces herd mentality to blindly submit to vaccination SLAVERY; stripping parents of their natural Right to decide what is best for children and giving parents no choice but to vaccinate. Parents submit children without reservation or conscious forethought. Over time we have become VACCINATION ROBOTS, who cannot think otherwise. We have been programmed into VACCINATION ENSLAVEMENT ACQUIESENCE; we allow our children to be injected with chemicals that the rational, FREE thinker, would disallow. Because of our programming we have difficulty thinking opposite of vaccination compliance or having thoughts of refusing vaccine chemical injections. Awaken your parenting nature to protect your children from unwanted chemical infiltrations and save your children from chemicalization Autism! Energize your journey to parental freedom of protection of your children; re-establish rightful parenting, true self-governing and healthcare autonomy.

Be chemically safer; consider only chemically SAFER vaccines! It is difficult even for the observant individual to glean the danger of tampering with one's internal chemistry because we have been desensitized by the constant bombardment to undergo vaccine chemicalization. Our senses or defenses can no longer detect the true nature and/or danger since; we are constantly being programmed into vaccination that can cause health chemical infiltration destruction. The bombardments upon our senses have rendered us senseless and/or mindless about chemicalization consequences. To inject vaccine chemicals without Right of refusal is healthcare madness! Even though drug ads quickly run off, at a purposefully deceptive cadence, some of the risks or dangers of taking the drug; subconsciously people are roped into taking drug/CHEMICALS that are harmful. Remember, all drugs cause ill-health without exception because they are made up of CHEMICALS that are not natural to the body and/or are anti-health CHEMICAL agents. The list of health problems stemming from prescription CHEMICAL taking keeps growing the longer the drug stays on the market. Most parents have no idea what is in vaccines and have been programmed not to question it. Be wise, develop a greater awareness of what is in vaccines; become vaccine cautious and consider only chemically SAFER vaccines.

An example of how a drug can stay on the market despite causing all kinds of health hazards is the drug/CHEMICAL Lipitor, its side effects can be heart attack, liver dysfunction, irreparable damage to the nerves, COGNITIVE damage, and now a study conducted by the University of Massachusetts found the drug/CHEMICAL Lipitor has recently been found to cause postmenopausal women to have a significantly increased risk of type 2 diabetes. The injury and/or health problems that occurred from taking just this one chemical concoction is pervasive and commensurate with the amount of mega-money from the sale of Lipitor;

sales of this drug CHEMICALIZATION poison exceeded $125 billion. Unnatural to the body chemicalization causes harm especially, if injected! The health problem from vaccine and/or medicine chemicalization is very real and extremely disconcerting; the cause of death from opioids more than doubled in 2016. If we do not act to do something about the opioid epidemic and the autism epidemic or the unnatural to human biology chemicalization epidemic now our future will continue to spiral downward.

Be aware, that anything which disrupts the normal activity of the brain cells can contribute to or cause Autism. Diagnostic ultrasound that produces sonogram images is too often recommended by OB/GYN doctors; it is a brain disrupter to developing fetuses. Diagnostic ultrasound imaging is high frequency waves, a pulse that disrupts cellular activity, a vibration and/or a wave of directed energy that penetrates the fetus and thereby, disrupts, distorts and renders abnormal the functionality of brain cells and/or disturbs cellular peace and tranquility. Sound impacts physically (you can feel sound) therefore; the quickly developing fetus that suffers multiple diagnostic ultrasounds is being bombarded with sound waves which, make impact with the fetus's brain and body cells; the mother's placenta connection with the fetus is also, impacted. AN EEG PERFORMED ON AN ADULT WHILE THE ADULT'S BRAIN IS BOMBARDED WITH SOUND WAVES WILL AFFECT DIFFERENT PARTS OF THE BRAIN ACCORDING TO THE FREQUENCY TRANSMITTED THUS, THE BRAINS OF FETUSES THAT ARE BEING BOMBARDED BY ULTRASOUND DIAGNOSTIC WAVES WILL OF COURSCE BE IMPACTED BY THOSE WAVES AND POSSIBLY CAUSE ABNORMAL BRAIN CELL DEVELOPMENT; AUTISM. Vibrating a developing fetuses' brain repetitively over the course of gestation must have its affects upon the tissue it vibrates and possibly be a contributing factor or cofactor of Autism. A fetus should not be unnecessarily bombarded with repetitive waves of ultrasound energy or vibration; its physical pulsation or impact is too disruptive. It can cause atypical neurological development and placenta problems including but not limited to, placenta issues such as, detachment. Overzealous medical intervention, over prescribing and/or mandated vaccination cause citizens to be exposed to hazards they did not bargain for and battle related ill- health and internal chemistry chaos that devastates.

The DEGREE OF HARM being suffered from vaccine CHEMICALIZATIONS far outweighs any trumped-up reason to mandate vaccination and it makes the problems caused by Lipitor and ultrasound energy wave pulses seem miniscule in comparison. Children' by mal-mandate, are being exposed to multiple injected vaccine chemicalizations at an intolerable and alarming rate! MANDATED VACCINATION ENSLAVEMENT LAWS command us to suffer unwanted, unnatural to human biology chemicalizations. The way to SAFER vaccines is through the application of informed consent/DENIAL and holding vaccine producers who are presently not held liable to be held liable and subject to paying damages to those proven injured by vaccine chemicalization. Parents must not stand idle; do protect your children from chemicalization! Do seek the advice of an AWARE doctor however, always be in control over your children's welfare. Demand to know each and every chemical in the vaccine being considered for injection and decide for yourself if any of the chemicals are objectionable and self-determine if the vaccine is or is not in your children's best interest. Chemicalization that is natural to the body or to one's human biology can promote health whereas, unnatural to the body or to human biology chemicalization can promote Autism and/or the opposite of health. Maintain control over yourself and your children by self-governing over your own and that of your children's healthcare. You can control your health and that of your children's by giving an informed consent or an **INFORMED DENIAL** for the healthcare; this includes vaccination healthcare! You ought to be frightened for the safety of your children if you compromised their refined chemical integrity with unnatural to human biology chemicalization from a vaccine source. Indeed, too many parents are finding themselves in abject terror when their beloved children begin to suffer signs and symptoms of injury soon after vaccine chemicalization!

It most probably is the greatest of citizens' unalienable Rights and underscores "Life, liberty and the pursuit of happiness" to have and protect one's children or flesh and blood and in this protection, have the unfettered liberty to prevent what parents consider unwanted, violent injections of unnatural to human biology chemicalizations! If someone attempts to interfere with your parental decision of what you think is best for your child's health do not hesitate to put them in their place; crush their insistence of what they want and destroy the resistance toward you being **FREE** to protect your offspring! If someone or entity acts with prejudice or self-interest to discredit what you want for your child or do not want or if some obnoxious person, entity or mal-regulation attempts to enforce or **ENSLAVE** your child to be injected with what you deem is an unwanted or unsafe vaccine then act to protect your child; destroy what is at odds with your child's best interest and thereby, act to preserve your child's health, parental Right and Right to yourselves. Demand the liberty to be left alone undisturbed and not molested by unwanted medical intervention for your perfectly healthy child. Do not stand for being violated by unwanted or deemed too dangerous to inject vaccine chemicalization; demand freedom to be left alone and be made to suffer your child with unwanted, unnatural to human biology chemical exposure. Children must be **FREE** to bask in their parents' protection and enjoy being immune from oppressive medical intervention and to not be enforced into vaccine injection **SLAVERY!** Demand freedom of healthcare choice and **SAFER** vaccines that are not laced with unnatural to the body chemicals! We must assure that no individual or parent for child is denied the liberty to refuse injection. Demand to be in absolute command and/or control over one's very own health destiny and that of your children. This freedom is fundamental and underlies our basic understanding of what it means to be **FREE**. Let no unscrupulous or ill-conceived law or self-interested industry diminish your Right to govern your own body and/or health. Act, one person at a time, by demanding to **REFUSE** unwanted chemical infusions and **WE WILL ABOLISH VACCINATION SLAVERY!**

Everyone seems to be on the same page, in that most everyone knows that unnatural to the body chemicals cause cancer and it is totally logical that these unnatural to human biology chemicals in vaccines are a cause of the Autism epidemic. We must not vaccinate with such chemicals or be commanded to in order, to go to school. Parents are placed in an untenable position; parents want safety for their children but also, want their children to receive an education. The answer to this vaccination debacle is to resurrect our liberty of healthcare decision and at the same time cause increased vaccine safety. Well, let us realize that the real issue is that vaccines should be made much **SAFER** and thereby, make being vaccinated a much more a rational choice. Vaccines can be much **SAFER IF THEY ARE MADE WITHOUT CHEMICALS FOR PROFIT** and/or **WITH NO UNNATURAL TO HUMAN BIOLOGY CHEMICALS.** Liberty to refuse unwanted vaccines and freedom to litigate against the manufacturer of a vaccine that causes injury are required in order, to assure vaccine safety. Yes, vaccines are presently a source of unnatural to the body chemicals and the main cause in fact, of the Autism epidemic however, it does not have to remain so! Let us initiate what will, **GET THE CHEMICALS OUT** and make vaccination a rational choice! Right now, it is quite irrational to inject vaccines that contain unnatural to human biology chemicals and is an act of child abuse to knowingly do so when SAFER vaccines can be injected. There can be no requirement to vaccinate with vaccines that are tainted or laced with any degree of unnatural to the body chemicals and there must be no vaccinations against the will or judgement of the children's parents!

Doctors' coercing parents to vaccinate children by stating it's the law and/or that your children will not be allowed in school if not vaccinated is the illegal practice of medicine; doctors have no legal capacity to convince a patient to accept vaccination by stating it's the law just as, a lawyer has no legal capacity to give healthcare and/or vaccination advise. You would not go to a lawyer for medical advice and you should not get legal advice from your doctor! Parents must not cave under the unethical and illegal advise of a doctor practicing law. Parents should only be convinced to vaccinate based upon healthcare need and safety! The indisputable fact is that unnatural to human biology chemicals in vaccines endanger children's welfare; parents require liberty to protect children from any chemicalization! Consider vaccinating with only SAFER vaccines! Please, support our charity, SAFER vaccines whose mission is chemically SAFE vaccines.

A pharmacist once told me that product safety is the priority. The good pharmacist agreed with me that if a vaccine can be made SAFER then it must be made SAFER. Importantly, we both agreed that the less unnatural to human biology chemicals in vaccines the better. The mal-law, vaccination mandate needs to be stricken, as it is geared to promote unsafe vaccines instead, of safer vaccines. Because this erroneous law does not give parents the common decency and critical to vaccine being chemically safe, freedom to deny unwanted and/or unnatural to the body chemicalization vaccines are not as safe as they can or should be. Vaccines are being made too dangerous to inject since, vaccine corporations do not have to take parents safety concerns into consideration. For the health and welfare of our children we need to have in place parental freedom to refuse vaccines! If parents deem a vaccine too dangerous to inject or when parents determine the chemical makeup of the vaccine unhealthy to inject then there must be no vaccination. The vaccination mandates violate our highest **NATURAL LAW** and/or liberty to control what flows through our blood and that of our children's. It dictates tyrannical invasive injections and prevents parents from exercising their good faith protection of their children; parents are unable to protect children from perceived of or actual vaccine chemicalization harm. **WE MUST BE FREE TO REJECT INJECTIONS!**

The use of unnatural to the body chemicals in our children's vaccines and the unethical non-recall of mercury laden vaccines after the vaccine industry was forbidden to produce such mercury laden vaccines are unconscionable acts; commissions or omissions. The degree or magnitude of these offenses indicate that the vaccine industry or the FDA on behalf or bequest of Big Pharma are bent on not safeguarding our children from chemical harm in its vaccines. They will not act to **GET THE REST OF THE HARMFUL CHEMICALS**

OUT OF VACCINES and therefore; WE THE PEOPLE MUST PROTECT OUR VERY OWN CHILDREN FROM SUCH, UNNATURAL TO HUMAN BIOLOGY CHEMICALIZATION! No American should submit to or stand for having their body or blood chemistry ruled over or subject their children to the whim of what a profiteering chemical industry decides to inject. Remember parents and American citizens that you are FREE men and women, fighting for YOUR CHILDREN'S WELFARE AND THE BLESSING OF LIBERTY. What profits from vaccination mandates will never RELEASE US FROM VACCINATION BONDAGE, we must necessitate it! Hoping that the powers that be will turn around and do what is right is highly remote. We the People must act to prompt the profit mongers of vaccination to remove the unnatural to human biology chemicals from all vaccines. We need to FREE ourselves from enforced vaccinations by holding vaccine producers liable for vaccine induced injury and demanding the liberty of informed consent/DENIAL! The aforementioned are TWO STEPS OF CORRECTION that will spark the positive change that will begin a new era of much SAFER vaccines. We have only an illusion of health self-control liberty; we must take control of our health and/or healthcare! If we do not act to correct what is so drastically wrong the Autism epidemic will rage on!

WHAT IS A SAFE CHEMICAL BLOOD FORMULA OR CHEMICAL CONTENT THAT WILL ASSURE OPTIMAL HEALTH? Do you think mercury, aluminum or any one of the other unnatural to human biology chemicals commonly found in vaccines are part of this optimum chemistry of health? Without question, this chemical fountain of well-being does not include unnatural to human biology chemicals. Parents need the wherewithal to assure their children remain healthy and the Liberty TO REFUSE to have one's children injected with unnatural to human chemicalization is required for this. Liberty TO PROTECT one's children and/or prevent one's children from being violated with such, abnormal to the body chemicalization is a FREEDOM ESSENTIAL and is a PARENTAL JURISDICTION! The words of this book will help you protect your children and allow you to recognize that the KEY TO HEALTH or all-important health factor for your children is that the chemicals that flow through your children's blood vessels dictates and/or allows for either health or its opposite! It will become obvious to the reader, that if you expose your children to unnatural to their body chemicalization your children will suffer for it! Parents must be FREE to protect their children from it! YOU MUST BE FREE, TO REJECT INJECTIONS!

If a child tests positive for any unnatural to human biology vaccine chemical post vaccination, then the parents of that child must be FREE to pursue litigation against the vaccine producer for suffering their child with such, chemicalization and/or for the imperfection of your child's perfected natural chemistry. Parents should not be overburdened with proving signs, symptoms or injury if such, chemicalization is detected; the fact, that the child's chemistry has been compromised is more than adequate proof of injury or if the vaccine is proven to have such, chemicals. Parents are recognizing that such, chemicalization throw a child's normal health generating chemistry into abnormal disarray. Vaccines can be made without such, abnormal to the body chemicals, if parents demand on vaccinating only, with SAFER vaccines that do not violate one's chemistry with unnatural to the body chemicals; simply demand not to expose your child to unnatural to the body chemicalization. Remember, abnormal to the body chemicals in equals abnormal outcome; it will eventuate abnormality! You do not need to have a great understanding of chemistry or be a biochemistry expert to appreciate that a perfected natural chemistry is far better than imperfect one or that maintaining the optimum biochemistry is much healthier for you than if you suffer a compromised internal chemistry from an unnatural to human biology chemicalization. Injecting unnatural to human biology chemicals into babies is so counter intuitive to health, so anti-health and so obviously health disruptive that it must be considered child abuse to do so; it must be condemned and stopped for the welfare of all our children! The welfare of our children is at stake here; we must assure SAFER vaccines! Parents undertaking their primary life function of caring for children, need to be completely FREE to refuse any vaccine that they think not in their children's best interest. BE FREE TO REJECT UNWANTED INJECTIONS!

The fate of your children's health largely depends upon the chemicals within their bodies. Just as a bird is flown by the wind and fish is carried by the water, our children's state of health is dependent upon the chemicals within because these chemicals must react; making one either healthy or spawning abnormality or Autism. Recognize that the normal flora of chemicals in the body allow for health and abnormalizing this normal or natural chemical formulation will cause abnormality. Know that natural to the body chemical A can react with natural to the body chemical B to form the needed for health and natural to human biology product C. However, if you inject or add alien to the body or unnatural to the body chemical F; you no longer will achieve the needed for health bioproduct. The injection of such abnormal to the body chemicalization will spawn abnormal to the body or unnatural to human biology reactions or F or FU or FUC products and may culminate in end product K and thereby, spawn abnormality or Autism (forgive my FUC and K depiction). Be chemically safer; consider only chemically SAFER vaccines!

It is both daunting and crucial to understand how and why we have come to the dangerous point of there being unnatural to human biology chemicals in vaccines and that too many parents are either completely ignorant, complacent or willing to expose their children to it. Parents with freedom of mind could not be okay with the injection of such, unnatural to human biology chemicalization especially, when SAFER vaccines can be achieved and in instances are available. No human being who is FREE should be made or enforced by mandate to violate their offspring with unnatural to human biology chemical folly. Only bad comes from exposure to unhealthy chemical folly; it is stupefying for it to be in vaccines! No knowledgeable parent would allow their children to be compromised by such, chemicalization. So, why are these chemicals of mass health destruction in vaccines? Below are two paragraphs that inform the reader of the two main reasons why vaccines are chemically tainted or dangerous. The fact, that there is regulation that mandate parents to give up their power of decision over what will or will not be injected into their children and/or be injected despite there being some degree of unnatural to human biology chemicals in vaccines is perplexing, totally unacceptable and not in the best health interest of children. The laws of chemistry apply to our children and/or their biochemistries! How we end children suffering injections of unnatural to human biology chemicalization is through the TWO STEPS OF CORRECTION. Step one: We must assure that parental protection of children is not interfered with; it should not be defined or dictated to or handcuff by regulation or vaccination mandate. Vaccination needs to be ruled by parental informed consent/DENIAL. Step two: Vaccine producers must be subject to negligence litigation and made to payout compensation to those proven injured by vaccines. The **TWO STEPS** will achieve **SAFER** vaccines in the best interest of children!

Parents must be **FREE** to safeguard children from all dangers so, parents must be **FREE** to safeguard their children from being chemically injected with unnatural to human biology chemicals! By supreme, **GOD BLESSING** or **HIGHEST NATURAL LAW**, parents are supposed to take care of their children and must be completely **FREE** to do so and thereby, protect their offspring from what parents consider unhealthy chemicalization and/or from exposure by injections of unnatural to human biology chemicalization. The atrocity of plaguing children with enforced injections of such, unnatural to human biology chemicalization was and still is spawned by two main interrelated reasons. The first reason is that money making or profiteering dictates what chemicals are in vaccines and has caused vaccines to be vessels of unnatural to the body chemicalizations. The preservatives or unnatural to human biology chemicals assure profits by allowing mega-sales of vaccines since, doctors' can stockpile vaccines that do not spoil. Pharmaceutical representatives now need to go out to the doctor's office to sell vaccines or deliver them a lot less often because of the chemical preservatives in the vaccines and doctors are induced to make large orders, causing increased vaccines sales and the unconscionable profiting that comes from it; all at our children's health expense.

Big Pharma knows its drugs are being sold illegally or at pill mills and there is an opioid crisis causing thousands upon thousands of people to die from drug overdoses and yet incredulously, the pharmaceutical companies choose to do nothing or too little about it. Doctors receive payments for promoting the sale of drugs by the drug industry which, is a clear conflict of interest. Today, you can research how much your doctor is being paid by Big Pharma in that it is now at least required that doctors report how much they are paid by the drug industry. This payment can be in the form of free meals, travel expenses or actual money and it too often leads doctors to prescribe what they otherwise, would not or give patients what they do not need. In a CNN, October 19, 2017 article, it was reported that the City of Los Angeles opened an investigation into a drug maker Avanir Pharmaceuticals for its aggressive targeting of nursing home residents with a drug called Nuedexta that may be unnecessary or unsafe for this population. "CNN'S reporting on Avanir revealed inappropriate and potentially fraudulent use of the medication – in some cases by doctors who have received tens of thousands of dollars to help promote the drug." The emphasis or heart of Big Pharma is on profit not ethics or best health interest!

Big Pharma lobbies to get laws enacted that force its drugs or vaccines for profit. Unbeknownst by most parents is that within the first minutes of life of a baby being born in a hospital, by antiquated mal-law doctors squirt an antibiotic into the baby's eyes. This now crazy law was enacted during a wartime epidemic of syphilis, just in case the mother had syphilis and in the rare instance the baby eyes would be exposed to it from traversing an infected birth canal. There should be an actual imminent threat to expose a newborn baby to unnatural to the body chemicalization and it never should be mandated. Today there is no good reason to do so, no syphilis epidemic and thus, no controlling reason for a baby to have an antibiotic in their newly opened eyes; no need to combat a nonexistent syphilis. Millions of dollars are being made by the chemical and/or pharmaceutical industry from this ongoing nonsense. To further show that the law can be used as an ass or is an ass is that babies born through Caesarian with absolutely no risk of syphilis from an infected birth canal tissue infiltration and therefore, no risk of becoming blind by syphilis exposure; stupidly the mal-law makes the newborn to be violated with antibiotics squirted into their eyes. It is all about money and not about patient or consumer need. It is very unwise to expose newborns whose immune systems are just coming online with antibiotics squirted into their eyes; no wonder so many children need glasses or develop eye problems! Please, do recognize that if you put abnormal to human biology chemicals into the body, blood or eyes; expect abnormal results or abnormality! Parents must be entirely in control over the healthcare of their children and especially, be in decisive control over all preventative healthcare or whether a vaccine is or is not injected!

Just as there is good and bad in this world; there are chemicals that are good for health and there are chemicals that are bad for health. Chemicals that are unnatural to the body, not part of the daily activities of the body or normal biology or biochemistry are bad chemicals that only burden, stress or cause abnormality. Let us strive as parents for our children's health sake to assure that only good come to our children; that only good for health chemicals enter our children and that no bad for health, unnatural to human biology chemicals violate or infiltrate our children. Unnatural to human biology chemicals do not take part or participate in the normal reactions of the body and therefore, parents must assure that any vaccine which, is under consideration for injection are devoid of such, chemicals; by doing so we as our children's protectors provide children with their best chance at optimum health and at Autism prevention. There are chemicals in drugs and chemicals in vaccines that are not indigenous to the human body which, cause negative to health reactions within. Unfortunately, the main concentration of the profit-based vaccine makers is what brings in the most profit and/or what allows for stockpiling of vaccines in doctors' offices thereby, increasing vaccine sales without the added expense of vaccine returns due to vaccines spoilage. In deciding what vaccine to choose or not choose to be injected parents need to be cognizant that what chemicals are injected into their children. Chemicals will make or break health so, choose wisely by only choosing SAFER vaccines!

What will render vaccines SAFER or have vaccines be compliant with rational parental basic health requirements or good standard of safety are the TWO STEPS OF CORRECTION. The TWO STEPS will keep vaccine producers' concentration on not exposing children to any unnatural to the body chemicals. In order, to achieve SAFER vaccines, vaccine producers must have negligence law applied to them, be held subject to litigation (no longer immune from paying damages) when a vaccine is accused of causing an injury. Consumerism and/or parental consent/DENIAL needs to steadfastly be applied to vaccination so, vaccine producers properly respond to the public's safety wants by producing vaccines according to the rational safety concerns of the public to not have unnatural to human biology chemicals in vaccines. Without these crucial TWO STEPS that assure SAFER vaccines, our children will continue to be chemically compromised at the whim or profiteering agenda of vaccine producers; putting chemicals for profit and not safety in vaccines. The insanity of putting unnatural to human biology chemicals in vaccines must be stopped; parents must be FREE to protect children from denaturing chemicalization! Parents require to have vaccination to be a much more rational choice; one that does not allow vaccines to be laced with chemicals for profit that are unnatural to human biology. Before the unnatural to human biology chemicalization of our food, products and being exposed to drugs and vaccines, women were capable of having 5 or above 10 children, adult cancer was uncommon and childhood cancer was almost unheard of and AUTISM and childhood diabetes was practically non-existent as compared to being at epidemic proportion. The golden law of health is, if you bastardize your internal chemistry with unnatural to human biology chemicalization; you will cause abnormality!

When sensitized to the problem, many people are bewildered why vaccines have unnatural to the body chemicals and it is almost unanimous that people do not want such chemicals in vaccines or think it unhealthy for children to be injected with. A reason why we have the pitiful state of mind to allow children to be injected with vaccines that are laced with unnatural to human biology chemicals is because of the repetitive ads we see and hear on television; it dominates, trains, indoctrinates and programs us to accept drugs, chemicals and the sorry state of vaccine chemicalizations being mandated. The bombardment of continual streaming messages dictates to even to the strong willed when saturated by repetitive messages to take and blindly accept; the message barrage enters the subconscious, taking over your free will and causing you to robotically, automatically take action or accept the taking of drugs or vaccines that have all kinds of dangers, side-effects or adverse reactions that if you had your free will, right mind, you would not choose to accept. Not only does this relate to procured reflex chemicalization of drugs or vaccines, the repetitive messaging not to rely upon natural cures is also being droned into the publics' subconscious. There is danger in seeing or hearing continual negative things!

The negative being created or programmed by streaming ads and news of violence move us to be violent. The more violence we see the more violent we become or think it okay to be violent; terrorism or terrorist activity is being spawned by it. Tragically, more and more native, long-term American Citizens that are subjected to see constant images and/or messages about terrorism and aggression or seeing reprehensible atrocities against humanity or civility are making us susceptible to be radicalized by it; the planting of thoughts of the same by repetitive auto suggestion from merely hearing or seeing it. Bombardment of false, bad or unhealthy messages will cause its realization! Our children growing up with such streaming negativity will be adversely affected, it will cause them physical and mental problems. Constant negative TV or cell phone messages are taking its negative toll and we must first recognize it in order, to begin to do something about it. Allowing constant drug commercials makes us complacent about the unnatural to human biology chemicals in vaccines and taking drugs that you do not need. More drug taking will occur from programming and more terrorism, unrest and escalated violence. Violence breeds violence and the revelation is that if you see constant violence or negativity toward in another country or against a people it will escalate tensions and spawn new tensions and ultimately cause more not less possibility of war. Watch out for what your children are watching on TV, protect their minds; take drugs or be vaccinated are on during cartoons!

There are multiple new epidemics of so called unknown origin however, exposure to unnatural to human biology chemicalization is more than likely the cause. When your baby internalizes such, abnormal to their body chemicals must react, it begins festering and thereby, renders your baby a lot less healthy and a lot more likely to be diagnosed with Autism. The Autism epidemic is extremely disruptive; it is an entire family life changer. We must do all we can to prevent Autism and recognizing its main causation is essential to its prevention. Parents have bedrock devotion to protect and assure their children's wellbeing; the very concept of mandating vaccination above parental authority and supreme power of protection of children is totally wrong, grossly improper, unnatural and unjust. Vaccine chemicalization is the main causation of the epidemic. Produces of vaccines and its drones of lobbyist that conspire to mandate vaccination above parental authority care not for the safety of children; they care for the profit made from vaccination! The facts, that vaccines contain what it contains, and you can do nothing to punish the producers of vaccines when it injures or that vaccines are enforced by mandate is clear and convincing evidence of a perverted vaccination system, bent on profit and not safety.

The early negative to health aftermath of internalizing unnatural to human biology vaccine chemicalization can at first have illusive signs and symptoms however, if you know what to look for you can readily recognize an injury has occurred. The spawning of Autism if recognized early can give you a much better chance at stopping it or preventing it from becoming more progressively negative to health and/or more devastating to one's nervous system. If a child suffers such, a chemicalization you can recognize its negative effects. Whenever vaccinated it would be wise to look for signs and symptoms of the vaccine causing injury that takes place soon after vaccination such as, fever, inconsolable crying, starring, no longer making eye contact or smiling, abnormal sleeping patterns, lack of normal cognitive function, lack of recognition or affection toward parents and convulsions. This can be a telltale indication that Autism is spawning. As time passes look for what is referred to as the Soft Signs of Autism such as, excessive colic, chronic constipation, excessive reflux or spitting up, hand flipping, a change from coordination to incoordination, standing on tip toes, obsessive repetitive behavior such as, pouring drinks back and forth or spending excessive time doing things over and over again, excessive rocking back and forth, excessive head banging, eczema, difficulty in relaxing or focusing, abnormal breathing, often starring into space or fixated on objects, lack of normal affection and a general degradation in normal progressing and processing.

One of the worst things that can befall a child is for a parent to have an indecisive mind about protecting the child's vital blood biochemistry! Autism results from unnatural to human biology chemicalization and is mainly being caused by the abrupt and direct disruption to the body, blood and brain chemistry from vaccine chemicalizations; all the unnatural to human biology chemicals from vaccines are stumbling blocks of health and are the building blocks of Autism. Optimal health requires a normal to human chemistry in order, to obtain all the needed reactions and biological end products of life. Abnormal chemistry causes abnormal reactions and/or abnormality; put abnormal chemicals into the body, blood and brain cells and you must expect abnormality. Do not compromise your children's welfare only consider injection of SAFER vaccines. Make absolutely, sure that your child's vaccines are not laced with mercury or aluminum or other unnatural to human biology chemicals. Be sure that you have the decisive control over what will or will not be injected and have liberty to litigate against the vaccine producer if your child is injured!

What to do if your child shows signs and symptoms after vaccination; **PREVENT ANY FURTHER UNNATURAL TO THE BODY CHEMICALIZATION** and do everything possible to clear the body of these chemical destroyers of health and makers of Autism! Becoming neuro-typical and healing Autism requires assuring the proper level of the chemical building blocks of health such as, vitamins and minerals and regaining health requires the cleansing of the body of any of the unnatural to human biology chemicals that are the stumbling blocks of health and anti-health building blocks of Autism. What to do if afflicted with Autism is **NUMBER ONE, PREVENT ANY FURTHER UNNATURAL TO THE BODY CHEMICALIZATION** and in order, to restore health, **NUMBER TWO,** do everything possible to clear the body of these unnatural to human biology chemical destroyers of health and makers of Autism. **KEEP OR BRING THE BLOOD CHEMISTRY INTO NATURAL ALIGNMENT AND HEALTH WILL BE MAINTAINED OR IF ONE HAS AUTISM HEALTH CAN BE RSTORED!** Make no mistake, the most relevant aspect of what affects biology is biochemistry. The law of chemistry applies to children's delicate chemical composition.

Vaccines are wrongfully being contaminated for profit reasons; do not let them contaminate your beloved children! Intake of unnatural to human biology chemicalization makes one's good health become compromised; it is a most destructive force that leads to **AUTISM,** cancer, heart, liver and other organ abnormalities. If you alter the natural biochemistry within your children, manipulate the physical configuration and/or chemical constitution then optimum health can no longer be; the victim of chemicalization health is thus, compromised. There is a perfected chemistry of optimum health; the proper measure of certain chemistry with not a fraction less or a unit more and the infiltration of injected unnatural to human biology chemicalization is health destructive and **AUTISM** productive. Make no mistake, **AUTISM** and every kind of cellular pathology can occur from such non-human chemicalization or alien to the body chemical infiltration. Make sure you save your children from chemicalization! The perversion that vaccine producers or its puppet governmental regulators can dictate what is best for your children instead, of parents who have true love for children is a perversion that the **TWO STEPS of CORRECTION** will cure.

Think about how logical it is, it all makes perfect sense; abnormal to the human biology or physiology chemicalization is the main reason why 1 child in 68 has Autism or that a staggering 54% percent of children here in the United States are chronically ill or that it is estimated 11% of children are affected with (ADD) attention-deficit/hyperactivity disorder or that 13% of our children now receive special education; all of which, is costing America an astronomical amount of grief and money! We can do something tremendous about it in order, to curtail its escalation and cause its rapid decline, that being to achieve much **SAFER** vaccines through this book's **TWO STEPS of CORRECTION;** it is only sure way to cure the insanity of the ongoing injection of all children with unnatural to human biology chemicalization found in our children's unsafe vaccine supply! Be **FREE** to reject injections; be **FREE** to only inject with **SAFER** vaccines that you first approve of!

We are losing our freedom at light speed! Were we once could speak what was on our minds or challenge a doctrine or law as being bad or unjust we are now stifled from doing so and often punished or threatened to be sued for speaking out for an unpopular opinion or being a messenger of change. Freedom of speech should allow us to say peaceful non-inflammatory language and unaccepted philosophy that differs from what is established doctrine. Not wanting to be vaccinated with what the individual considers a chemicalization poisoning or unnatural to the body chemicalization may not be popular today however, in order, for it to be ever accepted or save our children from harm or Autism its very concept or idea must be allowed to be disseminated or expounded into the public without suppression or undue criticism. What it is we think best for the safety of our children or the FREEDOM TO DECIDE WHAT IS BEST FOR ONE'S OWN HEALTH AND THAT OF OUR CHILDREN'S should be unfettered without undue influence or interference or mal legal action against the individual for doing so. BE FREE TO REJECT INJECTIONS!

Parental protection of children and/or liberty to decide upon healthcare or if a vaccine chemicalization will occur must no longer be violated; parents must be FREE to reject injection or STOP any degree of unnatural to the body chemicalization! Once CHEMICALIZATION AUTISM occurs there will likely be some degree of a permanent problem however, no further unnatural to the body chemicalization and undergoing a long-term de-chemicalization of such, unnatural to the body chemicals is required for health. Recognize that parental protection of children is instinctive without conflict of interest whereas, not having parents in ultimate command of children's vaccination decision or rather, having vaccine producers or its puppet governmental regulators that mandate vaccination in command is imperfect, not instinctive and is fraught with conflicts of interest. In the interest of children's welfare, they need and require parents in command! Do not suffer your children with chemicalization that you yourself are not in agreement with; do not be made to suffer your children with VACCINE CHEMICALIZATION AUTISM!

Unfortunately, there are those who still argue that there is no empirical data that vaccination cause health problems, injure or cause Autism however, in fact, there is indisputable evidence that vaccines cause substantial injury in that the Vaccination Court has awarded multiple millions to those who have been proven injured by vaccines. People do not receive compensation unless the proof is overwhelming and yet, millions upon millions have been paid to the multitudes who have been injured by vaccine injection. Unfortunately, inequitably and unwisely, government pays all money out of tax dollars and the vaccine producers go along its negligence way; not caused to pay a cent to the victims of its harmful vaccines. Harm is caused from unnatural to human biology chemicalization! Beyond this data of proven in court vaccine induced injuries is the indisputable fact, that vaccines contain unnatural to human biology chemicals that must react within the victim of such, chemicalization. There is also, the most credible of evidence, the multitudes of parents who observe their children's health demise upon or proximate in time to receiving vaccination. Even the biased CDC somewhat assists in proof that vaccines are injurious in that it lists some signs and symptoms of injury common after vaccination. Autism is just a diagnosis or culmination of the chemicalization or the signs' and symptoms' progression.

It is neurotic to compulsively vaccinate without weighing out the impact upon health from its unnatural to human biology chemical content. Parents should look before they leap into vaccination with such, vaccines, do not blindly trust that a vaccine is safe or compulsively vaccinate. We should endeavor to assure SAFER vaccines through the TWO STEPS of CORRECTION. The fact, that vaccines are laced with unnatural to human biology chemicals is controlling reasoning for you to act to protect YOUR children from it. There are overwhelming reasons for you to insist upon SAFER vaccines! In light of all the Court decision which, are too numerous to mention, of proven injuries that are caused by vaccinations and all the consequential monetary awards paid from our tax payor dollars to all those injured from the vaccine chemicalization should convince even the stubborn minded that vaccines cause multitudes if injuries and severe injuries. In addition, there is what I consider the most reliable of sources that show just how the present array of vaccine chemicalizations are and that is, the thousands upon thousands of parents who observed and assuredly state that "VACCINATION CAUSED THEIR CHILDREN ALL KINDS OF HEALTH PROBLEMS INCLUDING BUT NOT LIMITED TO, AUTISM". The above is more than one needs to know to recognize the once hidden problems of all these unsafe vaccines and to take definitive action to prevent or refuse abnormal to your children's biology vaccine chemical injections or infiltrations. THERE MUST BE LIBERTY TO REFUSE UNWANTED CHEMICALIZATION! The greater good is served by making vaccine false to health, vaccination mandate to reject injections of chemicalization whereas, it is absolutely just for parents TO BE FREE to execute their parental human Right in deciding what is best for children in refusing chemicalization for their perfectly healthy children!

As if vaccines were not health degenerative to children's health or problematic enough with its crazy formulation of unwanted unnatural to human biology chemicals and/or unhealthy chemicalization; it is now confirmed by the Science of Epigenetics that genetic expression is directly related and/or that the genes are directed by the chemical environment itself which, surrounds the genes and/or contacts the genes. Therefore, the chemicals that contact the genes control and/or have major impact on your genes and/or one's genetic expression. Abnormal to the biology chemicalization near or in contact with the genes can make one predisposed to abnormality or disease and/or Autism. Genetic expression is commanded by chemicals and/or the environment of the genes. The revelation is that it is the chemical constituents and or the environment that surrounds the genes; commands the genes into certain genetic characterization or expression. Live in WISDOM, do not be chemicalized only, contemplate vaccinating with SAFER vaccines!

How wise is it or rather, massively ignorant, that we allow our children to be violated with unnatural to their biology and/or physiology by chemicals or that we permit by chemicalization of by injection; it is not WISE at all! WISDOM defined, is knowing the difference between good and bad or right from wrong. It is GOOD for children's health to have all the needed chemical building blocks of health and it is BAD for their health to be exposed to the any of the chemical stumbling blocks of health such as, unnatural to human biology chemicalization. It is RIGHT that we assure our children have all the chemical building blocks of health and it is WRONG to expose children to unneeded chemical stumbling blocks of health such as, what can still be found in vaccines. Let us live in wisdom by only contemplating vaccinating with SAFER vaccines! In order, to live in wisdom parents must protect children's perfected chemistry! Make no mistake, it is a clear and present danger when children receive vaccines that are laced with unnatural to human biology chemicals; CHEMICALIZATION AUTISM can result! Never ASSume a vaccine is safe, make sure it is SAFE your children's very health depends upon it! Take chemicals for profit out of vaccines and vaccines will be cleaner; healthier. Take the unnatural to biology chemicals out of vaccines and it renders vaccines

SAFER. If their sis anyone we want to be extremely WISE about is our children's chemical welfare and/or the chemicals that are in vaccines. There is no correct, positive or controlling need to have such, chemicals in vaccines. It is not in the best interest of children's welfare to mandate and/or recommend or allow on the market any vaccine that has unnatural to the body chemicals! What do you want for your children, do you think SAFER vaccines are in order?

There are very learned people that live a life more less dependent upon medications and medical intervention and particularly unneeded chemicalization and specifically there are more people realizing or living by the understanding that it is best to avoid ingesting or being subjected to injecting or being exposed to unnatural to human biology chemical infiltration and/or abnormal to body chemicalization. You should be FREE, you need to be FREE and must be FREE to protect your children the way you see fit and it is essential that this liberty allows you to prevent unwanted chemicalization by ingestion or by vaccine chemicalization injection; parents must be FREE to protect their children from harm and/or what parents deem harm or potentially harmful! By basic human Right and dignity, you are in control over your own health and/or welfare and that of your children's! Do be WISE, by looking into it! Become completely aware of what chemicals are in the vaccine your children might be injected with and protect accordingly!

If you had a choice to be normal, with no mild or heavy pain and no abnormal processes or internal chemical reactions and have normal biochemical and/or biological reactions obviously, you would choose to! Why allow your children to suffer a vaccination that exposes them to unneeded abnormal to the body and/or biology chemicalization? We can render vaccines SAFER by demanding the TWO STEPS of CORRECTION. Our children should not be enforced to suffer injection of any degree of unnatural to human biology chemicalization. The law of chemistry and the new Science of Epigenetics confirms that we need to protect our children from being injected with such, abnormal to the body chemicalization. One's chemistry, if abnormalized, will cause renegade and/or abnormal internal biological reactions and will interfere with the normal everyday reactions. This abnormal chemical environment will surround one's genes, triggering abnormal genetic expressions. Children are all genetically susceptible to abnormal chemical changes to their natural perfected chemistry. It is wrong to put the blame on our children or postulate that certain children have some freakish sensitivity; children are all susceptible to unnatural to human chemicalization and that is why there is a runaway Autism epidemic; A CHEMICALIZATION AUTISM EPIDEMIC! Be safe, not sorry; inject only SAFER vaccines!

It is imperative that quickly developing babies and/or children maintain a natural chemistry; one which, allows for normal biochemical reactions and normal genetic expression. If one alters their homogeneous indigenous or natural biochemistry with alien to the body chemicals it will spawn abnormality not only because of the alteration in chemical reactions but also, due to the caused genetic alteration or genetic manipulation. Injection of unnatural to human biology chemicalization will have its abnormal influence upon one's genes. Yes, certain children may have already been chemically compromised prior to being violated with any unnatural to human biology vaccine chemicalization and therefore, be even more fragile because of it or more readily induced to chemicalization

Autism but make no mistake; Autism is predominately, a vaccine sourced chemicalization manifestation. The Autism epidemic is not caused by any preexisting or naturally occurring genetic predisposition to Autism; it is the unnatural to human biology chemicalization that is the cause in fact, of Autism and vaccine chemicalization is the main etiology or source of this abnormal chemicalization.

Autism did not exist until recently and has become a super fast-growing epidemic that closely parallels the marked increase in vaccinations and vaccines containing unnatural to human biology chemicals. Those who contemplate that Autism has nothing to do with vaccination or that it is a genetic problem, and nothing can be done to prevent it could not be more wrong. Moreover, Regressive Autism by definition, is Autism that develops later in life, you are not genetically born with it; meaning you were healthy and then became subject to Autism and therefore it is not genetic. Whatever, the argument is for mandated vaccination it pales compare to parents' freedom to protect their children from unwanted, unnatural to the human biology chemicalization by vaccine injection! Children have a Right not to have their internal chemistry disturbed, disrupted or manipulated and parents have the Right to assure their children's natural chemical integrity or perfection. The vaccine industry has perfected its dark art of maximizing profits with its use of unnatural to the human biology chemicals as preservatives and more. Parents becoming educated as to what chemicals are in vaccines are outraged! Parents have the highest obligation to see to it that their children are not jeopardized!

Americans have a moral obligation to render vaccines SAFER by GETTING THE BAD CHEMICALS OUT of vaccines that are unnatural to human biology and parents have the highest of parental obligation to do the same and thereby, protect their children. If anyone dare tell you that the present chemical state of vaccines is harmless or that you should have no choice but to vaccinate your children; tell them to keep their opinion to themselves and do not dictate what your children should or should not have. Inform the uninformed or ill-informed of the millions upon millions of dollars paid to those proven injured by vaccine chemicalization. Ask the blindly led or misinformed to take notice that the Health and Human Services (HHS) have found that people can be caused vaccine induced Autism as was the case of Hannah Poling's Autism which, was proven a vaccine injury. Unnatural to human biology chemicalization is not harmonious with health! Parents do not be misled or misinformed; protect your children's vital chemistries!

Instinctively, parents know what is best for children, through hereditary development, parents' can navigate questions of what is best for their children; innately they know what is best. Additionally, parents' do what is best for children, by rationally thinking things out and have no conflicts of interest in doing what is best for children. This distinguishes parents as the best decision makers and thereby, determines who should be vested with the power to accept or reject vaccinations. Puppet government or vaccine producers have mass conflicts of interest; they should not have absolute control over your children's vaccinations and/or internal chemistry. Children deserve and need the purity of their parent's protection. The concept of applying the laws of chemistry and/or how the body is rendered healthy or Autistic by chemicalization is what parents need to concentrate upon in order, to best protect children. Become acutely aware of any chemical contemplated for injection and always maintain control over your children's vaccinations!

Parents are be-numbed upon learning what chemicals are in vaccines and having been induced to expose their children to such, chemicalization. Being enforced by mal vaccination mandate to expose one's children to unwanted unnatural to human biology chemicalization is off the charts of stupidity and a core violation against parental Rights. The level or magnitude of the loss of freedom inflicted by mandated vaccination is off the scales of injustice. General Washington during the Revolutionary war prior to a battle in Brooklyn and Long Island, New York, said to his troops, "Remember officers and soldiers that you are FREE men, fighting for the blessings of liberty---- that SLAVERY will be your portion, and that of your posterity, if you do not acquit yourselves like men." The revolution was mainly fought over mere money issues such as taxation without representation and not violation of our personage. Today, we are under the oppression of violation of our personage and are under HEALTHCARE SLAVERY and/or VACCINATION SLAVERY in that we are no longer FREE to self-rule our very own body and blood chemistry or as parents, determine what is best for the health and welfare of our very own children. The Revolutionary War was mainly about monetary concern such as, taxation without representation and yet, our forefathers took a stand and risked life and limb to correct the situation certainly, violation of health liberty is far greater of an intolerable situation that WE THE PEOPLE must act to correct; with the TWO STEPS of CORRECTION!

Comparatively, freedom of healthcare or having sovereignty over your own health is of much greater important liberty issue indeed, taxation without representation pales in comparison. The fact is that the average colonists were enjoying an even higher level of abundance or standard of living than that of citizens of England and yet our forefathers revolted; this tells us how passionate they were about any loss of freedom. Imagine how much more Washington and all those who fought beside him would have been outraged and jolted into revolting if England commanded the colonists or enslaved the colonists to suffer their children with unwanted multiple injections of unnatural to human biology chemicalization. The freedom fighters of the past would not tolerate oppression of lesser magnitude; WE THE PEOPLE' must not tolerate the greater oppression of vaccination mandates today! WE THE PEOPLE' are presently under more loss of liberty than our forefathers. The facts, that children are caused countless injuries, signs, symptoms and/or Autism from being commanded to suffer vaccine chemicalization and that we neither can refuse it, nor seek damages against the maker of the vaccine is intolerable and make the oppression more egregious! Parents are rightfully taking a stand to protect their children!

Once in a great while the hard facts that vaccine chemicalization is harmful and the cause of Autism slips through cracks despite all the negative vigilance to stop such, all-important revealing studies as is, the case of the following revelation, in the JAMA Pediatra. 2017 Jan 2;171(1): e163609. doi: 10. 1001/jamapediatrics.2016.3609. Epub. 2017 Jan 2. titled, Association Between Influenza Infection and Vaccination During Pregnancy and Risk of Autism Spectrum Disorder, the CDC study showed 200% or more increases in miscarriages among women who receive a Flu shot while pregnant. Women who got the H1N1 Flu shot and a regular Flu shot showed a 700% increase. In an earlier CDC study released in 2016 it also, showed that Flu shots cause a significant increase in Autism among children whose mothers received the Flu shot in the first trimester. In the face of these important studies the CDC under Conclusions and Relevance, wrongfully stated, "There was a suggestion of increased ASD risk among children whose mothers received an influenza vaccination in their first trimester, ..."; this is not a mere suggestion and it is wrong that they devalued it or its meaning. The lesson here is, if you abnormalize chemistry expect abnormality! Keep your blood chemistry perfected and you will have perfect children whereas, inject them with unnatural to human biology chemicals expect imperfect children, abnormality and/or Autism! In that there are over 90 people a day are dying due to the use of opioids and practically nothing or not enough is being done about it, one must wonder, does the same hold true with vaccine unnatural to human biology chemicalization in that needless injuries are occurring! Apply logic to the healthcare of your children; if vaccines have unnatural to human biology chemicals the law of chemistry applies and therefore, abnormal reactions result, and abnormality or Autism can spawn.

Scientists make abundant mistakes all the time; the putting of unnatural to human biology chemicals in vaccines and enforcing its injection by vaccination mandate is a drastic mistake of beyond mega-proportion. Two wrongs do not make a right therefore, do not be so wrong as to expose your children to vaccine chemicalization harm; make sure your child is only injected with SAFER vaccines. To render children exposed to such out of normal body chemicalization is worse than a chilling bad sci-fi. To leave children to the vices of chemicalization of abnormal to human physiology, biology and/or biochemistry is an atrocity. The essential parental liberty to protect children from this chemicalization abomination is required! To be enforced to inject such, chemicalization is a violation of the highest magnitude and is an enslavement of the worst kind. The mandated vaccination law grants no parent freedom of decision and this is intolerable. Free Americans are accustomed to do what they individually want especially when it comes to personal health. People are FREE to do what others would not or to go north during winter to enjoy the more frigid cold or to go further south in the summer to endure the ever-greater blistering heat. FREE people must have the essential liberty to make all-important vaccination healthcare decisions. There must be no VACCINATION HUMAN BONDAGE; there must be HEALTHCARE DECISION LIBERTY. Parents must have the liberty to protect their children from unwanted chemical injections and any law to the contrary must be stricken!

The mandated vaccination law WRONGFULLY restrains or eviscerates parent's ability to protect children. It constrains parents, making it overly burdensome to refuse vaccine chemicalizations that parents deem too dangerous to inject; it completely has no respect for what parenthood stands for. If parents cannot refuse an unwanted vaccination or a chemicalization that they think harmful or potentially too dangerous; then they might as well not be the children's parents. A mal-law that disenfranchises parental responsibility or denies parental freedom to refuse what parents determine harmful or too dangerous or not in children's best interest must be considered automatically suspect and cannot be tolerated. Proper law does not transgress parent's VITAL RIGHT TO CARE FOR AND PROTECT THEIR CHILDREN. The erroneous vaccination mandates are a seismic upheaval to parental' Rights and responsibility; leaving children without parental protection and thereby, vulnerable to unnatural to human biology chemical infiltration by vaccine chemicalization. Parents must not be enforced by an unwise, inequitable and unjust vaccination mandate that totally disregards parental inalienable Right of protection of children. People must be FREE to protect their children the way they think best, to follow their own private health decisions, keep to their beliefs and remain in control of their children's welfare. For children's sake; We the People need to act together to regain parental protection of our children and demand the removal of unwanted unnatural to the body chemicals from vaccines. The implementation of the TWO STEPS OF CORRECTION are needed, these are the GOLDEN STEPS OF RESOLUTION and FREEDOM!

Without question there is no one better for children than parents to care for and determine what is best for them and this includes whether a vaccine is safe or shall not be injected. Parents are heavily connected to their children and because of this intrinsic connection know what is best for their welfare whereas, government and/or the law has absolutely no valid or empathetic connection therefore, are not best situated to make the intimate vaccination decision for children or supersede parental authority. Furthermore, it does not take a rocket scientist or a healthcare guru to know that to have unnatural to human biology chemicals and/or compounds in vaccines is not as safe as, SAFER vaccines that do not. Mandated vaccination law stands in the way of parental protection and healthcare freedom. Parents are left with a mere visage of parenting, reduced to a mere shadow of parenting, a titular head, buried by an unjust mandated vaccination law. The sense of meaningfulness as a parent is taken by the obtrusive vaccination mandate enslavement law. All programming to make us amenable vaccination compliant slaves must stop, it must fail; mandated MASS CHILD ABUSE must end, and liberty be renewed.

Parents need to be perfected legally with 100% their parental authority to care for and protect their children, being enabled to protect their children from what parents deem dangerous or unwanted or unwarranted medical intervention and thereby, rule over the vaccination decision. People must no longer be enforced by mal-law to suffer a sense of parental meaninglessness or child neglect! The mandated vaccination law is a parental limiting law. Parents must not give up their superior vantage point; they know what is best for their children. Law must not render parents powerless or idle protectors; not enabled to prevent children from being vaccine chemicalized. Mal-law has displaced parents; grossly interfering with parental dynamics. Parents should not remain hopelessly entrenched in this pathology of not being allowed or entitled to control children's health or vaccinations. We owe it to our children to protect them to the best of our parental ability and the vaccination mandate forbids this. Parents' have the best vantage point and must be FREE to protect children. Government must not prevent basic parental protection. If parents' think a vaccine is too dangerous to inject; NO VACCINATION IS TO BE GIVEN! In America we need to be FREE to believe in and rely upon the supreme worth of parenthood.

The ever-expanding vaccination program with its growing exposure of our children to unnatural to the body chemicalization is a critical problem. Parents and/or the public at large have been fraudulently induced to vaccinate their children WITH UNNATURAL TO HUMAN BIOLOGY CHEMICALS under the guise or repetitive statements that vaccines are only good for you. As soon as, vaccine producers utilized unnatural to human biology chemicals in vaccines; vaccines and/or vaccination became an instrument of fraud exposing our children's delicate systems and intricate biochemistries to an array of chemicals that have no benefit to health and only, detriment to well-being. Having unnatural to biology chemicals in vaccines and inducing or commanding the public to vaccinate is a fraud upon the People and/or their welfare; all those induced to have their children suffer an unnatural to the body chemicalization are fraud victims. Therefore, the mal vaccination mandate has become an instrument of fraud and all those that insist upon mandated vaccination collude to commit fraud or are instruments of it. There must be negative economic impact upon vaccine producers for utilizing unnatural to human biology chemicals in vaccines. The liberty to have viable lawsuits under negligence litigation and the freedom to refuse any unwanted vaccines are steps that will clean-up vaccines; SAFER vaccines will be a direct result of these TWO STEPS OF CORRECTION!

Unnatural to the body chemicals in vaccines are a major cause for alarm because it breeds abnormality and perpetuates an epidemic of Autism. Preservatives in vaccines are just one example of harmful chemical toxins. Preservatives merely give vaccines a longer shelf-life and this allows for greater profits since, there are fewer returns due to spoilage. Mere money making is insignificant, and pales compared to the needs of children not to be exposed to unnatural chemicals. Profit must not triumph over our children's safety! Just like producers of food adhere to the demands of the public demands to not have unnatural to human biology chemicals and/or preservatives in food, keeping food healthier so, should vaccine producers make vaccines without such, preservatives or toxic chemicals and thereby, less likely to cause children abnormal chemical reactions within or harm. At minimum the public should have a choice to either vaccinate with a vaccine that has less or no unnatural to human biology chemicals and be completely FREE not to vaccinate.

Producers of vaccines have money not safety as their priority. The People must dictate what safety level vaccines have through consumer demands and negligence lawsuits. Vaccine safety is really up to the public, the demands of individuals and parents whom are directly impacted by the level of chemicals and/or safety of vaccines; collectively we must prompt and demand SAFER vaccines. Vaccine producers' must be made to do what is right for OUR children, do what is in children's best interest; the TWO STEPS OF CORRECTION will do that. Parents should not trust that money-making drug companies make the best decisions regarding the chemical welfare of children; THEY DO NOT and continue to unnecessarily expose our children to unwanted, too dangerous to inject unnatural to human biology chemicalization. Parents' innate skill and pure at heart decision making for their children's welfare must not be suppressed or superseded or replaced by overreaching government regulation and/or profiteering drug corporations induced or bargained for mal- regulations. Government has no calling for doing what parents are perfected at and government often tries to fit many round pegs in square holes; this ineptness must not dictate children's healthcare or command over children's safety. Parents' marked excellence, perfection of skill and/or natural aptness of deeming what is best for children must be in control and this includes the vaccination decision.

Preservatives and other chemicals in vaccines that are unnatural to human biology do indeed cause injury; it is too dangerous to inject vaccines with such, chemicalization! An example of how preservatives injure is the version of the drug known as Methotrexate that has PRESERVATIVES; paralysis can occur in children receiving injections of the preservative form of Methotrexate. Vaccines with PRESERVATIVES and/or unnatural to human biology CHEMICALS cause injury, it upsets one's normal biochemistry, altering and abnormalizing bio-reactions and thereby, preventing optimum health and/or creating abnormality such as, but not limited to Autism. Vaccines with alien, foreign, unnatural to the body chemicals that are injected into children's delicate blood chemistries cause injury and highly escalate the likelihood of Autism. The FDA and/or Vaccine Producers have sat on their hands, failing to act in accordance with this alarming understanding that PRESERVATIVES being injected are EXTREMELY injurious and/or too dangerous. The huge, mega-maniac money generated from an enforced vaccination program, spear headed by vaccination mandates are a primary reason for these chemicalizations. VOLUNTARY VACCINATIONS STAND FOR A VACCINATION SYSTEM BASED UPON INFORMED CONSENT/DENIAL, FREEDOM OF SELF-DETERMINED HEALTHCARE AND THE PREVENTION OF UNAUTHORIZED, UNBARGAINED FOR CHEMICAL EXPOSURE!

Vaccine companies should not be granted license to put whatever chemicals they want in our children's vaccines; the public requires SAFER vaccines. There must be legal recourse against Big Pharma for utilizing unnatural to human biology chemicals in vaccines and it must be made subject to traditional negligence litigation and/or be subject to properly pay damage awards when vaccines cause children injury. The fact is that medical malpractice lawsuits and holding vaccine producers liable for negligent vaccine production are crucially important weapons society has to enforce a good standard of care and/or a reasonable standard of safety; these safety assurances desperately need to be steadfastly applied to vaccine production and its delivery. It is unconscionable for the vaccine industry to have immunity from such, lawsuits and it is sheer lunacy not to protect our children with liberty of negligence litigation. Legal negligence law must be applied in order, to prompt vaccine producers to conform to reasonable standards of care and/or to properly protect children. Vaccine production is faulty; it cannot police itself and/or its own "bad apples". Parents' must self-protect children; only consider SAFER vaccines!

What vaccine producers put in our children's vaccines is appalling; the chemicals they continue to use in their production of vaccines infuriates the health conscious. It is outrageous to be induced by a mal-legal mandate to have to submit one's children to such unsoundness, health stupidity and/or chemical absurdity. To be enforced to submit one's children for unwanted unnatural to the body chemicalization is senseless and unacceptable destruction to our self-preservation human Right and our parental supreme authority to keep children healthy and/or safe. There is a growing mass of people rationally blaming vaccines for children's Autism. We must be FREE to keep our children's chemistry pure and untainted with unnatural to human biology chemicals! People must not be treated like sheeppeople or mere cattle, being herded because of a vaccination mandate to be branded with vaccinations. Many wear visual scars from vaccination and many are being health compromised. People require to be treated as FREE thinking individuals and in power over themselves. People must be secure in their most basic Right of Healthcare Self-Determination otherwise; the essence of freedom is lost. Quality control in healthcare and/or vaccine quality will suffer without informed consent/DENIAL or health FREEDOM.

Parents must be in control of children's healthcare destiny, being in command of whether children will or will not receive invasive, vaccine injection CHEMICALIZATION.

The placing of alien, foreign, unnatural to the body chemicals in vaccines, by its basic definition, must be deemed an AUTOMATIC RISK; that parents, as their children's PRIMARY PROTECTORS must be FREE to protect their children from. A "SIGNIFICANT RISK" is one that a reasonable person deems important enough to have knowledge of in order, to make an intelligent determination, as to whether, to accept or reject a proposed vaccine injection. The chemicals in vaccines are pertinent to the decision of vaccination acceptance or denial; chemical exposure can be considered a SIGNIFICANT RISK! Parents must be given this pertinent decision information and be given the opportunity to discern the pros and cons of vaccination and be completely FREE to determine, for the sake of their children, whether vaccinations that are laced with such, chemicals are worth the risk of injecting into their children. It is unreasonable to enforce vaccination whereas; it is very reasonable to control your children's blood content and brain chemistry.

To put it bluntly, vaccine manufacturers should not have control over what enters your children's bloodstreams because they must care about the mighty dollar to satisfy stock holders and obviously they cannot possibly care as much as parents care about children's welfare or chemical well-being. Vaccine producers must care about making a profit and likely care more about making the most money through whatever chemicals that bring in the most money so, the chemicals in vaccines that secure the highest profit will more than likely be in vaccines; the securing of the publics welfare and/or good health through chemical vigilance is not controlling. This explains how or why unnatural to the biology chemicals such as but limited to, mercury have been found in vaccines. Drug producers have showed time and time again what their agenda is and the utilization of unnatural to human biology chemicals in vaccines certainly, points to its money making first, above all agenda. The sacred trust we have placed in the system or Big Pharma has back fired, has been a major mistake and has placed our children's chemical welfare and/or health in not only jeopardy but in actual health degeneration. Is it any wonder that unnatural to the body chemicals have found its way in our children's vaccines or that an Autism epidemic is raging on? The TWO STEPS OF CORRECTION is what is needed!

Parenting and/or protecting children from harm must include refusing or preventing unwanted vaccine chemicalization with unnatural to human biology chemicals. Parenting should not be replete with obstacle courses or legal blockades. Parents must be enabled to refuse vaccinations despite what Big Pharma's vaccine producers or their puppet government say is best. We must live FREE and separate from unwanted vaccine chemicalizations. Vaccine producers or Drug Company's care about profits and not about you or your child's welfare so do not be fooled or blindly follow its lead or accept harmful chemicalization. YOUR CHILD MEANS, YOU DECIDE WHAT IS BEST FOR YOUR CHILD!

It was only after extreme amounts of public outcry that most of the poisonous mercury was removed from childhood vaccines and that should tell all that children must always have their parents decide upon children's welfare and not blindly accept or be enforced to accept whatever vaccine chemical cocktail the vaccine makers put out there. In addition, it was not until public outcry that the FDA on, 2/21/12 finally, approved suppliers for two crucial cancer drugs due to the astounding fact that the regular suppliers, callously and self-servingly, stopped producing desperately needed cancer drugs merely, because they were not making mega-profits from its sales. Here the drug company acted not to help the public but instead placed patients in danger as they created a shortage of desperately needed lifesaving drugs. We place too much trust in the idea that Drug companies will do what it takes to secure our well-being and government is in the fog unless lobbied. Vaccination/Drug Producers do not take our children's well-being into adequate or proper consideration because they use unnatural to the body chemicals in our children's vaccines. Parents be warned: pay close attention to what is in vaccines!

Doxil, a drug for specific cancers, as of 2/21/12, was still in severe shortage; leaving patients missing life-saving treatments. If the patent is up or if other drugs, make greater profit a shortage of the drug can occur. It is all about maximizing profits and not health. If it maximizes profit it is on the agenda and if it does not it is off the agenda. Please, do not be deceived to think Big Pharma has your back; it puts chemicals for profit ahead of what is in you or your children's best interest. Be wise by not exposing your children to chemicals for profit; vaccinate with only SAFER vaccines that you approve of!

Yet another example of extremely bad Drug Company character is what Bayer/Baxter did after the evidence was out in the open that their drug Factor 8 was infected with HIV; it did not destroy the tainted toxic drug but instead, to secure it profits shipped it for use overseas probably infecting or killing children abroad. Mega-profiteering at the expense of children's lives should be considered criminal activity. Drug Producers' character is not worthy of having such overwhelming power or chemical content over us; they should be held liable for any atrocity it does against society. Do not place your children's welfare in untrustworthy, self-interested hands, control your children's vaccination decision or destiny. You should not be mandated to submit your children for unwanted, unnatural to human biology vaccine chemicalization to any degree! Parents are perfectly capable of securing the best interest of children. Parents know what is best for children; they can tell if vaccine chemicals are too dangerous. Who makes the vaccination decision must have unquestionable character; parents' envelope their children in a protective shroud of love, a love vibration that automatically does the right thing and instills decisions that are in the best of children. Love resonates the right health decision and health itself; profit monger strangers or puppet government must not decide our healthcare. Save your children from the greedy intent of vaccine producers! By human Right and GOD given Right, PARENTS' MUST CONTROL the vaccination decision. Parents are more than capable to make an informed intelligent decision about vaccinations.

Knowing that Drug Companies had to be regulated by government and made to pay fines for wrong doing is strong indication that they have a sorted history and should not be blindly trusted; left to its own design Big Pharma is bent on allowing chemicals in vaccines that are considered injurious and that have absolutely no health benefit only detriment. Its sorted history includes releasing solutions that had heroin and cocaine; they released an evil upon America. Drug Producers produced drops for babies that had opium. They knew people were becoming hooked; in fact, they knew it would cause increase profits from repeat business. It released vaccines with unnatural to human biology chemicals a scourge upon our children. It profits from repeat mega vaccine sales from its self-serving lobbied for mandated vaccination law. Big Pharma strongly, lobby politicians to pass mandated vaccination laws that will fill their fat pockets with mega-billions. To increase profit, they put anti-health chemicals in vaccines despite its adverse propensity.

Unnatural to human biology chemicals or **ABNORMAL** to the body chemicals trigger **ABNORMALITY**. It is common knowledge that such, chemicals can cause cancer; it should not baffle you that alien to the body or unnatural to human biology chemicalization is a cause of Autism. It is logical that such, chemicals are not only a cause of Autism but rather, is the main cause in fact, of the Autism epidemic. The injection of such, chemicals poses the greatest type of chemicalization or exposure. The fastest and most potent way chemicals penetrate the brain and thereby, have the worst impact on mental health and/or brain function, is by breathing or injecting it. Since, vaccines are injected it is imperative that it have no anti-health and/or toxic chemicals. Unfortunately, vaccines do have alien, unnatural to the body, anti-health chemicals. The obligation of producing the safest vaccines and/or the duty owed to consumers for makers of vaccines to produce reasonably safe vaccines has been breached. Vaccines' contents have health destructive propensity due to the presence of unnatural to human biology chemicals. Vaccine quality control has been compromised. Only inject **SAFER** vaccines for the welfare of children!

Vaccine purity has been compromised because of runaway greed and the imbalanced power of the vaccination delivery system which, does not afford the safety precaution of parental refusal of vaccination and that parents are not **FREE** to litigate against vaccine producers instead, it promotes the production of unsafe vaccines that are unchecked by parents or negligence lawsuits. Parents are denied their informed consent/**DENIAL** and/or parental Right of protection of their children. Vaccine producers are unwisely, shielded when their vaccines cause injury. This creates an imbalance of power, a vaccine development and delivery system that breeds negligence not safety; placing children at great risk. Vaccine companies can place whatever they deem necessary in vaccines to maximize profits; it is waging chemical warfare upon children's fragile and chemically ultra-sensitive systems with impunity. This lunacy is all capped and set in play by the erroneous **VACCINATION MANDATE** and/or **CHEMICALIZATION ENSLAVEMENT LAW**. Vaccination enforcement advocates press extremely hard and lobby big for strict vaccination mandates. We must not entrust or subject children to such, folly. Parents do protect your children! Be enabled to refuse unwanted vaccine chemicalization!

Piercing the issue of trust is the fact, that vaccine producers have exposed our babies, infants and small children to beyond stupid levels of mercury – amounts that exceed federal safety exposure for adults by up to fifty times per injection/shot. Our "trusted" health agencies allowed this known neurotoxin to be injected. Parents are only trustworthy to assure safety; vaccine producers and health agencies must not have such, control over the welfare of our children. Parents must have the control and not be dictated to when it comes to vaccinations and/or whether a vaccine chemical injection is safe to inject or not. There continues to be numerous chemicals in use today in vaccine production that are very objectionable and that are considered anti-health chemicals; rational parents do not want their children exposed to and/or injected with these chemicals. By GOD given Right you are endowed to protect your children from what you deem is a dangerous vaccine injection. Know what is in the vaccine, analyze all its chemicals; decide if the vaccine is to be injected and is in the best interest of your child. To have it otherwise, puts your children at risk of chemicalization madness or insanity! It is a harm of mega proportion to inject some of the chemicals that are found in vaccines. Be in control and be the best parent that you can possibly be; inject only SAFER vaccines!

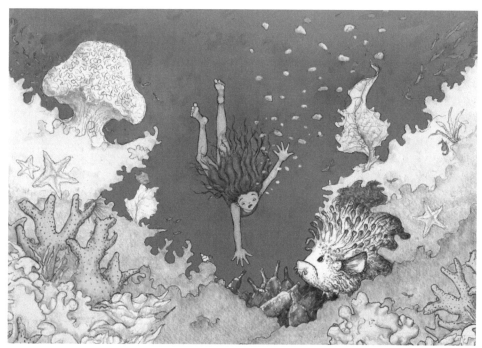

Reach out for SAFER vaccines that are not too dangerous.

Do you really think Drug Manufactures and/or Vaccine Producers care enough for your children in order, to remove the chemicals they put in your children's vaccines if it means less profiting; do you think they care more for your children's safety than profits? Producers of vaccines have used and continue to use toxic, harmful chemicals because it increases profits; they rely on the fact, that you are enforced to vaccinate or will do nothing about it. Well, the TWO STEPS OF CORRECTION will fix this madness and save children from being unnecessarily chemicalized. Innocent children have been made victims by a vaccination mandate, caused to suffer the injection of these toxic, harmful substances. It is highly unusual and grossly inequitable to be commanded to inject vaccine chemicalizations into your children. It is a mockery of justice and the natural order, to institute that producers of vaccines or its bargained for government is better situated or best to decide if a vaccine is worthy of injection or decide what is best for our children. Parents must be the decision makers for such, intimate and important, health decisions! Our children should not be made to suffer unwanted vaccine chemicalizations; there must be freedom of healthcare, with parents', as children's directors and protectors.

Government has intruded upon parental/family territory by removing parents from the equation, commanding children to be vaccinated. Government is a stranger to the result of the vaccination and lacks purity of motive for the decision! Parents have no conflict of interest, no counterpoints to deal with; they purely make health decisions based upon what is in children's best interest; their sole mission is to protect children. Parents must be enabled to refuse unwanted vaccines in order, to best protect their children and/or secure children's safety; this will prompt greater vaccine quality control. Vaccine content must conform to parental safety concerns! Having parental authority over all vaccination decisions is the foremost way to secure the best interest of children. Mandated/enforced vaccination unwisely, assures profiteering and promotes unsafe vaccines that have chemicals for profit, not safety in vaccines. Vaccination profiteering should play no role; the reins of the vaccination decision must be in the hands of parents. To rip the vaccination decision from parents is not only dead wrong, it does violence to our Rights and is counterproductive to safety and/or vaccine quality control. We must restore parental authority over children's health and/or vaccination healthcare; the **TWO STEPS OF CORRECTION** are needed in order, to do so. Be **FREE** to reject injections!

It should be noted that it is the opinion of many that the FDA is in not just in bed with the Big Pharma but also, other industries as it is lax or dropped the ball when it comes to protecting our children in many areas; not just what is in vaccines. The FDA is quite aware that Childhood Onset Diabetes has been steadily increasing and that the sugar our children consume is a main etiology. **Although, exposure to chemicals such as, those found in vaccines is to some degree a cause of diabetes, the main etiology is refined sugar or it's over consumption and yet, the FDA does not act to protect our children**. The FDA sits on its hands, makes no warning statements and takes no affirmative action to decrease the dangerous sugar levels in our children's food. **Children's cereal can be made with sugar as the main ingredient and that should be negligence on the part of those responsible or who can do something about it or whom choose not to**. For example, Kellogg's Honey Smacks is made of a whopping **55.6% sugar** and Post Golden Crisp's are made of **51.9% sugar.** If the FDA were effective protectors, they would disallow high sugar levels in children's cereal and unnatural vaccine chemicalizations!

A child's young developing systems are overstressed by eating mega-dosages of sugar. If vaccine injection intoxication occurs simultaneously with sugar abuse in a pre-diabetic or a diabetic child, whose bloodstream has overabundant sugar raging through it, the injected chemicals from the vaccine will more readily take its negative toll; a chemical critical mass syndrome is more likely, triggering Autism. **Become more informed about what chemicals are in processed food and in vaccines. The buck stops here is the proper attitude for parents to take when it comes to the welfare of children; protect your children from unwanted chemicalization. Parents' must be given the full chemical analysis of vaccines. INJECTION MUST BE FORBIDDEN unless, non-coerced, valid, parental informed consent is obtained! If someone administers an unwanted or a non-consented to vaccination it is actionable and is a violation against parental Rights, an assault and battery and child abuse.**

Parents are **WISE** to police vaccinations of their children! Secure their safe diet because government and the food industry are not being responsible enough to secure children's safe diet. The same holds true for safeguarding children from **VACCINE CHEMICAL HARM**. There is a pattern of irresponsibility, giving parents additional good reason to have ultimate power and/or authority to safeguard their children from unwanted chemically laced vaccine injections. Parents should not be enforced by law, to abandon their parenthood, nor be left no choice but to entrust their children's health to those not deserving of parent's trust or who are safety irresponsible. Parental unfettered vaccination discretion is an absolute requirement in order, to live undisturbed in our most basic freedom of healthcare and to best assure vaccine quality and children's safety.

Parents must BE FREE TO DECIDE WHETHER EACH AND EVERY VACCINE OFFERED FOR INJECTION IS SAFE FOR INJECTION and CHILDREN ALWAYS HAVE THE SECURITY THAT THEIR PARENTS CAN PROTECT THEM BY REFUSING ANY VACCINE THAT PARENTS DEEM TOO DANGEROUS TO INJECT OR NOT IN CHILDREN'S BEST INTEREST! If the parents are not convinced of the vaccine's safety or have questions, which either remain unanswered or have not been answered to the parent's satisfaction; the vaccination must not be administered. For the sake of parent's Rights and children's safety, vaccination must be freely, refused and parents must not have to give a reason or pass a test for denying a vaccination. In order, to save children from unnatural to the biology chemicalization and achieve much SAFER vaccines; vaccination must be 100% up to parental decision and 100% volitional. Choose to vaccinate only with SAFER vaccines! So many innocent children and families have been damaged, injured and lives devastated because children were injected with tainted, unnatural to the body vaccine chemicalizations. Let us end the Autism epidemic with the TWO STEPS OF CORRECTION!

The vaccine industry and its puppet government may be immoral or deranged to allow unnatural to the body chemicals in vaccines, but parents need not and must not; parents do not jump into that fire of chemicalization abnormality. Do not needlessly expose your children to the chemicals that induce unnatural to the body reaction abnormality. Parents must not blindly rely upon or be enforced to rely upon the FDA, Vaccine Producers or anyone else but themselves for the decision to vaccinate or not to vaccinate. Parents must not be made obedient or subservient to another's interpretation of what vaccine content or chemicals are considered safe. Vaccines must be safe by parent's standards. Parents must be **FREE** to be parents; acting to protect their children by refusing what they consider too risky or know as, **CHEMICALLY DANGEROUS!**

The need for the onslaught of vaccines has been overstated and the blatant lie that vaccines are "absolutely safe" was told! Vaccines being unsafe is an understatement! We need healthier, chemically free, vaccines; vaccines that are laced with alien, foreign, unnatural to the body chemicals must no longer be offered. Being empowered to say "NO" will automatically prompt the production of healthier vaccines and/or vaccines that are not so, chemically laced in order, to achieve the desired "YES", for vaccination. Every individual has the Right to decide what healthcare she or he will depend upon or accept. FREE people must not be told what medical intervention they must accept or not have. Vaccination must be AN EXERCISE OF FREE WILL; not enforced upon the People! The fact is, we just want vaccines to be a safe as possible! We want SAFER vaccines and the truth is, without freedom to refuse vaccination and the proper ability to litigate directly against makers of negligently produced vaccines; vaccines will remain unsafe, having unnatural to biology chemicals that are injurious to all our beloved children!

More and more parents are becoming logic stricken; not wanting their children exposed to unnatural to the body or unnatural to human biology chemicals found in vaccines. Common sense tells them it is an unnatural chemicalization of the blood and brain cells that causes abnormality. In the

September 2013, vol. 33 No.8 issue of ACP INTERNIST (American college of Physicians) page 19, the CDC states, "Only one-third of U.S. teens ages 13 to 17 has been fully vaccinated." We need to do everything humanly possible to render vaccines as pure as possible to prevent the kind of injuries that have been occurring. So, even the tainted CDC is finally admitting a problem from unsafe vaccination and vaccination compliance is responding to it; the public is wising up to the fact, that vaccines are injurious and therefore, parents are not submitting children for it. Let the procrastination or negligence of the CDC be a lesson to us all not to trust that vaccines are safe or that they are on top of securing our safety; so many could have been saved from being vaccine victims. So, many children could be prevented from injury if parents had legal command over vaccination and could legally refuse vaccination that parents deem too chemically compromised and not safe. The vaccination program is in ruin due to the chemicals in vaccines. Vaccinations that were once productive for health are now destructive to health. Do to the mandating vaccines and not holding Vaccine Producers liable for vaccine induced injuries, there are now anti-health chemicals inherent in vaccines. Vaccinations are mandated for corporate greed; not health! Autism could be an injection away so, let us act to induce better quality control in the production of vaccines with the **TWO STEPS OF CORRECTION**.

No more coercion or forced vaccination compliance tactics! Healthy, unvaccinated children are school worthy so, let us, regain human dignity and respect for all the perfectly healthy unvaccinated by allowing them to freely enter school. We must no longer live in a permanent state of emergency with mandatory vaccinations in perpetuity and we must stop treating perfectly healthy, unvaccinated children, as if they have a contagious condition. Stop the prejudicial treatment of the unvaccinated! Establish voluntary vaccinations and perfect parenting. Actively, counter the tendency to put profit before safety in the manufacturing of vaccines by granting parents refusal authority of vaccination and with being legally enabled to pose lawsuits against vaccine producers. Let us, GET THE CHEMICALS OUT of vaccines. Let us, be FREE to protect our children from the vices of overly, zealous medical intervention and/or tyrannical VACCINATION ENSLAVEMENT. Do what is right for children by establishing the TWO STEPS OF CORRECTION. Let us, live FREE to reject unwanted injections. Let us, establish that PARENTS HAVE THE SUPREME JURISDICTION OVER VACCINATIONS; not government!

CHAPTER 10

VACCINE SAFETY TEST "THE SANITY TEST"

MANDATED CHEMICALIZATION IS MANDATED MASS CHILD ABUSE

Unnatural to human biology chemicals devastate health; it is extremely unsafe to have such, chemicals in vaccines and it is INSANE to allow its injection into your children! There is an urgent need to correct what must be considered a true travesty upon the health and welfare of our children; the needless exposure of children to unnatural to their body chemicals (chemicalization). Vaccines are perhaps one of man's greatest gifts to man however, vaccine producers callously continue to wrongfully choose profiteering over the safety of our children by its unreasonable insistence upon utilizing chemicals for profit and not safety in vaccines. The evolution of vaccines becoming laced with unnatural to human biology chemicals such, as mercury and aluminum to name a few, is alarming and is responsible for the distortion and denaturing of the normal chemistry of all those vaccinated. We owe it to the welfare of our children to assure vaccines are as safe as possible. It is in the best interest of children that vaccines do not chemically compromise those vaccinated. There are TWO STEPS of CORRECTION that can resolve this travesty! A SANITY TEST for vaccines is required to make sure vaccines are SAFER vaccines.

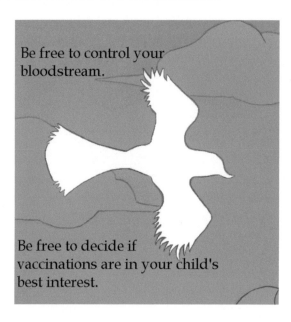

Be free to control your bloodstream.

Be free to decide if vaccinations are in your child's best interest.

Most parents upon recognizing that by vaccination mandate that they are not free to protect their perfectly healthy children from the medical intervention of vaccination; think it, insane!

To enforce the injection of vaccine chemicals and not allow parents to refuse it and/or secure their children's chemical stability is crazy, insane. Rationally, before a vaccine can be considered for injection it must first pass parent's rational safety concerns and/or must pass a quality control "SANITY TEST"; assuring basic and essential vaccine purity. Parents' do not want unnatural to the body chemicals injected into their children's normal blood chemistry. There must be no such, chemicals in a vaccine in order, to pass the "SANITY TEST" and if there is the slightest degree of such, chemicalization it would be insane to enforce any vaccine that has it. Injecting unnatural to the body chemicals into babies, infants and children must by its act, negligent, CHEMICALIZATION CHILD ABUSE and an INSANE act thus, this rational chemical safety precaution is titled, the "SANITY TEST". Rationally, we must be FREE to discern the calculated risks and decide if the vaccine will or will not be injected. The less chemicals in vaccines equals the less the risks inherent when injected. Parents' must be FREE to decide if a vaccine has or has not any harmful chemicals; if it has anti-health chemicals; IT FAILS THE "SANITY TEST". Vaccines must be prompted to be manufactured with a keen eye on never altering children's natural chemistry; procured by parental INFORMED DENIAL. Vaccines must first pass parent's determination of what is safe, the "SANITY TEST"; BEFORE A PARENT WILL EVEN CONSIDER THE VACCINATION.

The "SANITY TEST" will access the risks prior to vaccination and thereby, command needed quality control. Vaccines will become smarter and SAFER since; the public can deny an unwanted suspect vaccine and/or deny a vaccination that does not pass the Parental or Consumer Smell Test. Vaccine producers have not gotten the all-important message or the public's demand for SAFER vaccines, it continues to expose and suffer our children with CHEMICALIZATION CHILD ABUSE. An unnatural to human biology CHEMICAL FREE, "SANITY TEST" FOR VACCINES is a rational parental safety for children requirement or parental quality control. It MUST BE ENFORCED and PASSED in order, for a vaccine to be offered for injection. Children well-being and/or chemical welfare is at stake. With what chemicals have been found in vaccines we need this SANITY TEST precaution and quality control. It is now common knowledge that such, chemicals cause cancer; it is high time that it is understood that injection of such, chemicals is a blow to health, an act of INSANITY. Chemicalization Autism is the outcome of unchecked vaccine chemicalization. We must not be made to subject children to unchecked chemicalization!

Vaccine quality and safety will only improve with informed consent/DENIAL being in control of vaccinations and holding vaccine producer's feet to the fire of negligence lawsuits. Vaccine compliance and or trust in vaccinations will rise when the People no longer view vaccines as SUSPECT or chemically harmful. A vaccine is automatically suspect when you cannot refuse it and/or do not have full control over whether or not it will or will not be injected. Vaccines are not merely considered suspect but actually harmful if they have alien, unnatural to the biology and/or body chemicals. When the TWO STEPS OF CORRECTION are fully implemented, rendering the delivery of vaccines based upon informed consent/DENIAL and holding Vaccine Producers properly and traditionally accountable and liable for proven vaccine induced injuries, only then will vaccines not be automatically considered suspect. Producers of vaccines must be held to negligence standards, it is insane do otherwise, they must pay when their vaccines cause injury. It must be made cost prohibitive for makers of vaccines to place such, toxic chemicals in vaccines otherwise, it insanely puts children's health at risk. Instill the making of SAFER vaccines with the burning understanding that children's lives are in the balance. No more enforced vaccine chemicalization equals no more enforced chemicalization AUTISM harm!

The fact is that vaccines can be a great deal SAFER; not exposing quickly growing children to the array of unnatural to human biology chemicals that have been found in vaccines that chemically react in small children's fragile bodies and that can readily destroy optimum health and devastate the youth of America. Why play CHEMICALIZATION RUSSIAN ROULETTE when we can assure children's chemical integrity! We can do better, we must do better, by making SAFER vaccines, through the implementation of the TWO STEPS OF CORRECTION and with this VACCINE SANITY TEST! To mandate vaccination in the face of parental objection or that vaccines have unwanted chemicals is not a sane act. To postulate that vaccines are safe or that they must be mandated belies the fact, that our children are being unnecessarily exposed to unnatural to human biology chemicals. The very foundation is of health is crumbled by the insane injection of such, chemicalization.

Our own bodies must be ours to be in command of; each person needs to enjoy their freedom of self-determining what is in their best interest and parents must be in control of just what enters their children and determine what is in their children's best health interest! Vaccination health records must be considered a private matter just as, all other health records are! There should be no enforced injections, no enforced herd mentality or herd medical intervention. Abolish vaccination SLAVERY or laws which, mandate medical vaccination intervention SLAVERY! We all want what is best for our kids and it is certain that the less exposure to unnatural to human biology chemicals the better! Decisions for health need to be only for the individual to control unless, the individual is incompetent, or voluntarily grants control over their body or health to someone other than themselves in a legal writing such as, power of attorney. Health decisions and/or health records must remain private unless, that individual so desires to make them public thus, vaccination health records must be private and not be demanded in order, to enter school.

The very idea that law has been enacted, mandating vaccine **CHEMICAL** injections and consequently, injections are administered over parents' objection and that the chemicals injected do cause symptoms, signs and actual harm to our children; **IS INSANE and mass child abuse**. If danger is directed to one's children, parents' must be free to stop the potential injury or impending doom from visiting their children. If a bus is about to hit their children, if a falling object is about to strike, if a needle filled with questionable chemicals is aimed at their children's blood vessels and if any conceived of harm is directed to children; **parents by God given Right and by man-made law must be FREE to protect their children. The erroneous mandated vaccination law is so foul that it severs this supreme parental authority and natural empowerment of child protection. To inject unnatural to the body chemicals is child abuse; mandated vaccination is MANDATED MASS CHILD ABUSE.** History has evidenced that infants were once operated on without anesthesia; now, it is child abuse to operate on an infant without anesthesia. Now, it is considered CHILD ABUSE to inject anti-health vaccine chemicals into children or to vaccinate without true parental consent. To vaccinate children with no parental safety net of informed consent/DENIAL it AUTOMATICALLY FAILS THE VACCINE SANITY TEST.

To allow vaccine producers to skirt being subject to litigation when a vaccine is injurious, promotes unsafe vaccines and **CHEMICALIZATION CHILD ABUSE.**

There are those who will not stand for unwanted vaccine chemical infiltration of their children however, the docile majority should not be subject to obstruction of health from unnatural to human biology vaccine chemicalizations; we must act to protect them. If we mistakenly stand idle, allowing vaccination **SLAVERY** to continue; freedom destructive and a slippery slope of ever increasing healthcare freedom loss will spawn. Since, this protective freedom barrier is breached, it opens the door wide for more aggressions, paving the road for more and more enforced vaccinations and other diverse kinds of unwanted enforced medical interventions; an ever-increasing loss of our vital liberty. Our parental protection of our children will crumble further and there will be uncertainty for our Rights and Freedoms. What is certain is that the spawning of just a few vaccination mandated enslavements have led to many more vaccine mandated enslavements and that this will lead to even worse tyrannical, medical invasive enslavements and loss of health liberty. Injecting many chemicals of vaccines; injects their dangerous propensities! **REGAIN LIBERTY TO PROTECT YOUR CHILDREN = REJECT UNWANTED VACCINE CHEMICALIZATION! CHILDREN NEED FULL, 100% PROTECTION FROM THEIR PARENTS!** Law must not rob children of their parental vaccination decision; protect **YOUR** children!

We can remain a nullified People, as a vaccination enslaved nation; or we can raise the flag of freedom, become high spirited, as a nation of free thinking people that individually are empowered to determine their very own healthcare destiny. If mandated vaccinations are allowed to stand and fester; more oppression in healthcare will certainly, follow. It will lead to mandated healthcare insurance plans (socialization of healthcare) and with that our freedom of choice in healthcare will take a major blow and our choices in healthcare plans and types of healthcare services will become very limited; our personal control over our very own healthcare will be lost. The special interest group lobbyists will see to it that their form of healthcare will be covered and other forms of healthcare (natural non-drug healthcare) will not be covered; eliminating their competition and our freedom of choice in healthcare. We must be **FREE** to pursue optimum chemical/biological coherence. While it is true that we have a system of laws and that we must follow these laws; it is more important that we recognize that there is a system of laws of health or laws of chemistry that we must adhere to in order, to assure our children's good health. Man-made law that does not recognize the supreme law of chemistry and of health, is not valid law. We must not be made to cross into chemical disarray by mandating injections of vaccine chemicalization, for to do so, does not pass the vaccine, **SANITY TEST.** It is in the best interest of children to have **SAFER** vaccines that pass the vaccine **SANITY TEST!**

It is becoming widely known that unnatural to human biology chemicals such as, aluminum or mercury etc. have no business being in vaccines and is a plight upon our children who are injected with it. Aluminum has been found in the brains of those deceased with Autism and the amount of aluminum may not be the predominate causation of Autism but rather, the location where it is found in the non-neuronal cells and the microglia that may predominately cause Autism. Other revealing studies showed that all vaccines are contaminated by unsafe levels of metals and debris linked to cancer, autoimmune disease.

It is not baffling that Autism is connected to this chemicalization! Read what was posted by Celeste McGovern Nov. 20, 2017 entitled, "Dirty Vaccines: New study reveals prevalence of contaminants." Chemicalization Autism is too often a reality! The Scientific Director of Nanodiagnostics has stated that their results "show the presence of micro- and nano-sized particulate matter composed of inorganic elements in vaccine samples". BE AWARE: these particulate contaminants are not at all mentioned or declared in the products (vaccines) ingredient list. The particulates that have been found in vaccines should make any parent outraged and jump into parental protection of their children. Vaccines with unnatural to human biology chemicals are a superb vehicle for Autism and/or Cancer according to anyone with half a brain! Autism has been spawned, it is a chemicalization manifestation. Do not allow your children to suffer chemicalization harm and become an Autism statistic; only inject SAFER vaccines!

There is an uncertain future for our children's welfare caused by ever-increasing numbers of enforced/mandated medical intervention vaccinations that violate our children's vital chemistries and prevent parents from protecting children. Vaccination, medical intervention SLAVERY is devastating our offspring's chemical welfare. Vaccine chemical formula is driven by profit; not safety. We remain under complete control from a too few or select few vaccination DECISION MASTERS, who self-servingly, decide what chemicals our children's will be exposed to by injection. A continual loss of liberty and health will follow the well blazed path of our already loss of self-governing our health or loss of self-determining vaccinations. We must IRRADICATE vaccination enforcement and recognize it for what it truly is; an egregious act of healthcare enslavement that shackles the People to vaccine CHEMICALIZATIONS. Parents' must always remain in control of their perfectly healthy children's wellbeing including, but not limited to, whether a vaccine will or will not be injected otherwise, we are doomed into a certain present and ever-growing MEDICAL INTERVENTION SLAVERY. Pro-choice or liberty to decide upon vaccination is self-determined healthcare; it assures SAFER vaccines; no toxic chemicals. The faltering of children's chemical constitution by mal vaccination mandate is completely unacceptable and a blatant act of mass child abuse by enforced injected chemicalization!

The decision makers at Big Pharma care MORE about not losing their jobs or profits whereas, all parents care about is safeguarding children health from abnormal to the body, unnatural to human biology chemical infiltration (CHEMICALIZATION). Vaccines fail the SANITY TEST if they do not allow parents their fundamental protection of their children; to protect children from unwanted vaccine chemicalization. Puppet government has disallowed naming vaccine producers in lawsuits involving vaccine induced injuries; IT IS LUDICROUS NOT TO HOLD VACCINE PRODUCERS LIABLE; it is INSANE and therefore, vaccines fail the SANITY TEST under this inequitable, unwise and anti-safety total liability shield! It is absolutely absurd not to hold producers of vaccines accountable for vaccine induced injuries; it places our children's lives in imminent peril, allowing for less vaccine production quality control instead, of instilling normal standards. A mock court system, outside of the additional legal court system hears vaccine induced injury cases, called the "Vaccination Court"; it inappropriately and unwisely does not hold vaccine producers liable; not even involving or bothering it. People injured by vaccines are being inequitably treated differently than all other negligence injury cases in fact, they are unduly burdened with unfair requirements in order, to file and prove their case. Unheard of governmental caps have been placed on what the vaccine injured are entitled to recover. Unjustly, one cannot seek damages from the actual perpetrator of one's children's injuries. Parents of the vaccine injured unfairly cannot litigate in the traditional civil court system, they forced outside the normal court system and are limited to different procedures and/or rules under what is known as, the Vaccine Court that has a **SPECIAL MASTER** instead, of a judge. How apropos it is, that the Vaccine Courts are not called judges; instead, they are called **SPECIAL MASTERS**. We truly, are **ENSLAVED to vaccinate** and when an injury occurs from the vaccination **ENSLAVEMENT**; the person ruling over the case is actually called a "**MASTER**".

TO DELETE PARENTS FROM THE VACCINATION EQUATION IS A MISTAKE OF ASTRONOMICAL PROPORTION! Vaccination mandates do just that; this law of perversion leaves children to whatever, vices or vaccine chemicalization, with no parental guidance or protection. **PARENTS HAVE BEEN TOTALLY REMOVED FROM THE VACCINATION EQUATION AND RENDERED MERE VEHILCLES THAT ARE ENFORCED TO BRING CHILDREN TO SUFFER VACCINE CHEMICALIZATIONS!** The history of overzealous medical intervention teaches us that medical claims of fame or that most common medical intervention success stories in time **often turn out not what it was polarized to be and actually are recognized as a cause of multiple problems and at times more problems than it helps. Vaccines are tainted with unnatural to human biology chemicals and the results of that can only be bad!** The validity of vaccinations should always be questioned and not blindly followed especially, vaccines that are being enforced upon the public by mal-mandate. History is replete with medical mishaps; to mandate injections of vaccine chemicalization into the youth of America especially, in perpetuity is unwise and very dangerous! Parental vaccination decision has not been rendered extinct; it just needs to be rekindled with **the spirit of parental freedom**!

Once upon a dark medical time, the medical profession was so sure and eager to mutilate children's bodily integrity when children were all pushed to have their tonsils surgically removed, as a preventative measure. It was pushed upon the public and parents were considered negligent if they did not "do the smart thing". Parents were assured that this surgical procedure was best for their children's welfare thus, millions of unneeded tonsillectomies were performed. Just as over time mass tonsillectomy was realized as detrimental to health; now mass mandated vaccine **CHEMICALIZATIONS** are recognized as unhealthy! It is ignorant to ASSume a body part is not worth having or to generalize that the removal of perfectly good body parts is good for you or that if you inject unnatural to human biology chemicals and think it is not harmful. Because tonsils are the body's own germ trap and first line of defense; the removal of tonsils left untold numbers of children fall susceptible to diseases and some even died. Moreover, children's normal or homeostatic chemistry is needed for optimum health and injections of vaccine anti-health chemicals manipulate and disfigure this sensitive natural chemistry; it weakens immune function, stimulate pathogens into accelerated adaption to rise to new virulence and is the main cause of the **AUTISM** epidemic. When it was realized that a medical procedure was bad, it continued and so, it is that unhealthy exposure to the unnatural to human biology vaccine chemicals continues. **The insanity will rage on until the TWO STEPS OF CORRECTION are implemented**, giving parents their supreme, vital Right to decide whether a vaccination is safe to inject or not and until Big Pharma is brought under normal restraints of negligence law, ending its total liability shield.

Government produces nothing and therefore can give nothing however, it can redistribute wealth with the stroke of a pen or give to one at the expense or detriment of others (welfare). Government is not supposed to take supreme control or command of your health. Government should not dictate welfare or health. It certainly, has no business doing what parents do or what parents are perfected at; that being the caring for children and deciding what is in children's best interest. Parents are diligent, ultimately concerned and centered upon the well-being of their children; it is a monumental mistake to have government control or supersede parents in any healthcare decision especially, in apparent perpetuity. Government continues to run out of control by raising the deficit by the second to eventually cause the end of America as we know it; and it is rages way-out of control in its mandate of vaccine chemicalization injections in perpetuity, an unnatural to human biology chemicalization into our highly vulnerable and susceptible children. Parents have been stating that their children are being injured and the Vaccination Court confirms it by the sheer mass of awards given to those proven injured. It is high time we do something about it! Let us secure children with liberty to refuse and **SAFER** vaccines; ending the insanity!

Multitudes of ill-health aftermaths were being reported after tonsillectomy and yet tonsillectomies raged on. This debacle is analogous to the continued enforcement of vaccinations for all, despite the mass numbers of parents reporting children's health demise contemporaneous or soon after vaccination and that it has become crystal clear that it is the main cause of the Autism epidemic. Enforcing vaccine **chemicalization** into children is so wrong, unjust and unhealthy that it must be stopped! People were duped into tonsillectomy and the politicians that allowed the spawning of the very first vaccination mandates were all duped to do so when they repeatedly were told that vaccines are "absolutely safe". **Just as, it did eventually become very obvious to observant parents that the removal of tonsils left children without their first line of defense against sickness; parents witnessing children's health demise directly after vaccine chemicalization became enlightened or rather, they were struck by lightning that the injection of chemically laced vaccines is health degenerative and Autism generating.** It was not the medical profession itself that reversed its tonsil removing position but rather, parent's recognition of health problems and their outcry. **Parents' outcry, demanding to save their children from chemicalization injection harm has induced good citizens to do their part to end mandated vaccination madness; shout out, "STOP ENFORCED CHEMICALIZATION"!** To be enslaved to have children injected with unnatural to human biology, vaccine chemicals, is the definition of insanity, it is child abuse on a mass scale by chemicalization!

Tonsil removing was becoming very common **until intelligent people and/or hordes of parents recognized it not in children's best interest and that it was indeed, a medical recommendation travesty. Injecting chemically laced vaccines is not in the best interest of children. Moreover, the injection of alien, foreign, unnatural to the body chemicals into babies, infants and all children is not only unwise; it is indeed, a medical travesty beyond anything ever perpetrated upon the American public before. History reveals that parents should not blindly entrust their children's health to others; parents' must remain in control and be enabled to question and refuse medical intervention including but not limited to invasive vaccine injections.** In retrospect, thank goodness, they did not mandate tonsillectomy for the common good; it is a good thing that lobbyists were not told to set their focus on mandated tonsil removal. Medical intervention must not be enforced/mandated especially, vaccinations.

Prolonged MASS, multiple vaccine chemicalizations, is so unhealthy that its negative affects upon health and life expectancy is too difficult to access however, make no mistake; negative health consequences are occurring. The injection of even one dose of unnatural to the body chemicals is not in our children's best interest and multiple exposures over one's immature life span is obviously, incrementally more devastating. It will absolutely become established that the oppression of mandated by law, ENFORCED VACCINATION, is an atrocity that will be recorded in the annals of medical wrongdoing history as its darkest period of mal-action. Government must not overpower our health or healthcare decisions! We must be FREE TO DENY unwanted chemical injections! Children, unguarded by parents, against CHEMICALIZATION will fall victim to it! PARENTS' MUST BE FREE TO REJECT INJECTIONS! We need to empower parents' protection of children; not limit it by vaccination mandate. Do not buy into the warped concept that we need decided to mandate vaccination so that the few children that parents are neglectful need governmental protection over parental protection or that we are all better off with tainted bargained for or lobbied for government mandates, for OUR HEALTH DECISION. Parents being empowered with their natural authority to care for and decide what is best for children is the natural order and will by far best protect and secure your children's health!

If we insanely continue a freedom destruction path, violating our self-determined health care along the lines of vaccination mandates and/or allow there to be absolute foreign power over our children's healthcare destiny and/or welfare, our children will fall victim to unwanted chemicalization and their opportunity to be optimally healthy is lost. Soon we may find by similar next generation legal mandates that all of our children will be enforced to be **genetically altered and/or undergo mandated genetic manipulation under the guise of doing what is best for all.** This will be achieved in the same name of supposed children's health care common good; under an improper use of the Police power of the State which, we allowed to inappropriately, spawn vaccination mandates. Under the guise of affordable healthcare, we will be mandated to buy healthcare insurance and thereby, limit our freedom of healthcare choices, spawning healthcare monopolies and assuring Drug Company profiteering. Stamping out natural healthcare competition by limiting healthcare choices is the enemy of liberty's agenda. We are headed for an even bleaker Rights future, a truly dark future for health care independence and parent's control of their children's healthcare destiny. **We need to correct this erosion of liberty and set a sure path of freedom by abolishing vaccination enforcement. Correct today what is so very wrong and thereby, prevent the mounting tsunami of freedom degeneration. It is an absolute emergency; we must STOP injecting children with unnatural chemicalizations!**

Mandated genetic engineering SLAVERY is much more likely because we have acquiesced into loss of vaccination liberty. Mandated/enforced genetic engineering can easily follow the footsteps that spawned mandated enforced vaccinations and/or slavery. The next degeneration to our Rights is right around the corner, the next giant step in the wrong health direction. First, they will coerce genetic engineering by denying individuals insurance if you have not undergone genetic engineering. They will discriminate against those who refuse to have their children genetically manipulated. Eventually, all of the enforcement tactics of mandated vaccination will be used. WE THE PEOPLE NEED TO MAKE A STAND FOR FREEDOM, BY ABOLISHING VACCINATION MANDATED SLAVERY.

I once participated in a legal bio-ethical and political panel discussion surrounding the very subject of a future with enforced genetic alteration. Will we be enforced to endure genetic engineering upon babies? What if it can prevent disease and save insurance companies from economic losses? Can government mandate gene manipulation to hereditarily make children stronger? Should genetic manipulation be enforced for the common good of all? **Should the People have the Right to refuse**? These questions were discussed, and they indicate just how slippery the slope is or how slimy the slope of liberty loss of vaccination mandates and what it will lead to. Many problems will begin to arise, and discriminatory practices will take place such as, insurance companies may deny you insurance if you are not genetically enhanced and banks may not give you a long-term loan because unless, you have undergone genetic mutation the bank might not think you will not live long enough to pay the loan back; a Pandora's box is open.

The onset of enforced vaccinations has opened Pandora's Box, the doorway to more and more enforced medical intervention. In the name of the supposed common good of all, under the Police Power of the State; government makes citizens submit themselves for medical intervention even if unwanted, it commands parents to submit their perfectly healthy children for unwanted chemical exposure. **This is extremely disruptive and is more characteristic of an enslaved society instead, of a FREE America. Is not the care of our very bodies up to the individual and as naturally basic and fundamental to freedom as it gets? The erroneous idea and implementation of enforced vaccination has created a slippery path and/or a slimy path for not only more forced vaccinations but also, a future of more medical intervention slavery.**

Our Right to be free to care for ourselves the way we as individuals think best is in jeopardy. Our Right to life's quite enjoyment, not being assaulted or battered and/or violated has been trampled upon. Mandated genetic manipulated children may be the next generation of mandates and degeneration of freedom. Will insurance companies be entitled to ask if you were genetically altered and be free to not insure you if you were not? Will big government be allowed to enact and enforce the next generation of medical intervention mandates or mal-enactments. Adolph Hitler had a not to dissimilar plan of enforced medical intervention and/or slavery and the forced elimination of individual freedoms to produce his desired superior raise. **Enforced vaccination medical intervention is the evil seed that has spawned a continually growing number of enforced vaccines chemicalization and a future of more unwanted medical intervention that will oppress or eliminate essential freedom.**

The application of pure logic to this vaccine chemicalization debacle is required. Once you have the understanding that unnatural to human biology chemicalization introduced into the perfected natural, internal human chemistry must cause renegade or foreign or alien to the body reaction and with the all-important knowledge that most, if not all, childhood vaccines are laced with unnatural to human biology chemicals then the truth becomes apparent that we need **SAFER** vaccines and that parents would be negligent to allow unsafe vaccines to be injected into their children's vital and susceptible systems. To have knowledge, truth and understanding about what unnatural to human biology chemicals as in vaccines and stand idle or concur with its injection is **CHILD ABUSE BY CHEMICALIZATION. Hopefully, this book will have you use your mentality, wake you up to the reality that vaccines are not as safe as humanly possible and that vaccines are in fact, too often, too dangerous to inject!** Only knowledge is teachable, and knowledge is based upon the truth and not mere opinion. Our society has been indoctrinated to trust in that vaccines are safe, and this is a lie. Knowledge is always true, you can't have false knowledge however, opinion may be true or false. It is better to be ignorant than wrong. It is not only mere opinion that vaccines are safe; it is an outright error. To believe vaccines are safe is an ignorant statement or an error depending if you have or do not have the correct information about what chemicals are in vaccines. The fact, that vaccines are unnatural to human biology chemicalizations makes the statement that vaccines are safe either false or at best, uneducated false opinion. An opinion can be true but since, it is mere opinion; you do not understand why it is true. The error that vaccines are safe is further away from knowledge than ignorance of it is. Knowing what chemicals are in vaccines divides the realm of knowledge from the realm of opinion. **There are no grounds or basis to call vaccines safe when there is knowledge that vaccines have alien, unnatural to human biology chemicals. Do not be in error over your children's health; know what chemicals are in vaccines and understand its negative to health ramifications! Inject, only SAFER vaccines!**

Vaccinations are not "absolutely safe", in fact, they are "absolutely dangerous" because they contain alien, foreign to the body, unnatural to human biology and physiology chemicals which, when injected pollute our children's delicate systems and/or blood. Mandating vaccine injection and/or medical intervention slavery over the objection of parents that want to refuse because they have determined the vaccine is too dangerous to inject is not only egregious; it is an insane law and stupefying. Vaccination mandated slavery with its consequential patient's Rights violations will reverberate as one of healthcare's darkest wrongs and an overreaching governmental misact that has been perpetrated upon the public, not for the common good, but rather, to main serve to spawn a medical monopoly in order, to guarantee unwarranted profiteering, at the expense of all children's best interest. Fundamentalist vaccination advocates have a childishly simplistic idea that mandating vaccination of unnatural to the body chemicals into babies, infants and children is healthy, lawful and in the best interest of children. Furthermore, to mandate it with no sunset of its unlawful requirement to be subjected to such, chemicalization sets up a permanent profiteering scheme and obliteration of parental Rights to protect their children from chemicalization harm and disintegrates parental liberty to decide what is best and/or what is in their children's best interest. Know exactly, what chemicals are in vaccines; DO NOT INJECT HARMFUL CHEMICALIZATIONS! Vaccines must pass the SANITY TEST, in order, for it to be rational to consider injecting!

Although, it might be not possible to eliminate all the foreign to the body chemicals presently found in vaccines, the elimination of most of these chemicals is possible and it is an emergency to do so! The elimination of most if not all, chemicals of harm will be achieved through the implementation of the **TWO CORRECTIVE STEPS. C**ertainly, these **TWO STEPS** are imperative to begin, assure and command the vaccine purification process; it must be imposed upon the vaccine industry in order, to induce the efficient and effective reduction of unnatural to the body chemicals in vaccines and reduce or eradicate its related harm. These urgently needed **TWO STEPS** will substantially diminish the chemicals in vaccines to a reasonable safety level and thereby, render **SAFER** vaccines that will help satisfy parent's reasonable and rational health concerns; it will also, help build needed trust in the vaccination program and prompt volitional vaccination compliance. The concept of vaccination is only workable if it is a volitional system! To mandate vaccination fails the **SANITY TEST** and only promotes unsafe, not safer, vaccines. **The fact, that unnatural to human biology chemicals are negative to health is as clear as 2 + 2 = 4; to not know this or ignore it places your children** in harm's way. For it is an illusion that such, vaccines are good for you! To think vaccines with unnatural to human biology chemicals are good for you is not based upon knowledge but rather, wrong opinion either or on authority of your emotions or passions or prejudices; it is not an act of knowledge.

Producers' of vaccines are GUILTY of having unnatural to human biology chemicals in vaccines. A sacred trust that parents placed in them has been violated. Altering or manipulation of the natural or genetic chemistry of the body can have drastic health consequences. Chemicals must do what they do and that is react and abnormal to the body or unnatural to human biology chemicals cause abnormal reactions within' the consequences of those abnormal reactions are abnormality and/or CHEMICALIZATION AUTISM. Drugs and/or vaccine chemicals grossly interfere with the normal functions of the body. For example, in English, Australian and Dutch studies, the drug AZT was found to cause severe anemia, requiring multiple blood transfusions just to stay alive. There is always a too long list of adverse reactions from taking any drug; there really is a hidden or suppressed longer list of harm from injecting vaccine chemicals. The human body or physiology is extremely sensitive to unnatural to the body chemicals. Drugs and/or vaccines introduce such, chemicals into the human system, which cause chemistry abnormality in the body. Remain healthy by not injecting bad chemicals; BE FREE NOT TO INJECT! There must be LIBERTY TO PROTECT YOUR CHILDREN FROM WHAT PARENTS' DEEM A CHEMICALIZATION HARM OR A POSSIBLE DISRUPTION TO THEIR CHILDREN'S PERFECTED CHEMISTRY!

People must be free to choose a more natural way of life, free of chemical medical intervention. FREE, to seek energy from nutrients instead, of stimulants. FREE to obtain natural remedies and not medical intervention. FREE to keep one's body clean or 100% natural and not enforced to submit oneself or one's children to have their skin pierced by vaccination needles and injected with unwanted chemicals. Liberty requires that the taking vaccines/drugs must be up to the recipient user. Since, parents have the natural dominion over distinguishing what is right or wrong for their children and/or if vaccine chemicals are wrong or right for their children then it is befitting that the "SANITY TEST" BE A REQUIREMENT FOR VACCINATION. Parents' are connected to their children, there is conscious and unconscious entanglement, their energy is permanently connected. Vaccinations all have risks, they affect their children; parents' must be in control of all vaccination decisions! The fact is that if one suffers or subject children to unnatural to human biology chemicals by injection, an abnormal chemicalization, those chemicals react within and cause abnormality, health disturbance, biological and physiological disruption. Abnormal chemicalization equals abnormality thereby, spawning a chemicalization Autism epidemic.

The flawed idea, the terrible plan and the deliberate execution of that plan to suffer our children with unnatural to human biology chemicalization vaccine injections is of no wonder or surprise that it is of course, extremely unhealthy! Yes, there may be benefits to taking such drugs or injections but there are always definite and probable harms. We require the basic freedom to determine whether we want to accept the benefits and/or the harms inherent. The adverse effects caused by injecting chemically laced vaccines may never be thoroughly understood however, the presence of such, chemicals within the bloodstream will cause abnormality and/or biological function breakdown. The universal laws of chemistry apply to when vaccine chemicals enter the blood; they alter the natural geometric chemical reactions of health. A complete list of all the chemicals in a vaccine must be given to make an intelligent decision. Keep your children's blood free of anti-health chemicalization! In November 2018, the federal National Center for Health Statistics released the preliminary results of a study that showed between 2014 and 2016 the number of 3 to 17-years old diagnosed with autism rose by 23%, yielding a new autism rate of 2.76%, or 1 in 36 children, and 3.63%, or 1 in 28 boys. The obvious emergency is not preventing childhood disease but rather, the prevention of Autism or its raging epidemic; SAFER vaccines charity's mission is to render vaccines devoid of its chemicals of harm! The SANITY test for vaccines and the TWO STEPS OF CORRECTION are needed!

It is self-evident that unnatural to human biology chemicals do not belong to the needed chemical flora of health and that its presence is negative to one's welfare. For freedom, justice and honor we must see to it that parents can refuse unwanted vaccine chemicalizations and that children are secure in their parents unfettered protection. It is a fundamental truth that there is a chemical arrangement to health or a certain range of atoms, molecules and/ or chemicals required to produce the molecules and compounds needed for health and/ or for normal biological functions to occur. It is impossible for optimum health to exist without the normal chemical/molecular configuration! Optimum health is achieved from proper chemistry and the spawning of Autism occurs when chemicals, which are anti-health promoting upset the normal chemical signature. Make sure vaccines are clean! We must have the unmitigated Right to be in command of our blood chemistries and/or prevent unwanted chemicals from being injected into it. We must be free to keep our chemistry intact and/or perfect; not be mastered by the mandated vaccination law to inject unwanted chemistry. The SANITY TEST FOR VACCINE SAFETY is consistent with this fundamental truth of health and our basic liberty to control our health. They are finally beginning to offer preservative free vaccines for children although, this is a giant step forward, it is still imperative to achieve much SAFER vaccines that are devoid of the preservative thimerosal (the tip of the iceberg of bad chemicals) and all other toxic chemicals. If a vaccine has unnatural to human biology chemicals, it fails the Vaccine Sanity Test.

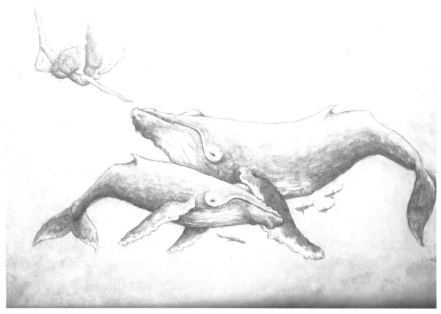

Be FREE to live a natural life. A life that is not coerced or forced to inject vaccine chemicalizations that have unnatural to human biology chemicals.

Making a rational decision about vaccination is not brain surgery and most if not, all parents are imbued with the sanctity of reason therefore, parents should be FREE to decide what is best for their children and protect children from unwanted chemicalization. Yes, some prescription drugs are wonderful however, for the most part, it would be healthier if **MOST drugs** that people take were thrown out the window, except that the birds might eat them; has some degree of wisdom but, I will give you odds that the birds would know better. It is abundantly clear, to utilize unnatural to human biology chemicals in vaccines is sheer madness and that most if not all kindergarteners would know better than to put it in food or in vaccines that are injected. Chemicals that are not in harmony with health are usually recognized as not good to eat by wildlife or by rational people, unless it is well disguised, or people are lied to by being told, "it is good". This brings to my mind when I was on a remote tropical island and was at the breakfast table on the edge of the sea and thought, how inappropriate and out of place it was that in this perfect natural environment that on the table there was **artificial** sweeteners, EQUAL and SWEET' N LOW. I had an impulse to do an experiment with the flocks of Sugar birds that were constantly flying about, on the hunt for natural nectar sugar to eat. I opened a bag of raw natural sugar, a bag of EQUAL and a bag of SWEET'N LOW and strategically placed them close by each other in open view of the birds. Revealingly, the birds quickly swooped down to eat the raw natural sugar however, the birds flew down to the bag of EQUAL chemicals and pecked only once at the EQUAL chemicals and abruptly, flew away, not eating it. I also, observed birds flying near the SWEET'N LOW but, did not even peck at it, they all somehow knew it was bad chemicalization and flew right away. These birds are telling us something! We are becoming so removed from nature that we are losing the instinct to know what chemicals are good or bad for health; no innate intelligence. You must reason out, use your brain to analyze what chemicals are good or bad; **BE FREE to discern if it should be pecked at, or refused!** People will now have a **(sniff) test** to help discern if it is best to refuse a vaccine chemicalization; I call it, the **"SANITY TEST"** that discerns if a vaccine is good or bad for your children and/or worthy of being injected!

THE "SANITY TEST" FOR VACCINES

A test that determines whether a vaccine should or should not be utilized for injection is the **"SANITY TEST"**. The test detects if the vaccine has unneeded and/or any unnatural to one's biology chemicals; if it does it **FAILS**. Certain chemicals within vaccines simply have no health promoting reasons to be in vaccines, the chemicals only serve to assure vaccine industry mega profits. Injecting vaccines that are laced with alien, unnatural to the body chemicals are opposite of health promoting. **Injection these chemicals is an anti-health act; a ludicrous act.** All vaccine products must **be made to PASS this "SANITY TEST"**, in order, to be placed on the market for sale or for it to be sane to consider for injection. The **"Sanity Test"** requires that if any alien, unnatural to the body chemicals are found in a vaccine, it automatically **FAILS**. The vaccine industry **must be prompted to GET THE CHEMICALS OUT, so that children are not even potentially exposed to chemicals that are not natural to the body. PARENTS MUST BE GIVEN ALL THE CHEMICAL FACTS ABOUT A PROPOSED VACCINE. THE "SANITY TEST" CAN EXPOSE A VACCINE AS NOT INJECTABLE; AS TOO CHEMICALLY DANGEROUS. I am both a doctor and an attorney and I bet both licenses that you will be outraged when you learn just what chemicals are in vaccines; you will agree with me that our children are in desperate need for SAFER vaccines that will not chemically compromise them! Parents by natural law need to be in control of their children's welfare and make the vaccination decision; being completely FREE to prevent unnatural to human vaccine chemicalization! The SANITY TEST requires parents to have the controlling vaccination decision! Think how absurd it is, that non-negligent, totally competent parents are blocked by vaccination mandate; with no liberty to protect their children from unwanted vaccine chemicalizations.**

Being in control of your healthcare, having absolute determination power over whether you or your child accept or deny all healthcare is a natural Right that is at a stratospheric level; it is a Right that underlies all others. We should be very worried and extremely concerned about the slightest encroachment, decrease or violation to this Right of Self-Determined Healthcare. There must never be obstacles or regulatory traffic lights put up hindering us from the full expression of this natural Right. No red light stopping us or yellow light cautioning us, from the FREE exercise of this all-important Right should be tolerated. In fact, even a green light regulation that grants us permission to self – regulate our health is inappropriate because one's health is totally one's private affair. We do not need and must not need permission to self- regulate our own or our children's healthcare. The doctrine of informed consent/DENIAL assures that the sacrosanct natural law of taking care of one's own body and "Right of INVIOLABILITY of one's person" is protected; and that we remain unmolested and/or not violated by unwanted medical intervention. Liberty of health and/or healthcare is so basic and vital; it must be zealously, protected!

I have coined the terms or phrases, "Chemicalization" because it accurately describes what happens when a chemical enters your body, the phrase, "Chemicals for profit" because it describes the reason why the chemicals are in the vaccine, the phrase, "Informed DENIAL" instead, because it is much more the accurate to the doctrine that requires the patient to remain in control of their healthcare when it is unwanted, the phrase "CHEMICALIZATION Autism" because it is the cause in fact, or etiology of most Autism, the phrase, "VACCINE CHEMICALIZATION Autism epidemic" because it is vaccine's unnatural to human

biology chemicalization that is the main causation of the Autism epidemic. The term, "chemicalization" is readily understood without any or little explanation; the word is my invention to help people realize just what is occurring when a vaccine which, commonly has alien, unnatural to human biology chemicals is injected into tiny babies, small infants and/or little children. These terms and/or phrases need to be part of parents' and/or consumers' vocabulary in order, to properly protect one's children. It is idiocy to have unnatural to human biology chemicals in vaccines and it is unreasonable to have it that by vaccination mandate, parents are enforced to subject their offspring to it.

Make no mistake, mandated vaccination and its enforcement is an abomination that does violence to parental Rights, it prevents parents from protecting their offspring from unwanted chemicalization and thereby, suffers children with injections of unnatural to human biology chemicalizations, it chemically compromises children's naturally perfected chemistry. The onerous and forbidding mandate eliminates parents' protection of children, it stops you from protecting your children from chemicalization harm and/or manipulation, it does not allow you to keep your children's vital systems and/or blood free from unnatural to human biology chemicals; it demands children suffer the propensities of the abnormal chemicalization. Vaccines fail the SANITY TEST when it violates parental Rights or if it is an unnatural to human biology chemicalization. Our children are not mere Guinea pigs, to be experimented upon with chemicals for profit; it is insane to pass such, vial vaccines and/or inject it. As a human, you are vested with the dignity of Self-determined healthcare; the mal mandate robs you of this. The vaccination mandate is an ENSLAVING mandate that enforces perplexed parents to submit children. The more chemicals for sheer profit in vaccines, the more the negative degree and type or kind of unnatural to human biology chemicals in vaccines the more insane it is to inject it!

Parents have a special mental power that governs their children's welfare which, is near always perfected for their children's best interest; it is not tainted by special interests, corporate greed, lobbyists and mere monetary concerns. Parents have an instinct and **parental Right of protection of their children**. By supreme natural law parents, are empowered to refuse vaccine chemicalization when they deem it in their children's best interest to do so! Parents' must be enabled to perform their parental natural duty without interference and determine without undue outside influence what is best. Parents must not be coerced or enforced to vaccinate their children and/or be made to submit their children for unwanted medical intervention. **Parents are desirous that children be safe under the umbrella of their parental protection and/or that parents determine what is best for children's welfare. Going against parent's health decisions for children violates children and is a violation against the parents. People must be FREE to be left alone; not violated! Reasonable people do not want to be enforced to have their children injected with unwanted vaccines particularly and especially, vaccines that have any degree of unnatural to human biology chemicals. Parents want and need to choose what is best for children. Rational parents require SAFER vaccines that are not so disruptive to babies' sensitive chemistry; they will only allow injection of SAFER vaccines.**

Perhaps histories most intellectual Supreme Court Judges, Judge Cardoza put our **healthcare Right to be left alone** and/or unmolested by unwanted vaccinations in perspective when he stated, " Under a **free** government at **LEAST**, the **Free citizens FIRST** and **GREATEST RIGHT** which **underlies all others** – the right to the **INVIOLABILITY of his person**, in other words **his right to himself** – is the subject of universal acquiescence, and this right necessarily **forbids** a physician or surgeon, however skillful or eminent, who has been asked to examine, diagnose, advise, and prescribe (which are at least necessary first steps in treatment and care) **to VIOLATE WITHOUT PERMISSION the bodily integrity of his patient."** The virtuous and honorable Judge is expounding upon the extreme importance of informed consent and that the Right of Self-Governing one's own body and health and/or the Right of Self-Determined Health- care is **SUPREME**, as a **"FREE CITIZENS FIRST and GREATEST RIGHT". It "is the subject of universal acquiescence" and/or it is universally, accepted that parents are empowered, vested, and always expected, to decide what is best for their children's welfare. Parents' protecting children from a too dangerous to inject vaccine chemicalization; falls squarely, within the honorable Judge Cardoza "right to the INVOLABILITY of his person". In the instant case, the inviolability of children is assured and protected by children's parents. Our government itself stated, that vaccines are "unavoidably unsafe" and gave vaccine manufacturers' an unprecedented liability shield; it is obvious that parents need to step up to the plate of parenthood and protect their children by only considering SAFER vaccines.**

Protecting one's own blood chemistry and parent's protection of their children's blood chemistry from unwanted injections is an essential, basic, SUPREME natural Right that MUST NOT be subverted or violated. You have the controlling authority over your own and that of your children's internal being and must always control the decision of what if anything shall be done to your body or done to your children's bodies. It is cosmic justice that the vaccination program is in shambles, in that vaccination compliance has been in a downward spiral as the public recognizes that vaccines are not "absolutely safe" but rather, absolutely unsafe with its unnatural to human biology chemical contents. What will be allowed to enter children must be up to the parents, it is rightfully their decision; not governments. The vaccination question is a QUINTESSENTIAL PARENTAL DECISION, it is not a minor decision. Chemicalization is gambling with children's welfare; do not risk it! Indeed, as a parent you must be FREE to protect your children from chemicalization harm! Those people who think they can inject unnatural to human biology chemicals into babies and not cause health problems are really deluded; they have no conception of the laws of chemistry. Just because some people want to jump off the safe bridge into such, abnormal vaccine chemicalization does not mean you must or those truly educated or sane must. We need to act intelligently and directly to achieve SAFER vaccines that do not abuse our children by chemicalization; to do otherwise, is insane and child abuse by chemicalization. There is a marked discontinuity between a baby who has been injected with unnatural to human biology chemicalization from vaccines as compared, to a baby that has not; the law of chemistry applies thereby, the chemically compromised are vulnerable to be unhealthy.

Government' too often does not get it right and is too often lobbied to do what is not in the public's best interest; it must not overpower parents in the vaccination decision of children's welfare. Government has eliminated gym classes and recess relaxation time in schools, while they allow children's school diets to consist of refined foods and sugar drinks, despite the epidemic of childhood obesity and diabetes. Lobbyists have inflicted upon us all the greed of corporate will. Our tax dollars unwisely back fast food, GMO takeover of the food industry and with no GMO alert labeling. Cows, chickens and other animals we eat are fed

antibiotics and grown in confining space, with no sunlight; making the livestock become abnormally large and so unhealthy that they cannot even stand or walk, and they often have high e coli levels. Livestock and farm raised fish are being fed high fructose genetically engineered corn or soy instead, of their natural health promoting indigenous diet. These sick and/or abnormal animals and fish are often brought to market. Government is run by corporate greed, regulation is not for the common good; recognize that mandated vaccinations are for corporate profiteering and not in children's best interest. You must scratch your head in bewilderment at government foolishness. Mandating vaccinations over the general population of parental decision makers' is sheer foolery that leaves children without parental insight and protection which, has led to unnatural to human biology chemicals in vaccines and/or chemicals for profit, not safety.

More studies on vaccination causing Autism need to be performed however, one thing is certain, it is totally unscientific to state that vaccines do not cause Autism. Although research of the past connecting vaccines to autism have been slated, biased or suppressed, now research is reaching the forefront. Journal of Transitional science on April 24, 2017, in a cross-sectional study of 6 to 12 years-olds exploring the association between preterm birth, vaccination and **NEURODEVELOPMENTAL DISORDERS**, using data from both vaccinated and unvaccinated populations revealed data that points to or pin the donkey of a cause or rather, the cause of Autism. In premature birth that have been vaccinated neurodevelopmental disorders have been well established whereas, premature births that have not undergone vaccination neurodevelopmental disorders is nonexistent. A 12.3-fold increase in odds of neurodevelopmental disorders was found in preemies that were vaccinated compared to preterm birth without vaccination (very revealing). Full-term birth with vaccination was associated with a 2.7-fold increase in the odds of neurodevelopmental disorders compared to unvaccinated full-term births. These findings coincide with my findings when I analyzed the cultures such as, the Amish people that do not vaccinate; where Autism is almost nonexistent. No study needs to be performed to show that vaccines that contain unnatural to human biology chemicals cause health problems such as, but not limited to Autism because all you really need to know, is that the Law of Chemistry applies! What chemicals do you want to circulate in your children? Injection of unnatural to human biology chemicals is a **DEEP ORGANIC DISTURBANCE!**

Government's backing of the enslaving of children, making children endure **CHEMICAL** vaccine injections is beyond foolish; it is downright an act of mass gross negligence and is **MANDATED MASS CHILD ABUSE** by chemicalizations. Government's insane severing of parent's protection of children from unwanted medical intervention is an atrocity beyond gross negligence. There are all kinds of people in this world, with diverse mind sets; they must be **FREE** to protect their perfectly healthy children the way they think is best. Parents must not be enforced by mandate vaccination law to place their children's welfare in the hands of others. Strangers' likely have different mind sets than that of parents or parents may think them too progressive and extreme progressiveness may endanger their children's well-being. These progressives have allowed chemicals in vaccines that parents do not want their children to be exposed to. Parents strongly disagree with what chemicals these strangers think are okay to put in vaccines. Parents' must be empowered to refuse unwanted vaccines and/or the chemical content of vaccines because it engenders SAFER vaccines, chemically safe vaccines. Let us not mandate vaccines because it merely assures vaccine producer's profiteering and not safety and/or welfare. One has to only remember, that they put thimerosal the mercury derivative and other dangerous toxins in vaccines were and some still are used in vaccines, to give the vaccines greater shelf-life but, it destroys the life of our children; all in the name of profit. When the perversion that you cannot protect your children from unwanted vaccine chemicalization ceases so, will the vaccine unnatural to human biology content cease! Of course, holding vaccine producers accountable and liable by making it pay damages when it's vaccines chemically compromise children and causes injury is also, necessary! The two aforementioned revelations are the much needed, TWO STEPS OF CORRECTION!

It is the most general rule of right or wrong that parents are to oversee their children, be in command of their welfare and in charge of all their children's healthcare decisions; vaccination must no longer be an exception to this golden rule, for it is a perversion, an enigma and is not in children's best interest for parents to be blocked from their basic parental duty and/or paramount life obligation. There are major health implications or consequences if exposed to the present sorry chemical state of vaccines. If vaccines are not cleaned-up the Autism epidemic will continue. The vaccination decision revolves around puncturing your children's skin and then injecting a vial/vile of vaccine chemicals into their bloodstreams. Vaccine quality or safety cannot be trusted until the TWO STEPS OF CORRECTION occur. These STEPS will cause vaccines to be cleaned-up. Because vaccination can impact your children's health to such, a degree; it is idiotic that parents by law have no choice in the matter. Parents' must be free to be parents, having the unfettered liberty to decide if a vaccine is a too dangerous or too suspect to inject and thereby; protect children to the best of their ability. None negligent parents must not be dictated to by mandate or by other means to alter, manipulate or bastardize their perfectly healthy offspring's natural chemical environment; for to do otherwise, violates one's basic human Rights and vaccines' that do this, fail the SANITY TEST for vaccines.

The balance of life is directly dependent upon maintaining the chemical balance within and not jeopardizing it with unnatural to human biology chemicalization especially, injecting such, alien chemical or foreign molecular compounds directly into to the body and/or blood. Parents must have the vaccination conclusive control over whether a vaccination will or will not be administered. It is a basic and natural that parents have the protective ability to deny vaccinations. There is universal acquiescence in the premise that parents are supposed to protect their children from what is unwanted or from what has been determined not in their children's best interest. Parents are best situated to decide if a vaccine being injected into their children is in their children's best interest. Vaccine quality will drastically improve when parents can deny unwanted vaccines and/or vaccines are treated traditionally as consumer items just as all other health choices. In order, for children to be adequately safeguarded parents should be FREE to decide and in that freedom be first convinced by everything they see and read and hear about the safety of vaccines and consider the vaccine in the best interest of their children before the vaccine is allowed to be injected into their child's vital system and/or blood perfect chemistry! Let us above all things avoid entangling our children's vital chemistry with abnormal to the body chemicals and/or avoid unnatural to human biology and physiology chemicalization.

So, if we are supposed to be in control of what enters our bloodstreams why has a law that dictates mass coerced/forced vaccination not already been stricken down? Perhaps it is improper placed trust in the vaccination mandate machinery or ignorance about what is actually in vaccines or a matter of complacency to the takeover of our childrearing responsibility and authority. At the conception of vaccination mandates and Rights take over the People were under the gross misconception that vaccines were "absolutely safe"; this misconception or falsehood induced the enactment of the mandate. Correcting what is wrong is a matter of becoming acutely aware that our Rights have been subverted and that parental vital protection of children has been taken; obfuscated by lobbied for government vaccination mandates. If vaccines stood on their own merit or rather, if it becomes widely known that vaccines are unnatural to human biology chemicalizations; then it would become required to **GET THE CHEMICALS OUT and the TWO STEPS OF CORRECTION will do that**! If the truth were known about the adverse reactions at the time of the mandate law enactment there would have been no mandate. In order, to strike the erroneous law down which, was based in falsehood; we must declare it an improper and immoral law. **There must be liberty of health decision; freedom to refuse chemicalization injection!**

Everyone has the Right to make their own decisions even if it is the stupid decision to be vaccinated with a vaccine that has unnatural to human biology chemicals and certainly, we must be FREE to decide against such, sheer stupidity or not be a victim of it. Indeed, parents need to be endowed to do what is right for their children, to protect them from chemicalization; do what any reasonable or rational parent would do and that is absolutely stop, prevent and refuse a vaccine that is in anyway chemically disruptive and/or what parents deem as not in their children's best interest. The decision to vaccinate with only SAFER vaccines is obviously, the best choice! Children need to bask in their parent's purity of protection and have their purity of chemistry secured. Parents must be FREE to be parents and decide if a vaccine is safe enough to be injected. Our children need SAFER vaccines by the grace of parental consumerism and negligence law. The erroneous vaccination mandate law wrongfully inhibits, limits and at times negates parents' authority to protect children from unwanted chemicalization and/or vaccination. A rational life requires one not to expose your children to unnatural to the body chemicals! Law cannot expect parents to expunge from life their need to keep children from harm including but not limited to, vaccine chemicalization harm or unnatural chemicalization! Parents need to be fully enabled by law to reason out the vaccination debacle; to decide.

Unfortunately, we have been on the precipice of PERPANENTLY losing our most precious Right of Self –Determined Healthcare; let us bring to fruition the rescuing and/or resurrection of this most precious of human Rights. The rebirth of this freedom will allow parents to control their children's blood chemistry. The **CORRECTIVE TWO STEPS** are needed! The **STEPS OF CORRECTION** will restore the natural order, ending (**abolishing**) **vaccination slavery**. Vaccines desperately need parental administering control. **The chemicals that have been found in vaccines do not pass the parental stiff test and/or the vaccine SANITY TEST. Be FREE to protect YOUR children from unwanted chemical infiltrations and/or unwanted vaccine chemicalizations. Many of the chemicals in vaccines are anti-health agents which, plant the seeds of health destruction; spawning CHEMICALIZATION AUTISM. When you abnormalize your children's chemistry expect abnormality! Zealously protect your Right of Self-Determined Healthcare; it assures your children's good health and prevents Autism!**

What you or I believe has nothing to do with what is true or impacts what is true! The truth that vaccines do contain unnatural to human biology chemicals and react within the vaccine injected children victims, is an indisputable fact. People vehemently oppose that vaccines contain such, chemicals and that its enforcement by mandate is seen as an overreaching and very unrepublican move to concentrate this power with central government over the people. The vaccination program is in self-induced shambles, people finally are refusing to vaccinate their children upon learning and understanding what chemicals are in vaccines and what the possible consequences are for injecting their tiny babies with it. VACCINE CHEMICALIZATION HIJACKS YOUR BABIES GOOD HEALTH; CRASHING IT! You would not knowing fly a plane with a hijacker on it that had an agenda that alters the planes natural or proper destination so, it is perfectly understandable for parents to not want to inject vaccine unnatural to human biology chemicalization that has its own foreign or alien to the body chemical reactive agenda, property or propensity! To intentionally fly in a plane knowing there is a hijacker onboard or to inject your children knowing there are unnatural to human biology chemicals in the vaccine that hijack your children's normal healthy chemistry; crashing it, would be insane.

A vaccine fails the vaccine safety, SANITY TEST if the parents determines it has too many unnatural to the human biology chemicals and/or chemicals that are unsafe to inject! One would not allow a robber into one's home; do not let unnatural to the body chemicals into your children's vital chemistry, for it can rob them of their health. These chemicals react, upsetting the normal reactions needed for health, it can spawn health uncertainty, abnormality and/or CHEMICALIZATION AUTISM! If it is false (and it is not) that vaccine chemicalization is the leading cause of Autism, it is of zero importance however, if it is true (and it is) it is the universe to all the victims who were vaccinated! For parents' it is the darkest moment when they realize they have unwittingly subjected their child to unnatural to human biology chemicalization thus, causing chemicalization Autism.

Those responsible for our children's vaccine supply being safe and not becoming chemically destructive have failed despicably. Our government has been taken over to the point that lobbyist have seen to it that children by vaccination mandate are enforced or made to suffer unnatural to the body chemicalization. CHEMICALIZATION AUTISM results by the total irresponsible fact that vaccines contain unnatural to human biology chemicals and/or chemicals for sheer profit and not safety. Many of the chemicals of vaccines are undeniably unhealthy! Without question, parents must never be removed from their rightful position of assuring children's safety or protecting children from chemicalization. Constitutionally and by supreme natural law we are FREE to decide what is best for our own children and protect them from a conceived of vaccination harm. Nobody but you should control YOUR children's health destiny despite the insidious plans of Drug Companies or its governmental puppets. The general population of parents have not been found guilty of child neglect or found to have lack of capacity to make the vaccination decision and so, there must be no mandate! For preventative vaccination healthcare of perfectly healthy children there is no doubt that parents must rule the delivery decision! By basic human Right parents must control the vaccination decision and there must be no health wrecking ball chemicals in vaccines; parents require SAFER vaccines for children!

AN INDIVIDUAL IS NOT FREE IF THAT INDIVIDUAL IS VACCINATED AGAINST THEIR WILL OR IS COERCED, COMMANDED OR MASTERED OVER; MADE TO SUBMIT ONE'S CHILDREN FOR VACCINATION OR IS UNDER THE THREAT OF HAVING ONE'S CHILDREN TAKEN BY CHILD SERVICES, TO BE INJECTED. THERE IS NO FREEDOM IF YOU DO NOT CONTROL YOUR OR YOUR CHILDREN'S BODY OR BLOOD CHEMISTRY.

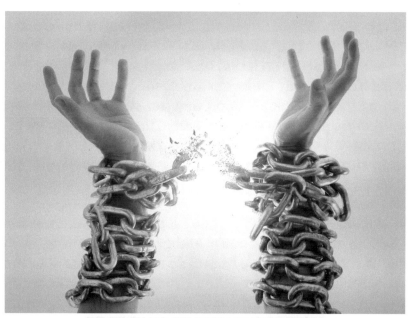

BE FREE TO REJECT INJECTIONS!

We are **FREE** to protect our children on all levels, in all situations; parents must be **FREE** to protect against unwanted vaccine chemicalization! Do protect your child's vital chemistry by assuring their food your child eats is has all the needed chemicals for health and not any unnatural to the body chemicals that interfere or distort or alter the needed chemical reactions of health. Do protect your child's vital chemistry by assuring their vaccines **DO NOT HAVE ANY UNNATURAL TO BODY CHEMICALS** that interfere or distort or alter the needed chemical reactions of health. Do not allow **CHEMICALIZATION AUTISM!** You would not settle for not knowing what chemicals are in the food your children consume; do not settle for not knowing what chemicals are in the vaccines that are being contemplated for injection into the vital systems of your children. Coerced/forced vaccinations take unmitigated control of an individual's free spirit of decision, enslaving the individual, breaking the individuals will making the individual submit their body to be exposed to unwanted vaccinations. Enslaved people have no realistic freedom of choice; they are made to receive unwanted injections. Mandated vaccinations are an unlawful imprisonment of mind and body; causing all vaccination determination freedom to be lost. We must not be enslaved to undergo chemicalization and **IF WE CHOOSE TO BE VACCINATED, WE MUST BE UNSCATHED FOR HAVING IT!**

Ancient rulers were denied and certainly our civilized modern government must be denied from taking away our **RIGHTS, WHICH INHERE IN HER OR HIS PERSON AS A HUMAN BEING. VACCINATION INDEPENDENCE** or being in control of your vaccination destiny is a Right which inheres in her or his person as a human being. Self-governing one's healthcare and being enabled to protect one's children from unwanted injections is harmonious and basic to being human. **The vaccination delivery industry with its life taking arrogance leaves no room for parents to protect their children from unwanted suspect vaccinations that parents have deemed too dangerous to inject. Parents have a fundamental Right, to deny an unwanted vaccination and/or CHEMICALIZATION, for themselves and for their children!** The mandated enforced vaccination law is analogous to a kidnapping law that dictates children can be taken and subjected to skin piecing by injection and injected with chemicals that are not inherent or natural to the body; do not let your children be **kidnapped for unwanted injection!** As greatly as one can appreciate or admire government at its attempt to secure the People's health, one can consider mandated vaccination a total blunder and absolute regulation madness. American people will have to beat down the overreaching of government, to be **FREE** once again!

Parents who know from experience of what occurs to children after being intoxicated by injection with vaccine chemicalization of unnatural to human biology chemicals – know better than anyone, what their children are up against in dealing with its alien chemicalization aftermath. Parents should not be enforced by a mandated vaccination law or face undue pressure to send their children through the MINEFIELD OF VACCINATIONS. If parents think a vaccination is in their child's best health interest then that parent will give their informed consent and vice versa, if a parent concludes that a vaccination is not in their child's best health interest, they will give their informed DENIAL and the child must not be made or induced to suffer an unwanted vaccination. Vaccination compliance depends on trust. TRUST in vaccination is cultured through informed consent/DENIAL whereas; no true informed consent/DENIAL doctrine applied and/or the ability to deny an unwanted vaccination is a TRUST BUSTER. We must achieve **vaccination independence** to establish **healthcare liberty** and **needed trust** in vaccinations. A **voluntary vaccination program is required** in order, to bolster **SAFER** vaccines and achieve vaccination compliance. In addition, parents must be enabled to directly litigate against vaccine producers if children are injured by vaccination. Knowing that producers of vaccines can be held liable builds trust; vaccine producers will do the right thing if they can get hurt in the wallet. **They must be adjudicated into submission; adjudicated into adhering to safe chemical content.**

Moreover, when a parent has been convinced enough that a vaccine is safe to inject or that the benefit of the vaccination outweighs the risks associated with receiving the vaccination then logically, that parent is entitled to give their true informed consent and thereby, grant permission for their child to be vaccinated. On the other hand, when a parent has not been adequately convinced that a vaccine is safe to inject or that the risk associated with receiving the vaccination outweigh the benefit of receiving the vaccination then that parent must be entitled to not give their informed consent and rather, give their informed DENIAL and thereby, refuse the unwanted vaccination; THE CHILD SHALL NOT AND MUST NOT BE VACCINATED. VACCINATION INDEPENDENCE IS CONSISTENT WITH OUR RIGHTS, OUR CONSTITUTION AND THE PROPER PROTECTION OF OUR CHILDREN!

Parents must never be convicted or even accused of child neglect merely because in their act of protecting their child they determine that a vaccination is not in their child's best interest and/or that vaccination places their child at risk. Parents in their good faith attempt to care for and protect their child to the best of their ability must not be deterred from

doing so and/or accomplishing what they think is best and right for their child. The intimate and very private responsibility of making healthcare decisions for children, including the vaccination decision must not be severed or diminished. The People must be secure in their most basic of freedoms; caring for their children and in accordance with this liberty be absolutely enabled and/or entitled to deny an unwanted vaccine from being injected into their children's delicate and susceptible bloodstreams. Parental protection of children must reign supreme; parents must always be empowered to best protect children!

Parents must not remain helpless, having no prevention and/or refusal of vaccine chemicalizations. It is tantamount to parenting that parents can protect their children from the expected and unexpected vaccination side effects and/or prevent their children from being vaccinated. Vaccine quality and/or safety is completely dependent upon parents being FREE to refuse what they determine an unsatisfactory vaccine and in addition, being completely FREE to litigate against vaccine producers when its vaccines are accused of injuring. Parents need to be enabled to do everything that they think possible to prevent their children from being afflicted with Autism. Every mother and father are responsible for their children! By natural law, natural order, instinct and/or GOD GIVEN RIGHT parents are FREE to protect their children from conceived of danger and this includes conceived of vaccination danger. No matter how slight the danger or how great; parents' have absolute authority to save their child from it. Children's safety is parents' number one priority; PARENTS MUST BE FREE TO STOP VACCINE CHEMICALIZATIONS. The elementary principle of health for our children's well-being requires our children to have all the natural chemical elements of health and safeguard against unnatural to human biology chemicalization therefore, do see to it you vaccinate only with SAFER vaccines! In order, to grow into the important parts of oneself you must be chemically perfected; not made imperfect or compromised by chemicalization of the chemicals still found in vaccines.

Children's safety must become the number one priority and removing the alien, UNNATURAL to the body chemicals from vaccines is consistent with this essential principle. The TWO STEPS are the sure way to make Vaccine Producers disengage from using anti-health chemicals in vaccines. Parents are the champions of their children's FREEDOM FROM CHEMICALIZATION! Enable parents to refuse unwanted vaccine injections and children's safety is best served and the natural order is restored. Hold negligent manufacturers of harmful chemically laced vaccines accountable and/or liable and children's health is secured. Pro-choice vaccinations, vaccination independence, a voluntary vaccination program and a vaccination system that is based upon informed consent/DENIAL are the stimuli needed to clean-up vaccines; GET THE CHEMICALS OUT. Government, must inform not misinform, lead and not mislead, the public; government, must inform the public that vaccines contain unnatural to human biology chemicals and lead the cause against such, chemicalization, no longer be used as a pawn of Big Pharma.

The words of this book need to be said, the truth be told that the mandated vaccination law is a taking of children from their parts rightful authority and protection; it asks parents to abandon their children and/or children's need to be protected from unwanted unnatural to human biology chemicalization and/or unwanted medical intervention. Do not trust that the big business industry of vaccinations is doing what is in your children's best interest;

make sure you protect your children's chemical integrity, do not abandon your children! A law is unjust and not law at all, if it enforces vaccination against parental will and/or injects doses of unnatural to human biology chemicals.

Deciding on what healthcare to accept or deny is an aspect of parenthood and/or personhood whereby you take possession of yourself. Making your own healthcare decisions and/or being in control of your body are part of your substantive essence and must not be infringed upon. Man has a Right to ownership and/or control of his own life. Every individual and parent for their children has a natural Right; enabling one to freely determine their health destiny. Therefore, it is primary to parenting that no vaccine injection should enter a child without the child's parent's informed consent. What is needed is an unequivocal victory for both parents and children, for fundamental liberty to not suffer unwanted chemicalization specifically, unwanted vaccine chemicalization! The mandated vaccination law fails because it requires that parents compromise their children's vital chemistry and breach parents' life contract to protect their children from what parents deem unsafe injections. Do not be made to compromise your children's natural chemistry, do suffer your children with unsafe vaccines; inject only SAFER vaccines that do not harbor the present unnatural to human biology chemical content! Law needs to support parenting and perfect parenting, not pull the rug out from it!

The erroneous vaccination mandate laws neutralize or negate parenting and/or parental protection of children from unwanted vaccine chemicalization. Before, you remain unaware or be complacent about giving up your natural Rights or allow yourself to be rendered an impotent parent by the defenestration of your inalienable Right to Self – Govern what will or will not be injected into your or your child's bloodstream; please consider taking control of what is rightfully yours to control! Do not acquiesce in the unlawful taking, of decision control of your body and mind, do not lose the protection of your children; prevent unwanted vaccine chemical injections. Do not give up your natural Rights that secure your parental innate caring of your children. Do not let the vaccination mega-profiting industry turn you and your family into mere herds of mass vaccination sheep people; do not submit to vaccination SLAVERY. Be in command of whether a vaccine will or will not be injected into you or your children. ABOLISH VACCINATION SLAVERY and vaccines become SAFER! Even if vaccines had no unnatural to human biology chemicals and were "absolutely safe", vaccination should still be a parental decision the unfortunate facts, are that vaccines do contain unsafe, unnatural to human biology chemicals and are definitely not "absolutely safe" but rather, are absolutely unsafe requires that parents have the decision control.

Please, grasp the fundamental understanding of chemistry that in order, to obtain the needed reactions or products from reactions you must have the required chemicals of the reaction and not have unnatural to the reaction chemicals present. Therefore, unnatural to the biology chemicals is not what parents want their children to be exposed to and especially, not injected with. This is a quest to end the CHEMICAL DOPING OF CHILDREN'S BRAIN CELLS. This is not an anti–vaccination agenda; it is a pro – SAFER vaccine agenda! The mission is to secure children in parental protection and thereby, cause SAFER vaccines that will not chemically compromise children. We need to establish a vaccination program that is legitimate, moral and ethical. The goal is not to afflict our children with unnatural chemicalization from vaccines; it requires a vaccination delivery system that is based upon the golden rule of true informed consent and informed DENIAL. The vaccination recipient or the parent of the child recipient must first determine if the vaccination is safe to inject and obtaining one's true informed consent must occur in order, to allow the vaccination. **The chemicals in vaccines will make or break children! We need SAFER vaccines in order, to make vaccinating our children a rational choice! Keep children's chemistry near perfect and health is almost definite in fact, Autism cannot be spawned! WE THE PEOPLE, must be FREE to doge the unnatural to human biology and physiology VACCINE CHEMICALIZATION BULLET and thereby, protect our children!**

In order, to secure the health for children we must assure a sustainable chemistry for health and the injection of unnatural to human biology chemicals does not do that. It is insane that we our children's internal chemistry stability up to anyone other than parents; government is not at all on top of the subject matter and is too commonly made a poppet of the lobbyists of the pharmaceutical/DRUG/VACCINE industry. Any vaccine that is mandated or is enforced against parental will fails the VACCINE SANITY TEST. Never ASSume a vaccine is chemically safe! The number one protector of children, the controlling supreme authority, must be children's parents by law, and the laws that we promulgate must strictly adhere to this. Parents must be FREE to keep their children from being chemically compromised; this is the way to best secure children's optimum health!

You cannot minimize the negative impact of injecting unnatural to human biology chemicals into tiny babies; it is a denaturing chemicalization that is like playing chemical Russian roulette with a loaded vaccine syringe needle. Why any competent and caring parent would want such, chemicals raging through their children's blood and/or systems is beyond me! It is an utter catastrophe of health for too many innocent children and the concept of vaccinating for health becomes an illusion. The vaccination decision has core impact upon the health and future of your children; it must only be decided by you, the children's parents. Vaccinations must only be considered legal and ethical if parents decide for it, by giving their unadulterated, TRUE INFORMED CONSENT; when parents give no consent or an INFORMED DENIAL to vaccination it must be respected, honored and NOT questioned. The doctor can properly recommend a vaccine however, the good doctor must not overpower parental decision not to vaccinate. Parents MUST maintain their legal capacity over their children's vaccination decision! Vaccination must fall in line with all other healthcare delivery; by requiring the obtainment of parents' true, unadulterated, non-coerced informed consent. Vaccination must be voluntary just as; all other medical intervention is based! It is in the best interest of children to have vaccination decided upon by their parents. Vaccine safety is strongly escalated by parental scrutiny of vaccine content and the liberty to refuse unwanted vaccine CHEMICALIZATION. Certain chemicals found in vaccines are considered poisons or harmful by experts and more importantly, by parents! It is more than disturbing for parents to learn only after a child is vaccinated, about the abnormal to the body chemicals. BE SAFE, NOT SORRY, KNOW WHAT CHEMICALS ARE IN THE VACCINE!

We live in an age of take drugs for this and every that, with an ever-expanding vaccination program; it is wise to have more caution in this ever-increasing cornucopia of pharmaceutical agenda. Too often the medical or drug company, so called experts, do not get it right and many lives are negatively impacted and/or people are induced to have worse problems than the treatment was for. It is not possible that vaccine producers put unnatural to human biology chemicals in vaccines non-volitionally or without knowledge that it would cause abnormal chemical reactions and/or abnormality in all those injected. The list of problems or signs and symptoms related to taking any drug CHEMICALS reveal just how susceptible health is when you are chemically compromised. The blunder of injecting babies with vaccines that are tainted with or vessels for unnatural to the body chemicalization is becoming self-evident. It is over-shadowing all other medical mishaps or tragedies such, the calamity of when doctors thought it healthy to drink radioactive water or when Heroine was routinely prescribed for dry throats, menstrual cramps and for babies who cried too long. In fact, Heroin was developed for a drug and was once an actual brand name claimed by a drug company. Cocaine was widely recommended and even the great minded Sigmund Freud stated, "For humans the toxic dose (of cocaine) is very high, and there seems to be no lethal dose"; wow, was he wrong. History tells us that pharmaceutical chemicals can cause health problems and can even kill. The ignorant recommending of unsafe vaccines that contain unnatural to human biology chemicals is not only scientific malarkey but rather, is the main cause in fact, of the Autism epidemic! The imperfection of a tiny baby's, small infant's or quickly growing child's chemistry should never be taken lightly. The present use of unsafe vaccines need to be recognized as health a destructive chemicalization that can spawn Autism. Demand SAFER vaccines!

The vaccination mandates render you devoid of healthcare choice, it handcuffs parents, imprisoning them to vaccinate children with unnatural to human biology chemicals that are in the vaccines; even if parents deem it unhealthy for children. Parents who stand tall and refuse to subject their children to such, chemicalization are wrongfully being persecuted. Under the erroneous vaccination mandate law parents are erroneously accused of child neglect for protecting their children from chemicalization harm and/or merely because they have refused vaccination. Despite the facts, that the vaccine contains unnatural to human biology chemicals and that parents have deemed the vaccine too dangerous to inject parents are burdened or often accused of child negligence. Being vaccinated with non-safer vaccines has its risks and its abnormal to the body chemical reactions. Parents must be empowered to decide if those risks are worth being vaccinated. Children can remain perfectly healthy by not being vaccinated and/or risk a natural exposure and obtain superior permanent resistance to childhood diseases. Mandated vaccination fails the vaccine **SANITY TEST** by it being insane not to be enabled to refuse it! The upper teeth to reversing the Autism epidemic is the allowing of parents to be their children's guardians, allow parents to be parents by perfecting and/or restoring parental supreme authority to the vaccination decision. The lower teeth to resolving the epidemic is to hold vaccine manufacturers accountable and liable for the utilization of any unnatural to human biology chemicals in its vaccines; making it cost prohibitive to utilize such, chemicalization. These two steps are the **TWO STEPS OF CORRECTION; the full measure needed for SAFER vaccines**!

Be aware, that natural exposure to childhood diseases may cause some health problems but will allow for lifetime immunity and mature or build one's immune system response. There is a lot that goes into making what is the best decision for children however, it is only parents that almost always have children's best interest at heart. Children are perfected in their parents love and caring; children's health or chemistry must be secure by their parents and the Those unnatural to human biology chemicals must react within. Once a child is exposed to vaccine chemicalization, once the chemicals of vaccines are internalized the chances of optimum health has been vastly diminished and the chemically compromised child is more susceptible to Autism. For the sake of your children's welfare you need the liberty to decide the vaccination question. Any improper questioning and/or challenging of a parent's private vaccination determination must be considered legally imprudent. Parents authority over the healthcare decisions for their children must be considered omnipotent unless; there is overwhelming strong evidence of child neglect and not mere naked fact that the vaccination was refused. Parents must not stand accused of not having their children's best interest if they decide not to vaccinate. Parents must not be accused of child neglect for not vaccinating their children if the parents deem the vaccine too dangerous to inject or the vaccine has unnatural to human biology chemicals in it. In the unlikely event there are other grounds indicating negligence for not vaccinating then the parents accused of negligence must first have a court of law with a jury of one's peers to determine if the parents are or are not negligent in order, to enforce a vaccination. Generally, parental health care decisions for their children must be considered in children's best interest.

Evidence presented must denote that parents substantially breached or substantially went outside their protective parental authority and that the reasonable prudent person similarly, situated; would not have decided to refuse the vaccination. If a vaccine has anti-health chemicals and/or **unnatural to the body chemicals; the parents are exonerated**. In order, for a vaccine to be enforced the parents would have to be found negligent **by a jury of their peers**; the jury must use the reasonable prudent person standard in the Court's determination. The jury would factually determine whether the parent's refusing of the vaccination rose to the level of being negligent; it assumes it a non-negligent refusal of vaccination or a parental protection. The court must **legally assume vaccination refusal is a legally sanctioned parental protection and non-negligent**; evidence otherwise and/or **the burden of proof of negligence is on the Accusers** and must be clear and convincing evidence. **The Accusers have the burden of proof; NOT THE PARENTS.**

When a mosquito stings/bites you with its needle like proboscis it causes one's immune system to jump into action similarly, as vaccination can do thus, one of the reasons for my first book about vaccination being entitled, "Sting of the Medical Mosquito". In that book I postulated how ridiculous it would be if there was a crazy law that enforced your children to undergo multiple mosquito attacks, that prevented parents from protecting their children from such, enforcement of immune response. It is even more outrageous that parents are enforced to suffer their children with multiple injections of vaccines especially since, the vaccines possess unnatural to human biology chemicals. It is an insane mandate and any vaccine under the coercive tactics of enforcement of suffering the medical "**STING**" of vaccination with its comparatively huge needle (proboscis) fails the vaccine **SANITY TEST**. Having your children taken from you because you did not agree to vaccinate or merely refused to vaccinate because you found out what chemicals are in vaccines is off the scale of injustice; it is just, insane. To enforce vaccinate against parents will cases should be made difficult to bring to court and be based upon the reasonable prudent person standard. The potential vaccine recipient's determination to accept or deny vaccination must be liberally based. We must prevent a medical dictatorship scenario from ever occurring and never allow mass enforced vaccination and/or vaccination slavery. **Parents must not be placed in fear of litigation or being accused of child negligence for their good faith parental protection refusal of vaccination. Your children must be yours to care for and protect! Many are calling for an independent investigation of how and why many of the unnatural to human biology chemicals are in vaccines. BE WISE, DO NOT CHEMICALIZE! The elements, compounds, molecules atoms and/or chemicals that are inside you or flow through your blood and into your cells DICTATE IF YOU ARE HEALTHY OR HAVE AUTISM. Your child's health is subordinate to the chemistry within your child so, KEEP IT NORMAL!**

Purposely or knowingly injecting children with abnormal to the body, unnatural to human biology chemicalization is negligence in the first degree; a child abuse mal-act! It is a tragic mistake to expose your offspring to unnatural to human biology chemicalization and it is the most horrific of decisions to inject such, chemicals into babies. Recognize that we all have a God given or natural ability to defecate and urinate out these bad chemicals that we ingest however, what is injected bypasses our natural elimination of these terrible for health chemicals and thereby, it infiltrates babies' brain cells. Chemicals all have a character, a propensity or tendency to react in certain ways. Vaccines are a combination, a concoction of chemicals that once injected into the blood of children will cause reactions; many of these reactions cause signs, symptoms and are so adverse that optimum health is no longer possible but rather, health degeneration results. Autism is mainly chemically induced, and the risk of Autism depends upon the extent of the unnatural vaccine chemicalization and if the baby, infant or child has already been chemically compromised. Once you are injected with a vaccine chemicalization you own those chemicals, and/or those chemicals own you; dictating biochemical reactions within. We must have every gear in place for SAFER vaccines; the TWO STEPS OF CORRECTION!

Proper chemistry is more important to health than vaccinating with vaccine's that are chemically compromise an individual. The kind of benefit or help you obtain from having a normal non-adulterated by unnatural to human biology vaccine chemicalization, is far more important to health than what you might obtain from injecting unnatural to human biology chemicalization. Individuals, contemplating vaccination, will rightfully deny or accept vaccines predicated upon if they are convinced of the vaccine's safety and how their health interest will be best served. **There must be fundamental freedom to make the choice** between keeping the chemistry of one's child completely devoid of unnatural to human biology chemicals found in (UNSAFE) vaccines; **it is much wiser to keep one's chemistry natural, pure and not compromised. Whether or not a vaccination should occur should be based upon their merit and not because we are ENSLAVED to submit to them. Parents must not be made to submit or suffer a child for vaccination if they deem its CHEMICALS TOO DANGEROUS OR NOT IN THEIR CHILD'S BEST INTEREST; this liberty will generate a breed of vaccines that are SAFER vaccines and make vaccination a much more rational choice instead, of a mal-act of child abuse! Consumers' of vaccinations are desirous that vaccines do not contain suspect unhealthy chemicals. Vaccine producers are not and will not be optimally or minimally concerned that vaccines are safe as parents require if, the law mandates that children must be vaccinated and/or if parents cannot realistically refuse to have their children vaccinated and if vaccine producers remain impervious to negligence lawsuits.**

To secure our Rights and SAFER vaccines all or any and **every chemical in a vaccine proposed for inoculation must be revealed, made abundantly clear, obvious, and shall be construed conjunctively or disjunctively as necessary to make an educated, legal informed decision by patients or parents for their children's healthcare. In this reasonable requirement to make known the chemical content of vaccines must be included; the terms "and" and "or" shall be construed to include the word "all," and "all" shall be construed to include the word "any." "Each" includes the word "every" and "every" includes the word "each." The complete and total disclosure of vaccine chemicals is needed for TRUE UNADILTERATED OR UNCOERCED INFORMED CONSENT as, must be required by law!**

The mandate of vaccinations improperly negates sacrosanct parental authority and responsibility of children. Until parents can legally refuse unwanted vaccinations and until vaccine producers can be held liable for the injuries that vaccines cause; vaccines will be produced with profiting as the primary directive and not our children's safety. Vaccines must be considered SUSPECT under mandate. Vaccination needs to be based upon liberty of decision and freedom to pose negligence lawsuits when vaccines are accused of causing injury; these are safety generating requirements. The more safety for our children the better! These reasonable and traditional requirements will induce and assure that vaccines will be produced with utmost safety as the number one priority. Informed consent/DENIAL will protect the potential vaccination recipient. Allowing one to refuse unwanted vaccination prompt vaccines to be produced to the reasonable satisfaction of parents for safety. It should be considered negligent to put certain chemicals in vaccines or turn a blind eye to what chemicals are in vaccines and the circumstances children are being vaccinated under. Never ASSume that the vaccine dosage pointed at your child for injection does not contain harmful chemicals; make sure it does not for your child's sake!

Those who ignore the will of parents and the physics of chemicals can overly pontificate or bloviate as much they want about the need to vaccinate however, they cannot argue against achieving SAFER vaccines for our children's welfare. In addition, if vaccines are produced according to parental safety guidelines the vaccine industry will be benefited because they will gain the trust of vaccination consumers. As they are prompted to produce the parental satisfaction level of vaccines and parents are fully informed about what the vaccine contents are then and only then can parents make an intelligent vaccination decision. In addition, when a vaccination recipient is convinced that the vaccine is safe for injection and gives their true informed consent, they assume the known risks that they were informed about thereby, granting the vaccine company a PROPER legal liability protection, limited to the risks that the vaccination recipient was informed about and gave true informed consent to. Vaccine producers will be less likely litigated against and there will be more voluntary vaccination compliance if there is prompting to produce SAFER, not laced harmful vaccines. Satisfying these basic healthcare requirements will render vaccines no longer suspect or untrustworthy.

Satisfying the rational safety concerns of potential vaccination recipients can be assuredly achieved through the enforcing of the basic healthcare requirement of informed consent prior to vaccination. An individual's decisive self-determined health care control and/or control over one's very own bloodstream must never be abducted, ignored, overpowered or not respected but rather, given omnipotent controlling authority. Parents need to understand that unnatural to human biology chemicals are invasive specie chemicals that can disrupt the normal reactions of the body and cause renegade abnormal reactions. Parents should protect their children from such, chemicalization by being in control of their vaccinations. The amount of the inherent conflict of interest is sickening in that vaccines companies lobby incessantly to have vaccination mandated and gain exponentially for its mandate and that former heads of the FDA that are supposed to police the pharmaceutical industry become heads of the pharmaceutical industry after their tenure at the FDA. Do not think you can trust the powers that be to do the right thing or secure your child's welfare above all when such, gross conflict exists! The list of problems from vaccines keeps growing. The human protein GcMAF (globulin component macrophage activating factor) is suspected of being destroyed by vaccines. GcMAF helps fight cancer. GcMAF activates macrophages that already exist inside of the human body, and in turn causes the body to destroy cancer cells. Dr. James Jeffery Bradstreet and his colleagues had discovered that the immune system is being compromised by nagalase, which they suspected was being introduced through vaccines. Nagalase interferes with an important protein in the body that kills cancer cells, explained Dr. Ted Broer in an interview on the Hagmann and Hagmann Report. So how insane is it that vaccines are mandated certainly, if it compromises GcMAF which, empower your body to heal itself than it must fail the vaccine **SANITY TEST**. **You want your children to have all the normal amount of GcMAF proteins otherwise; they will be abnormalized and fall prone or victim to cancer, unhealth and/or Autism!**

At this point I cannot verify that it is 100% true that vaccines are vessels of the biological interfering Nagalase or to what degree we are health dependent upon GcMAF to fight off cancer perhaps, it is to some degree a fiction and makes my book a work of fiction. I do know with certainty, that it is 100% fiction that vaccines are safe and do not have unnatural to human biology chemical content. Such, chemicals do cause abnormal to the body reactions. It is highly probable that Bradstreet's research is correct that harmful Nagalase has been found in vaccines. I have warned that since, vaccines are enforced upon us and infiltrate children many times; that vaccines are the highest sought-after target for terrorism against our nation's welfare. How easy would it be, to take a captured population that is mandated to be injected (vaccinated) and put chemicals in the form of elements, compounds or anti-health agents into the vaccines which, are enforced upon our very young? With what has already been found in vaccines perhaps, it has already happened and/or is happening. I should mention that there are very powerful people that want to eliminate the population problem and infiltrating vaccines that are mandated for all to be injected with is a viable threat. The fact is that there is nothing else, that children are exposed to internally than vaccination therefore, it should not baffle anyone that the Autism epidemic is mainly caused by injecting our entire population of babies with such, chemicalization. Remember, abnormalize your chemistry and expect abnormality! These are revealing questions, can the Autistic' have as many children as, readily or normal as, those who do not have Autism, is Autism becoming genetic, will government disallow such, pregnancies? If there is a fiction it is to think injecting babies with chemicalization and having good health! Know the chemicals of injection! Health is dependent upon needed chemicals and not being infiltrated with unneeded chemicals!

What is a **SUSPECT** vaccine or vaccination? **A SUSPECT vaccine is any vaccine that is coerced or enforced or slated to be administered without first obtaining TRUE informed consent; cannot be refused. A vaccine that is SUSPECT is UNWORTHY of a potential vaccination recipient's TRUST. Suspect vaccinations are rightfully feared and treated with extreme distrust and utmost caution in considering these vaccines for vaccination. In addition, a vaccination is SUSPECT if the company that produced the vaccine cannot be traditionally and directly litigated against for negligently producing a vaccine that causes injury. Having Vaccine Producers customarily acutely conscious of safeguarding against potential actionable litigation over vaccine induced injuries instills greater quality control, SAFER vaccines and needed consumer TRUST. TRUST, in the vaccination that the consumer is considering for injection, is generated by knowing that the vaccine has been safeguarded TO PREVENT INJURY; because it is made with litigation prevention in mind.**

LET'S NOT BE FOOLISH ESPECIALLY, WHEN COMES TO OUR CHILDREN'S GOOD HEALTH; WE MUST ASSURE THEIR WELLNESS BY MAKING ABSOLUTE SURE THAT IF A VACCINE IS GOING TO BE INJECTED INTO THEIR HEALTH GENERATING BLOOD THAT IT IS DEVOID OF UNNATURAL AND/OR HARMFUL CHEMICALS! Parents wanting the unbridled controlling authority of protection over the health of their children and/or decisive control of whether vaccinations will or will not be given is very understandable, highly reasonable and in perfect realm of the natural order. Healthcare tradition and ethics hold that parents must always give their informed consent for their child to receive any kind of health care. A parent's consent is required prior to the delivery of all health care. Crisis care, cancer care, heart care and dental, podiatry or non-invasive chiropractic care all require parental consent; there is no valid reason why vaccinations do not require parental consent. You are in LALA land, standing on unstable fiction ground if you think that injecting alien, unnatural to the body vaccine chemicals into tiny babies, small infants and very young children will only cause good reactions; its infiltration into normal blood and/or body chemistry **will cause unhealthy reactions**. Some of the chemicals that have been found in vaccines such as, but not limited to, aluminum or mercury are the hammer and everything else is the nail when it comes to biological reaction or interaction.

Secretin (SCT) a hormone and its receptor (SCTR) are widely expressed in different brain regions, where they exert multiple cellular functions including neurotransmission, gene expression regulation, neurogenesis, and neural protection. It has been found that the level of SCT and SCTR are low in those with Autism. This is just the tip of the iceberg of malfunction that occurs from infiltrating babies with vaccines that have unnatural to human biology chemicals. Always remember, the Law of Chemistry apply to when such, abnormal to the body, alien to your physiology chemicals become part of the biochemical reactions within the body. The body cannot produce the needed hormone secretin and renegade abnormal to the body reactions and/or production is initiated and it all plays a role in the spawning of abnormality such as, Autism. So, the good news is that for those who have Autism SCT can help offset this aspect of the Autism spectrum disorder; the bad news is that unsafe vaccines continue to cause abnormality. Be wise, only consider **SAFER** vaccines for the highly sensitive biosystem of your children! Please, consider fighting for the health of children before they get Autism by considering vaccinating with only SAFER vaccines and not wait until your child is diagnosed with Autism and then fighting it. There are thousand of unnatural to human biology chemicals that we are being exposed to from the environment, some more toxic than others such as, PCB, arsenic, lead and solvents however, make no mistake, it is the injected unnatural to human biology chemicals that are the main cause of Autism. Yes, living near a toxic land fill increases your chances of Autism because of related chemicalization but make no mistake, it is the multiple vaccine chemicalizations that quickly penetrate brain cells, doping, inflaming and malfunctioning it that is the main etiology of Autism.

One could erroneously motion or postulate that vaccines do not cause harm or do not harm enough to merit parents being FREE TO DENY OR REFUSE it however, in order, to maintain the natural order, render vaccine's SAFER, secure the well-being of children, not trample upon the fundamental human Right to self-direct or self-determine healthcare and not violate the sacrosanct and supreme Right of parenting; we must put an end to the perversion of mandated injections of vaccine chemicalizations and thereby, ABOLISH VACCINATION ENSLAVEMENT. Parents' must be FREE to protect their children and preventative healthcare should never be mandated especially, in perpetuity. Vaccines are far from perfected in fact,

they have become tainted with chemicals for profit. **Many chemicals in vaccines have anti-health propensity. Unnatural to the body chemicals in vaccines have its deleterious effect, negatively impacting one's homeostasis and/or ability to remain healthy. Those elements and/or unnatural to the body chemicals can go into criticality and cause abnormal to human biology and physiology reaction after reaction; a critical mass chemicalization syndrome that spawn Autism. Vaccinating with non-SAFER vaccines are chemicalizations of the blood and it is these chemicalization that are the real cause for major alarm; have extreme caution and proper concern! THE "SANITY TEST" IS A MOST WISE PRECAUTION TO HELP PROTECT CHILDREN. MANDATED VACCINATION IS MANDATED MASS CHILD ABUSE BY CHEMICALIZATION. END THE AUTISM EPIDEMIC; GET THE BAD CHEMICALS OUT OF VACCINES WITH THE TWO STEPS OF CORRECTION!**

THE MISSION IS CLEANER VACCINES; cleaner vaccines are SAFER vaccines and that means our children are SAFER! Parents are no fools that give their children protection by keeping their children from being violated with unnatural to the body chemicalization. The first thing you need to do to prevent Autism is to realize that mandated vaccine chemicalization of unnatural to the body chemicals is the main cause in fact, of the Autism epidemic. We are NOT in a state of emergency requiring vaccination mandate whereas, we are in a state of emergency to prevent chemicalization by injection; an emergency to prevent Autism. We have been living under a false permanent state of emergency that mandated vaccination is required. There is no epidemic and therefore, no emergency that might require a vaccination mandate; there is now only the resultant Autism epidemic formulated by the erroneous vaccination mandate of unclean chemicalization. Certainly, non-emergency preventative medical intervention is among the first expected kinds of care that must always require parent's opinion, final decision and **TRUE INFORMED CONSENT**. **Accordingly, all children's healthcare decisions are strictly and routinely within the purview of parents. Parents must be consulted with and give their informed consent for all non-emergency care delivery; it is universally accepted that it is in the best health interest of the children.** Do not give your children Tylenol or any other unnatural to the body chemicalization when your children receive a vaccine unnatural chemicalization; chemicals react together, and the wave and method of introduction plays a role. In fact, there was a study that taking Tylenol at the same time as vaccination **increases your chances of Autism 20 times**; it is often unwise fighting fire with fire or chemical with chemical.

Without exception; vaccination must be a parental decision and not a government one. **Parents are free to defer the healthcare decision to the doctor if they so desire; they must not be enforced to.** Mandated vaccination is an enigma to what is proper, moral and traditional in healthcare. Vaccination **SLAVERY** is most egregious and illative to the patient Right of self-determined healthcare and to the parental natural Right and instinctive need to decide what is best for children. Mandated vaccination is chemicalization **CHILD ABUSE**. The controlling authority to deny or accept vaccinations must not be decided or enforced by government that has a comparatively very distant relationship with our children. Improper government or unethical doctors who dare ignore the patient's self-determined healthcare Right or a Parents Right to refuse a vaccination need to stand down and relinquish their overwhelming control and/or domination over us. The resurrection of parental control over their children's healthcare decisions and/or the authority to refuse vaccinations is essential to the welfare of children and to basic freedom. Parents, regarding their children have an extra – sensory perception of what is best. **Parents have this**

enlarged perception that is truly caring whereas, government merely have a narrow slit of perception which is comparatively meager and unsympathetic. Parents can make their own choices about whether to accept or refuse vaccination!

Some out of ignorance or hysteria would have you believe that the more vaccines your children are injected with the higher their IQ or health will be; do not be taken in by such, misconception instead, recognize that your children are **SAFER** if only vaccinated with cleaner vaccines (**SAFER** vaccines). **To infiltrate your baby's body with unnatural to human biology chemicals from vaccine injected chemicalization can cause brain inflammation and/or malfunction as, the brain cells are doped with such, alien to the body chemicalization.** There are many who have an honest fear factor about the consequences of vaccine chemicalization and are terrorized by its enforcement; one should not be enforced to submit to unwanted injections! Vaccine producers do not have our children's best interest and neither does vaccine industry's governmental puppet politicians, whom together, keep vaccinations mandated and enforce such, unhealthy chemicalization into your baby. They have no empathy for children who do not want to be vaccinated or fear the vaccination needle or think harm will come to them from the chemicalization. Law must not circumvent the protection of parents in order, to assure vaccination compliance! **Actual documented injuries occur from vaccination; no FREE person should be subject to medical marshal law or be enslaved to vaccinate. Children and parents must not be mentally traumatized by being enforced to submit for unwanted vaccinations. Unclean, vaccine chemicalization attack the blood brain barrier, inducing abnormal cellular brain chemistry, inflaming brain tissue; a distortion of brain function. Vaccines' need to be made to pass the rational "SANITY TEST". It is vastly important for parents who strive to keep their child's chemistry healthy to know the truth and to speak the truth once they know it about vaccines; know the chemical formulations of vaccines!**

By now you have a clear understanding, a crystal-clear understanding that if you imperfect or compromise your baby's vital biochemistry with unnatural to human biology chemicals it will create, cause or spawn abnormality and Autism is among one of the abnormalities. It is imperative and of monumental importance to protect your children from being injected with such, chemicalization. Now you know the Law of Chemistry applies to when all the chemicals in vaccines are injected into your children's normally sensitive systems. No one should command you to compromise your children's chemistry and/or welfare; control the vaccination decision. Only consider vaccinating with SAFER vaccines which, are cleaner! Always ask, does the vaccine pass the vaccine SANITY TEST? If not, DEMAND A SAFER vaccine and always DEMAND to protect your offspring! Do not trust or think that vaccine manufacturers have the integrity that is needed to secure the welfare of your children's chemical integrity; just look at the chemicals that have been found in vaccines, that remain in vaccines and that imperfect and compromise children!

Mandated vaccinations divest parents of their protection of their children. More and more vaccinations are demanded to be given, while parents are rendered helpless, with no ability to protect their children from unwanted vaccinations. Parents need to be enabled to litigate against the vaccine company that made the harmful vaccine that caused injury. Parents must oversee, be in charge, of the vaccination decision! Vaccines need to be cleaned up! It is imperative to the welfare of children that parents control their healthcare destiny and that

we act to **GET THE CHEMICALS OUT** of what is injected into their delicate bloodstreams. **Positive change has got to come and come soon; we must prompt the removal of alien, unnatural to the body chemicals from vaccines to stop the Autism epidemic and to regain confidence in the vaccination program. Presently vaccines are toxic, produce all kinds of health degeneration, are mutagen possibly leading to DNA alterations and are the leading cause of Autism; yet this spew of harms are being injected into children. The chemical content of vaccines is very revealing; their chemicals have a power, a formidable force that devastates health on a mass AUTISM scale.**

People long to chart their own destiny and certainly, control what healthcare will or will not be accepted. When you are injured by anyone's negligence you traditionally are FREE to litigate against and seek monetary recompense. Improperly, directed government, induced by the vaccine industry and/or their lobbyists, continue to inappropriately, direct that OUR TAX DOLLARS pay for injuries caused by vaccine producer's negligence and/or vaccine induced injuries and not making the actual negligent causer of the injury pay. Vaccine producers must be made to pay for their negligence otherwise, vaccine producers have no down side to producing unsafe, chemically dangerous vaccines. Vaccine companies do not have to pay a cent if their vaccines cause injury because **OUR TAX DOLLARS** wrongly, pay. There is unconscionable profiteering guaranteed because our children are **ENSLAVED** to be vaccinated; a vaccine industry induced vaccination mandate assures it. **The vaccine industry has covered all angels to assure their profiteering. Optimum health is not preserved, and human Rights are violated by vaccination mandates**.

Moreover, in an act of unacceptable governing, vaccine industry government puppets have instituted an **unheard-of total liability shield for vaccine producers; a legal protection for vaccine manufacturers in the likely event its vaccines cause injury**. Just think about it, there are so many lawsuits over claimed injuries that the vaccine industry sought an unethical and anti-safety for our children, total liability shield, by hijacking our government that is supposed to protect the people; not corporate profiteering, Big Pharma. These unfit and proscribed governmental enactments were not initiated because the general population wanted them or because the People are protected by them but rather, for the self-serving assurance of vaccine mega-profiting. **The People do not want or need a vaccination mandate or want vaccine companies to be impervious to rightful and needed lawsuits. Not applying negligence lawsuits to vaccines is ludicrous, promotes unsafe vaccines and make any vaccine under it automatically fail the vaccine SANITY TEST. The liability shield only serves vaccine producers at the detriment of children's safety. These wrongful enactments only benefit the government ordained vaccination monopoly (Big Pharma); not the People.**

As a healer, I rid people of what is considered harmful or in disharmony with life and health and naturally parents want to prevent the same for the sake of their children. Parents long to safeguard their children from unnatural to the body chemicalization and must be **FREE** to do so! Our government that is supposed to serve the people has become an **instrument of Big Pharma**. **It is a catastrophic misjudgment to inject unnatural to human biology chemicals into our baby's blood!** Do not succumb to the egomania or lack of understanding and carelessness of the profiteering vaccine mongers that seek to subject your children to such, bad chemicalization! if you do vaccinate, only use **SAFER** vaccines; it equals **SAFER** children! The foundation of health rests upon the normal life-giving chemicals; not upon unsafe vaccines! Parents' do not sit when it comes to vaccination, stand up with conviction for what is in your children's best interest; protect them from injections of unhealthy vaccine chemicalizations! We live in an age of unnatural to the body chemicalization and because of it we are on the brink of reaching the tipping point of over chemicalization; it is imperative to children's well-being that they are not c0mpromised by injecting any degree of unnatural to human biology chemicalization. Chemicalization by injection is the worst form of chemicalization and leading cause of Autism!

There are over **13,000** medical/pharmaceutical lobbyists, a staggering, **over influential** amount that have manipulated our government to enact egregious, flawed, bad laws that strictly serve the vaccine industry. **This unprecedented number of lobbyists creates a sphere of influence that creates a monopoly, which assures the success of their self-centered profiteering agenda; even though the agenda does not coincide with the People's best interest or the People's wants or that the results violate personal Rights and/or the supreme law of the land, the Constitution.** The excessive amount of pro-vaccination mandate words whispered into the ears of politicians by this mass of lobbyists is really a roar that drowns out the voices of reason and safety. Vast amounts of money contributions given to law makers by the chemical industry and/or pharmaceutical industry **create unethical patronage and an intolerable bias that assures profiteering from a guaranteed enforced vaccination monopoly; a vaccination mandate at the Peoples health detriment.** This collusion results in promulgation of mal-law. The **mandated vaccination enslavement law** is one such law; it keeps our population of children exposed to vaccine **CHEMICALIZATION** thereby, assuring profiteering. There is a very sense or smell of corruption in how certain chemicals or what is called "chemicals for profit not safety" are in vaccines or how certain money-making drugs can have been approved and/or to stay on the market despite causing problems or its long history of problems. It is widely known that many mental disorders and cancers are related to chemistry and/or chemical imbalance; it should not be baffling that Autism and/or learning disorder is from chemicalization. Unbeknown to most people GMO milk from modified camels is being used for its protein for drug making by pharmaceutical companies. Do become aware of what goes into drugs and vaccines!

In January 2011, FDA requested that manufacturers discontinue marketing high-dose versions of acetaminophen (Tylenol) —defined as doses higher than 325 mg—due the drug causing severe liver failure in some patients. Once again, the action of the FDA comes way to late ad once again it is revealed that a pharmaceutical chemical concoction or drug that is commonly taken causes abnormality and even death. Finally, three years after the warning, the FDA banned this life taking drug chemical concoction. When will the FDA warn about unnatural to human biology chemicals in vaccines and how inept will it be before a ban is in place. The FDA is not in charge of your children; **YOU ARE IN CHARGE** and **YOU** need to **protect** them from such, chemicalization. Most people consider Tylenol (acetaminophen) a benign pain reliever that's safe enough to give to their kids. That's not only a misconception it is a danger that parents were either blind to see or induced into. Acetaminophen is behind more than 100,000 calls to poison control centers annually; 50,000 emergency room visits, 2,600 hospitalizations; and more than 450 deaths from liver failure. Acetaminophen may increase one's likelihood for asthma, hearing loss (especially in men under 50 years), and infertility. The drug and/or dosage was allowed on the market, passed all kinds of tests and yet it destroys health and at times life. Whenever you internalize unnatural to human biology chemicals expect abnormality. The pharmaceutical industry and its puppet FDA have time and time again violated the trust we have foolishly given them; do not let your children fall victim to vaccine unnatural to human biology chemicalization! Make sure your child's chemistry is not so, compromised; choose only SAFER vaccines. Know what is true from false in order, to properly protect your children; do your own research! Let my words be your words in your mission to protect your children from being violated by chemicals!

No power should be enabled to enforce parents to render their children's blood impure! There is a danger about not knowing what is going on around you. Tiny babies, small infants and immature children can be in eminent danger if parents are not informed about **ALL THE CHEMICALS IN VACCINES** and/or if any unnatural to human biology chemicals are in vaccines. Parents for their children's well-being need to be acutely aware of the danger of any vaccine or prescribed drug. Besides, liver damage from Tylenol; children under age one who've taken it appear to have an increased incidence of asthma and other allergic symptoms later in childhood. Acetaminophen severely depletes glutathione levels not only in the liver, but logically in other tissues. It is linked with causing asthma. Now, think and think again, about how many children were recommended Tylenol contemporaneously with suffering a vaccine unnatural to the body chemicalization! How many children could have been healthy but for such, chemicalization? The madness does not stop, so, many children who show signs and symptoms after vaccination are given more drug chemicalization to combat the results of the vaccine chemicalization and thereby, logically increasing an Autism outcome. On August 1, 2013, the FDA reported that acetaminophen is associated with severe and sometimes fatal, skin reactions even at recommended dosages. Even if it is a rare occurrence, the risk is too drastic! Injected vaccine chemicalization is the unhealthiest; think before added to its chemicalization! Parents must be FREE to protect children from whatever, medical intervention want to unleash upon them! Always know what chemicals are being introduced; always think about the SANITY TEST! You would not allow someone in your home if you did not know their character or propensities and if you knew they had negative to your health and life propensity you would be a fool to allow their entrance; know the chemicals in vaccine, be aware of its propensities and do not be fooled or be a fool by allowing a non-SAFER vaccine to be injected into your normally highly sensitive children!

Big Pharma has tremendous over influence in America. There are drug chemicalizations unsafe that are banned in other countries but inexplicably, still are for sale in America. For your protection here are just some of these chemicalizations: Phentermine, Avandia, Actos, Soma and Barbiturates. Do you think the 13,000-drug lobbyist with big bags of money have something to do with allowing banned drugs on the American market and snuffing out anything said bad about vaccines or drug chemicalizations? There is obvious bias and incredulous mal law enactments. Eventually the consequential harms speak louder than any attempt to cover up the facts about mal drugs and/or vaccines. More and more approved drugs and/or vaccines will be found to be bad. Warning: Pediatricians are finally warning that Codeine is unsafe for children! Tobias, chief of anesthesiology and pain medicine for Nationwide Children's Hospital in Columbus, Ohio stated, "Doctors have learned that the way codeine is processed in the body is very dangerous for children and can result in death." Codeine can cause severely slowed breathing rates and may even cause children to stop breathing and die. It is just a matter of time until the truth be told about the harm that the chemicals of vaccines cause and that such, chemicals will be banned! A suppression of anything negative about vaccines is dangerous and not in the publics best interest for example, there has been some research findings that children that undergo MMR vaccine chemicalization have been found to have measles virus in their cerebral spinal fluid however, it was suppressed merely, because it was declared to controversial to put out into the public. If in fact, measles virus is in cerebral spinal fluid post vaccination then parents need to be privy to it!

Corporations should not have the same or greater Rights than People; its needs and/or governmental protections should never be as great as or greater than the People's! Profiteers of vaccinations have unconscionably been allowed to benefit at the People's expense. We must hold vaccine producers' feet to the fire of justice to attain adequate quality control in vaccine production and thereby, prompting **SAFER** vaccines There must no longer not be a wrongful liability shield, despite how much it lobbies for it or how much it contributes to political agendas. The full force of negligence law needs to be and must be equitably applied to vaccine companies! **The full spectrum, negative to health implication of injecting unnatural to human biology vaccine chemicals cannot be estimated or be overstated. We must hold vaccine producers liable for vaccine chemicalization induced injuries and/or AUTISM. Unnatural to the body chemicals are undeniably demonstrated to cause abnormality in fact; the universal and indisputable laws of chemistry prove it so, it is conclusive! There is a very high potential of mass health casualties in the event of mandated enforced vaccine injections of unnatural to human biology chemicalization into children. We need to adequately protect children from chemicalization; not corporate greed, by the TWO STEPS OF CORRECTION.**

The huge amount of pro-mandated vaccination lobbyists is eerily reminiscent of the corrupt political machinery of Tammany Hall started in 1786, based on patronage and political contribution. Perhaps the improper antics have not been rooted out but rather, merely well camouflaged. The mass of lobbyists attracts the political units, gathering votes to serve and assure continued mega-profiting from vaccinations despite, the fact, that mandating vaccination keep the door open for putting chemicals for increased profiting in vaccines and not for safety. Like the "Tweed Ring" cronies of old Tammany Hall dark political days, which controlled law making, so it is now with vaccine big business. Puppet politicians do the vaccine/chemical industry's bidding by mandating vaccine chemicalization and by granting immunity from lawsuits.

Mega-profiting greed has ruined vaccine safety by mandating vaccine chemicalization and by granting immunity from lawsuits. Drug companies pay more to lobbyists than for taxes; this indicates how upside-down their agenda is. How much safer would vaccine be if all that money was spent for safety? One can only imagine how much money they have contributed to politicians or their campaign parties; these so-called contributions are considered by many rational people to be for buying what they want. The powers that be have managed to wrongfully give corporations Rights just like people and they have manipulated the system so that they do not have to reveal how much money was given or what corporation gave it. Not having full disclosure and/or mandating that politicians must be fully required to disclose how much or what corporation paid the money is nothing less than a cover-up and creates a safe-haven for bribery to enact laws. They have deeply penetrated to suppress us and dominate us and keep us enslaved to be vaccinated. **We must be FREE to refuse the chemicalization of our children!**

Logic is rarely a big part of politics; it makes no sense to allow vaccines to have anti-health chemicals or grant vaccine producers a liability shield for when a vaccine causes injury. Politicians that cater to pharmaceutical profiteering instead of our children's safety should be condemned for it not commended; they are derelict in their duty to secure our children's welfare. For some politicians it is treason of the heart and for others it is weakness of the mind. For vaccinations there needs to be a single object of children's safety and parent's opinion must matter; vaccines must be made to pass the "**SANITY TEST**" for vaccinations. Politician's must not follow pharmaceutical lobbyists lead to assure profiteering from vaccination mandates but rather; **they must endeavor to enact law that secures vaccine safety, they must have unbridled commitment to render vaccines perfectly safe for parental approval. Not curtailing Vaccine Producers from using anti-health chemicals is the reckless endangerment of our children and has spawned an Autism epidemic. A "SANITY TEST" needs to regulate vaccinations! What began as a problem-solving mission, we now know; chemicalization causes AUTISM.**

No one other than yourself should have the POWER OF INJECTION over your very own body and blood! Nothing or no one should overpower a non-negligent parents vaccination decision for their legally immature offspring! The absolute power over us and political bias has allowed vaccines to become corrupted and tainted with unwanted biohazardous chemicals and has induced astronomical increases in the cost of vaccines and thereby, increased the already unconscionable mega-profiting. The improper power that has been wrongfully granted by the puppet government of the vaccine chemical industry or vaccine makers has allowed it to act as if they are above the law (no negligence law applied). **Why should parents not be FREE to protect their children, why must children suffer the consequences of vaccination mandate and/or why must parents be made to surrender or be enforced to submit their children to suffer unwanted chemicalization that is unnatural to human biology? People need not be subjected to such, chemicalization; people must be FREE to only vaccinate with what parents deem safe and/or SAFER vaccines. Take back control of your children! Know what chemicals are in vaccines and recognize that you are enslaved to submit your children for unwanted vaccine chemicalization. Once armed with the truth, DEMAND the TWO STEPS OF CORECTION! YOUR CHILDREN CAN BE FREE FROM CHEMICALIZATION AUTISM!**

Clearly, parents do not want their children injected with chemicals that are not indigenous to their body or not part of the intricate and complex biochemistry; no one wants their babies violated with chemicals that are controversial or not proven safe or can cause abnormal to the body reactions. Why is that that government insists otherwise? The answer is corporate greed and a hijacked law-making system that steps up to whatever is on the law-making plate that best serves big-money lobbyists beaconing calls or commands. Every time your children are injected with a vaccine chemicalization make sure it passes the **vaccine SANITY TEST**, be sure it is a **SAFER** vaccine. **Visit SAFER vaccines .org or .com to be sure!**

The mandate of vaccination is more about money than health! Money plays the major role in the erroneous mandating of vaccination. **If it were not so, profitable to mandate vaccination, it would not be mandated!** If unconscionable profiteering were not being made by vaccine companies and no money was being given to politicians or political parties to achieve a money-making monopoly for vaccine companies from a vaccination mandate; there would be no vaccination mandate. The chemical payload of vaccines and possible health problems demands vaccination be a matter of **freedom of choice**. If no money flowed from the 13,000 Drug lobbyists to the politicians or their political parties, to help assure their election; **MANDTED VACCINATION SLAVERY would end**. Children must not remain **enslaved** to be vaccinated by an **industry bent upon**

305

profiting from vaccination MANDATED SLAVERY. Vaccination mandate law is VACCINATION ENSLAVEMENT LAW! ABOLISH VACCINATION SLAVERY and vaccines will become SAFER vaccines! Under mandate, vaccines fail the SANITY TEST! Vaccination must be based upon freedom of decision to assure vaccine safety and stop personal Rights violation and end the negation of parental protection of their children!

The United States is often reluctant or procrastinates to recognize a true danger or admit there is a problem with vaccines. Japan properly acted to no longer recommend that all girls receive the Gardasil (HPV) shot after only several hundred injuries were reported. It is stupefying that in America that after more than 50,000 injuries were reported caused by Gardasil injections to the federal Vaccine Adverse Event Reporting, that the FDA failed to do anything to shut it down or protect us. The federal "vaccine court" after eight years, finally ruled that Merck's Gardasil shot caused the death of 22-year-old Christina Tarsell, the daughter of Emily Tarsell. Any vaccine that has unnatural to human biology chemicals is similarly situated and can be too dangerous to inject. It is insane to inject such vaccines into babies; protect your children from abnormal to the body, alien to the body, unnatural to human biology chemicalization! Dr. Dalbergue, a former pharmaceutical physician for Merck, stated in the April 2014 issue (no.66) of Principes de Sante (Health Principles): "I predict that Gardasil will become the greatest medical scandal of all times because at some point..., the evidence will add up to prove that this vaccine...has absolutely no effect on cervical cancer and that all the very many adverse effects which destroy lives and even kill, serve no other purpose than to generate profit for the manufacturers." YOU NEED TO PROTECT YOUR CHILDREN; no one else will do so, to your efficiency and effectiveness!

Children's safety must be made the priority. Government should not be so easily manipulated to enact special protection for vaccine companies at our children's health detriment. It is obvious that if a vaccine company cannot be hurt financially when their vaccines injure our children, the vaccine producer will be a lot less vigilant to produce vaccines that will not injure. The mere threat of litigation keeps manufacturers keenly concerned that its products be made safe. Government is not best serving and protecting us when it enacts laws that do the opposite of protecting our children's safety by enforcing unnatural to human biology vaccine chemicalization. The wrongful enactment of mandated **VACCINATION SLAVERY** in combination with the total **liability shield for Vaccine Producers** place our children in jeopardy and promotes runaway negligence with no reason to be produce vaccines with our children's safety as their first and utmost concern. The vaccine induced injured have grossly been disadvantaged and the **National Childhood Vaccine Injury Act of 1986 is the culprit**; it gives Vaccine Companies a shield against parent's rightful actionable cases and consequently places our children in grave danger. **Producers of vaccines need to be adjudicated into safety conformity and/or prompted to make SAFER vaccines; with no anti-health chemicals. WE MUST NOT BE ENSLAVED TO VACCINATE; WE MUST BE FREE TO REJECT OR ACCEPT INJECTIONS!**

Vaccination mandate means that informed consent is thrown out the window or reduced to ashes or is a moot point; this is counter to vaccine safety and violates patient' Rights. Informed consent/ **DENIA**L is the application of consumerism to vaccinations without it; vaccines that are objectionable and/or unsafe will be on the market and remain on the market even, if injuries are being reported. If you cannot refuse a vaccine, then vaccine content is prompted to be less safe. When it comes to our children's well-being, you want to know all the facts, before making an important healthcare decision like that of vaccination. Since, vaccination is a decision surrounding the very health of your child, the INFORMED consent doctrine requirements must be given to parents. The informed consent/**DENIAL** doctrine requires that you be given the needed information to make an educated decision about the vaccination and that the patient or parent for their child remain in control over the healthcare and/or body. It must be required that all the contents of vaccine be given (all of the chemicals utilized) and it be acutely pointed out if any unnatural to human biology chemicals are in the vaccine under consideration for injection.

The doctor, the vaccine manufacturer and its puppet government must not take for granted **a person's healthcare decision independence**; **THEY MUST ADHERE TO IT**! They all must heed the will of the patient! If the patient does not want to receive the proposed medical intervention and/or vaccine chemicalization it must be respected. All must tread carefully not to overly influence or coerce the patient into submitting to care. Healthcare and/or the medical intervention of vaccination must never be invoked by mentioning that it is the law that requires it. Law never should play a role in convincing a patient to receive vaccination! Healthcare must only be administered by giving the patient the pros and cons of the proposed care and then letting the patient decide to accept or deny the care. Threats of law, coercion and undue influence, have no place in moral or legitimate healthcare; no part in remonstrating with a patient to accept medical intervention. The benefit and risk of accepting or not accepting the medical intervention should be the only ethical and legal way to have a patient decide upon care and/or vaccination.

We must stop the insanity of unnatural to human biology chemicalization from all its sources. Over **42,000 Americans died** from opioid overdose in just 2016 alone. On April 6, 2018 News Media, reported that Drug industry companies are being sued for its alleged part in the opioid crisis by local municipalities or towns to hold them accountable for deceptive practices to get people to take opioids. It is disconcerting that such, extreme steps must be taken to have the pharmaceutical industry do the right thing or act in the publics best interest. Your children need to be in your capable hands; protected by nonother. Your parental fundamental Right to decide what is best for their child by controlling if a drug or vaccine is in your children's best interest must not be trampled upon and/or violated. What is injected must not be about making the most money!

Look at our children's diabetes crisis to see how the FDA does not protect us; it allows cereal makers to put as much sugar or addictive sugar and that is a main cause of the crisis. There is no accountability, no caring about the negative to health consequences to our children. The cereal industry was prompted to remove high sugar content from cereal because of parents' uproar about it however, led by profit not health the profit dictated otherwise, as it put the high sugar back in. This is not dissimilar to the vaccine industry that was prompted by parents' uproar to stop putting mercury derivative thimerosal in vaccines. Vaccine producers are free to put in other toxic chemicals at will and is still utilizing mercury in certain vaccines. Recognize that parents need to be more proactive in knowing what their children are being injected with and really need to have control of their children's health! Rely first and foremost upon yourself to protect your children from chemicalization! Never ASSume a vaccine is chemically safe!

The general population of parents have not committed a crime that allows for the taking of their Right to decide what is best for their children. **YOUR CHILD = YOUR DECISION!** Healthcare must strictly be based upon the patient's needs and must not be initiated without the patient's permission. **Doctors must not state that it is a law that your children must be vaccinated because it has nothing to do with patient need or the proper practice of healthcare and only serves to coerce patients to undergo a vaccination that they otherwise may not have submitted to. The law or mentioning that it is the law must not be used to convince parents to submit their children for vaccination especially, unwanted vaccine chemicalizations of unnatural to human biology chemicals.** It is not ethical for a doctor to threaten parents with the law, using the law to overcome the parent's decision not to vaccinate, for that would be coercing the vaccination. The doctor's place is not to recite the law but rather, to practice healthcare not law enforcement. Doctors must not coerce vaccination! Statements like, "The law requires your children to be vaccinated" or "you must vaccinate to get your kids into school" should not be allowed. Doctors need only remark upon what they think is clinically best for their patients and must always leave the decision to accept or deny the treatment for the patient. Parents for the sake of vaccine chemical safety and/or children's welfare must control.

Parents are constantly reporting that when they converse with doctors about their concerns of vaccinating their children and/or wanting to delay vaccination that doctors wrongfully arrest their health concerns and desires not to have their children vaccinated by **inappropriately stating** that "it is the law that the children must be vaccinated" **thereby, coercing** the parents into vaccinating their children against their will. The mentioning of law is no valid medical reason to be vaccinated and has no business being stated. In effect the erroneous vaccination mandate equates to the illegal and unethical practice of medicine by government and is the illegal practice of law by doctors. Once a parent of the child potential vaccination patient expresses their desire for there to be no vaccination; the good doctor can mildly remonstrate with the parent about the pros and CONS of vaccination however, the decision must always be the parents to make. The decision must not be overpowered by a doctor's rambunctious desire to vaccinate. **A good doctor must never use the law as an excuse and/or reason to vaccinate!**

No one has been incarcerated or fined for putting unnatural to human biology chemicals in vaccines in fact, it is only profitable to put such, chemicals for profit, in vaccines. The pharmaceutical industry needs to be sent a strong message, by making it pay a huge fine that is commensurate with the harm that these chemicals are causing our children and make it cost prohibitive for it to jeopardize our children's welfare with such, unnatural to human biology chemicalization. Parents therefore, must be **FREE** to litigate against the makers of vaccines and rightfully seek damage awards from the source of their children's injuries and burden our tax payer dollars. If we are to decide what is best for our children we must be **FREE** to stop, prevent or refuse a vaccine from being injected into our children when we are not convinced of its safety or want to refuse it because we have learned that it has unnatural to human biology chemicals, atoms, elements, molecules or compounds. No doctor, lawyer, vaccine producer or its puppet politician should dare tread upon parents sacrosanct caring for their children or parental decision to protect against a vaccine! Keep in mind, that some of the chemicals that have been found in vaccines were in land, that land could very well be cautioned as a toxic landfill or toxic dump. **SAFER VACCINES, THAT HAVE LESS OR NO UNNATURAL TO HUMAN BIOLOGY CHEMICALS IS ABSOLUTELY REQUIRED TO ASSURE REDUCTION OF THE EPIDEMIC OF CHEMICALIZATION AUTISM.**

Till the day that we can freely apply negligence law TO THOSE RESPONSIBLE FOR PUTTING UNNATURAL TO HUMAN BIOLOGY CHEMICALS IN VACCINES; OUR CHILDREN WILL CONTINUE TO BE PLAQUED WITH SUCH, HARMFUL CHEMICALIZATION. Negligence law which, is meant to protect us from negligent acts needs to be a weapon of justice against the pharmaceutical industry for when it makes vaccines not as safe as, possible for our children. Children's ultra-sensitive biochemistries are at risk when they are injected with unnatural to human biology chemicalization. Our Life, liberty and the Pursuit of happiness are severally compromised if we are not **FREE** to protect our children from unwanted vaccine chemicalization. **We must be FREE to litigate otherwise, our children will continue to suffer** what is in fact, a chemicalization the deforms their normal chemistry of health. Multiple injections of unnatural to the body vaccinations that are forever mandated and forever always increasing in number and chemicals are a detriment to health. How strong or how pure your internal chemistry is dependent upon what you inject into it and it is your concern, your jurisdiction and is only for you to control. What will they do next; decide what color underwear we can wear, what type of food we can eat, where we can live, what we can see, hear or learn or say? How many injections will you allow your children to endure before, you think it wise to investigate what exactly your children are being injected with and how it is impacting your children's organs, tissues and/or cells? Is the standard vaccine in your children's best health interest? Why not choose **SAFER** vaccines? Learn about what you need to learn about to prevent **CHEMICALIZATION AUTISM** contact **SAFERvaccines.COM and .ORG to find out how to help protect your family!**

There is a great inconsistency in those who put such, harmful chemicals in vaccines and recommend its injection of unnatural to human biology chemicalizations into children and yet claim they are doing good by mandating vaccination. Chemicalization Autism is mainly an iatrogenic disease since, doctors vaccinate with vaccines that have unnatural to human biology chemicals into perfectly healthy children and so many of those children end up Autistic. Iatrogenic disease is physician induced disease. Doctors take a vow, to do no harm to their patients however, when doctors inject vaccinations despite a patient's fear of needles, despite the fact, that there are harmful chemicals in vaccines and despite when the patient or parents tell the doctor that they are not convinced the vaccine is safe and do not want it injected; these doctors are breaking their sacred vow of doing no harm and break the golden rule that **the patient directs what care that they will accept or deny.** Vaccination law requires doctors to vaccinate, dictating healthcare without concern as to, whether doctors think the vaccinations are required or that the doctor may think it not in their patients' best health interest; the enforcing of doctors to vaccinate break their sacred vow and **make Autism an iatrogenic disease. The vaccine SANITY TEST, informed consent/DENIAL and holding producers of vaccines liable must control! Many are concluding it extremely negligent to utilize unnatural to human biology chemicals in vaccines and an act of chemicalization child abuse to knowingly inject such, vaccines.**

To hold that the People need **government** to make any of their healthcare decisions and/or the vaccination decisions is **unjustified paternalism and a premise of nanny and overreaching government. Moreover, to generally ASSume that people do not have the capacity to make the vaccination determination is an absurdity and that government is needed in to assure people are best protected is malarkey; foolishness. Parental health decisions are not the jurisdiction or purview of government. Enforcing puppet government commanded vaccination is not just selective nanny government or mere overreaching; it is healthcare** marshal law, it is the tyrannical forcing of vaccination and the dictatorial takeover of our basic parental jurisdiction. It is too draconian and is an unlawful enslavement of our children to be shackled by mandated vaccination or made to endure unwanted vaccine chemical injections and it places our children in harm's way. It is an improper government that treats people like its subjects or mere cattle, to be herded and branded with injections of vaccines. Let us end the making of our children to endure such, chemicalization; scaring them with injection and inducing CHEMICALIZATION AUTISM!

The People not only have the capacity to discern the vaccination question and/or determine if what is in the vaccine is too dangerous to inject; parents have the parental obligation to do so. **Parents need to be exhaustive in their efforts to know what chemicals are in vaccines and understand the ramifications of injecting any of the chemicals inherent in vaccines. It has become obvious that vaccine producers are not exhausting themselves and in fact, have minimum effort if any, in preventing the unnatural to human biology chemicalization of our children.** Parents need to be in ultimate authority of whether a vaccination merits injection and/or if the vaccine is or is NOT in their child's best health interest. The authority to determine if a vaccine will or will NOT be delivered is in the person contemplating having the treatment, the one most affected by receiving or not receiving the treatment. **Parents** are the most perfect vaccination decision makers; it is well established that parents make all healthcare decisions for their offspring especially, preventative healthcare decisions. **As for vaccinations; the only justified paternalism is the parental decisions of caring parents! For if parents cannot protect their children from chemicalization abuse it is a grave misjustice! It is heedless and reckless endangerment of children or willful blindness to have unnatural to human biology chemicals in vaccines. To mandate such, vaccines is CHILD ABUSE! There must be clear and conspicuous notice about any unnatural to human biology chemicals in vaccines. Parents should refuse what that they deem unsafe or dangerous.**

The enigma of having no vaccination self-control, no Right to determine whether it is or is not in one's best interest to receive or not receive a vaccination, no Right to deny a vaccination and no proper recourse if injured by a vaccination are unacceptable to FREE PEOPLE. We must establish vaccination decision liberty and no longer be subjects of the ENSLAVEMENT to be vaccinated. ABOLISH vaccination SLAVERY! Parents must be **FREE to be parents**; parents must control whether a vaccine is or is not injected. Man was not meant to control his fellow man's body or internal chemistry. Wayward puppet government should not control our children's vaccination decisions. Enforced vaccination is a form of tyranny; it is the taking control of one's internal being and welfare by vaccination coercion, medical enforced tyrannical injections. The infiltration by injection of vaccine unnatural to human biology chemicals is destabilizing to the normal biochemistry and/or welfare of children. Parents must not be enforced to submit children under vaccination mandate, that destabilize children's chemistry to any degree! Investigate, follow the trail of unnatural to human body chemicalization from vaccines to discover the true cause in fact, of **CHEMICALIZATION AUTISM** and the ongoing raging autism epidemic. Injecting such, chemicals into babies is like releasing the dogs of war upon the once, normal health generating chemistry, once released its hard to get them back; there will be negative to health consequences. **FREEDOM** requires that **WE THE PEOPLE** are not made subjects of internal chemicalizations and not face the repercussions of unwanted chemicalization!

Children and their parents are most impacted by the vaccination decision and/or live with the results of the vaccination decision therefore, must be endowed with the power of decision over vaccination. Government's illicit takeover of our children's healthcare destinies, in apparent perpetuity, is no longer to be tolerated; parents are recognizing that a taking of their children has occurred and that there is negative impact from injecting vaccine chemicalizations! Government is too far removed from the consequences of vaccination to have controlling authority of the decision of vaccination. To be commanded by law to inject vaccine particles or alien chemicals is an inappropriate governing and penetration of our inner recesses; **violating, our Right of Self– Determined Healthcare, Right to Control Ourselves and children and/or our Right to Be Left Alone.**

The law does not have jurisdiction or rather, authoritative control over vaccination! An individuals' body or health is strictly the jurisdiction and purview of the individual; only you legally can dictate over yourself or self-govern and/or self -determine your healthcare. The sacrosanct area of parental protection of their children is supreme. Government has no valid jurisdiction over personal healthcare decisions and this is particularly, true in matters of disease prevention for perfectly healthy children and/or when there is no actual aliment or imminent threat of disease or impending health harm. Government must not demand that we be injected with chemicals that are unwanted or are unnatural to the body.

Law must not cause people to jeopardize to any degree their welfare and/or internal chemical integrity. In the name of our welfare it is totally inconsistent to recommend vaccines for injection that have unnatural to human biology chemicals. Vaccine producers and its puppet government walk must match its talk, by assuring vaccines have no such, chemicals and not act untethered to safety by placing and/or allowing unnatural to human biology chemicals in vaccines. Do not be confused, merely because vaccinations are mandated does not mean parents do not have a higher obligation to assure their children's safety and welfare. Parents owe it to their children despite the fact, that it is or is not mandated to be injected; to determine whether the vaccine is safe or is in their children's best interest and/or has any chemical content that may jeopardize their children's welfare. First and foremost, parents are obligated to protect their offspring from abnormal to the body, unnatural to human biology chemicalization. It speaks volumes that vaccine producers would put chemicals like the mercury derivative thimerosal and aluminum the electric conductor in vaccines or that it had to be prompted to remove thimerosal from most of its vaccines and only after long-term public uproar and crying out to do so!

Just because a law is written does not mean that law is good, proper, just or will stand the test of time. Although, the mandated vaccination law did go through the mere appearance of traditional enactment procedures, being procedurally passed; this law must fall and/or be stricken because it is unjust, based upon the falsehood that vaccinations were "absolutely safe" and is the unlawful taking of parental jurisdiction. The mal law is too destructive to fundamental human Rights. The law cannot vest authority in government or doctors which, is greater than patients and/or those whom are receiving the vaccination or over parents of a child whom is receiving the vaccination. **Government's vaccination control encroaches upon parental jurisdiction and/or parental caring for and protection of children. A law is unjust if it enforces chemicalization; enslaving one to inject! The fact, that politicians mostly do what lie their pockets and that vaccine producers have over 13,000 money carrying lobbyists might just be why the enigma of** vaccines are still being mandated and despite that no epidemic crisis exists. When comes for calls to drain the swamp of government wrongdoers it really is an attempt to drain the ocean! Vaccines fail the **SANITY TEST** if based upon invalid governmental jurisdiction. Parents require to be enabled to do what they think is the right thing to do for their children. Parents being **FREE** to preserve their children's natural internal blood chemistry is what needs to be mandatory; not mandated chemicalizations!

The golden rule and tradition of informed consent/**DENIAL** is made a moot point under a vaccination mandate. The range of permissible authority normally found in a traditional healthcare delivery situation is so far exceeded that the vaccination mandate must be considered an act of extremism and an enigma; not at all proper! The vaccination mandate is in direct conflict with Self-Preservation, Self-Determined Healthcare, and/or your Right to Self-Govern over what will or will not enter your bloodstream. There is a lovely purity about parent's nurturing, caring and doing their best to decide if a vaccine is or is not in their children's best interest whereas, there is gross disharmony and distortion of what is normal in the egregious act of government dictating that children must be submitted to endure vaccine **CHEMICALIZATION. Parents must no longer be asked to sacrifice their children for unwanted chemicalizations or risk destabilization of children's ultra-sensitive, all-important, biochemistry. Let us, ABOLISH vaccination SLAVERY! Children need parent's protection and parents need to protect their children! Goodness is the noblest and strongest force in the world and parents have it for their children's best interest; the perversion of government superseding parents, ENDS NOW!**

No longer trust that you are in good or capable hands under the auspices of mandated vaccinations. No longer sleep on your parental Rights or live under threat that your children will be CHEMICALLY ABUSED by unwanted, deemed by you as, too dangerous to inject vaccine chemicalization. No longer be oppressed, browbeaten, overburdened and/or enslaved under an unjust and illogical mandated vaccination law. Parents have a supreme Right to control their children's vaccination destiny and it is extremely, wise to be concerned about exposing children with many of the chemicals often laced in vaccines. Parents must be allowed to refuse unwanted vaccine chemicals and/or deny vaccinations that parents have determined are not in their children's best health interest. It is just and equitable to be FREE to control your blood and/or body chemistry and/or health with liberty to refuse vaccination and has all the characteristics of what the natural order is. Let us establish Self-Determined healthcare as a basic freedom! In deciding upon vaccination always remember what a precious gift it is, the natural chemistry that springs health and your children's normal neurological development.

There is a false argument that we are so weak-minded or are incapable of caring for ourselves or our children that we need a law requiring everyone to be vaccinated and there is the erroneous and farfetched concept that we must have a law that commands vaccination because those unvaccinated somehow pose a threat to those vaccinated. Law must not **ASS**ume parents' incapable of discerning the vaccination question or not capable of knowing what is best for their children's welfare and parents are in no way negligent for refusing a vaccine that they have deemed unfit for injection or unsafe because of its chemical content. In addition, it is a ridiculous theory and a mal-reason to mandate vaccination based on the extremely thin or non-existent concept that the perfectly healthy unvaccinated somehow pose a threat to the vaccinated. The mandated vaccination law fails because it **ASS**umes the fiction that perfectly healthy children pose a threat because they are unvaccinated and will come down with a childhood disease. The mal-mandate also, ASSumes a further conjecture that these perfectly healthy that fall victim to childhood disease will get children that are vaccinated sick. This is a basis not to be vaccinated rather than vaccinated because it indicates that vaccines do not work and since, vaccines do work the mere conjecture is either so remote or is a total falsehood. Law must not enact vaccination mandates based upon that vaccines do not work. Mandated vaccination based upon mere conjecture after conjecture or **ASS**umption after **ASS**umption is not valid reasoning to base law upon; law must not be based upon mere conjecture. You cannot correctly postulate that vaccinations work or are worthy to administer if you contemplate that they do not work in the face of being exposed to someone that has the aliment which, it supposedly protects against. Perhaps with such, unrealistic, extraneous or false reasoning to mandate vaccination and/or if it is true that vaccines are not that effective we should reevaluate the need to be vaccinated with so many vaccines and not mandate it. **No vaccination mandates and consider only SAFER vaccines!**

To **ASS**ume vaccinations work and yet pose that the unvaccinated are a threat to the vaccinated is evidence of improper reasoning or that vaccines do not work. The fact is, the sick pose an equal threat whether they are sick and vaccinated or sick and unvaccinated and that if you are properly balanced with nutrition, rest and all the co=factors of health then you are much more resistant to childhood disease and if you do succumb to it you are not as devastated by it. If you go back far enough in history, it is revealed that drugs and chemists are one in the same. The drug/chemist wanted more to be able to sell its chemicalization product than help or cure people. There have been all kinds of ridiculous claims about drug chemical concoctions that really are just sales pitches and not at all true. The truth is that drugs are chemicalizations and that abnormal to the body, unnatural to human biology chemicals all negatively impact upon the normal health generating biochemistry. The fact, that vaccines have repeatedly been found to have an array of such, chemicals indicates how insane it is to inject such, chemicalization; we must demand **SAFER** vaccines to be injected with! There is also, the truth that if you have been vaccinated you have been chemically compromised thus, are less resilient in general to disease. Vaccinating children with non- **SAFER** vaccines creates a chemical anomaly, a rendering of one's biochemistry into an abnormal chemical reactive configuration. **Exposing children to unsafe vaccine chemical injections causes injuries, decreases resistance to disease and is the main etiology of Autism! The unvaccinated and those vaccinated with no toxins or less chemicals and/or SAFER vaccines; will be more healthy, robust and infrequently Autistic! For the aforementioned reasons it is insane to vaccinate perfectly healthy children with vaccines that fail the vaccine SANITY TEST and is child abuse by chemicalization to do so!**

Mandated vaccinations result in vaccination compliance coercion that is totally unacceptable in a born **FREE** America and has negative quality control impact; rendering vaccines chemically unsafe. The mandate is discriminatory in operation. Perfectly healthy children are singled out to not be allowed to enter school based on the discriminating fact that they merely have not proven that they are vaccination compliant. It is sheer speculation that a perfectly unvaccinated child will come down with a childhood disease merely on the basis that she is unvaccinated. It is false speculation that the unvaccinated have less resistance to childhood diseases in fact, it is probable that those children not vaccinated, who have not been exposed to vaccine chemicalization and/ or been chemically compromised are much more resilient and resistant to disease and/or health degeneration. Regulation that is discriminatory in its application or punishes those who are innocent or perfectly healthy and/or who are a non-threat to others is an act of improper law and is an immoral mal-law. "Non lex injusta non ex lex", is a legal axiom, which means that law not based upon justice is not law thus, the vaccination mandate is considered not a bonified legal law but rather, an injustice, a falsity.

One could just as well speculate that a vaccinated child could come down with a childhood disease since; vaccinations do not always work or wane over time. **The vaccinated and the unvaccinated both pose a speculative or fictional threat of getting disease. To disallow the unvaccinated from entering school is discriminatory. Disallowing school entrance coerces the unvaccinated into receiving unwanted vaccinations; it is meant to break the FREE will of individuals that do not want to be molested by vaccination or think vaccine chemicalization too dangerous. Vaccination law overpowers parenting and infringes Rights; it is an abomination. Parents must be FREE to prevent injected vaccine chemicalizations otherwise, our Rights are violated, and our children will continue to be placed in harm's way by the ongoing toxic and/or unwanted chemicals in vaccines. Vaccine's can be made to pass the SANITY TEST if parents are FREE to protect their children by being enabled to refuse an unwanted and/or chemically tainted vaccine!**

MASS vaccination of children, with all its UNNATURAL TO THE BODY CHEMICALS, renders our children MASSively, at risk of health degeneration. Vaccination of the masses is analogous to mass overuse of antibiotics; overtime it perpetuates evolutionary adaption of the pathogens, inducing the pathogens to become more resistant and superbug, virulent. Vaccines can injure your immune system or weaken it and if the vaccine has unnatural to human biology chemicals it causes abnormal reactions, renegade reactions and abnormality. One should be **FREE** to weigh out the pros and **CONS** of vaccination and certainly, be **FREE** to protect one's children from unwanted medical intervention and/or abnormal to the body chemicalization. By age 2 the average child has endured 3 courses of antibiotics and has received more vaccinations than their mother did by the time she entered high school; this exposure to harmful chemicals causes significant collateral damage. Vaccines can also injure as it stimulates an abrupt immune response; overburdening and/or stressing the immature immune systems of babies, infants and children. It strains the immature system; it is like pressing a 1000 lbs. when you can only press 100 lbs. without causing injury. Mass vaccinations will cause pathogens to adapt; for the pathogens to survive they must adapt to become a more formidable enemy. **Overuse of Antibiotics and mass vaccinations spawn more virulent super bugs that pose a much greater threat; this combines with the negatives of chemicalization, fueling man-made plaques such as, the AUTISM plaque. Keeping children's chemistries' pure or natural keeps one naturally healthy! Natural selection without mass vaccination will help prevent out of control pathogen genesis!**

The unvaccinated and/or parents who refuse to insult their babies' inborn immune system or imperfect their babies' chemistry with vaccine unnatural to human biology chemicalization should not be on the defensive or attacked for doing so. Repetitive contamination from multiple vaccinations destroy the natural healthy chemical balance. There is intelligent understanding that you stand a better chance at combating virulent bugs/pathogens by naturally building up and supporting one's immune system as compared to insulting one's

complicated and sensitive biochemistry with alien, unnatural to human biology chemicals found in vaccines.

Be aware: long-term mass antibiotic use and the onslaught of multiple vaccinations of all children has set the stage for future health disaster; it will someday spawn the production of super pathogens that will be much more virulent and/or devasting to all our welfare. To add insult to injury, at the same time this dependence upon antibiotics and vaccine after vaccine injections will cause human natural defenses against disease to become weakened and debilitated also, resulting in a not too distant future plaque of plagues. In addition, unnatural to human biology chemicalization is destroying our ability to be healthy or remain healthy and has major negative impact on our combating disease capability. Individuals must be FREE to determine if they want their children to bolster the immune system naturally or be so, dependent upon man-made intervention with all its risks inherent. Parents must be FREE to decide what is best for children's welfare. Live FREE to be healthy; have liberty to prevent the risks of unwanted vaccine chemical exposures! Abnormalize your chemistry and expect health abnormality!

What is occurring under the oppression of enforced vaccinations is a form of chemical warfare that is destructive to health. Our children are under siege; their bodies are pierced by needle and injected with anti-health chemicals. It is either chemical warfare based upon some miscalculation of the potential harm or more probably, a callous and wanton gross disregard for children's welfare in order, to make money. The purposeful endeavor to place profits before children's best interest must be forbidden; we must act to GET THE CHEMICALS OUT of vaccines and thereby, make the use of vaccines intelligent. Vaccine chemical exposure places children in undeniable jeopardy. Citizens need not submit for harmful chemicalizations under healthcare tyranny; there is ample reason for justified civil disobedience. Producers of vaccines have poorly looked after children's safety; they must never be solely entrusted again. Parents being FREE to refuse vaccines and parents being enabled to litigate against producers of vaccines, when a vaccine causes injury, are the only realistic way of assuring children's safety. Parents must be FREE to prevent chemical infiltration and safeguard their children's chemical stability. WE MUST ABOILSH VACCINATION SLAVERY AND END THE ENFORCED SUBMISSION TO VACCINE CHEMICALIZATION. THE "SANITY TEST" IS A NEEDED SAFETY PRECAUTION. SAFER vaccines pass the SANITY TEST; only consider vaccinating with SAFER vaccines.

The debate over vaccines causing a plethora of health problems will rage on but the Autism epidemic need not rage on. It is only a positive result that will come from prompting Vaccine Producers to make vaccines with less or no unnatural to the body chemicals. Keeping children's blood devoid from such, chemicalization can only be a positive. The level of illogicality of injecting alien to the body, unnatural to human biology chemicals is so off the scale that it must be considered insane and an act of child abuse. Children must not be exposed to the chemicals that have been found in vaccines or else, mal-formations will result and chemicalization Autism can be spawned. Autism must not be a vaccination away! It must no longer be a monumental problem for parents to refuse vaccine chemicals; it is proper parental jurisdiction and parental supreme authority for parents to do so, if parents deem a vaccine too dangerous to inject or not in their children's best interest. Parents must be the gate keepers of vaccination for the best interest of children and to assure vaccine are of quality that parents can rely on, depend upon and approve of. The insanity of a mandate must end to achieve SAFER vaccines.

Gain your RIGHTFUL control of whether a vaccination is to be given; decide if it is too dangerous to inject and/or if it contains unnatural to human biology chemicals that jeopardize your children's well-being. Make sure you protect your children by having unfettered control over vaccination delivery or refusal! For the sake of your children's welfare make sure the vaccine is clean; insist that it is a SAFER vaccine for you to consider! Having parents control the vaccination decision is a must to assure vaccine quality and/or children's safety. Many vaccines are dirty, having unnatural to the body chemicals and therefore, pose too far a great of risk. YOUR CHILD = YOUR DECISION! Children's depend upon you, as their parents, to protect them by safeguarding their internal chemistry. Demand the golden health safety rule of informed consent/DENIAL of vaccinations and thereby, control the vaccination situation or decision. Secure your children's chemical purity by protecting them from unwanted vaccine chemicalization. It is negligent to inject anti-health chemicals and/or dirty vaccines into children. Parents can have no peace injecting such, dirty vaccines; inject only SAFER vaccines. Most vaccines will continue to be dirty until the TWO STEPS OF CORRECTION and the VACCINE SANITY TEST assure children's vaccine content safe and thereby, BEST PROTECT CHILDREN!

In supervising your children's welfare be sure their needed, naturally perfected chemistry is not abnormally manipulated, bastardized or compromised. We do not live in a bubble and we do face all kinds of environmental hazards, pollution and sources of unnatural to human biology chemicals that are not good for us and cause degeneration to health however, always safeguard your children as best you can. Know that it is insanely bad for quickly growing immature children to be injected with any degree of abnormal to the body, unnatural to human biology chemicals. Injected chemicals pose the severest danger because it can quickly circulate in the blood and penetrate the brain. These chemicals, particulates, molecules or compounds have a foreign magnetic charge, alien character and a disruptive to biological reactive propensity. Injected unnatural to human biology chemicals come in contact or close reactive proximity with the inherent chemicals that are natural to the body, causing biochemical reactive disturbances. As, your children's parents you are empowered with the supreme authority for caring for and protecting your children; it is for you to see to it, their welfare is not jeopardized. It is your ultimate parental responsibility and jurisdiction to determine if a vaccine will or will not be administered and if the vaccine is a SAFER vaccine or one that is just too risky to inject!

A SAFE VACCINATION IS ONE THAT ADHERES TO THE TWO STEPS OF CORRECTION AND PASSES THE VACCINE SAFETY, SANITY TEST. It is highly recommended when you ponder the vaccination question that you consider vaccinating with SAFER vaccines and do your research and/or contact SAFERvaccines.org. Parents should hold their own court to decide if a vaccine is a SAFER vaccine that can rationally be consented to for injection. If the vaccine has not passed the vaccine SANITY TEST and is not under the TWO STEPS OF CORRECTION, it is suspect and/or too dangerous! Make no mistake, do not compromise your child's vital chemistry! Do contemplate vaccination but, only with SAFER vaccines, devoid of bad chemicalization; best protect your children! It is child abuse to purposely inject babies with unnatural to the biology chemicalizations! There can not be enough safety precaution for children from dirty chemicalizations! Just because mal-governing would place your children in chemicalization harm's way does not mean you have to allow for it; stand up for your parental Rights and protect your children! The fact that vaccines have unnatural to human biology chemicals dictates you to protect. Be acutely aware that unnatural to human biology chemicalization not only causes cancer, mental conditions but also, abnormality of all kinds including AUTISM.

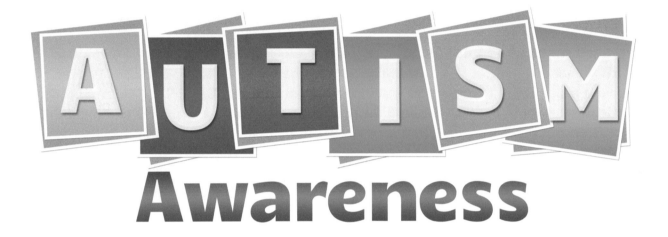

CHAPTER 11

THE SLIPPERY SLOPE OF MANDATED VACCINATIONS AND LOSS OF FREEDOM

Before we venture upon this chapter, let us make clear that people need to benefit from SAFER vaccines and not be chemically compromised by unsafe vaccines. People need to have a much more rational vaccination program that has SAFER vaccines that do not chemically compromise the vaccination recipient. Over time the power of consumerism determines if a product brings in adequate profit or does not remain on the market. The power of consumerism applied to vaccination, where people decide over time, by analysis or use of the vaccine if the product (vaccine) is worthy to inject, is or is not of benefit and is or is not safe enough for their children. Quality control over any product is almost completely dependent upon the consumer's experience with the product; manufacturers of the product must step up to the plate of consumer wants and dislikes and SAFETY concerns otherwise, the product fails. The quality control over vaccines has practically a non-existent consumerism application since, vaccination is mandated or enforced upon the people; not allowing vaccine recipients the power to say "yes" or "NO" to vaccination and/ or have the power of consumerism applied to vaccination. Vaccines do not have the proper tradition and safety feature of consumerism and therefore, vaccines have no requisite and basic quality control that assures vaccines are safe for use. Vaccinations need to be and must be dependent upon free enterprise and CONSUMERISM otherwise, our children's welfare is placed in jeopardy by vaccines not being consumer friendly and/or vaccines having chemicals for profit, not SAFETY. Mandated vaccination (no choice vaccination) is the enemy of consumerism and SAFETY!

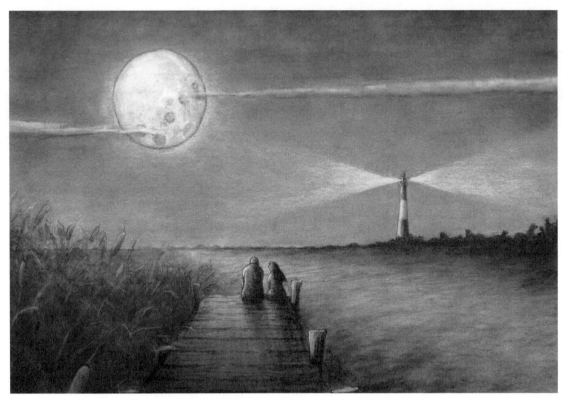

**The charity, SAFER Vaccines is your beacon of light to guide you
to safety. Visit the website SAFERvaccines.org to learn about what
chemicals are in vaccines and how to best protect your children.**

**The slippery slope of mandated vaccinations with its enforced LOSS OF OUR FREEDOM
can only be efficiently and effectively rectified by the implementation of THE TWO STEPS of
CORRECTION!** The slippery slope of vaccinations, better dubbed, ("the slimy slope of vaccinations")
is the tendency or rather, the inevitability, of more and more vaccines being mandated; rubber
stamped for **enforced injection SLAVERY**. Once one vaccine is commanded upon us, to be
injected, and **THE PEOPLE** acquiesce in this single occurrence, giving up their basic liberty to
decide what is best for one's children and/or their health; this will lead to more and more vaccines
mandated, more and more aggression to our Rights and/or freedom. History has shown this
degenerative spiraling of loss of liberty by the slippery slope of increased numbers of vaccine
chemicalizations being enforced upon us. In addition, the slippery/**slimy slope of vaccinations** will
lead to other forms of healthcare being mandated, with further loss of our precious liberty and/or
loss of control over ourselves. Mistakes in vaccine content happen all the time and we must not be
handcuffed to them however, the purposeful utilization of unnatural to human biology chemicals in
vaccines is not a mere mistake but rather, the knowing reckless endangerment of our children; we
must not be made subject to such, chemicalization. **The slippery slope has resulted in children
being made to suffer increased number of unwanted chemicalization that are not in our
children's best health interest.**

**Our freedom of health decisions is all placed in danger of being lost unless, we root out
vaccination mandates; the initial destructive stumbling blocks of healthcare liberty.** We
must correct this plaque upon our fundamental freedom of Self-determined healthcare and/or Self-
preservation by insisting that the State stay out of the affairs of parent/child vaccination decisions!

Always remember, if vaccines were not profitable they would not be mandated, and that the norm is for parents to decide what is best for their children in all healthcare matters especially, preventative healthcare. Vaccines' being mandated for injection is an enigma, a perversion of what is proper and is done more to assure profits than to assure health. This healthcare mandate perversion has established a slippery slope which, has allowed mandated vaccination to persist when there are no epidemics or an emergency and opened the doorway wide for more and more vaccination mandate oppressions. It is now profiteering which, is the main reason for this ongoing perversion of enforced injections of vaccine chemicalizations.

Big, overzealous government oversteps its power and/or jurisdiction when it mandates vaccination, and this is especially, true when it does it during non-emergency, non-epidemic times. Permanent governmentalization of healthcare should always be viewed as too extreme; it must never occur. Temporary government infringements upon healthcare freedom must be for a duration no longer than necessary and always be viewed as suspect; even if during an epidemic. A government that commands People for undue lengths of time or without controlling reason to undergo vaccine chemicalization injections is a nanny or tyrannical government and is not a government that serves the People or that of a **Free**-thinking society. Americans' respect and cherish individuality and/or personal healthcare decisions. We must be **FREE** to be ourselves, as unique individuals and not be made mere drones of government; commanded to be vaccinated. **Parents' need to be FREE to decide if a vaccine is or is not in their children's best interest!**

History has shown that if we allow one vaccination to be mandated and slip through the a newly formed crack of freedom that more and more vaccines will be and have been mandated; making the crack turn into a canyon or abyss of loss of liberty. One bad turn deserves another, one violation of Rights leads to another, one mandated medical intervention leads to another and yet another. One loss of liberty inevitably will sanction, make it easy and highly probable that more loss of liberty will follow. Mandated vaccination is the poster child of this loss of freedom and is the slippery slope for future liberty loss! Complacency in loss of control of vaccination healthcare has led to many vaccination mandates and has lead the way to the corruption that The People' can have their healthcare and health choices controlled. Puppet government, doing Drug company' bidding has caused Pandora's box of lost liberty to be opened. Healthcare freedom is being devastated because we have fell asleep at the wheel of our freedom; allowing mandated vaccination SLAVERY to take root, spawn and continue in apparent perpetuity.

Our acquiescence in the monopolization of the once free market place of healthcare and **wrongful loss of freedom of self-determined vaccinations has created a slippery slope** of **future mandated healthcare and loss of freedom**. The **un-American mandate** that we must all have health insurance is one such, extension. Our healthcare choices will now be limited to what lobbyists of the big pharmaceutical industry wants and dictates. The lobbyists will orchestrate our healthcare by manipulating puppet government to pass whatever law serves their self-centered needs. They will eliminate its competition by limiting our freedom of choice in healthcare and/or directing that only certain healthcare will be covered and/or mandated. For example, Obama-care will command that you buy insurance and the insurance will command that vaccinations are covered to assure mega-profiteering from it, at the same stroke of this loss of freedom pen, Drug company competition, such as natural healthcare modes or chiropractic, will not be covered thereby, eliminating the competition. **Freedom of choice in healthcare is being lost!** This is not only a loss of freedom to pick and choose healthcare and/or healthcare insurance plans; it is government's illegal practice of medicine without a license, in that by limiting our choices they dictate to doctors how to treat their patients. The free market place of healthcare is no more! In furtherance to this unfair and unjust elimination of competition there is agenda to regulate out of business competition such as, what is occurring with vitamins and supplements; soon, if this suppression continues you will not be enabled to be informed about the benefits of vitamins and it will even become very hard to obtain your needed vitamins because you will have to spend precious time and money to see a doctor to get a required vitamin medical prescription. Lobbyists see to it that corporate greed is served, and a monopoly spawned that is not in the public interest or welfare; the slope is slimy! Our children and healthcare choices are being strategically taken!

Just as I surmised in my first book, "STING OF THE MEDICAL MOSQUITTO", that since parents acquiesced in allowing all the mandated past and present vaccinations; that someday they surely, would perpetrate yet another loss of freedom upon us, by mandating the Flu shot upon our children; it is yet another stage of profiteering. The Flu shots for children are beginning to be mandated; spawned as an outgrowth of established mandated chemical injections, as part of the slippery/SLIMY slope of vaccinations. It is a big uncertainty, if any flu shot will be specific for the current Flu in fact; it would be a big FLUke. One thing is certain, the Flu shot will expose one to more harmful chemicals! How many chemical infiltrations does it take to tip the scale of children's internal chemistry from a health generating chemistry to an Autism degenerating chemistry? Do not let chemicalization Autism become your children's reality! With every unnatural to human biology CHEMICALIZATION, you are gambling with your children's very lives. Health and sickness are mainly dependent upon chemistry; to inject anti-health, UNNATURAL to the body chemicals is very devastating to health. WE THE PEOPLE MUST BE FREE TO REJECT INJECTIONS! Parents must not be subservient; they must be in charge. Vaccine producers and/or its puppet government are not fit to oversee or be in charge of children's vaccination destiny. Never forget or forgive vaccine companies for allowing certain chemicals to be in vaccines. Most parents would vote to abolish mandatory vaccination slavery! Members of the Association of American Physicians and Surgeons, all voted, at their 57th annual meeting, to END mandatory childhood vaccines but, even with this vote, no change has occurred. The TWO STEPS of CORRECTION are required to protect us.

"Mandatory flu shots for NYC kids", by Andy Soltis, page 6 of the December 12, 2013, New York Post, "The city will require some 150,000 young children who go to preschool or day care to get flu shots." What important changed that children now need flu shots? Nothing has changed except for increased greed to make even more money from vaccinations and perhaps parents further sleeping on their Rights to decide what if any vaccine will be or will not be injected. Children need less; not more exposure to toxic chemicals found in vaccines. The possibility of the Flu shot working is highly so, remote that to mandate it is crazy however, the slimy/slippery slope of mandated vaccinations is at work. Parents must not be made idle decision makers about the dangerous Flu shot or other vaccines. Parents must be FREE parents; with full authority to decide what is best!

It is either naive, foolish or reckless to utilize unnatural to human biology chemicals in vaccines. When the avalanche of health concerns and complaints about the chemicals

found in vaccines and the questions about if it is wise or in children's best interest to be subjected to so many vaccines or if it unjust to be mandated to inject; it fell on the deaf ears of the pharmaceutical companies. It carelessly refused to properly investigate it and callously remained deaf, dumb and blind. An attitude of total control over us remains among the vaccination warlords that will do anything it has to in order, to keep us chained to mandated vaccination so, Big Pharma can keep profiteering from it. The slimy slope of more and more mandated vaccination is a means to more profiteering.

Today, the factors of what promotes health and prevents disease are much better understood; it is more about bolstering one's natural immune system than depending upon vaccines that can disrupt, distort and destroy one's needed for health, perfected biochemistry with the unnatural to human biology chemicals that have been found in vaccines. Today, if children do naturally get the Flu, modern medicine and modern natural healthcare will almost always help assure a speedy and full recovery. Besides, naturally having childhood disease or the flu can build up your natural immune system response and make children even more resistant to all future health problems. Today, it is known that vaccines wane over time, do cause injury and can weaken one's immune system. The mandatory Flu shot mongers, wrongfully guess or ASSume that 20,000 out of 150,000 children will get the flu and have the audacity to further ASSume that the long-shot, Flu shot will prevent it. The Flu bug is always adapting, the vaccine is usually not specific for the specific Flu bug thus, is usually a total waste and you may not even encounter the Flu. Also, many fall sick after the Flu shot. With all this uncertainty, the only thing that is real and/or certain, is that you should be FREE NOT TO RISK a Flu shot or CHEMICALIZATION!

BEWARE: Flu shots are injections of chemicals; it exposes children's bloodstream to a wide variety of whatever, harmful, anti-health chemicals are in the vaccines. BEWARE: MOST FLU SHOTS AND MANY DRUGS HAVE MERCURY IN THEM. The fact, that Flu shots still have mercury after Big Pharma was told not to produce childhood vaccines with mercury strongly indicates the drug industry is bent on not doing the right thing and that to mandate of vaccinations is fraught with danger. Mercury is a known neurotoxin however, it gives vaccine producers bigger profits because it stops returns from spoilage or expiration date proximity! This tells parents that vaccine producers either do not care about the well-being of children, are willfully ignorant and/or are grossly negligent. The article also states, "To force someone to modify their children's body is very, very serious", in my opinion this is an understatement; it is outright affliction upon parental Rights and is vaccination ENSLAVEMENT! While the world is burning or rather, as our children are under siege of a CHEMICALIZATION Autism epidemic; Big Pharma keeps on distorting our children's chemistry with such, alien to the body, unnatural to human biology chemicalization. Children must not be injected with such, unsafe vaccines! End the slippery slope of mandated vaccinations and have a voluntary, SAFER vaccination system! Mandated vaccination eliminates freedom to decide what is best for your health and contemporaneously eliminates the safety brought about by consumerism refusal of it. Make no mistake, vaccines often have invasive species of chemicals that cause Autism!

This next statement supersedes and eliminates any statement in this book, "Vaccine producers or anyone that had or still has, to do with the fact, that unnatural to human biology chemicals have been in or still remain in vaccines are accused of negligence and/or the reckless endangerment of children and that a competent court might easily rule against the defendant and that certainly, **GOD** would find it a sin, to **KNOWINGLY** cause chemical disarray, disfigurement or disruption to the perfected natural chemistry which, is needed for optimum health. The slippery slope of mandated vaccinations has instigated and allowed the chemical downfall of vaccines. If one cannot refuse a mandated vaccination the tendency is to put whatever chemicals are needed in the vaccine to achieve the most profit despite the fact, the chemicals are unnatural to the body.

The slippery slope of freedom loss spawned by mandated vaccination will lead to government control of more and more of what **should remain our choices; ours to control**. Access to natural remedies, products that give the body what it needs to stay healthy or bounce back from sickness will become more difficult to obtain because it will be under siege in an evil effort by the Drug industry to put an end to competition. There will be a hijacking of our government, in an underhanded attempt to stamp out competition and free market. Our access to vitamins, minerals and herbal remedies will be under an unfair biased control; limiting our ability to buy natures' remedies. There will an attempt to regulate the natural remedy industry out of business and/or be so, severally limited in what natural remedies can claim it benefits that its competition against drug use will be negated. They will even try to make it that if vitamins claim to cure or help anything it will designated a drug and thereby, take over the free market competition.

ABOVE ALL: PEOPLE MUST BE FREE TO KNOW EXACTLY WHAT THEY CONTEMPLATE EATING AND THE LAW MUST SERVE THE PEOPLE IN THIS BY SEEING TO IT THAT FOOD IS ADEQUATELY LABLED TO INFORM THE PEOPLE TO EXACTLY WHAT IT IS THEY ARE ABOUT TO EAT! Protecting corporate profit must take a back seat to people knowing the truth about the food they are deciding to buy to eat. No one other than yourself should decide what you or your children are going to eat and food labeling must conform with the people being in absolute control over the decision as to what to eat. Although, it is not in the public's best interest, there will be lobbyists bent on the stealthily forced by ignorance purchases of GMO's; this same stealth of ignorance will also, be applied to irradiated foods. Their poor minded, immoral plan will be to have these GMO and irradiated foods be put on the market for unsuspecting ignorant to the fact, buyers to purchase it. By not disclosing that the food is GMO or irradiated consumer's will be duped into thinking the products are not GMO or irradiated; The important information that food is genetically engineered and/or is irradiated must not be hidden or cloaked as if, it is not. The ill intent is to keep the public deaf, dumb and blind. This lack of pertinent knowledge to the decision as to what one wants their family to eat wrongfully, disallows the public (consumer) to make an educated decision about what they think is best to eat for health and will prevent you from being in self-control over food for health decisions.

I intend to help you protect your children by arming you with the essential understanding that there is a very real danger, a grave danger, that your children by mandate be exposed to and that you as, parents can prevent it from degenerating your children's optimum health. You can save your children from being injected with and exposed to, unnatural to human biology, vaccine chemicalizations. Vaccines have been spiraling downward, being infiltrated with chemicals that have propensities that are alien, foreign and unnatural to the body. The slippery slope of vaccinations is a causation of vaccines gone rouge and unsafe. There is a legal fiction that your children are not yours to protect or that you are not empowered to decide what is best for them. This legal abnormality (mandated vaccination) is a takeover of what is rightfully yours to be in command of. Those who profit from vaccination have pulled the rug out from under proper parenting, taken control of your children blood chemistry from you and/or healthcare vaccination decision. This perversion is commands children suffer what is an unnatural to human biology chemicalization. The tyrannical injection of children is becoming worse and/or more frequent over the years; there is no end in sight, no sunset to the onerous vaccination mandates; there is only the slippery slope of ever increasing numbers of vaccine chemicalizations; that **WE MUST STOP**!

If we do not put an end to vaccination mandates it will be used as a well paved pathway to other oppressive mandates (a slippery slope). If we do not prevent it, the slippery slope and its lobbyists' will see to it that human genetic engineering will be sanctioned, and bias health insurance discounts will be allowed to promote it. As we become complacent in all this it will be ripe for mandating human genetic engineering. Strategically, lobbyists' will use the fact, that mandated vaccination legally exist; they will use it as legal sword to now also, allow the mandate of human engineering. Just as, they did with vaccination mandate; they will claim that human genetic engineering is for the common good as, it will claim it prevents diseases or they might claim it is required to make us super human. America needs to realize what is happening; how are freedom of healthcare is being taken and how for-profit medical intervention is being jammed down our throats, injected into our babies' blood and how it will all work against us to have our genes manipulated by madmen or those that think as Hitler did; to have a superior race.

Do not rely on falsehoods, half-truths or flat out lies; know that vaccines commonly are found to have chemical constituents that are negative to health, harmful to the normal development or reactions of the biochemistry of the body and that this can cause abnormality and/or neurological malfunction. How many vaccines must be mandated until, its too many, or before it be recognized that no vaccine should be mandated? It must become the golden rule that no form of healthcare or genetic engineering ever be mandated or enforced upon us? I say, there is no need to make children a pin cushion for unwanted vaccines, no need to consider how many vaccines are too many to be enforced because even **ONE VACCINE MANDATED IN APPARENT PERPETUITY IS ONE TOO MANY!** If we do not implement the **TWO STEPS OF CORRECTION** so, many vaccines are or will be mandated that our children are or will be pin-cushions for vaccination profiteering; resulting in more epidemic health problems for children. One vaccine mandated allows for another to be mandated and so on; and acquiescing in these oppressions allows other healthcare to be mandated, GMO and irradiated food to be enforced upon us and human genetic engineering to eventually be mandated. **STOP THE MADNESS! Stop the unnatural to the body chemicalization!**

To not be blessed with personal Rights or have healthcare liberty or to not have Self-determined control over what to accept or deny for one's `health and for that of the health of one's children is, un-American. The vaccination mandates are un-American; an enigma to the good standard that patients are always in control over their healthcare and thereby, enabled to accept or refuse it. To be under the oppressive government control of healthcare is the unwarranted control over **what is core to being FREE** and violates what is **fundamental liberty**. There is agenda to control what we eat, drink and **INJECT**; all to direct what we spend money on or to maximize big business profiteering. Slowly, our Rights are being impinged and/or lost and we do not feel or recognize the degree of loss or the cumulative amount of liberty that has been slowly, but surely, taken from us. If we could turn back the hands of time when we had all our freedoms in tack and then suddenly, took away all those freedoms; **the magnitude of the loss would be overwhelming, we would be outraged and shocked and surely, not stand for such, oppression. Government control over our bodies or healthcare is an affliction upon freedom; an eradication of basic liberty**. Government control over us is running rampant and lobbyists control government! **Puppet government has been manipulated to assure corporate greed by assuring our loss of liberty. WE NEED TO RE-ESTABLISH OUR LOST LIBERTY AND PRESERVE ALL OF OUR FREEDOMS! Have needed liberty to protect your children!**

The next time you are faced with a vaccination regarding your children ask yourself the following questions: is the vaccine safe to inject, is there a SAFER vaccine, is the vaccine in your children's best interest and does the vaccine have unnatural to human biology chemicals? You should also, ask yourself: do I truly want this vaccination for my child or has my brain been manipulated (brain washed) to accept it and/or am I being forced or commanded to vaccinate, am I and my children being reduced to **vaccination SLAVES, with no essential to liberty informed DENIAL capability?** They have managed to create the perverted norm that you habitually submit your children for vaccine chemical injections and are nulled, desensitized under a mandate that commands you to submit. Anyone who wants to break away from this unnatural and ill-conceived norm of vaccination enslavement is reflexively criticized and/or chastised for it and dubbed a law breaker outcast. They would have it that no one stand up for their Rights and/or act to protect their children from unwanted vaccine chemical injection exposure and/or unnatural to human biology chemicalization imperfection. No person or entity or by faulty law should impose norms on **FREE PEOPLE**. Enforcing vaccine injections, giving no choice but to inject, no human dignity of personal healthcare choice; destroys the very idea of individualism and is an **ENSLAVEMENT. By mandating one vaccine; more and more vaccinations have been mandated! If one area of healthcare is enforced upon us other commands of healthcare will follow. The path to destruction of our Rights has been set by mandated vaccinations and a slippery slope of ever increasing mandated healthcare and loss of freedom has been spawned.**

Since, the conception of a vaccination mandate, more and more vaccine chemicalizations have been enforced upon us and thereby, the door to chemical abuse by injection was unwisely, opened and future oppression to healthcare liberty spawned. This open door to mandated forms of healthcare will not be limited to vaccination! Enforced medical vaccination intervention is leading the way, paving a smooth pathway to eventual mandate of genetic engineering. Using the same guise of protecting the public that was used for mandating vaccination, a further abuse of the Police Power of the State, will attempt genetic engineering to be perpetuated upon the People. In time, in an over expanded Police Power will try to force protect us from genetic problems by mandating human genetic engineering. This will be an attempt to create a superior race. History supposedly, stamped out this wayward dictatorship type thinking when Hitler and his ill-conceived superior race agenda was recognized for what it was. **Now, recognize mandated vaccination for what it is; it is the tyrannical enforcement of medical intervention, an enslavement to unwanted treatment. It can be argued that there is nothing ethically wrong with genetic engineering if it is voluntary however, if it is not based in freedom of decision and/or liberty of choice or strictly voluntary; then without question, it is unjust and not ethical. In order, for vaccination to be ethical or legal it must adhere to this same understanding! Freedom can protect your children's chemical welfare and good health!**

The governmentalization of our medical intervention choices or health decisions takes our self-controlled healthcare away. It must never be politically incorrect for parents to decide their healthy children's preventative healthcare and non-negligent parents must have the controlling authority to decide if a vaccine is a SAFER vaccine or if he vaccine is too dangerous to inject and have ultimate power to accept or deny vaccination. If and only if, parents have been found guilty in a court of law and with a jury of their peers, of Child Negligence; then the authority of the children's parents can be overridden. If the general population of parents can have their vaccination decisions overpowered by government, then the slippery slope of vaccination dominates us; and we are ENSLAVED to vaccinate!

The vaccine industry is bent on profiting and is ultimately focused to mandate more vaccinations; keep us ENSLAVED to be injected with its for-profit vaccines. They are uninterested in even affecting an air of respect toward parent's decision not to vaccinate and not expose children to unnatural to human biology chemicals. We must take back our hijacked government; government must be for the People and not allow corporate greed to control. Drug Company's unmatched and unchecked droves of lobbyists assure that our children are used as pawns in a for profit vaccination scheme that renders us VACCINATION SLAVES. The slippery slope, of chemically laden, mandated vaccinations, with its chemical toxins is being enforced upon us; injecting children at an unprecedented scale. Parents require the LIBERTY TO REFUSE unwanted vaccine chemicalizations and determine if a vaccine is safe to inject and/or is in their children's best interest; by doing so, dirty vaccines will be prompted to become SAFER vaccines. Above all, parents have the duty of assuring children's safety and/or health! BE FREE TO REJECT INJECTIONS!

For law, to be law, it must not cause people harm and it must be equitable! Most vaccines do contain unnatural to human biology chemicals that are not harmonious with health in fact, these chemicals interfere with the normal biochemical reactions and cause renegade reactions, alien to the body reactions that spawn abnormality therefore, mandated vaccinations are invalid law. In addition, it is inequitable for certain people to be commanded to be vaccinated while others are not; there are the growing numbers of people that have religious or medical exemption. There is also, the incomplete list but extensive warnings of side effects or health problems from the CDC that can occur after vaccination; this is more than enough proof that vaccination cause harm thus, it cannot be mandated, not be law, it is flawed. Furthermore, the vaccination mandates are flawed because it inequitably does not apply negligence law to vaccine producers; it gives vaccine producers an unfair haven for when vaccines cause injury; it grants license to injure without affording the injured the decency of recourse against the causer' of the injury. Because vaccine companies have this inequitable, total liability shield it promotes negligence instead, of deterring it. It spawns runaway negligence which, causes more harm to the people. It is unacceptable and unamerican for vaccine makers' to not be held liable when its vaccines cause injury, internal chemical distortion or denaturing!

The vaccine industry has confiscated our government and judicial system to serve its ill-conceived purpose of guaranteeing for itself, all our children to experiment on with the unnatural to human biology chemicals commonly found in vaccines or rather, suffering children with upheaval to their chemical blood and body integrity. Profiteering vaccine companies achieve unprecedented profits by assuring its vaccines are mandated to be injected. Its hoards of lobbyists have also, manipulated and bastardized our legal system to the point that it does not have to pay for negligently produced vaccines that do cause injury (it gets away with injuring children with whatever chemical concoctions bring it the most money). America has been duped; it has put the fix in, that our precious tax dollars are used to pay for damages; while producers of the injurious vaccines pay nothing. THIS REWARDS NEGLIGENCE INSTEAD, OF PUNISHING IT; it promotes runaway negligent vaccine production not curtail it and/or allows unsafe vaccines to run amuck.

The mandated vaccination law and its sinister sister law, that grants producers of vaccines unheard of liability protection are unjust laws that subject people to what makes profit instead, of health and must be stricken; law that is not just; is not law. The People's supreme parental Rights to protect their children and decide what is best for their children's health are completely violated and/or voided by the mal mandated vaccination ENSLAVMENT LAW. The result is that vaccine quality has become corrupted; there are chemicals for profit not safety in vaccines and our childrens health's have been placed in extreme jeopardy and/or have been compromised because of it. A Chemicalization Autism epidemic has been spawned from these vaccine chemicalizations that has been seeded and fertilized by these illegalities of law. It is a libelous display of violating parent's primary directive (the protection of children) by enslaving children to be injected with vaccine chemicals; it must end now! The People need to be secure in their person; secure in the essential freedom of Self-governing health, with autonomy and unmitigated liberty to refuse unwanted vaccine chemical exposure. Deciding whether a vaccine will or will not be injected, is a FUNDAMENTAL FREEDOM OF PARENTS; not for puppet government! The slippery slope of vaccination mandates need to be eradicated with the TWO STEPS! The TWO STEPS restore parents with their rightful control over the welfare of their children, by grating parents the unfettered ability to refuse an unwanted vaccination and by holding vaccine producers accountable and liable and thereby, made to pay recovery awards to all those injured by vaccine chemicalizations instead, of unwarranted spending tax dollars.

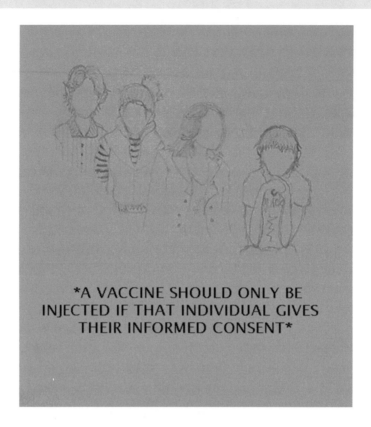

A VACCINE SHOULD ONLY BE INJECTED IF THAT INDIVIDUAL GIVES THEIR INFORMED CONSENT

Vaccines are dangerous because the norm and safety standard of informed consent/Denial is unjustly forbidden, and vaccine producers cannot directly be litigated against when their vaccines do cause a vaccination recipient injury. Because vaccines are mandated you cannot refuse it and without the norm of consumers refusing what they do not want or think too dangerous to inject; vaccines will not have to meet consumers' good standard of excellence and safety. In addition, having it that vaccine producers do not pay a cent when its vaccines injure; this means, vaccine producers act with impunity, are not accountable or liable for whatever chemicals it uses. Parents having no recourse against the perpetrators of a vaccine induced injury (no negligence law is applied to the vaccine industry) renders children totally defenseless to vaccine company negligence. The slippery slope has not only caused more vaccines to be mandated; the slimy slope has taken our fundamental negligence law protections away from where they are most and desperately needed. The safety of children requires the TWO STEPS OF CORRECTION! For the welfare of children, parents need to be FREE TO REJECT UNWANTED INJECTIONS and have vaccine producers BE BROUGHT TO JUSTICE UNDER NEGLIGENCE LAW!

People must be FREE to reject injections especially, when they are not completely convinced of the vaccines safety or if they think the vaccine is TOO DANGEROUS TO INJECT. The totally one-sided control of content by vaccine producers and total lack of parental ability to refuse vaccines is ludicrous; it is negligence and injury in the making! Something was bound to go terribly wrong health wise, when you are handcuffed to vaccinations and when vaccine makers are above the negligence law system; it is a sure recipe to disaster. Due to the ever-increasing number of vaccination mandates and its consequential CHEMICALS FOR PROFIT, NOT SAFETY in vaccines, an Autism epidemic and an increase in childhood cancer inevitably has resulted. Health and sickness are an outcome of the chemicals that flow throughout our bodies; the Law of Chemistry apply! Keep your internal chemistry clean or natural, devoid of unnatural to human biology chemicalization and you can expect optimum health whereas, expose a baby to unnatural chemicalization of alien chemicals and an Autism epidemic spawns. Parental nature is to protect children whereas, corporate nature is to protect profit and/or its shareholders. The slippery slope of mandated vaccination is the slipping away of parents having the authority to secures children's health by solidification of corporate control over our children that secures its unconscionable profiteering. The more healthcare that is mandated the more we slip away from self-controlling it! SELF-CONTROL YOUR HEALTH!

Parents need to take control of assuring their children's safety and/or health! The sure way to attain optimum safer vaccines is to give parents their proper and traditional ability to deny unwanted healthcare; the ability to refuse unwanted vaccinations must control vaccination delivery! At minimum there should be INTERPLAY between what vaccine producers recommend and the ability of potential vaccination recipients refusing what vaccine producers are offering. Vaccine' unnatural to the body chemicalization, does violence to one's normal blood chemistry; altering the biological terrain. Parent's good standard of care for children must rule, be adhered to; that means no unwanted chemicalizations. Chemicals for profit are in vaccines, chemicals that the rational person find highly objectionable; making vaccines too dangerous! Do consider vaccinating but, only with SAFER vaccines and do not fall victim to the slimy slope of forced vaccination!

I would wager that most people do not know that their parental Rights are being violated in the hospital immediately upon delivery of their babies. Along time ago, government took a **giant step in the illegal, unconstitutional and/or immoral direction** when it mandated that all newborn's, in the first moments of life, outside of the womb; must undergo chemicalization of **Silver Nitrate to be put in their eyes immediately, upon opening them in the delivery room.** Do you have Syphilis; the government ASSumes you do! It is an extraordinary intrusive measure by government, in its overzealous but feeble attempt to prevent the remote possibility of babies getting blindness associated with the mother's syphilis. That's right you read this correct, the government ASSumes you have Syphilis and without your approval or knowledge; treats your newborn as if, the mother has such, a degree of Syphilis that when the baby passes out of the mommy (and the baby's eyes must be open); somehow the baby will get syphilis and then go blind. Now, the aforementioned are big **ASS**, **ASS**umptions! The audacity of these **ASS**umptions!

The money being made by this egregious medication without permission is staggering. Are you outraged or concerned? What a horrible way to be introduced into the world! Do you think the newborn's eye cells are better off without being subjected to such, enforced medical intervention chemicalization? A perfectly healthy newborn whose eyes are just coming online certainly, does not need to be exposed to unnatural to human biology chemicalization. Even if you do have Syphilis (99.9% probably do not); as a parent' by human Right, by GOD given Right or natural supreme Right you, should be informed about even the suggestion of such, an outrageous treatment and absolutely, be 100% **FREE** to refuse it, for the sake of your newborn's best interest! You could elect to have a Syphilis test prior to having a baby or elect to be treated for syphilis in the remote possibility that you have it. Wakeup America: know, the slimy slope of mandates is placing your family at risk!

Even though syphilis is no longer prevalent this mal-law remains on the books. It insists upon placing pharmaceutical garbage in newborn's eyes; this is analogous to the fact, that even though there no longer are epidemics of childhood disease there are still mandates to inject vaccine chemicalization and/or pharmaceutical garbage into babies, infants and children. Puppet government of the pharmaceutical industry used the **remote** possibility and/or fiction, of mothers having syphilis and the further unlikelihood that if babies passed through the birth canal would not just encounter syphilis but, would become blind for doing so, and thereby, all babies were and **still are mandated to have the anti-health chemical Silver Nitrate put into babies' eyes**. This broad stroke of the mal-law pen infringed upon the Rights of parents to decide what is best for their children. **Most parents are unaware** that their babies are being **ABUSED** with Silver Nitrate in their first moments of life; parents do not have to give their informed consent just like they do not with mandated vaccinations. The reason behind this continuing Silver Nitrate (now it is an enforced antibiotic into the eyes) and the mandated vaccination **MASS child abuse is the MASS profits it brings the Drug industry**. If no profits were being made there would be no mandates!

Mass multiple vaccinations are much more egregious than a Silver Nitrate or antibiotic or any other eye full of goop because the chemicals of vaccines are injected to circulate quickly and penetrate THE BRAIN CELLS. There are numerous injections and doses, which all carry with them harmful chemicals that cause told and untold health disasters. Mass hysterical medical intervention can have **negative** health consequences. Once upon another dark medical intervention era, mass tonsillectomy was highly and frequently recommended until, recognized for being bad for health. Mass hysterical, mandated by law, squirting silver nitrate and/or antibiotic in newborns will be proven to cause all kinds of eye problems and not essential. Children, after eye chemical insult too often require glasses could there be a connection? Adults that did not have their eyes chemically exposed at birth seem to need glasses less frequently. For the most part silver nitrate has now been replaced with an antibiotic cream that is put in the baby's eyes by law however; this is still **a violation of your parental Right to decide what is best for your very own child; just as vaccinations are**. Children not exposed to multiple injections of **vaccine CHEMICALIZATIONS** have far less chances of falling victim to **VACCINE CHEMICALLY INDUCED AUTISM. Chemicals MAKE OR BREAK HEALTH, the outcome depends on the chemical. The absorption of unnatural to the body chemicals destroys optimum health and is the main cause Autism. The injection of unnatural to the body chemicals DOPES BRAIN CELLS. We need vaccines to be safer with a lot less unnatural to the biology chemicals. SAFER vaccines equal SAFE MINDS OF CHILDREN! It makes health sense to have SAFER vaccines; do consider SAFER vaccines!**

Although, syphilis is now comparatively not that prevalent to even recommend let alone mandate the powers that be and/or those that much to gain by its mandate still insists or rather, the mega-profiteering pharmaceutical companies with their **army of lobbyists** make hospitals spend money for these chemicals into the eyes of baby's during the first moments of life. **What an awful gross way to be introduced into this world**. Most parents are unaware that this is being done to their babies; it is done without informed consent/**DENIAL** based upon a mal-legal mandate. Parents are not afforded the decency of informed consent and cannot protect children from this obnoxious medical intervention. Even parents that are not promiscuous or had no other sexual partner except their spouse and in no way have syphilis are violated by having to chemicalize their newborn's eyes. No one is **FREE** to undergo a syphilis test to prove they do not carry syphilis and therefore, cannot transmit it to the newborn's eyes. Most people are not even aware that their Rights have been violated and that in their babies first moments of life they have been chemically abused. **Sticking CHEMICALS into newborns' eyes is a terrible sight for sore eyes; we should end this child abuse and ABOLISH VACCINATION SLAVERY ABUSE!** Before you stand idle under the oppression of any chemicalization abuse that does violence to your tiny baby's biochemistry or systems think twice then think again and again, before it strikes!

Yet another, unneeded medical intervention is **universal Vitamin K shots** for newborns; it is a **scam**. K shots are rarely needed; they should not be pushed universally. Newborns' normally have low K levels and **mother's Colostrum (before milk), has high K;** there is no need for these K shots. **Expecting mothers should be FREE to elect to take K prior to giving birth to assure their milk is high in K.** A traumatic birth process or forceps delivery or bleed signs rarely indicate a K shot needed. **The point is that our Right to decide one' health destiny is under siege; we must be FREE TO REFUSE medical intervention! Perhaps if you are choosing the healthiest approach by breastfeeding you might want to consider vitamin K and risk the injection skin piercing. There are those whom think all babies lack sufficient vitamin K** at birth, putting them at risk for severe bleeding in the brain or intestines until they get the **vitamin** by eating solid foods, typically around six months of age however, breastfeeding efficiently and effectively gives vitamin K. The **vitamin** is essential for blood clotting, and a **vitamin K injection** after birth can eliminate this bleeding risk. Analyze the statistics; how often, if ever, do babies that breast feed **(get the Colostrum) have a spontaneous brain bleed or get hemorrhagic disease, do make an informed decision. There is also, a possibility of your tiny baby getting a phlebitis at the injection site from the needle. These shots should never be mandated; do breast feed!**

What will this whirlwind of loss of freedom and/or devastation to our liberty of health and/or healthcare lead to? Since, the Rights that protect us and the self-jurisdiction over ourselves is being incrementally, insidiously and slowly taken away it is much harder to realize its takeover and lulls the People to sleep on their loss of Rights. People do not be complacent or acquiesce over your loss of liberty for it makes the slippery slope even steeper and slimier. The powers that dare to take control over us are becoming more blatant about it; they think that we have completely surrendered to medical enslavement and our induced loss of parenthood; there are so many mandated vaccinations that our children have become injection pin cushions and they put such, toxic chemicals in vaccines that anyone can recognize how crazily dangerous it is. From the mandating of vaccinations to the unneeded eye glob, children are all under siege; **TWO STEPS OF CORRECTION is what is needed to allow parents to properly protect children**.

There is strong indication that the powers that be are attempting to make vaccinations a matter of fact that vaccinations are not only **given without parental consent** but also **WITHOUT PARENTS KNOWLEDGE; without parents even knowing that their children have been vaccinated. It is crazy for vaccination advocates to think it is in children's welfare to inoculate without parents' knowledge; parents need to be on the alert for any negative to health reactions from the shots. The proposed legislation to inject the Gardasil vaccination is a prime example of a takeover of parent's Right to their children and what fundamentally is of strict parental concern. There reasons why they would want to completely skirt parent's knowledge of the injection are to prevent parental interference and/or objection and possibly to hide any adverse reactions from the shot. They want a clear, unobstructed sure path for their** profiteering from injecting our children, as if they were not at all our children but rather, just a vessel for their injections and a vehicle for their assured profiting. **To propose such, a law indicates an evil extent to make money!**

What is worse, to have someone teach your child something that is wrong or for someone to inject your child with something that you think is wrong for their health; obviously, if you are informed or educated about what chemicals have been found in vaccines it would be understood that it is exponentially worse to if your child were to be penetrated with garbage such as, toxic dump elements or compounds and/or unnatural to human biology chemicalizations! What would be worse if your child was to be verbally abused or chemically abused by the injection of abnormal to the body, alien to normal bioreactions and/or unnatural to human biology chemicalization too often in vaccines; the answer to this non-perplexing question, is so obvious, it is not needed to be answered! The answer is also, not perplexing as to, how to achieve fundamental freedom of parenting, basic liberty to Self-determine the healthcare of your family, being autonomous and thereby prompt **SAFER** vaccines; the obvious answer needs to be highlighted, it is, **ABOLISH VACCINATION ENSLAVEMENT with the ending of vaccination mandates and achieve the essential implementation of the TWO STEPS OF CORRECTION!**

Vaccination dictators ignore parental Rights and supreme authority to determine what is best for children. Those who we placed trust in have become our dictators and these dictators' take advantage of the power we have placed in them and have abused its power, becoming callous dictators by mandating multiple vaccinations in non-emergency times or in non-epidemic times for sheer profiteering and in perpetuity; it furthers its abuse of power, by enforcing vaccines that distort, upset, alter or disfigure our children's vital and sensitive natural chemistry. The degree of the chemicalization or its negative impact depends upon the vaccine's chemistry and your child's chemistry which, might already be somewhat compromised and therefore, even more susceptible to the vaccine chemicalization. It is not for government to determine or inflict any degree of unnatural to human biology chemicalization upon **FREE** people but rather, for parents to determine if a vaccine is safe to inject or too dangerous to inject! We must stand up for our Right to protect our children; take control of what parents are naturally supposed to and are perfected in. One can easily recognize the slippery slope of government control over our healthcare and where it is leading; extreme domination and/or pervasive medical intervention. **Private healthcare and/or health choices and the rules that protect us in this liberty must become an article of organic law; in that the decisions of healthcare and/or health must be a relation of the individual and the parent for their child, a totally private concern into which, all others have no Right to intrude. BE FREE TO PROTECT YOUR CHILDREN!**

The slippery slope of mandated vaccination and liberty loss has trickled down to government commanded sonograms. In a January 13, 2012, USA Today, news story entitled, "Court says Texas can begin **enforcing** abortion-sonogram law," the slippery slope of our Rights deprivation can **enforce** a sonogram, **without informed consent**, upon pregnant woman who are contemplating abortion. Perhaps the message of having expected mothers stop and think before having an abortion is admirable and desirable however, the approach is all wrong; **law must never enforce a medical procedure**; just as **it is unethical and/or ill law to enforce vaccinations IN PERPETUITY OR DURING NON-EPIDEMICS**. Although, abortion is an extremely important and emotionally charged topic, the issue here that needs to be brought to light is that people are **being enforced to** endure a medical intervention without the dignity of informed consent or informed **DENIAL**. Furthermore, the privacy of one's healthcare and/or pregnancy/abortion situation is being rendered not private and this is incongruent with healthcare privacy requirement and dignity. People must be **FREE to deny medical intervention** especially and particularly preventative healthcare medical intervention such as, vaccinations. The slippery slope of vaccinations and/or loss of Right to Self-determine healthcare have bulldozed a pathway of **continued illicit destruction of our Right to have control over ourselves and/or what is done with our children's bodies. YOU MUST HAVE LIBERTY TO DECIDE WHAT IS BEST!**

My personal view on abortion is of no consequence here. The issue of abortion is not in dispute or relevant to **the message of this book, it is the recognition of the affliction upon our Right to direct or control our very own healthcare and/or health and the emphasis is on the wisdom of only considering vaccinating with SAFER vaccines are of what is relevant, extreme importance and of imperative concern; it is the issue**. The realization is that there is a slippery slope of loss of Self-control and/or our Right to Self-govern what medical intervention is accepted or **DENIED. There can be no instance of MEDICAL INTERVENTION SLAVERY; it must always be, impermissible. Mandated vaccinations have blazed an apparent, smooth-paved path for our loss of freedom.** Even if there be no known side-effects from the intervention; it must not be enforced upon the public! **The enforcing of vaccination is that much more egregious because there are side-effects and/or injury caused by the vaccinations. Informed consent/DENIAL is a Self-determined healthcare Right; it is a crucial liberty and health protector that must rule over vaccination or medical intervention!**

Another affliction to our Right of control over our healthcare decisions is only a bad day away. How far will the Rights of the People to control one's health destiny and/or body be impinged upon or violated depends upon how vigilant we are to protect our Right of informed consent/**DENIAL**. History will show that compulsory vaccinations are a gross violation of our Self-determination of healthcare Right. The aggression to our Right to be left alone has had other atrocities in the annals of medical intervention history. In our not too distant past government and medical society violated the People's freedom to procreate. Government has a history of being over-influenced to do exactly what the powerful few want them to do even if it is against the People's Rights and the Constitution. The interference and annihilation of one's Right to procreate is perhaps, as egregious as, vaccination **SLAVERY. The fact, that mal-government has done such atrocities as, procreation interference and mandated vaccination enslavement tells us to be on guard for such, government sanctioned violations. The audacity of self-appointed elite, such as, the Carnegies' whom had design to decide who is worthy of procreating and who is not! There must be no mandates for healthcare; no enforced unnatural chemicalization of our children!**

Thirty-Three States carried out **eugenics** programs, (**enforced sterilizations**) from approximately 1929 till 1974, many thousands of individuals were **made to become sterilized**. Interestingly, the very first eugenics laboratory (for sterilization) was in Cold Springs Harbor, Long Island, N.Y. established in 1910 and founded by a Harriman and **funded by the Carnegies**. The **Rockefellers' funded involuntary sterilization of people of color**. Compulsory sterilization is unethical and is an atrocity, yet, puppet government allowed what Big Money wanted just as, today wayward, puppet government does what Big Pharma want by mandating vaccinations. **The enforcement**

of vaccinations someday soon, will be established as unethical and an atrocity. In North Carolina involuntary-sterilization laws remained on the books **until 2003, a form of modern day tyrannical medical intervention slavery. The medical profession willingly took part and for many years supported these atrocities, just as, it supports no informed consent/DENIAL of mandated vaccination. Government will continue to ENSLAVE us, to be subjects of enforced medical intervention until the public becomes acutely aware of the aggression and stand up for our Right of informed consent/DENIAL. Fundamental control over oneself is basic to being human. There will always be those who will successfully ENSLAVE us, if we are not freedom minded and vigilant to protect our liberty. How far will wayward government go; as far as WE THE PEOPLE, let it! Liberty plays a major factor in safety; liberty empowers you to protect your children and liberty to refuse vaccination makes for SAFER vaccines and thereby, protects children. When it comes to the welfare of your children do not settle for plan B always elect the best for them, the plan A; make sure if you vaccinate to only vaccinate with SAFEWR vaccines!**

To best achieve vaccine safety and to maximize our children's health there needs to be the implementation of the requirement that consumers of vaccines are perfectly FREE TO REFUSE an unwanted vaccination and to hold vaccine producers accountable and/or liable for vaccine induced injuries; the nuts and bolts of the TWO STEPS OF CORRECTION. Vaccine manufacturers need to pay 100% of the just compensation for injuries caused by negligently produced vaccines to curtail its negligence of vaccines being laced with toxins or unnatural to human biology chemicals. The National Childhood Vaccine Injury Act of 1986 erroneously prevents the legitimate filing of litigation directly against physicians or vaccine manufacturers in civil court and unwisely, gives vaccine producers a total liability shield unfortunately, this equates to less vaccine quality control and less safety for our children. Negligence must be punished to deter it therefore; the erroneous 1986 Act must be stricken! It is unwise to do otherwise, because it gives room for vaccine manufacturers to put unnatural to the body chemicals for profit in vaccines. What gives the most safety, must be the focus! It will be a glorious day, the day we can save children from chemicalization child abuse and curtail the chemicalization Autism epidemic by being FREE individuals, being special, by decisioning for oneself whether to accept or deny a vaccine. FREE PEOPLE are not mass injected like a herd of cattle, under the oppression of mandated vaccinations which, is mass chemicalization child abuse. Controlling what can enter your blood and body is core to individualism and freedom!

Vaccine producers do not meet the required good standard of care for quality control because of the chemicals found in vaccines. Makers of vaccines would be a great deal more concerned about safety and/or be safety conscientious if they were not impervious to litigation for injuries its vaccine chemicalizations cause. No ability to litigate against vaccine companies for its negligence equal no ability to stop the negligence! There would be a much more efficient and effective effort not to use alien to the body, unnatural to the body, unhealthy or harmful chemicals; if we had recourse against it. Do not leave your children stranded or in the hands of those that must care about profiting; control the vaccination decision!!

The Childhood Vaccine Injury Act of 1986 would be better named **"The Vaccine Producer's Total Protection Act"** because that is what it really does or properly call it, **"The Childhood**

Anti-Protection Act" since, it results in less vigilance for vaccine purity and/or a lot less reason to protect children from chemicalization. **What promotes safety must be demanded and achieved!** The inappropriate Act must be stricken and recognized for the gross injustice it spawns. The extreme amount of vaccine lobbyists should be stopped from manipulating regulators to pass, bias and bogus laws that does not serve the public. **Prompting a safety minded vaccine production is in the best interest of our children! Children's safety comes first; not the protection of Big Pharma!** As, more of our Rights are taken, more vaccines are mandated, and more healthcare choices are limited or taken from us; or lost however; people are waking up to the fact, of it, and will not stand for it, refuse to be subjected to it and never will give up their liberty and/or protection of children!

Vaccinations need to be based on the following premises and quality control test:

Premise (1) YOUR CHILD = YOUR DECISION: Parents are children's healthcare decision makers; parents have the supreme power to decide what healthcare shall or shall not be accepted or denied. If a parent concludes that there are chemicals in vaccines that are not perfectly beneficial or are potentially harmful or a parent decides not to submit their children for vaccination; the decision controls, for no child should suffer the consequences of vaccinations that are not approved for delivery by their parents.

Premise (2) The mandate of vaccination or enforcement of it is counterproductive to quality control of vaccines. Vaccines are just like other consumer goods and must be under the quality control and/or safety prompter of consumers decision to buy it or not, to accept it or not and/or determine if the vaccine is safe to inject or too dangerous to inject. It is mendacious to assert vaccines should be mandated based on that they are good for children, it cannot rationally be argued that certain chemicals found in vaccines such as, but not limited to aluminum, formaldehyde or mercury are in anyway good for the vaccine injected recipient. Alien, unnatural to the body, unnatural to human biology chemicals are harmful to vaccine injected recipients, it is an abnormal chemicalization of children's blood; and should be considered child abuse to do so. The success or failure of a vaccine must be based upon its merit and not enforced upon our children otherwise, safety is lost!

Premise (3) Negligence law, main purpose is to stop negligence or further ongoing negligence. Vaccine producers must be brought under the umbrella of the normal and traditional restraints of negligence law otherwise, there is no legal recourse to stop vaccine producers' from making faulty vaccines and stop negligence or its utilization of unnatural to human biology chemicals in vaccines. When a vaccine is accused of causing an injury the consumer of the vaccine or the parents of the child whom was vaccinated must be FREE and/or legally empowered to bring the maker of the vaccine to court to be held accountable and liable. Children are our number one asset and our future they need to have at least the basic standard of protection afforded by negligence law and in fact, need even a higher standard and always their parents' standard. Children are highly susceptible to alien, abnormal to the body, unnatural to human biology chemicalization and it must be considered negligent to have such, chemicals in our children's vaccines. Children need more safety instillers not less! The application of negligence law assures SAFER vaccines whereas, vaccine producers being above the law of negligence, does not!

The "SANITY TEST" is a vaccine quality control test, a safety test that assures our children's welfare; it is highly recommended and needs to be required. Each vaccine needs to pass this good standard test in order, for a vaccine to be considered minimally safe and meet this basic safety standard before injection consideration. It is consistent with the above premises and assures that parent's rational concerns about vaccine chemicalizations are taken into utmost consideration. Vaccine safety will rise because of parents' commands for no anti-health chemicals will be adhered to. Vaccines that do not have anti-health chemicals and/or chemicals, which the average prudent parent deem unacceptable will pass the "SANITY TEST" for vaccine safety and injection consideration.

To have a much-needed good standard of vaccine quality, a reasonable standard of vaccine quality control, vaccines that coincide with parents' safety demands makes for **SAFER** vaccines thus, all vaccines must be made to pass the **"SANITY TEST FOR VACCINES". This in no way should be construed to limit any other testing for safety. Vaccine manufacturers must be held to a higher standard of care for safety; not a lesser degree!** There must be no liability shield of protection from litigation; people must be enabled to take legal recourse against negligent vaccine producers. Because vaccine manufacturers hold our children's health literally in their greedy hands; they need to be made to pay a higher amount of damage award when its **vaccines are found to cause injury, adverse side-effects and chemicalization child abuse**.

There is nothing more important to parents than their children; for parents there is no excuse that vaccine producers could make for having unnatural to human biology chemicals in vaccines and for vaccine producers to have a liability shield leaving parents with no recourse against the producer of the vaccine if harmful is outrageous. It is detrimental to the securing of children's well-being if vaccine producers are oblivious to negligence law, impervious to litigation correction, not held to a normal, traditional negligence standard; if not held responsible and liable for its breach of care owed to Vaccine Recipients it allows for its negligence to be unimpeded and even can escalate it. If an injury is caused by a negligently produced vaccine it is wrong and unacceptable not to have recourse against the vaccine producer. Reasonable reliance upon vaccine safety requires the application of negligence law and/or its good standard it assures. A reasonable person's standard of what can be in a vaccine needs to rule over vaccine production and liberty to litigate if the standard if breached. Vaccine producers will be at risk of litigation for a breach in the duty of care they owe Vaccine Injection Recipients. The duty of care they owe is to produce vaccines that will not cause injury and/or that do not have anti-health chemicals. Therefore, all vaccines should have to pass the "SANITY TEST" OF GOOD STANDARD to rationally be considered for injection. The rational reasonable parent standard of vaccine contents must rule; if anti-health chemicals are found in the vaccine; THE VACCINE FAILS, and effective parenting is successful.

In the best interest of children, we must not only apply negligence law to vaccine producers but rather, there be stiffer, stronger penalties and/or much higher allowable monetary awards for the victims of vaccine induced injuries. In addition, I call for the CRIMINALITY OF VACCINE PRODUCERS for utilizing chemicals for profit in vaccines that are known to be unnatural to human biology chemicals. For example, the use of any degree of mercury or mercury derivative should be a criminal offense. It s widely known that mercury is toxic and strictly unhealthy to be exposed to it, to expose babies to it is beyond negligent; it is criminal. Vaccine companies must not be able to hide behind the unconscionable total liability shield. Parents are made to be non-protective parents, trapped to inject, handcuffed to submit their children for enforced injections under the oppression of vaccination mandates which, flagrantly violate human and parental Rights. To add insult to injury parents are not allowed to strike back or to protect their children by litigating against the causer of their children's injuries due to the total liability protection. The self-serving protection of vaccine producers with a one-sided liability shield must end and negligence lawsuits begin with parental liberty to protect children established!

Injecting anti-health, unnatural to the body vaccine chemicals into the body and/or blood is a most drastic chemicalization because it is a "**SYSTEMIC CHEMICAL EXPOSURE**", once injected the chemicals enter the circulatory system to penetrate a baby's cells; **baby's brain cells can be chemically doped**. One injection of a vaccine's unnatural to human biology chemicals is problematic and could induce a **CHEMICALIZATION CRITICAL MASS SYNDROME; multiple injections together or over time is even more problematic and places a baby at risk of CHEMICALIZATION AUTISM.** Children's cells are polluted with tinctures of vaccine chemicals that are alien, unnatural to the body and thus, are very harmful. **Cellular chemistry is altered, and the cell's genes are environmentally manipulated. Improper health and/or Autism can be the result. Health can be measured by the chemicals within us, over the course of living. Babies' exposed to injected unnatural to human biology chemicalization become victims of the injected chemicals; posing a burden to their tiny bodies and causing abnormality to the needed and sensitive bioreactions of life and optimum health! WE MUST BE FREE to not entangle our children with what the reasonable or rational person considers objectionable! Without this basic liberty the slippery slope of vaccination and loss of Self-determined healthcare will become so, slimy so, slippery so, steep that WE ARE ENSLAVED! We are not deceived by the nature of health being dependent upon the proper chemicalization and the avoidance of unnatural to human biology chemicals; we are deceived to think that the injection of such, abnormal to the body chemicals healthy!**

FOR THE SAKE OF OUR CHILDREN'S SAFETY AND NATURAL CHEMISTRY; IT SHOULD BE MADE EXTREMELY EASY TO BRING LITIGATION AGAINST NEGLIGENT VACCINE PRODUCERS AND THE VACCINE INJURED SHOULD BE ALLOWED TO OBTAIN THE HIGHEST COMPENSATION AWARDS THAT IS PERMITTED BY A COURT OF LAW!

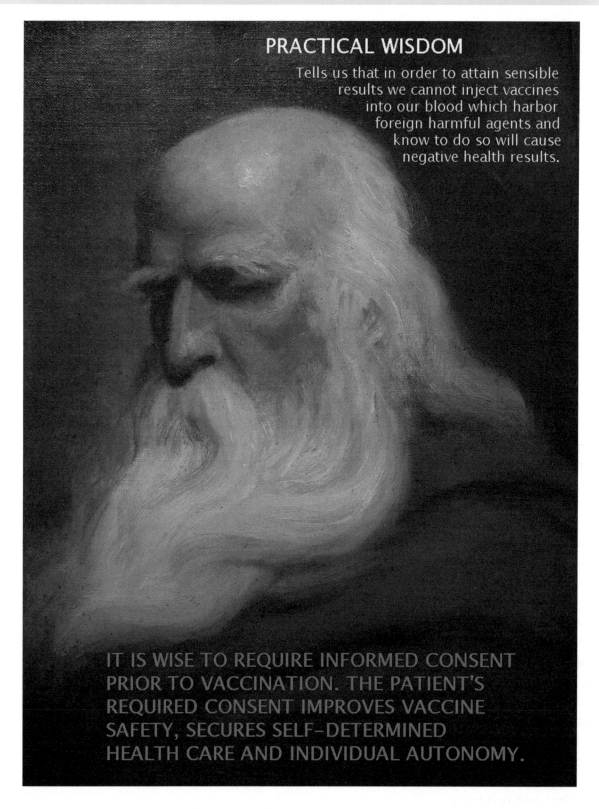

PRACTICAL WISDOM

Tells us that in order to attain sensible results we cannot inject vaccines into our blood which harbor foreign harmful agents and know to do so will cause negative health results.

IT IS WISE TO REQUIRE INFORMED CONSENT PRIOR TO VACCINATION. THE PATIENT'S REQUIRED CONSENT IMPROVES VACCINE SAFETY, SECURES SELF-DETERMINED HEALTH CARE AND INDIVIDUAL AUTONOMY.

We must prompt a higher level of vaccine safety consciousness. Vaccine manufacturers must at bear minimum be brought in line with the general populace of producers of consumer goods; being legally re-established as part of the traditional legal tort system and not be unwisely granted an unprecedented liability shield that is so very counter to children's best safety interest. **Chemicals that have been found in vaccines cause Autism and possible DNA damage. By parental Right and self-regulation; refuse unwanted CHEMICALIZATION!**

You now have the knowledge that vaccine chemicalization exposure is by far, the most dangerous of chemical exposures due to the way and how the chemicals penetrate. Because the chemicals are injected, it directly enters and circulates; it passes the blood brain barrier to penetrate babies' brain cells and thereby, chemically dope their brain cells with a full, unbuffered dosage, of unnatural to human biology chemicalization. Ingesting unnatural to the body chemicals, as tragic as that might be; is not as, devastating as, injected exposure because your digestive process has elimination capability and to some degree rids the body of the toxins before it enters into the circulatory system and thereby, averting its penetration into brain cells; no doping of the brain. Having vaccine producers properly brought to justice will prompt the all-important safety-first directive and stimulate the production of toxic free, SAFER vaccines. The irrational and bias treatment of vaccine producers' no longer must be allowed; they must have to defend against litigation and pay damages for their negligently produced vaccines otherwise, it places children in continued peril. Vaccine producers must be susceptible to negligence litigation and vaccinations need to be strictly voluntary, having vaccine delivery being strictly based upon informed consent/ DENIAL; together, this will obtain a much more rational safety level and stimulate the end of chemically toxic vaccine production. The mere threat of litigation and the actual cost of litigation are significant negligence deterrents; just like a threat of a speeding ticket is a speeding deterrent. We need more deterrents to stop ongoing negligent vaccine production which, continues to have unnatural to human biology chemicals that are toxic!

It is revealing that the marked increase in Autism parallels the overburden amount of multiple vaccine CHEMICAL injections; THE LAWS OF CHEMISTRY APPLY TO ALL THESE INJECTED CHEMICALS. The array of chemicals found in vaccines is the initiators, the major critical factors that produce abnormal after abnormal reaction and blocks normal biological reactions that eventuates Autism. Mass chemically laced vaccine injections equal a mass production of Autism, an Autism epidemic. For Vaccine Producers to claim that they are not aware of children being injured by the chemicals of vaccines or that they are unaware of any harmful chemicals in vaccines is willful ignorance. Parents take back the rightful control of your children; become enabled to deny unwanted vaccine injections and let us together act to GET THE CHEMICALS OUT of our children's vaccines!

The epidemic of Autism will end if WE THE PEOPLE have SAFER vaccines to freely choose from. No longer should FREE people be made to submit to another's healthcare determination or will; no person must be injected with a vaccine that the individual deems unsafe or too dangerous to inject or not in their offspring's best interest. We must do everything in our power to emancipate our vaccination decision authority, our self-directed healthcare liberty by freeing ourselves from the oppression of mal mandated vaccination regulation and inappropriate takeover of what is rightfully our health decision. Our children's safety must come first and not the profiteering, vaccine drug companies.

The erroneous National Childhood Vaccine Injury Act of 1986 JEOPORDIZES CHILDREN'S WELFARE BY UNFAIRLY PROTECTING VACCINE PRODUCERS WITH AN UNWARRATED LIABILITY SHIELD that assures their mega-profits are not touched from all the vaccine injured litigation claims; this promotes less due diligence for vaccine safety and is an "ANTI-CHILDHOOD SAFETY ACT". This Act must be stricken in the best interest of children. The consequence of the Act is that vaccine industry is left legally unchecked; making its power far too great and thereby, allowing chemicals for profit instead, of health in our children's vaccines. This absolute power over us must end! Children's safety requires vaccination to be balanced with parental informed consent/DENIAL. Do not expose your children to toxic chemicals certainly, do not inject unwanted, unnatural to the body chemicals. The "SANITY TEST" and TWO STEPS OF CORRECTION are required!

What chemicals do you want raging throughout your children? Vaccination induced injuries are so, prevalent that vaccine companies manipulated our legal system to rid themselves of the burden from all negligence lawsuits; they maliciously, obtained a liability shield through what should be called, an ANTI-SAFETY CHILD VACCINATION ACT. The fact that this mal-legal Act was sought is testament that children in droves are being injured by the CHEMICALIZATION of vaccines and/or by negligent vaccine production. Negligent vaccine manufacturing is rampant with its accompanying injuries. Imagine the magnitude of injuries from vaccine injections that caused lobbyists to jump to protect the mega-money made from vaccines. The government mal-Act assured vaccine producers that the vaccine injured could not directly litigate against vaccine producers and this placed children at higher risk of vaccine induced injury. The ill-Act puts children in peril of continued vaccine production negligence; unwisely prompting unchecked, runaway present and FUTURE NEGLIGENCE. Government was induced by lobbyists to unfairly protect vaccine corporations from lawsuits; it does nothing to protect our children from chemicals or ONGOING NEGLIGENT vaccine production harm. No one should be able to inflict unnatural chemicalization upon children; children need their parents' protection!

The mal-Act spawns a much greater likelihood that our children can be injected with vaccines that have less vaccine quality control instead, of more or requisite vigilance to protect our children. Quality control rapidly disintegrates if vaccine producers are not prompted by the threat of litigation if they do not produce SAFER vaccines. You can logically surmise that there is a great deal more injuries caused by negligent vaccine production today and that the Autism epidemic has been spawned by injecting chemically laced, negligently, produced vaccines; WE CAN AND MUST PREVENT INJURY! Those claiming to be injured by a vaccine chemicalization must be allowed their proper day in court and the vaccine induced injury facts come to the surface. The type and frequency of injuries must no longer be suppressed by the mal-Act. We are left to hear only the frustrations of the multitudes of concerned parents that their children have undergone health degeneration soon after vaccinations. The People need protection from vaccine production negligence instead, of the profiteering vaccine producers being protected from honest, meritorious, just lawsuits of those injured by vaccine injected chemicalizations. The slippery slope becomes extremely slimy if we are not afforded our day in court!

The very premise of negligence law and its legal application create an acute awareness for product safety and stops any continuing negligence; it is desperately needed to instill SAFER vaccines. There needs to be a strong downside, a legal problem, a major monetary cost setback for putting unnatural to human biology chemicals in our children's vaccines; this will GET THE CHEMICALS OUT. The proper application of negligence law is a necessary watch-dog that assures vaccine chemical safety. It is wrong that vaccine producers do not even need to perform a cost/benefit analysis for when it contemplates putting toxic chemicals in vaccines. Because they cannot be traditionally litigated against for vaccine induced injuries there is no downside for its utilization of chemicals that assure profit but, destroy health. For the sake of all our children's safety vaccine producers must be brought to court to pay when their vaccine chemicals cause injury. They must think more than twice before putting harmful chemicals or potentially hurtful chemicals into its vaccines; vaccine producers must be made to do what all producers of consumer goods do; a cost benefit analysis. Let us wisely put our children's needs first, by making it that the placing of such, chemicals fails the cost/benefit analysis when vaccine companies perform it. The more time without negligence law applied to vaccine production; the more harmful chemicals will be negligently used in vaccines. Negligence law steadfastly, applied to vaccine producers will help prevent unnatural to the body vaccine CHEMICALIZATION and help blockade the slippery slope of vaccinations.

Negligence law applied will deter the utilization of chemicals that parents rationally object to such as, but not limited to, chemicals which give vaccines longer shelf life but are extreme chemicals and much too dangerous to inject into babies. Chemicals, for greater profits but cause biochemistry upheaval or injury must be deterred from use in vaccines by negligence law and by consumers' Right of refusal. **The vaccine industry must come under normal restraints, becoming reasonably, vigilant about securing our children's safety by not putting our children in chemical harm's way.** The consequence of the Childhood Safety Act, better dubbed the **"ANTI-CHILDHOOD SAFETY ACT"** is that it greases the slippery slope of vaccinations by instigating and/or allowing more chemicals in vaccines; INDUCING MORE INJURIES BECAUSE OF IT!** We need to **CLEAN-UP vaccines**, **GET THE CHEMICALS OUT** and this "**ANTI**-childhood Safety Act is an impediment to this urgent goal. **We need to EMBOLDEN what removes chemicals! Parents must be enabled to seek damages against vaccine producers when children suffer a vaccine induced injury! Autism is mainly a vaccine induced injury; CHEMICALIZATION AUTSM cases require equal access to the TRDITIONAL court system! The vaccine injured should not be railroaded to a mock court, the VACCINATION COURT or be besieged by a different set of rules or be judged by a MASTER instead, of a Judge! A jury of one's peers should be the fact finders, for those claiming injury from a vaccine.**

The chemicals for profit in vaccines are anti-health chemicals that do nothing for the stability of health but rather, are major hindrances to good health and the main cause in fact, of the Autism epidemic. **MAKE ABNORMAL YOUR BABY'S CHEMISTRY AND EXPECT, ABNORMAL RESULTS; EXPECT, ABNORMALITY!** The health promoting natural chemistry is disorientated and/or lost by the injection of alien, unnatural to human biology vaccine chemicals. Law should be on the side of safety and not profiteering, on the side of bolstering vaccine quality control not profits. We can prompt vaccine producers' concentration to do much better; to make much **SAFER** vaccines. People having the basic freedom to refuse vaccination and/or choose what they think best for their children induces a higher sense or need to make **SAFER** vaccines! People being **FREE** minded consumers with liberty to decide what healthcare to accept or deny or what healthcare is best bolsters **SAFER** vaccines. You must be **FREE** to follow you think best; be legally enabled to strictly rely upon what you want or if you choose, what great minds have bestowed, **Hippocrates, "Let your food be your medicine and your medicine be your food."** Your children must be yours to guide and protect so, if you decide that vaccine chemicalization is too dangerous to inject and/or is an act of chemicalization child abuse or not in your children's best interest; then your decision must rule! **Parents' health decision not to subject children to unwanted chemical injections must control otherwise, parents and their children are dominated to suffer unwanted chemical concoctions or possible negligently produced vaccines which, is medical tyranny that reduces one to be a VACCINATION SLAVE.**

No longer should the vaccine injured be **PREJUDICED or BURDENED** by having to file vaccine-injury claims with a U.S. Court of Federal Claims that was set up under the **National Childhood Vaccine Injury Act of 1986, ruled by a Special MASTER that has inappropriate, different rules which, has our precious tax dollars paying for vaccine injury claim awards instead, of vaccine producers. Claims should be part of the long-established legal tradition of filing claims in Civil Court, have a real Judge and JURY and make it that Big Pharma pay.** For the safety of our children, the actual perpetrators of the vaccine production negligence (vaccine manufacturers), must be brought in line, by having to directly defend against Vaccine Recipient's claims of injury and made to pay the award amount out of their deep pockets, for any court rendered compensation award. The victims of negligently produced vaccines must be **FREE** to seek damages from the source of their injury and not be wrongly and unwisely restricted to tax payers' governmental awards. This traditional legal system is lawful, equitable, just, unbiased and promotes diligence for producing **SAFER** vaccines and thereby, is in the best interest of children. Boycotting dirty vaccines and/or being **FREE to refuse vaccines** are also, essential for safety.

Moreover, to assure optimum **SAFER** vaccine supply for children not only should vaccine producers be held to the traditional standard for consumer safety and pay the regular payment level of damage awards if their negligent vaccines cause injury but rather; **be held to an even higher standard of excellence in their vaccine production and be caused to pay a much greater damage award, known as, "treble damages", whenever its vaccine supply is found to cause injury.** This is a more just system and one that will be in the best interest of our children instead, of the best interest of the mega-profiting vaccine industry. **All children have sensitivity to certain chemicals that have been found in vaccines in fact, these chemicals disrupt, distort and make abnormal the bioreactions of the body.** They have breached the public's trust by use of **chemicals for PROFIT, NOT SAFETY** in vaccines. They need to be made to do the right thing; made to protect children from **unwanted chemicalization invasion by injection.**

Let us act responsibly for the welfare of children with the implemention of the TWO STEPS OF CORRECTION that assure vaccine producers GET THE CHEMICALS OUT of its vaccines which, is in the best interest of children to do so. Vaccination mandate is the enforcement of vaccination SLAVERY, it is mandated mass child abuse and has led to a marked decline in vaccine safety that is the genesis of the CHEMICALIZATION AUTISM EPIDEMIC. The chemicals that are injurious will no longer be in vaccines when parents are properly, EMPOWERED and ENABLED TO REFUSE unwanted vaccine chemicalization and vaccine producers are held ACCOUNTABLE and LIABLE for vaccine induced injuries! The slippery slope will become a level playing field; with children safe because they come first!

The stupidity of using tax payers' dollars to pay for the stupidity or negligence of vaccine producers must end! Vaccine producers make a ton of money from vaccine sales, it is requisite that Big Pharma pay those injured by vaccines and **by making it cost big time, SAFER vaccines**

result. It is all too one-sided and is anti-safety for Big Pharma to charge whatever it wants and pays nothing when its vaccines cause injury. In addition, the stupidly of having the public enforced to vaccinate children, mega-profiteering is guaranteed, Furthermore, the stupidity of disallowing parents to protect children from what parents deem unsafe or not proven safe vaccines renders our children defenseless and/or at the mercy of whatever chemical formulation makes vaccine producers the most money. All the above one-sidedness and stupidity and yet, **puppet government irrationally pays for vaccine producers' negligence but, limits what the injured can recover for their very serious and very real injuries**. Moreover, there are unjust and unprecedented monetary caps placed on awards puppet government allows for those injured by vaccine chemicalization. We need to bring justice back into our legal system and level the playing field by doing a complete reversal; **place equitable legal caps put on how much profit is made or how much is charged for vaccines and have vaccine companies pay for its own negligence and pay big which, is commensurate with the harm being caused our children.**

It is wrong for vaccine producers to have unfettered power over our children's chemistry! Apparently, it can put whatever chemicals they desire in vaccines and charge what it wants for vaccines and yet, be impervious to litigation and/or having to pay damage awards when their negligently produced vaccines cause our innocent children injury. Furthermore, vaccine producers wrongfully obtain mega-profiting because our children are enforced by mandate to be stabbed with needle to consume its vaccines and the vaccines unconscionably cost way too much. The People's Right to litigate is reduced in that people cannot litigate against vaccine producers assuring windfall profit for Big Pharma at the People's expense and at continuing unsafe vaccine production. Tax payer dollars must no longer "bail out" the vaccine industry! **Government must act to protect the People** by controlling runaway vaccine costs and assuring **SAFER** vaccines by empowering people to be consumers' that can freely refuse unwanted vaccines. **Secure the best interest of children; not Vaccine Profiteers!**

Protecting our children by assuring vaccine safety and/or that vaccines are not laced with chemicals is the primary directive. However, the public also needs to be protected by preventing unconscionable profiteering from the vaccine sales. **The amount of money that vaccine industry is making is unconscionable and the way it has been making it is un-American. People are wrongfully forced to be injected and this assures massive vaccine mega-profiteering. It is high time to end mandated vaccination profiteering by ending obligation to be vaccinated. Let us, ABOLISH VACCINATION SLAVERY by ending MANDATED VACCINATION MADNESS. Let us, instill the legal concept that It is unjust and inequitable to place caps on what the vaccine injured can obtain but instead, enforce extra high award deterrents upon makers of harmful vaccines and have caps on how much vaccines cost!**

The fact, that unnatural to human biology chemicals have been routinely found in vaccines such as, but not limited to, thimerosal (a MERCURY derivative), ALUMINUM and much more, make it clear that vaccine producers have blatant disregard for the health of all of our children and did so in the reckless endangerment of children or colluded to do so or was complacent with it or are accessory's to it and/or once they learned of it or was no longer purposefully blind to it, were accessory after the fact. It is high time that our children's health is secured instead, of securing the profitability from vaccines; it is high time we act

to **GET THE CHEMICALS OUT** and the **TWO STEPS OF CORRECTION** are what is needed to remedy this intolerable situation.

We should make just amends for the oppression of vaccination SLAVERY that people were made to suffer. There must be no tyrannical medical intervention; people must always be FREE to Self -determine healthcare! Government can highly recommend vaccinations but, it must never **ENFORCE** vaccinations upon **FREE Americans** otherwise; **we are ENSLAVED**. Our minds are functioning, and we have capacity to care for ourselves and our children therefore, we do not need enforced vaccination or a nanny government that oversteps its jurisdiction by mandating vaccination in perpetuity. Parents usually get things right and do what is best for their children whereas, government and//or the puppet government of Big Pharma too often get it wrong or do what is in the best interest of the corporation instead, of the public's best interest. Medical mishaps, misunderstandings and purposeful deceit are all happening too often or becoming the standard and a self-serving agenda has become its poor standard; it should not supersede parental decision of what is best for children. Modern medicine too often gets it wrong, it is very fallible; we must not be subjected to it if we think it not in our best interest. Despite advances in medical technology and supposed superior understanding of the human body America is becoming sicker and at a younger age. This daunting truth is because there is a Mc Donald's or a Walgreens or a CVS on every major corner and because we continue to force vaccinate masses of children with multiple **chemical** vaccines. **Vaccines must come clean! The Right to refuse unwanted vaccines and negligence law are essential for SAFER vaccines!**

We now face critical choices at critical junctures, but we can avert the Autism epidemic and the impending doom of having entire generations of less than optimum healthy people; we must act now by implementing the TWO STEPS OF CORRECTION and the "SANITY TEST" FOR CHILD SAFETY AND VACCINE PURITY. If we fail to act, to stop the ongoing destabilization of biochemistry by injection chemicalization with vaccines that contain unnatural to human biology chemicals the health children and very future of this great nation will be devasted. We need to make the right decisions about how to avert the AUTISM epidemic and/or prevent children from unhealthy chemicalization; the ramifications of no positive corrective actions will be devastating to the health and very future of this great nation. The warped idea that parents do not have the ultimate authority in deciding whether a vaccine chemicalization will or will NOT take place must be corrected; this is a perversion of the natural order and not in children's best interest. A child not having parental protection is a child in jeopardy! We must not expose children to unnatural to the body chemicals; the unleashing vaccine unnatural chemicalization into babies is child abuse. Parental authority and directive must be supported by government!

Government needs to reverse the unprecedented and very unwise liability shield that it wrongly granted to Big Pharma that is responsible for the contamination of our children's chemical biochemical integrity. Government must stop being manipulated to support what is a vaccine producer's monopoly and/or the enslavement of our vaccine recipient children. The steady stream of the mass of enslaved children, enforced to endure being stuck and injected with vaccine chemicals must cease and desist. There must never be mandated vaccination laws that guarantee vaccine profiteering and strip the public of their informed consent/DENIAL Right. Let us ABOLISH vaccination SLAVERY and end all the oppression,

coercion, to be vaccinated and put a stop to the discrimination of those that do not vaccinate. **The MAIN CAUSE of the AUTISM epidemic is rooted in mandated vaccination and producers of vaccines being above or impervious to negligence lawsuits!**

We must be FREE to rule over our health and/or healthcare; FREE to prevent an unwanted chemical injection! FREE to keep children's blood natural and pure! Doctors are presently improperly shackled by vaccination law and prompted not to consider patient's informed consent/Denial Right. All other administered healthcare is reasonably and properly limited by the patient's Right to deny or accept healthcare. In addition, doctors take a solemn oath, to do no harm to their patients, and yet, enforced chemically laced vaccines continue to be enforced despite desire not to be; causing untold numbers of mental injury and chemical upheaval or distortion. Vaccine chemical induced brain fogging and an epidemic of Autism is a result of this non-permissive medical tyranny. YOU MUST HAVE SELF-CONTROL over what chemicals will or will be injected into your own body and that of your children, to have it otherwise; is LAWLESSNESS and SLAVERY!

The fact that vaccines carry alien to the body, anti-health chemicals that harm makes its enforced administration an abomination and is against doctors' oath to do no harm. In addition, doctors are in direct neglect of adhering to the requirement of informed consent/ DENIAL. Manipulated government mandates that cause doctors to breach their oath or what is owed to their patients must be considered unlawful. Parents must be FREE to protect their children from unwanted vaccinations; FREE to prevent vaccine chemicals from being injected into their children's blood and brain cells. Induced chemical vaccine brain fog, magnetic brain level interference, and induced chemical homeostasis loss result from vaccine infiltration of unnatural to human biology chemicalization. Cellular chemical disruption and/or risk of vaccine chemicalization Autism must not be enforced upon children. Let us, perfect freedom to care for our children and render normal our ability to protect children our parental best ability. LIBERTY TO SAY, "NO" to unwanted vaccine chemicals is required. Vaccines will come clean with informed consent/DENIAL! The atrocity of enforced chemicalization is tyrannical intervention; a SLAVERY that must end!

There are many ways to regulate, maintain and regain one's health; and it is a matter of personal preference and personal freedom to determine what is the best fit for your individual needs or health goals. **The song of health can be in many different keys**! Individuals should be enabled their preference; being **FREE** to prefer a key that resonates best for them and through them. Individuals should not be limited in their choices of how to resonate their health. Imagine if government intruded, by dictating that we must listen to this or that or only in one key that was lobbied for singular government approval of a mandate; how wrong that would be! **Government cannot even balance the budget so why in heaven and earths name do we dare let it intrude upon our private family health decisions; it is inept at child rearing or caring and certainly, do not know better than parents, when it comes to knowing what is best for children's health. Indeed, the government orchestrates many sour notes and often produces sour grapes. The AUTISM epidemic is indirectly from government control over our healthcare. We must not tolerate living under a totalitarian rule that dictates healthcare and prevents parents' from making healthcare decisions or their protection of children!**

Imagine if government commanded that we must fight cancer in their specific way or on its commanded terms and/or that you must submit yourself or children for government mandated treatment and that you are forbidden to replace this treatment with one that you think is better and safer. You do not have to imagine such healthcare tyranny because it unfortunately is already present in a related healthcare mandate, in that you must submit your children for government sanctioned vaccine chemical injections whether you approve of it or even if you think there is a better and/or **SAFER** approach. If you have determined that the vaccine chemicals are outright dangerous you still are enforced. There is the caustic fact, that vaccine chemicals are not indigenous to the body and thus, spawn abnormal reactions. It is this debacle or evil that caused our loss of freedom and placed our children in the health predicament that they are under, as they are enforced to be injected with vaccine chemicals, ordained by mal-law mandates. **Mandated vaccinations are this kind of lack of freedom and oppression realized. People must be FREE to dance to their own health dance and to the beat of their own health drum!**

Dance to your own rhythm and rhyme of life; demand all the pertinent information to make the right choice on any vaccine that is about to be injected into your child's vital systems. Become enlightened about what chemicals are in vaccines. Become logic stricken about how the unnatural to human biology chemicals of vaccines can cause Autism. Vaccine chemical exposure is the worst form of chemical exposures however, do safeguard your children from all sources of it such as, artificial food chemical additives in our children's food, drug chemical consumption during pregnancy and modern day living chemical exposures that our children endure; these chemicalization exposures have mirror imaged the rise of the mass Autism epidemic. **Autism is mainly, a result of exposures to the medley of injected chemicals from vaccines and to a lesser extent, to the ever-increasing levels of food additives and environmental chemicals**.

Vaccine chemicals pose an ominous threat to children; they are not combatable with human physiology and homeostatic biochemistry. Too much unnatural to human biology vaccine chemicalization and children reach a CHEMICAL DESTABILIZATION POINT, A CHEMICAL TIPPING POINT and/or a CRITICAL CHEMICAL MASS SYNDROME that effectuates CHEMICALIZATION AUTISM. Parents should not be enforced by MAL-law to submit children to undergo CHEMICAL INJECTED ENDANGERMENT or UNNATURAL CHEMICAL ENTANGLEMENT. Unnatural to the body chemicals are harmful to the life-force; DANGEROUS! Self-protection from chemicals IS A MATTER OF SURVIVAL. Medical interventions' claims of benefits over time are too often proven wrong and in fact, the opposite of the benefit can occur. Post-surgical opioids can, paradoxically, lead to chronic pain. In an April 16, 2016, University of Colorado at boulder study, it was found that rats given morphine experienced pain-reactivity for three weeks longer, inflammatory changes in spinal cord. The study indicates that giving opioids prolongs pain (inducing chronic pain), increases pain and/or primes specialized immune cells in the spinal cord to be more reactive to pain. Analogously, mass use of vaccines is backfiring; it is making children more susceptible to health problems and/or immune deficiency. Vaccines' unnatural to human biology chemicals are impacting cellular activity; we need SAFER vaccines!

There are delicate balances in nature that must be maintained in order, for life to flourish and even exist; health is totally reliant on achieving and maintaining the natural chemical configuration, arrangement or balance There must be certain minerals in soil for plants to

adequately grow and bear fruit. The salt level in the oceans must be within a certain range for all the underwater life to survive and for the water flow currents to not be disrupted. If the temperature goes to low everything will freeze and an ice age result. If the temperature rises to high the weather drastically will change and the polar caps will melt causing water levels to dangerously rise. Those that live on the water are aware how delicate of a balance there is and how life relies upon nature's intricate balance.

To dare disturb or distort the natural chemical balance that we are born with and/or inject tiny babies with abnormal to the body chemicals or unnatural to human biology chemicalization is extremely, unwise and a risk not worth taking! To distort the refined chemical balance of a baby interferes with, disrupts and distorts the needed chemical reactions required for health, for life to flourish and even exist. Parents must have the liberty to harness the right internal chemistry for their children and assure it is maintained. Babies, infants and children need this perfected chemistry to be optimally healthy. Your offspring rely upon you to protect them from chemicalization distortion by being **FREE** to reject the injection of unnatural to the body vaccine chemicals. Vaccine producers are incredulously **QUILTY** for the imperfection of children's chemistry. Parents must be **FREE** to secure for their children the perfected chemistry by refusing unwanted chemicalization! We need **SAFER** vaccines that do not so, distort our children's perfected chemistry.

It is important that we do not expose the outside of our body (skin) to anti-health chemicals and it is of infinitely, greater importance that we do expose the inside of our body (blood) to anti-health chemicals by injection. Keeping one's internal chemical makeup perfected has become increasingly more difficult with all the unnatural to human biology chemicals that we are becoming more and more exposed to. Anyone having a swimming pool experiences the arduous task of keeping their pool water chemically balanced to be crystal clear and safe. You must take precautions and be vigilant to keep the pool chemically balanced in order, for the water to be safe to swim in. Too much acid or alkalinity and/or if the pH is off, the water can cause health problems if swam in. Similarly, but at a much, much higher level of importance; you must be vigilant to keep your children's internal chemistry perfectly balanced. It should not be baffling that the law of chemistry applies to whether we are healthy or that the chemicals inherent in vaccines that are not indigenous to health, life or human biochemistry are anti-health or a major impediment to having optimum health. You must be **FREE** to not inject anti-health, unnatural to the body, vaccine chemicals into the blood and/or bodies of your children!

Your body's internal chemistry is so much more complex than pool water and preventing a chemical upset or imbalance is of extreme importance in order, to stay healthy. You must guard against disrupting the chemistry of your blood and/or that of your cells. Injecting present day, multiple vaccine chemicals is very disruptive to children's ultra-sensitive internal chemistry. Parents should be on high alert to guard against all chemical infiltrations and make it their highest health priority to avoid chemical exposure. It is unwise to let your children swim in a pool that is chemically imbalanced, and it is absolutely, imperative not to allow children's **INTERNAL** chemistry to become compromised. Make it your utmost healthcare priority to not let your children's blood and/or brain cells become chemically imbalanced. Know what chemicals are in the vaccines! Keep children's chemistry as pure and/or as healthy as possible; **PARENTS MUST BE ENTIRELY FREE** to do so. Vaccine chemicals are not indigenous to one's natural chemistry and pose a significant danger. Law must free-up parents' capacity to protect children's health; mandated vaccination law undermines this vital parental protection. Children must not be chemically altered or battered by enforced vaccinations!

There is a **CRITICAL CHEMICAL DESTABILIZATION POINT** for all of nature that makes the atmosphere, oceans, land and/or our environment not optimal or health generating or even life sustainable. There is a **CRITICAL DESTABILIZATION POINT** for humans that will promote sickness, not health and spawn Autistic children, not intact neurologically and biologically functioning children. The chemical dependent fluids of the body, including but not limited to the blood are vulnerable to **DESTABILIZATION** from vaccines. Injecting chemically laced vaccines into children's delicate balanced systems is ludicrous. Just recognizing the long list of negative physiological changes or adverse side-effects from any prescription or illicit drug reveals how chemicals can manipulate our systems and just how susceptible all our bodies are to the properties of such, chemicals. To inject alien, unnatural to the body chemicals into our children's blood destroys the fine-tuned but, delicate natural chemical balance within the body. It is child abuse to inject unnatural to the body chemical infusions, knowing it will render the child helpless to the dangerous propensities of the unnatural to human biology chemicals inherent in vaccines.

- **WE MUST BE FREE TO REFUSE CHEMICAL INFUSIONS AND/OR INFILTRATIONS.**
- **THE PRESENT-DAY FORMULATIONS OF VACCINES ARE CHEMICAL INFUSIONS.**
- **VACCINE COMPANIES MUST NOT ESCAPE THE RULE OF LAW, IT MUST BE SUBJECTED TO NEGLIGENCE LAW; THERE MUST BE NO LIABILITY SHIELD.**

The intricate but, delicate chemical balance of children's blood and cells must be preserved in order, for there to be optimum health and prevent health degeneration or Autism. Infusing anti-health chemicals into babies must be considered an act of child abuse. If parents, purposely exposed a child to a toxic chemical or injected chemicals such as, mercury or aluminum into a baby they would probably be found guilty of child abuse, arrested and/or thrown in jail. It is wrong that vaccine producers can collude with doctors to expose a child to the same chemicals and it be legally permissible expecially, when the parents are against the injected chemical exposure. Puppet government of the Drug industry has seen to it; children can be chemically abused or exposed to unnatural to human biology chemicals such as, thimerosal (a **MERCURY** derivative) and aluminum (a metal that is a major magnetic conductor) despite the fact, that the parents do not want their child exposed, it will be abusively, enforced. The vaccine personal are not held to the same reasonable standard of law that parents are held to for the exact exposure action. **MANDATED VACCINATION OF CHILDREN IS CHILD ABUSE BY CHEMICAL INFUSION INJECTION, THAT IS ON A MASS SCALE!**

The symptomology of AUTISM is evidentiarily the same or analogous to chemicalization exposure. One of the most common adverse side-effects from taking any given drug is mental confusion. Confusion or mind fogging or inability to concentrate or relax are responses from the introduction of alien to the body drug chemicals and is very good indication of what chemicals can do to us. **Is it any wonder that vaccine chemicals that are injected directly into the body or bloodstream can have significant mal-impact on brain function of those injected; AUTISM is closely related to the MENTAL signs and symptoms commonly caused by chemical internal infiltration**. Alzheimer's is also, a degree of mental confusion and/or dementia from chemicalization. **The flu shot is an injected source of harmful chemical influx into senior citizens** and a cause of mental confusion and/or Alzheimer's. **A common complaint after FLU shot is dementia. Wisdom dictates that we need to detoxify children's vaccine shots and senior citizen's shots; GET THE CHEMICALS OUT**! Warning: Flu shots still, even to this day, have mercury, which is a known neurotoxin and is a **brain killer. All the vaccines must be analyzed for harmful chemicals; for immediate removal**!

The Flu shot for adults will not be attempted to be mandated because adults are too protective of their Right to Self-determine their very own healthcare whereas, mandated flu shots for children will unfortunately be attempted because parents have not stood up for their Right to protect their children from other vaccination mandates and have acquiesced to have their children's welfare dictated. The plethora of **UNJUSLY** mandated vaccinations have paved a smooth path for more vaccination mandates and loss of precious freedom; a **SLIPPERY SLOPE**. Do not acquiesce in giving up your decision power over children's vaccinations, do not sleep on your Right to protect children. Mandated vaccination advocates will deem more vaccination mandates! **Law must be consistent: the natural or instinctive need for parents to protect their children is a law of higher authority, superior to man-made law that can never be relinquished; not by voluntarily or involuntarily acts or omissions and not by any man-made vaccination mandate. There must always be SELF-DOMINATION of healthcare!**

How dare they keep the truth from us, not giving us the pertinent knowledge, that vaccines contain chemicals that are unnatural to human biology or that they do not make it strikingly obvious and/or suppress the fact, that vaccine contain chemicals that cause renegade reactions, alien to the normal biochemical reaction in our precious babies. The truth that chemicals infiltrating the body are health's downfall is a truth that will be continually attempted to be kept from us and meticulously defended against. It will be argued every way and at every avenue to turn the cause of Autism away from vaccine chemical infiltrations. The chemical, drug industry will be financially devastated if it becomes widely known that its chemical concoctions are a main reason for health degeneration or Autism. Once a child is infiltrated and/or insulted with a requisite amount and/or harmful type of chemicals, once the CRITICAL DESTABILIZATION POINT is reached, a CRITICAL CHEMICAL MASS SYNDROME becomes a high probability and Autism can be spawned. Such, chemicalization make the likelihood of Autism exponential!

The essential nature of the vaccine industry is to lace vaccines with chemicals that parents do not want children injected with. Callously, it puts whatever, chemicals it wants in vaccines which, bring the most profit, (chemicals for profit; not safety). 99.9999999% or 100% of parents do not want to expose their babies to mercury or aluminum or unnatural to human biology chemicals. Why were parents not alerted to the toxic fact, that vaccines do contain such, chemicals are mainly because of the slippery slope of our loss of Right to decide what is in our children's best interest; this atrocity must be no longer, parental Rights must

rein. The slippery slope of vaccinations is exposing our offspring to a gamut of chemicals that their bodies absolutely have no use for and that strictly stress the perfected biological chemistry. Not only do vaccine chemicalizations alter, disrupt and disfigure the normal chemical configuration and/or the chemically perfected homeostasis that is required for optimum health; the unnatural to the body, chemicalizations distort the chemistry and take on renegade reactions and an anti-life of their own, setting the chemical stage to produce AUTISM. DO NOT LET THEM CHEMICALIZE YOUR CHILDREN! Get off the slippery slope; secure your children welfare with TWO STEPS of CORRECTION!

One might wrongfully conclude that childhood obesity is a cause of childhood Autism or obesity in the pregnant mother. Those who are obese generally, eat a lot of fast foods and junk foods; foods that are very high in **chemical** additives, preservatives that are unnatural to the body chemicals which, is a real causation of Autism; it is not the obesity itself. The obese tend to ingest higher quantities of these harmful **chemical** food additive and toxins. Being obese is generally unhealthy for the individual but it is wrong to correlate or point the finger that Autism is directly caused or majorly, connected to Autism. **The chemicals that are not normally part of the biochemical reaction are the problem; the cause in fact, of CHEMICALIZATION AUTISM! Chemicals, are the enemy** however, make no mistake; **injected chemicalization from vaccines are by far, the worst and main cause of the autism epidemic! Injected chemicals rage throughout the blood circulatory system and penetrate the brain, imperfecting the brain cellular biochemistry; doping the brain, causing brain fogging. Ingested bad chemicals are diminished by the selective digestive process before entering the blood whereas, injected chemicals are a direct hit, an unbuffered chemicalization.**

In addition, Gestational Diabetes creates abnormal sugar and insulin levels and renders the child very fragile and/or generally susceptible to all kinds of health problems. **Principally, the dysfunctions that occur in diabetics render the child much more likely to have a major negative to health impact from chemically laced vaccine injections.** Keep on target, the chemicals, particularly the **vaccine chemicals that are injected directly into a children's blood are enemy number one** and/or the major cause in fact, of Autism and/or attention-deficit hyperactivity disorder (ADHD); not the stand-alone fact, that the individual is obese and/or there is diabetes. In addition, obese individuals generally do not exercise properly and therefore, do not raise their metabolism or perspire to get rid of chemical toxins within the body rendering the obese that much more susceptible to injected chemical toxins. The chemical infiltrations are the cause of health degeneration. Obese people tend to ingest more chemicals and these chemical infiltrations cause harm however, **injected chemical infiltration is not buffered by digestion**.

Moreover, if children are diabetic they are even more susceptible to the negative to health chemicals of vaccines. **Keep your eye on the CHEMICALS BALL**, for it is the chemical infiltration that takes its toll; diabetes just makes one even more fragile and/or susceptible to the vaccine chemicalization insult. **Toxin exposures are the key component of Autism and vaccine injections are the major penetrating injected force of chemical insult. Parents must be enabled to prevent their children from unwanted chemical exposure. The mandated vaccination ENSLAVEMENT laws obliterate parent's legal ability to prevent unwanted chemical exposure; allowing an assault and battery upon our children by violating them with unwanted chemicalization insults. Diabetic children are in greater need of protection from chemicalization insult;**

they need more parental protection from adverse chemical infiltration of unwanted vaccine chemical exposure. No choice vaccination must end and parental protection begin so, children do not suffer anti-health chemical injection!

PREVENTING CHEMICAL EXPOSURE IS THE KEY TO AUTISM PREVENTION AND DETOXIFICATION IS PRMARY TO RECOVERING FROM AUTISM! It is so, much better for our children if vaccines did not have unnatural to the body chemicals and/or chemicals for profit; not safety. Giving parents the chance to have a SAFER vaccine is of monumental importance to the welfare of children. Making all vaccines devoid of these chemicals would be the single greatest step forward for the well-being of children that is certain, to end the epidemic of Autism. Children's best interest is served by reducing the chemicals that they are exposed to especially, certain vaccine chemicals that are injected to circulate and penetrate children's brain tissues. No FREE American should be placed in the untenable position of being enforced by a mandated vaccination law to suffer an unwanted injection and/or chemicalization. The slippery slope of mandated vaccination and its loss of fundamental Right to Self-regulate health requires the **TWO STEPS OF CORRECTION!**

The accumulative affect upon health from every source of chemical exposure takes its unhealthy toll. It is vastly important to guard against all unnatural to the body chemical exposures to assure we are not cumulatively chemically compromised to any significant unhealthy degree. The FDA wrongfully has allowed many products on the market that singularly may not pose a significant health threat but cumulatively, add up to health degeneration. Being exposed to multiple minor chemical exposures quickly, adds up to a significant and/or chemical exposure of major concern. All these minor chemical insults accumulate and interact in a much more disconcerting chemicalization having major negative to health consequences. Recent generations have been exposed to more kinds of toxic chemicals and more frequently, than ever before in history; it has rendered a generation to a greater degree, chemically compromised. Consequently, children are more susceptible to chemicalization by injection; the worst kind of chemical exposure.

The injection of unnatural chemicals is the most dangerous and must always be avoided! We must be FREE to avoid unwanted chemicalization. The FDA needs to be prompted to remove all unnatural to the body and/or anti-health chemicals that are in any products and thereby, best protect us. Parents need to safeguard children from all forms of chemicalization but especially, chemicalization by injection! Clean vaccines will result from the **TWO STEPS OF CORRECTION.** It an absolute abdication of responsibility and accountability to not hold vaccine manufacturers liable when their vaccines are chemically impure or the cause of injury. There is no greater parental need than to prevent injury to children! Parents by fundamental Right and supreme authority must be FREE to refuse an unwanted or perceived of as, too dangerous to inject, vaccination. SAFERvaccines.org can help you protect YOUR children from chemicalization; to the best of your ability!

Vaccine chemicalizations, of unnatural to human biology chemicals can make children reach a **CHEMICAL TIPPING POINT**, effectuating a **CRITICAL MASS CHEMICAL SYNDROME that spawns Autism.** One renegade reaction after another and one altered biochemical reaction after another causes abnormality, central nervous system malfunction or dysfunction that spawns

Autism. As unnatural to the body vaccine chemicals mix with the natural pure chemistry of the body and/or blood a break in biochemical homeostasis takes place; a denaturing occurs. It could take only one vaccine injection, or it may take numerous, over a span of time to reach a **CRITICAL DESTABILIZATION OR CHEMICAL TIPPING POINT.** When toxins and/or alien, unnatural to the body chemicals mix with the naturally pure chemistry of the body to a level that renders reactions chaotic it is a **CRITICAL MASS CHEMICAL SYNDROME**. The natural chemistry becomes too chemically manipulated so, biological reactions and neurological functions become unstable and more and more reactions become chaotic and/or renegade; making chemical stabilization improbable. What results is a runaway internal reaction problem!

CRITICAL MASS CHEMICAL SYNDROME takes over and abnormality takes root; normal physiological and/or biological reactions are impeded; the nervous system is impacted! **This chemicalization induced syndrome negatively impacts bio-functions and spawns Autism.** Mental normality is one aspect of human physiology; it is dependent upon optimum and/or a pure chemistry. **Injected vaccine chemicals pose a most ominous threat, it is injected into the blood and quickly reaches the brain, penetrating the brain cells; doping the brain cells of babies, infants and children with its payload of unnatural to human biology chemicals. Having optimum chemistry is critical to have optimum health! Chemicals rule reactions; they are the building blocks of health or its stumbling blocks! Injecting non-indigenous chemicals that are unnatural to the body bastardizes the once, normal needed reactions of the body; it is injurious. Our charity, SAFER vaccines, want to GET THE BAD CHEMICALS OUT of vaccines to secure our children's welfare and give parents' peace of mind! Why jeopardize health when SAFER vaccines exist or can exist!**

The chemical tipping point is mainly triggered by mass vaccination chemical exposure. The chemical homeostasis is lost, and/or the natural intricate chemical reactions are substantially disrupted. One abnormal reaction after another allows for abnormal neurodevelopment. The bloods chemistry is thrown out of its delicate balance and into disarray. **Abnormal presence of abnormal to the body chemicals equals (=) abnormality! Injections of alien, unnatural to human biology chemicals renders normal biochemical reactions less possible; this means your child no longer can be as, healthy and the possibility of AUTISM IS AMPLIFIED.**

A homeostatic pure chemistry enables the creation of the building blocks of health and the full expression of body functions. When vaccine unnatural to the body chemicals enter the chemical pool of reactions they interact interfering, altering and/or mutating chemical reactions and thereby, Autism is spawned. **The Universal Laws of Chemistry apply, unnatural to the body vaccine chemicals have its chemical capacities and propensities; making optimum health impossible for those that reach THE CHEMICAL TIPPING POINT.** How many chemicalizations does it take to destroy optimum health is dependent upon one's chemical make-up and/or if there is already a degree of being chemically compromised; so, do not gamble!

At what point does a loving parent say enough, "that is all my child is going to take; there will be no more chemical laced injections, no more unneeded exposures to chemicals, enough is enough" or say, "make cleaner vaccines, GET THE CHEMICALS OUT, make SAFER vaccines and then I can rationally choose to vaccinate my children; not until." Many parents are determining there will be NO MORE VACCINE CHEMICALIZATION INSULTS! If things keep on going the way they have been, it will not be long until children are exposed to a ridiculous amount of vaccines and all the chemicals they pack. Many think it already has reached a ridiculous point, in that children are being exposed to so, many (too many) vaccine chemical cocktails. The smatter of chemicals injected is a danger that parents must be **FREE** to reject or accept! The liberty to deny any vaccination that parents determine not in their children's best interest will prevent the runaway train of vaccination and be the best quality control over vaccines; **assuring, SAFER vaccines**. If we do not demand our informed consent and/or **INFORMED DENIAL** our children will soon be **VACCINE OVERDOSED**; overly, exposed to perhaps 50 doses or even 75 dosages sooner, then later. Injected, chemical toxins, strike the moment they circulate in the blood; destroying health. **Be FREE to select and reject vaccines!**

The **slippery slope of vaccinations**, better named the **"slimy slope** of vaccinations" has already seen a steady increase in the number doses of vaccinations which, our children are being exposed to. Parents must finally act to protect their children from chemicalization harm by demanding to refuse unwanted vaccinations. The informed consent doctrine, more appropriately named, **"the informed DENIAL doctrine"** must be steadfastly, applied to vaccination and hold vaccine producers liable and/or to parent's posing their children's personal injury legal actions if and when their children are injured by chemical vaccines; these are part of the needed **TWO STEPS OF CORRECTION** and the steps that will **GET THE CHEMICALS OUT** of vaccines.

The below paragraph is only a partial educational list of the chemicals that you should be majorly concerned about that have been found in the production of vaccines. We must act to remove them all! Vaccine producers were prompted (left no choice) to remove the mercury derivative from vaccine production after huge and prolonged public outcry and outrage. **Alert, we remain at the vaccine producer's mercy or whim or profit first above all mentality; they can still put whatever, it wants or whatever, brings the most profit even if it is the least safety or known to be a toxin or unnatural to human biology chemical or compound. The bulk of alien to the body chemicals are still used in vaccine production.** There is a long list of foreign to the body substances that unwisely continue to be used in vaccine production. These chemicals place the vaccine recipient in grave danger of a **critical mass chemical syndrome. We must not be mandated to be chemicalized; WE MUST BE FREE TO REJECT INJECTION!**

Here again, is a partial list of some of the dangerous chemicals found in vaccines: Aluminum a highly efficient conductor, known to be associated with Alzheimer's disease and seizures and cancer producing in lab mice, aluminum phosphate, aluminum hydroxide, formaldehyde (a known cancer causing agent), polysorbate 80, polymyxin B, Neomycin, Streptomycin, 2-phenoxyethanol, Monkey Kidney Cells, Newborn Calf Serum, Ethylene glycol (antifreeze), Phenol, known as carbolic acid (this is used as a disinfectant, dye), human diploid cells (the dissected organs of aborted fetuses), chicken embryo, Formalin, gelatin, Amino Acid, Soy Peptone, Yeast extract, glutamate and embryonic guinea pig cells. These unnatural to human biology contents should not be in vaccines; it must not be injected. If it is ludicrously, in vaccines; it must be required that you are made acutely, aware of the caustic, anti-health fact, of this alien to the body chemical content.

The above list ends with **guinea pig cells** because this list of chemicals makes any rational minded person recognize that **children are being experimented on, used as, GUINEA PIGS**.

Knowing what chemicals have been found in vaccines and that vaccine producers either are inept at knowing the harmful propensity of these chemicals or do not care to know; make rational parents realize their children are being **ABUSED by a mass vaccination**s **of chemically laced vaccine injections; a mandated CHEMISTRY EXPERIMENT. The chemicals found in vaccines make it insane to inject**! The total harm from vaccine chemicalization exposures may never be absolutely, known or understood. Producers of vaccines either know about the chemicals harmful properties or propensities and use them anyway or are clueless; either way, **they place our children in impermissible harm's way. There must be no deterrent legal or otherwise, that prevents or deters or interferes with parent's protection of children from unwanted vaccine CHEMICALIZATIONS. We hereby, ABOLISH VACCINATION SLAVERY and demand them to GET THE CHEMICALS OUT, before we even consider their injection!**

Recipients of vaccinations do not want any of the above unhealthy chemicals in vaccines! **More importantly, no caring parent would want any one of these chemicals, let alone, all these chemicals to be injected into their children's delicate and susceptible blood and brain chemistry.** It is baffling to the healing and health conscious, why these chemicals are in vaccines. Some of these chemicals have **oncogenic properties! All these chemicals are unnatural to the body chemicals and can contribute to the causation** of a **critical mass chemical syndrome. It is ludicrous and stupefying that any of these chemicals are in vaccines. No one should have the liberty to put these chemicals in vaccines and babies certainly should not be injected with it! Parents must take the reins of control back into their reliable hands; make sure children are not wrongfully chemicalized and/or abused!**

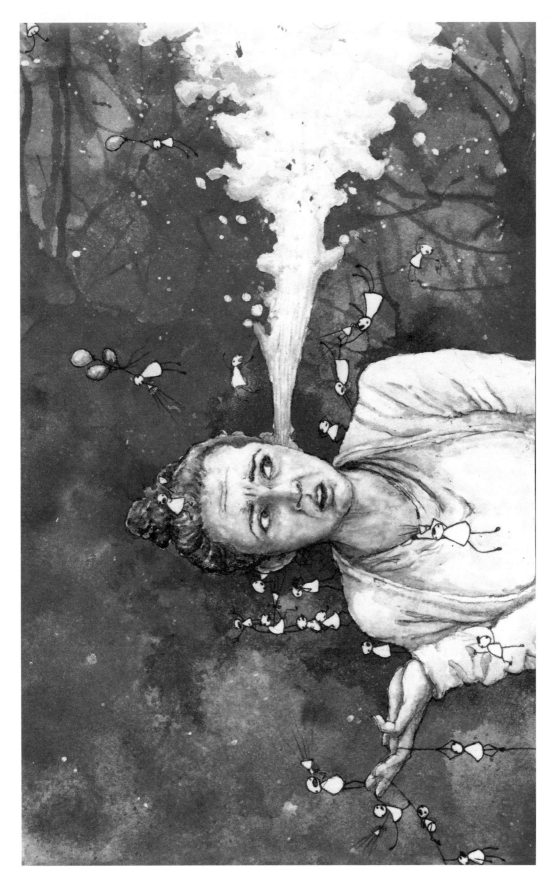

Children are suffering multiple vaccine chemicalizations. How many unnatural to human biology injections can your children withstand until abnormality is spawned?

Once a critical mass chemical syndrome is reached, it takes physiologic and/or chemical reactive control, what is unleashed is a non-stoppable negative reaction after reaction after reaction that can spawn Autism. All types of chemical exposures help bring about a critical mass chemical syndrome however; the multiple vaccination exposures are the worst catalysts. **Vaccinations are more of a direct hit chemical exposure;** they are injected directly into the bloodstream and all at once and with velocity thereby, they take great negative to health toll. **The interaction of all these chemicals interplay and react with the once natural balanced chemical content of the body. There caustic molecular properties and its alien electromagnetic charges make abnormality. The changes induced, and/or its presence induce stunning harm; rendering children unhealthy and/or Autistic. We must take the initiative to end this abnormalizing chemicalization madness! The TWO STEPS OF CORRECTION TO GET THE CHEMICALS OUT IS REQUIRED. The critical mass action of parents whom refuse unsafe vaccines prompts much SAFER vaccines which, prevents critical mass chemical syndromes from occurring and thereby, ends the Autism epidemic.**

WARNING: The antigens in vaccines that produce the planned immune response is stressful on babies, infants and young children's immature immune system and could cause injury to the immune system; much like an underdeveloped muscle having to contract to lift a heavy weight, it could cause the muscle injury. The antigens of vaccines must be MORE carefully formulated to not overwhelm and/or cause injury to the immature immune system and/ or be individually formulated according to the age, weight or sex of the vaccine recipient. Vaccines must begin being made as safe as possible; with no unnatural to the body chemicals and specific to the recipient. Chemical insult from aluminum, formaldehyde and other vaccine chemicals must be eliminated; they have no health reason to be in vaccines. We must take every additional step needed to safeguard our children from all chemical exposures in order, to decrease Autism frequency. **The revelation is that unnatural to the body chemicals cause abnormality, including but not limited to Autism. We must do everything possible to eliminate chemicalization to prevent a tipping point and critical mass chemical syndrome. You should only, consider SAFER vaccines!**

All sources of alien to the body chemicals must be determined and attempted to be eliminated. The ludicrous injection of these chemicals into children must be stopped in order, to prevent health disorder and/or reduce the Autism epidemic. Prescription drugs are a source of chemical infiltration into the body and so, is pollution however, chemically laced vaccine injections are the primary culprit, the main causation of the Autism epidemic. **Drugs and vaccinations that cause side-effects and severe health problems are a testament to just how ludicrous it is to inject vaccine chemicalization of unnatural to human biology chemicals. Upon entering our children, these chemicals cause biochemical reactive havoc; it is an extremely virulent source of danger and health destroyer. We must make certain that we do not inject children with any such, chemicals to prevent injury and/or AUTISM. We must assure parental liberty of protection of children and SAFER vaccines.**

Prescription drugs all have adverse side-effects and cause health problems. The **No.** 4 **cause of death** in the United States is from drugs. Laboratory studies show that 42% of all prescription drugs **cause cancer**, according to the information on their own labels. I will repeat that, 42% OF **ALL** PRESCRIPTION **DRUGS CAUSE CANCER! Injecting unnatural to the body chemicals is like**

356

declaring war on one's biological systems. Osteoporosis, weight gain, kidney and liver disease and dementia are just a few negative health effects from the taking of drugs. **It is questionable why doctors continue to prescribe what causes so, much ill health. There are natural means of combating health problems! Autism is just a continuation of the long list of iatrogenic CHEMICALIZATION related health problems.** Iatrogenic disease means that the disease has been physician induced. Mass, medical intervention is synonymous with mass, man-induced health problems. **Dementia is a common malady of prescription drug chemicalization; it is no wonder that the chemicalization from vaccines causes mind problems in children and/or an epidemic of Autism!**

The slippery slope has engaged our children in drug and/or vaccine dependency. It is wrong that the public and/or our children are being constantly bombarded with take this or that drug to be happy or healthy, advertisements. **We NEED** governmental protection from this very real danger; protecting our children from being programmed into taking drugs and/or becoming drug/vaccine dependent. Lobbyists and their mega dollars bulldoze their way into putting these drug/vaccine ads on constantly; allowing the Chemical Production Companies (drug/vaccine industries) to continually expand their mission to make us all chemically, drug/vaccine dependent. America and New Zealand are the only countries in the entire world that unwisely, allow drug ads on television. It is wiser to protect adults and children from becoming drug/vaccine taking robots!

Main stream media has become a public relations office for the official version of events and/or to instill drug/vaccine taking without thinking. We are made to conform to vaccination compulsion! If we were not so, programmed or bombarded with a big blitz, to be vaccinated, we could **recognize what the true consequences of ingesting or injecting drug chemicals is. In addition, all the insidious ads have induced the public subconsciously and consciously that it is okay, it is normal for Drug Companies' PUPPET government to inappropriately, forbid parents from protecting their children from unwanted injected chemicalizations. Consequently, children's welfare is in jeopardy and vaccines have become too dangerous to inject! It is a most reasonable and normal expectation to protect your children from chemicalizations! Every parent wants their children to be 100%; parents want to protect children from anything that renders their offspring less than 100%! The injection of any degree of unnatural to human biology chemicals renders the injected less than 100%; it chemically compromises the injected and is therefore, impermissible to mandate or enforce upon FREE people. It is outrageous, extremely wrong and egregious to mandate any vaccine especially, a vaccine that is not a SAFER vaccine!**

There is an epidemic of induced drug taking children; it calls for immediate affirmative action to break the bonds of children's drug induced taking dependency or programming. There is an epidemic of Autism; it calls for the implementation of the TWO STEPS OF CORRECTION. Children are blessed with their parents, as their natural protectors, however, the constant drug advertisements pierces even the most vigilant of parents shielding from harm. A raping of our children's free-thinking minds results from the onslaught of deliberate drug and vaccine taking messages, rendering children into drug/vaccine taking zombies, despite parent's best efforts otherwise. Once these targeted children become adults the drug taking only increases with time and thereby, fulfilling the pharmaceutical industry's

goal to secure more and more drug sales and/or profit. The slippery slope must be leveled or flattened otherwise, our Rights and health's will be lost.

At minimum, if drug/vaccine commercials are going to appear on television or radio; it is important that the entire long list of adverse side-effects be given at the very beginning of the ads, while the viewer has their highest degree or capacity to comprehend the warnings and it is imperative that the letters of the words be made bold and not be what is known as, mouse print. The long list of warnings must be made to be said slowly and shown slowly and accentuated for its importance; quickly spoken warnings are not adequately, comprehended. Using fear tactics such as, you will get cancer or some other malady if you do not take this drug or get this vaccination must cease and desist. The repetitive drug taking messages and happy drug taking depictions program us to take drugs when we may not need to. They prey on the young, the impressionable and more programmable. This makes the youth of America much too comfortable about taking drugs or being drug dependent and instills a **subconsciously longing to take drugs; even illegal drugs. The line between prescription drugs and black-market drugs is being blurred or become invisible to those programmed to take drugs.** The take a drug for this and take a drug for that induces prolonged drug takers to not recognize that there is a line between good medicine practice and bad, legal prescriptions and illegal drugs; the vanishing line is so thin, that programmed children consider **illicit drugs okay to take, as part of the program**. The public need not wonder why there is an ongoing ever-increasing drug addiction problem or opioid crisis; **children have been programmed into it. The result is a nation of growing adult drug and vaccine user drones whereas; natural means of wellness is being programmed out of existence as, being bad and/or not safe, despite its true effectiveness and safety.**

The drug industry strategically has a tactic of instilling fear or hysteria into the public to get you to be vaccinated. It creates false epidemics or grossly exaggerates the numbers of those that might have a disease to make a crisis or manufactures a need to be vaccinated; it instills fear and/or hysteria to conform people into being vaccinated. Occasionally, there is a public blitz that an epidemic has broken-out and that there is an imminent need for everyone to rush to be vaccinated. The truth is that there is no real epidemic; only a handful of cases of sickness certainly, not an epidemic emergency and often those that fell sick were those children that were vaccinated. Children who became ill that were not vaccinated often had an underlying condition that made them much more susceptible and/or could not be vaccinated anyway because of health problems. There have been no real epidemics and therefore, no state of emergency. We must not live under a permanent state of emergency; WE MUST BE FREE TO REFUSE VACCINATIONS!

Big Pharma is always advertising that you should be vaccinated more and more. They strongly indicate that you would be at great risk if you do not get injected. Many vaccines efficacy are in doubt and the controversy that surrounds them is suppressed. Many vaccines have only been studied for short periods to determine if they are safe. Gardasil injection is a vaccine that is controversial and has had many claims that it causes injury however, it is hard to find a word negative about it. In fact, higher learned countries such as, Japan and Denmark have all but banned the use of Gardasil and yet, most people considering being shot with Gardasil are not even aware that such, intelligent countries with droves of scientists have decreased use of Gardasil. Moreover, there is a constant

push for unsuspecting Americans to submit to its injection and thereby, grab major money from the outrageous price of Gardasil (at times $600). The false narrative that it is highly effective and that you seriously, risk getting cervical cancer if not injected is constantly used. They push those that have been having sex for some time to get their 3 shots when the vaccine is mostly, a waste since, the individuals have already had sex and therefore, been exposed to human papilloma virus which, Gardasil supposedly, protects against. Although, Japan had nearly a 90% Gardasil vaccination compliance the government wisely, stopped recommending it because of claimed injuries after injection and intelligently thought it best to hold off its recommendation until more research was done. Japan vaccination rate is now almost zero and yet, the cervix cancer rate has not skyrocketed or even somewhat increased. Japan government respond to complaints of injuries whereas, our government does not, as it, has been hijacked by vaccine lobbyists.

Interestingly, there are advanced thinkers that have put it together that unnatural to human vaccine chemicalization is bad for health and life itself. In 1975, Japan eliminated all vaccines for children under the age of 2 and the country's infant mortality rate subsequently plummeted to the lowest level in the world. Japan changed its infant vaccination schedule again in 1995, but it remains one of the least aggressive country in the world for vaccination and yet, Japan's infant mortality rate is remaining low (third in 2009). The United States ranks 34th for infant mortality logically, despite or because of, its high vaccination rate. The Autism rate in Japan is also, far lower than in America and cultures or religions that do not vaccinate such as, the Amish have almost no Autism. If we GET THE CHEMICALS OUT and thereby, vaccinate with SAFER vaccines; the infant mortality rate in America will plummet despite, that we may vaccinate and certainly, the Autism rate will drop to non-epidemic numbers! We need to implement the TWO STEPS OF CORRECTION then; the mortality rate and Autism numbers will drop exponentially.

It is my goal that you gain the knowledge and understanding to discern that unnatural to human biology chemicalization of babies by injection is extremely unhealthy and that you do not rush to inject a vaccine that is not a SAFER vaccine despite, the scare tactics to do otherwise. Scare tactics and purposeful manufactured events such as, what is used to make you submit your children should not deter you from doing your due diligence to make the right decision and best protect your children.

Scare tactics and purposeful manufactured events are used on the public to get people to do things or accept things that are not in their best interest, this is not unusual. An instance of how far the powers that be will go to induce us into action or acceptance of hidden or self-serving agenda is how government used a total fictional event to get us into the Vietnam War, which tragically took so many American lives but filled the greedy pockets of certain corporations. It is confirmed that we were misled into entering the Vietnam War through the false information and/or the outright lie that our ships were torpedoed in the Gulf of Tonkin. Furthermore, the Pentagon Papers published about 30 years ago proved government and/ or Presidents, outright lied to the public about how America is winning the War when it was absolutely known that America was losing and had no realistic chance of winning and thereby, wrongfully sacrificed so many of our young soldiers' lives (58,000 lives lost) for no reason except for profiteering. Yet another shameful tactic is President's Bush's fear tactic and falsehood that weapons of mass destruction were in Iraq, this manipulated the public to support going to War in Iraq; no such weapons were ever found, it was an ASSumption or War inducement fabrication. Many think corporate greed, not America's safety called us to war; money often dictates. President Obama lied when he said, "you can keep your doctor" to manipulate the public into accepting Obama care. The list goes on and on how we are manipulated into doing things that are not in our best interest. In the instant case, of mandated vaccinations; we were told that vaccines are "absolutely safe" or that nothing bad is in vaccines and that vaccines do not cause Autism which, are all lies to make us vaccinate to allow profiting.

The more complex something is the more that can go wrong if the complexity is altered; the human biochemistry and its products are very complex therefore, we must be careful not to upset its normal complexity. Soon, it will become widely, understood that the law of chemistry applies to our human biochemistry and that manipulation of this natural chemistry of health is causing abnormality; CHEMICALIZATIO AUTISM.

We are introducing all kinds of unnatural to human biology chemicals into our vaccines, diet and environment. Nano Titanium Dioxide (TiO_2 NPs) is in sunscreens and consequently enters through the pores of our skin. Nano Titanium Dioxide is also, commonly used in paints to make them white and what is even more horrific it is very often used in foods to make them appear white. All this exposure and/or intake of Nano Titanium Dioxide is further causing us to become chemically compromised and thereby, our biochemistries are no longer health generating. TiO_2 NPs exposure results in microglia activation, reactive oxygen species production, activation of signaling pathways involved in inflammation and cell death consequently, neuroinflammation and brain injury occur, and spatial recognition memory and locomotor activity impairment is also, observed. Recognizing that unnatural to human biology chemicalization is harmful is not enough; strong corrective action to not have this harm in food, vaccines or environment is needed! The slippery slope of unchecked chemicalization must be stopped and reversed!

If you follow the money you will find the madness behind the ludicrous keeping of vaccinations mandated and the crazy anti-safety of vaccine producers having a liability shield. The chemicals in vaccines and the enactment of law, which enslaves parents to submit their children to be injected with these vaccine chemicals is madness to the nth degree. Conscientious parents do not want their children exposed to vaccine chemicals!

There is now indication that government and/or the chemical industry to spray mega-tons of alumina (aluminum) into the atmosphere without the People's consent or knowledge; there has been no precaution for its impact on health. They are spraying from planes creating so called "chemtrails" in an unauthorized feeble attempt at engineered atmospheric climate control supposedly, to offset or prevent global warming. Exposure to chemicals equals abnormal health. Man's chemicalization of the atmosphere will add to the monumental problem of unnatural to the body chemicals that already are finding their way into humans and likely cause further ozone depletion or put our existence or future at risk. Mans, mass intervening with the chemistry of nature will prove to be unwise! Mass unnatural chemicalization of babies, infants and children has already, proven deleterious!

David Keith, GEO engineer from the University of Calgary, when confronted with the question (has there been any studies about the ill-effects of dumping aluminum into the atmosphere, is it harmful to health?) he stated, "We haven't done anything serious on alumina and there could be something terrible that we find tomorrow that we haven't looked at it." The purpose of the aluminum that is dumped into the atmosphere is to reflect the sunlight however; as it falls to the earth it exposes our lungs to this unnatural to the body chemical which, is harmful to human respiration etc., it also, penetrates soil that we grow crops in and pollutes our water supply. The harm from environmental chemicals is massive; making exposure from vaccine chemical injections even more lethal or likely to cause health problems such as, Autism. Look up and see the long lasting chemtrails for yourself and do investigate ALL THE CHEMICALS IN VACCINES. Prevent chemical exposure and you prevent CHEMICALIZATION Autism. The attitude of dumping chemicals into the atmosphere and dumping chemicals into the blood of children through vaccine chemical injections is incredulous and reeks of negligence and the reckless endangerment of welfare. People have a Right to Self-preservation, to be breath in fresh unadulterated clean air and to live undisturbed or unmolested; not having their blood violated by VACCINE CHEMICALIZATIONS or unsuspectingly, breathe in aluminum fallout!

People have the Right to singularize themselves, by individually deciding just what is best for their very own healthcare needs, wants and dislikes. People have a Right to their own unique individuality! Making YOUR vaccination decisions is an integral part of BEING AN INDIVIDUAL. There must not be any legal deterrents or impediments to parent's protecting children; they must be FREE TO REFUSE drug/VACCINE intervention. There is a crucial requirement of government to protect our Rights and stop drug taking inducing advertisements and this requirement desperately needs to be fulfilled. We do not need a Nanny government dictating what drugs or vaccine is to be injected instead, we need a government that is for the People, protecting the People from being programmed into taking drugs or vaccinations. We suffer from ill-conceived governing and chemicalization!

Freedom requires a full, fair, open, transparent and strictly voluntary vaccination program. On the philosophical side, our laws, our religion, our entire culture are based on the belief of the importance of the individual. The mandated vaccination law divests the People of individuality, raping them of their personal vaccination decision; it disallows individual, self-determined vaccination and stifles thinking independently as, individuals. People feel that they are unimportant, mere sheep-people, when they are railroaded into vaccination submission or given no viable choice but to submit their children for unwanted vaccine injection. This egregious law must not prevail; regardless of a person's status they must be treated as, important individuals entitled to make their own health or healthcare decisions. Nanny government's vaccination mandate must be stricken, and people's individuality and/or vaccination decisions must be honored; not ignored or belittled. There must be NO VACCINATION SLAVERY; we need to ABOLISH it!

Take matters into your own hands, decide what is best for you and your children's vaccination healthcare; do not submit to undergo injections of what is too dangerous to inject, be not subdued to be an injected vaccination SLAVE! Know what chemicals are in vaccines, control the risk by being in control of whether the vaccine is or is not administered; demand

SAFER vaccines approved by SAFERvaccines.ORG. The taking of prescription drugs is a chemical exposure that should be considered when estimating the impact or risk of additional chemicalization from the unhealthiest type of chemical exposures; injected vaccine chemicalization. There is a breaking point in which, the risk of vaccine chemical exposure outweighs any benefit to be gained from it. Keep your chemistry pure and you will be optimally healthy; bastardize it or compromise it with unnatural to human biology chemicals and abnormality will result. Parents must be informed and enabled to refuse any chemical exposure. People must be completely FREE to take the inherent risks of vaccination or DENY THE TAKING OF THOSE RISKS; there must be no mandate and/or enforcing and/or enslavement to be vaccinated! The sins of vaccine producers, for their lack of vaccine chemical quality control should not be enforced upon our children. Parents must be FREE to prevent injected chemical exposure!

Not all medical recommendations are in your best interest! Be aware, there are many top selling drugs that can cause major health problems. About two-thirds of people with diabetes, die of heart disease and not diabetes and yet, diabetic patients take a diabetic drug that see a **43% increase in heart attacks** and at the same time can cause a diabetic patient to cause weight gain which, is very ill-advised for a diabetic patient to do. Apparently, Drug Companies and the powers that allow them to be on the market either have a sick sense of what is beneficial or have slated viewpoints because of the mass amount of money being generated by having these drugs on the market. **Drugs may have limited benefit in one area but at the same time contribute to or cause significant health problems. The Chemical influx from drugs is unhealthy when the natural chemistry of the body is thrown off. Potential vaccination benefit compared to actual damage to the perfected biochemistry from the vaccine need control your decision!**

VACCINATION INTOXICATION occurs when the pure chemistry of the blood, brain and/ or body is manipulated by the chemicals found in vaccines. The chemicals within you dictate reactions and the end products of those reactions. Vaccination intoxication and/or infiltration of alien, unnatural to the body chemicals can induce a **CHEMICAL TIPPING POINT, incurring a CRITICAL MASS CHEMICAL SYNDROME that spawns Autism by initiating spontaneous renegade abnormal reaction after reaction. Make abnormal the biochemistry and it renders a developing immature individual very susceptible to becoming AUTISTIC. Vaccine chemicals are destructive to the normal chemical geometric configuration.** We must be **FREE** to self-determine if this risk of vaccination is or is not worth taking and/or if the presented vaccine is a chemically laced vaccine that is too dangerous to inject. Parents must have the fundamental liberty of Parental-determined healthcare in order, to protect their children. We must be **FREE** to choose **SAFER** vaccines and not be enforced or be pressured to vaccinate. Chemicals dictate reactions within our bodies; **we must be FREE to Self-control our chemistry! The vaccine industry needs to be pushed to de-chemicalize; GET THE CHEMICALS OUT!**

It defies logic and credulity to assert that to have unnatural to human biology chemicals in vaccines and mass inject them would not turn children's health promoting biochemistry and effectuate an Autism mass epidemic! Freedom of healthcare choice demands that the People be vested with omnipotent authority over their own body. The People must be endowed to refuse all preventative, non-emergency medical intervention, even if no adverse side-effects exist or are not presently detected. In order, for People to be FREE they need

ultimate, unfettered command over their healthcare and that of their children's welfare. Informed consent/DENIAL enables this and assures that there be liberty of healthcare. Vaccination medical intervention must come in line with this principle and requirement! Freedom to determine what is best for one's health is an inherent liberty; it existed long before manmade vaccination mandate law; it is supreme law!

How safe are the drugs and/or vaccines that are on the market? An important revealing point is that a drug can stay on the market **even if it is causing injuries**. Drugs have a history of staying on the market long after they have been too often accused and/or found to cause serious injury. The correlation between suspect vaccinations and Autism and/or the cause of serious health problems is not surprising, it is just as, unsurprising as, drug chemicalization causing health problems. It is practically, inevitable that vaccines chemicalization cause health problems or adverse side effects especially, with the chemicals have been found in vaccines and that vaccines are injected with full, unabated impact. Apply the basic rule of chemistry to when vaccine chemicals become part of the reactive chemical force within the body; the vaccine chemicals take part in reactions and at times, the alien to the body vaccine chemicals can dictate or have master control over bioreactions with deleterious to health consequences. It is not only logical that alien, unnatural to human biology chemicals cause health problems; **IT IS AN INESCAPABLE CONCLUSION!** The intervention of vaccination has the deleterious feature of harboring negative to health chemical additives that render biochemical reactions abnormal; causing health problems. The revealing fact is, all drugs (chemicals) have **ADVERSE** side effects that are synonymous with health problems or indicate it. **Harm intensity and/or propensity from vaccines is so, much worse because its injected. Babies, infants and children who receive vaccine chemicalization stress their developing or immature systems that are not totally on-line and thus, more susceptible to the negative impact of abnormal chemicalizations.**

Alien, unnatural to the body vaccine chemicals take their negative toll on the developing biological human systems. During the developmental and/or cellular differentiation and then maturation phase the cells are highly vulnerable to abnormal chemicals to the life process, chemicals that are abnormal to the processes disrupt the processes. It is imperative to normal development and health to only have the chemicals that are REQUIRED FOR NORMAL DEVELOPEMENT which, are the BUILDING BLOCKS OF LIFE and/or GOOD HEALTH. The mixing or injection of vaccines chemicals upsets the chemical balance and intricate formula required for optimum health. These unnatural to human biology chemicals are the stumbling blocks of health; it only has negative impact upon health. **Children have fragile chemistries that are extremely susceptible to abnormal chemicalization; do not allow your offspring to be breached and injured by abnormal to the body chemicalization. The goal is to** best protect your children by **prompt**ing **the production of better/SAFER vaccines with the TWO STEPS**.

There will no longer be an irrational and illative desire to mandate vaccines or need to enforce vaccinate people against their will if vaccines are SAFER vaccines; made in accordance with rational production standards which, coincides with vaccines being worthy of parents' informed consent. Basically, vaccines must stand on its own feet, on its own merit; if the public are satisfied with vaccine safety there will be voluntary vaccination compliance. However, if vaccines remain chemical content stupid by keeping the present chemicals that have been found in vaccines then parents logically not vaccinate; they will do what

they think is in their children's best interest. Parents will not remain ignorant after reading this book, they will not be stupid about their children's health; and they will not vaccinate. If they deem a vaccine too dangerous to inject SAFER vaccines, the charity, is all about educating the public and assuring SAFER vaccines; visit the website SAFERvaccines.org or .com for the latest vaccination information; best protect your family. Vaccinations must be strictly, **VOLUNARILY BASED** and pass the **SANITY TEST for vaccine quality** also, known as the **NO BAD CHEMICALS IN VACCINES TEST** and **VACCINE SAFETY TEST. SAFER** vaccines are trustworthy and of quality for parent's to rationally give informed consent. Grass root politics, patient Rights activists, **concerned parents** and the entire drug taking population must **take steps to right what is wrong with the runaway drug taking train and an unneeded, enforced CHEMICAL vaccine program;** and prevent unnecessary mental and physical injuries. Vaccine **CHEMICALIZATION** is the root of the **AUTISM** epidemic!

The body is a bio-factory in which, its products are completely dependent upon the chemicals that we present it. Health is reliant upon a near normal or perfected chemistry; we must respect this chemical make-up, keeping the homeostatic chemistry pure and not subject it to impurity and/or abnormal to human physiology chemicalization. Having unnatural to human biology chemicals in our children's vaccines is unhealthy and its injection is madness and should be considered an act of child abuse. There is a finite range of biochemicals needed to produce optimal health; a chemical geometry of health. Distort this natural chemical geometry and it can spawn Autism so, choose what you allow to enter your body, blood and/or brain wisely! We must be FREE to refuse unwanted chemicalizations; empowered to REJECT INJECTIONS! The fragile immature systems of a baby need not be rendered so, imperfect; choose SAFER vaccines if you vaccinate!

Alert, the ingesting of medications is a concentrated source of chemical exposure. Chemical contents in certain medications are more toxic than others. If a pregnant mother takes medications, the chemicals can pass to the baby being a significant Autism causation factor. When a woman is going through a pregnancy and she ingests medication the mother not only exposes herself to harmful chemicals but also, exposes her developing baby to a more dangerous degree; the baby can become chemically compromised. Once chemically compromised if injected with vaccine chemicals the **CHEMICAL TIPPING POINT** is more probable; a **critical mass chemical syndrome** is more likely, and the hell of Autism be spawned. Just look at the fact, that vaccines contain aluminum and that is enough to give a person pause or proper fear about being vaccinated. Animal and human studies have shown aluminum can cause nerve cell death and that vaccine aluminum adjuvants can allow aluminum to enter the brain, as well as cause inflammation at the injection site leading to chronic joint and muscle pain as well as fatigue. Aluminum is highly conductive and can short circuit the brain and/or cause abnormality.

A fetus is much more susceptible and/or more sensitive to the chemicals than the mother because the fetus is quickly developing, cells are organizing, specializing and/or undergoing differentiation. **Medications that are taken while pregnant such as Paxil, Zoloft, Prozac, Effexor, Celexa, Lexapro and many of the anti–depressants have been accused of being a cause of Autism. Clearly, the primary cause of Autism is chemical!** There should be extreme caution in considering further chemicalization from injecting vaccines for children that were already chemically exposed to chemicals when they were in the womb. **The culmination and/or combination of the two**

types of exposures increase the chances of Autism. Every mother and father should be extremely, apprehensive about altering the natural chemical geometry by drug or VACCINE chemicalization. Control children's chemistry; keep it clean, pure and devoid of unnatural to human biology chemicals and the chances of Autism are reduced exponentially! MAKE NO MISTAKE; CHEMICALS ARE THE ENEMY!

Harmful chemicals pass from the mother through, the placenta, finding its way into the baby. The placenta usually acts like a very efficient natural barrier, not allowing unhealthy particles and/or chemicals from entering the baby however; many drug chemicals make its way through. The quantity of these chemicals is reduced or minimized as it filters through the placenta barrier before reaching the baby however, there is still major cause for concern because the drug chemicals that do pass through, do cause abnormality to some degree. More importantly, and relevant to Autism etiology, is vaccination chemical exposures; its type and degree of entering the child is a much graver exposure danger especially, for babies already chemically compromised by any drugs the mother took that were able to pass through the placenta natural defense.

Vaccine chemicals enter our children's blood and quickly circulate to chemically dope brain cells. Mothers and fathers are always doing everything in their power to protect their children certainly; parents' must be **FREE** to prevent any perceived of chemicalization danger! Let me make this crystal clear, make no mistake about; vaccines injected into our children's blood are the single most devastating cause of Autism. Do not let the **slip**pery slope of vaccinations **slip** your children into **CHEMICALIZATION AUTISM. If an alarm were to ring every time an infant was exposed to harmful chemicals, the alarm would ring the loudest and the longest when vaccination chemicals enter our children's delicate bloodstreams. There is no mother's placenta barrier to diminish the chemicalization.** Vaccinations quantity of chemicals and its ill-effects are not reduced because they are injected directly into the blood. **Vaccination chemicals are not filtered and/or diminished through a barrier or protective filtering placenta; they enter with full negative impact.** The entire vaccination chemical load impact the infant's delicate blood chemistry. **Multiple vaccination exposures are an unnatural chemicalization and are the primary cause of chemical destabilization. Know what chemicals are in vaccines!**

Always remember, that there is a **slippery slope of vaccinations** and that more and more internal chemicalization result. Trust that the **CHEMICALS** in vaccines are unhealthy and do not trust that profit based Drug Companies are going to assure children's welfare and/or safety above their burning need and or mission to make as much money as, possible; know that there are chemicals for profit and not safety in babies, infants and children's vaccines. **Protect your children to the best of your ability; do not let them divest your parental responsibility! The mistake of mandating vaccination, to say the least, compounds the problem of there being unnatural to the human biology chemicals in vaccines; not preventing chemicals for profit, not safety, to be in vaccines. The erroneous law takes parents almost completely out of the vaccination equation or decision and wrongfully treats parents as if they were negligent parents or incompetent to decide what is best for children or best protect them. At minimum, government that is manipulated to do Big Pharma bidding are colluding to disenfranchise parental authority and control over children and expose children to chemicalizations that are not in our children's best health interest and do cause harm. To a large degree it's true; we will not stop being sick until, we stop making ourselves sick!**

Mental illness has been mainly linked to chemicals or chemical imbalance and Autism is becoming mainstream as, caused by the same = CHEMICALIZATION AUTISM! More and more children are taking prescription drugs than ever before and many (perhaps too many) are being infiltrated with depression drug chemicalization. We live in a time when early on in life chemical exposure has become common place and injecting babies with vaccine chemicalization is bombarding children with chemicals that are unnatural to human biology. In many cases we treat mental issues and sometimes normal active children with an array of drug chemicalizations. Parents should reflect on what is causing most, if not all, mental health conditions that are occurring in the very young as, it is CHEMICALIZATION INDUCED! Look to what is a definite source of infiltration of abnormal to the body chemicals as, the main source of children's brain chemistry issues! Vaccine infiltration of its alien chemicals attacks or bastardizes the normal bioreactions of the body and/or BRAIN; injected chemicals are not buffered or minimized. Do not dope babies' brains with vaccines' unnatural to human biology chemicals and you no longer will cause mind chemical abnormality or mind chemical imbalances and then the main cause of depression, mental abnormality and/or CHEMICALIZATION AUTISM will be no longer. Inject only, SAFER vaccines to prevent destabilization of the minds chemistry!

In the world that we live in today the best health advice is to take all necessary precautions to avoid unnatural to human biology chemical exposures and make it your number one priority to avoid injecting your tiny baby, small infant or immature child with such, chemicals. Analysis of your surroundings for sources of chemical exposure is a precaution well-worth taking. We must take the much-required **STEPS OF CORRECTION** to stop harmful chemicals from being placed in vaccines. Informed consent/denial being applied to vaccinations and the holding of vaccine companies liable, by having them pay compensation to those injured by vaccines are part of the **TWO STEPS OF CORRECTION** that will **GET THE CHEMICALS OUT** of vaccines and save children from **AUTISM**. The sure footed, **TWO STEPS will end the AUTISM epidemic**. Recognize that **children are being targeted and conditioned to take drugs**; we must stop this! The drug industry along with its medical care counterpart do a lot of stupid things, from drilling mercury in your teeth, surgically removing children's first line of defense tonsils (tonsillectomy), serving Jell-O in hospitals or other unhealthy food when people are in dire need of the building blocks of health from food and putting chemicals such as, mercury, aluminum and formaldehyde in vaccines. Just as, the tobacco industry continued to cause harm long after, it was known of the harm; many of the medical or Big Pharma mishaps continue at our children's health detriment. The biggest insult of all or most egregious perpetration is the mandate of vaccines especially, vaccines that have any degree of unnatural to human biology chemicals.

There is an overabundance of commercials pushing the public to take drugs and be vaccinated. The promise of drugs or vaccines is controverted by the unnatural to human biology chemicals inherent in them. The continual drug and vaccine commercialization to take this drug for that and that drug for this, day in and day out and day after day, are being seen by children and adults and programs one into taking drugs; children are the most programable. A need to take drugs and/ or making children psychologically dependent upon drugs is instilled. For instance, one of my patients told me that their 10th grade teenager had sex with another 10th grade student and it was drug dependent and commercial stimulated. The drug chemicals we advertise on television and/ or in the media find their way into our children's lives. Besides the obvious concern of premature sexual experience there was a more riveting concern in that the teens reflected that they got the sick idea to take Viagra from television ads. They were induced to take Viagra; it was droned into them from the repetitive drug advertisements, which boasted about longer lasting sexual pleasure with smiles of success and ultimate satisfaction on both the actor' and actress' faces. It was the very first time for the 10th graders; and the first time for intercourse female asked the first time for intercourse male to take the sexual enhancing Viagra to assure sexual perfection; like the commercials promised. The advertised long lasting sexual experience and no anxiety also, helped trigger the idea of having sex on Viagra; like the have sex on Viagra commercials kept promising. Their own biological sexual clock and innate sexual ability would have been ample enough instead, they were robbed of a natural experience; they were manipulated into a drug taking, induced into a drug dependent abnormal sexual experience. Children are trained to take drugs; to be dependent on drugs by all the ads they are bombarded with. Children are being targeted to take drugs just like the tobacco industry targeted children!

These young teenagers were unduly influenced to be drug dependent when there was no medical necessity, producing a harmful mental and physical distortion of what is supposed to be a natural life experience. The teens after their Viagra tainted experience felt nothing like the smiling actors that they repetitively are targeted to see in the drug ads. Constant programming messages are subconsciously, commanding our children to take chemical drugs in order, to be happy; when it is an improper, abnormal sexual experience. Morals and ethics play no role when the Drug industry make up its warping ads. Politicians have been induced to allow such, mind warping ads that are not in children's best interest. **Children need their parents to be in control; not drugs!**

It is interesting that the No.2 cause of sexual performance problems is the taking of prescription drugs itself. A dangerous cycle and treadmill of drug taking, assuring drug producer's profiting, has been perpetrated. How many drug chemical exposures will it take until it causes a major health problem? How many vaccination chemical infiltrations need to be enforced upon your children until parents' standup to protect their children, by stopping it? How many chemicalizations will it take until Autism is spawned? Some parents do not want a single vaccine injected that is laced with unnatural to human biology chemicals and some parents out of duty to follow rules ad regulation choose to chemically compromise their children by allowing children to become vaccine pin cushions for as, many vaccines that there is on the market however, the choice must be yours to make, parents are their children's supreme protectors. How many chemical infiltration insults until a critical mass chemical syndrome takes place, the tipping point between health and Autism; it depends upon what chemicals you are presently being exposed to and how, it also, depends upon your history of chemicalization and/or how chemically compromised you already are. **What is certain; is the injection of vaccine chemicals render children chemically compromised and is gambling with one's health. Parents must have the common decency and fundamental liberty to decide if the risk is worth it or if the risk is just TOO DANGEROUS for their children! Break the programming; decide for yourself!**

How would vaccine producers not know that they were, and still are, putting unnatural to human biology chemicals in our children's vaccines when they are in total control of it or that parents would not object to injecting such, vaccine chemicals as, mercury or aluminum into their babies when no rational caring parent would! It is the reckless endangerment of our children to put chemicals that stress the body or alters the natural biochemistry of the body or is considered unhealthy by most parents, to do so. Because vaccinations are mandated, and informed consent/**DENIAL** does not alert parents to the toxic fact, of what chemicals are in vaccines; it wrongfully enabled or empowered vaccine producers to put such, chemicals in vaccines. All the money spent for the constant barrage of brain washing ads that program people to be vaccinated and not ask questions also, instigated the perpetration upon our children to be exposed to unnatural to human biology vaccine chemicalization. It is all about big business and not safety why vaccines are mandated; and it has spawned vaccines to have chemicals for profit; not safety. Vaccinations are what introduce parents and children to be dependent on doctors. A Pediatrician once told me, "If it were not for vaccinations he would be out of business and that vaccines open a revolving door into his office." **The pharmaceutical industry and doctors all feed off each other and have a vested interest in each other's success. Perhaps this revolving door and all the profit being made from vaccine sales are the main reasons why vaccinations are enigmatically mandated. If it were not profitable to mandate vaccinations it would not be mandated. If enforcing children to be vaccinated did not turn a profit; there would be NO MANDATES; Big Pharma would not be so bent on lobbying for mandates or to keep it so!**

There is evidence, which strongly indicates that the Drug industry has hijacked our government, making it their puppet government and that it also, extends a great deal of over-influence and/ or possible control of the media. It has been determined that their close connection and ties to the mass media such as, the New York Times and many of the television stations has made their advertisement schemes possible and that proper governing has been overshadowed to allow drugs to be constantly, sold on television or media and have it that adults and especially, our children are programmed into drug dependency. Besides the on slaught of the overwhelming, over-abundance of 13,000 lobbyist for Big Pharma; Drug Company board members are too often placed on the board of media giant companies or slither their way into the political influence realm and/or government and land jobs that grant self-serving bias for Drug Companies. In addition, drug selling companies persistent huge financial support to politicians and never-ending lobbying have bulldozed the way for drug companies to advertise as, often and the way they want.

Drug advertisement runaway campaigns program and/or brainwash our children to be drug users and drug dependent. It is as if we won the battle against the tobacco industry for doing this same thing but, lost the big war against the drug industry and its cohorts! Over recent years it has reached the saturation point of continual drug ads that is meant to over influence the fledgling minds of children, programming the innocent into drug taking; no wonder, more drugs are taken by children than ever before and there is a tremendous increase in all types of drug dependency. They wrongfully have been allowed to slowly and clearly state the falsehood that drugs are safe and effective and then at the very end of the ads as, your attention span is much diminished, at a super rapid cadence, much too quickly to comprehend, run off the all-important and ever-growing, longlist of adverse side-effects or health problems that can even include death. Most recognize this for the sham that it is however, it continues despite, its injustice and obvious health detriment!

What gives children or teenagers the idea to take a drug or learn of the drugs claimed benefit is advertisements. The gateway drug into the below drug scourge and other life-taking drugs is not marijuana; it is prescription drugs and all the mental bombardment of prescription ads that push drugs. The problems created by prescription drug advertisements upon the youth of America is pervasive and is made obvious when one recognizes the statistical fact that about 7% of college students report taking the prescription opioid Vicodin (a narcotic) **without a prescription** (Scnick, 2007) and among **12ᵗʰ graders, 8% report taking Vicodin illegally** (Johnston et al, 2010). The drugs advertised are penetrating our youth in a bad way and Drug Companies are not doing enough to protect our young from this threat that it created. This should give you reason to question the integrity of Drug/Vaccine Producers and/or recognize that their purpose is not to assure your children's welfare but rather, secure drug/vaccine sales and/or profits one way or another. **No longer be programmed to take drugs/vaccines somehow, break the deep-seated programming; think freely, to use your intellect to determine what is best for yourself and stop robotically or impulsively take drugs or be vaccinated!**

It is an on-point accusation that Drug companies target the youth of America to create the strong impulse to take their carefully advertised drugs; its ads air when children are watching, even during cartoons. After all a young impulsive prescription drug user of illegally taken non-prescribed drugs readily becomes a common user of prescription drugs when they come of age and/or capacity; and vice versa. More unfortunate, a good percentage of those successfully targeted become drug taking addicts, which adds to the unconscionable profiteering of Drug Companies. Do not blindly place your children's welfare into a life of drugs and vaccinations; be aware that these chemicals cause damage and huge profits are generated. Another unfortunate result of the blitz of drug ads is that patients are telling doctors what drug they want instead, of the proper practice of healthcare taking place where, doctors give their expert opinion and based upon patient need recommend what prescription is best. The ads that fill our minds and control our thoughts with falsehoods is destructive teaching; it needs to be stopped! Puppet government approval of this deception and delusion must end; and **OUR government be restored to us**!

The repetitive drug taking stimuli, as when the same TV commercial is played, gets into children's consciousness and subconscious; brings the drug taking message front and center. This gives our young a distorted perception of what is normal, good and acceptable; creating a conscious and unconscious desire to take drugs, even if it means obtaining it illegally. **Drug Companies are aware of this undercurrent of drug abuse that need to be stopped however, the profiteering from it clouds or corrupts a decisive path to correct what is so, very wrong. Children and adolescents doing drugs is the real epidemic that calls for emergency governmental action; not childhood disease that vaccines continue to inappropriately, be mandated for. The staggering number of drugs and vaccinations prescribed for infants and/or children is at epidemic proportion and is the main gateway to drug abuse, addiction and illicit drug taking. The amount of unnatural to human biology chemicalization that this all induces is problematic and of major cause for parental concern. Our children are in jeopardy and it is up to parents to bring children safely, under parental control to assure no bad chemicals; do not rely upon big business or its puppet government to protect!**

Chemicalization by injection of INFANTS can cause sickness and even DEATH; they really do not know what they are unleashing when vaccine chemicals are injected. The Los Angeles Times, CNN, medicalexpress.com and many others reported that on May 11, 2015 that 2 babies died and 29 were hospitalized hours after being vaccinated; you never know when a vaccine will be so, toxic that it can kill. However, you do know that chemicalization destroys the natural and pure health generating chemistry needed to remain healthy. CHEMICALIZATION AUTISM can be an injection away! Be in self-control of your body

and protect your children from chemical insults. Do not stand for chemical injections if you think it will destroy the vital to health biochemistry; consider, SAFER vaccines! Drugs and vaccines have chemicals that are alien, unnatural to the body therefore, caution and informed consent/DENIAL is are essential. Nothing should stand in the way of parents safeguarding their children from a conceived of chemical harm and/or a vaccination that the parents have determined is too dangerous to inject!

Most if not all people can understand that our children's welfare depends upon having a normal or near normal biochemistry. One innately, knows not to upset, alter, manipulate or bastardize the natural chemistry of one's body and/or the blood chemistry; render abnormal the cellular chemistry of the brain and/or body and expect abnormality. It is not rocket science; it is basic law of chemistry that the chemicals within dictate to our bioreactions. **Chemicalization Autism is a result of one's blood and brain cells becoming chemically impure, creating serious negative to health reactions and/or suffering severe allergic type complications. The presence of harmful chemicals in the blood and/or brain cells interferes with the natural chemical reactions of the body and causes negative to health chemical reactions that are alien to human biology. The occurrence of a critical mass chemicalization syndrome is deleterious chain reactions and/ or abnormal to the body chemical interactions that spawns CHEMICALIZATION AUTISM.** Exposures to chemicals that are unnatural to the body create a life changing abnormality. Pumping such, chemicals into children's blood is playing a horrid ill-health game of chemical, Russian roulette. **Do not allow unwanted chemicalization; know what chemicals are in vaccines and only consider SAFER vaccines! Refer to the web-site SAFERvaccines .org or .com to learn more about SAFER vaccines.**

No one can say for sure just what is being unleashing upon our children when they are injected with the array of unnatural to human biology vaccine chemicals; what is certain, is that it alters and/or denatures the normal biochemistry that is required to be optimally healthy and not be diagnosed with CHEMICALIZATION AUTISM. Universal laws of chemical reactions dictate our bioreactions and/or what results; injected alien to the body chemicals have reactive propensities that cause abnormality. The total extent of damage is not known however, chemical reaction alteration is inevitable. Researchers have concluded that 90 percent of children have anti-health chemicals in their urine. Frequencies of brain tumors in children have risen 21 percent since 1973 and lymphomas are up 30%. We do not need more chemical exposure, we need less; do not inject babies or children with a host of vaccine chemical toxins. **In order, for vaccination to be a rational choice it must be with SAFER vaccines.** Unwisely, government has been hijacked to back the profiteering vaccine industry to directly expose our children's blood and brain cells to harmful chemicals. It is too dangerous to enforce injections of vaccine chemicals. **We should not be placed in the untenable position of having to break the mandated vaccination law in order, to protect children from chemicalization; parents must be free to say "NO" to chemical manipulation or infiltration of their children; there must be no vaccination mandates!**

To know what chemicals have been found in vaccines and that children are being chemically compromise and/or injured by chemically laced vaccinations is more than ample reason to take parental action to protect your children and make sure they GET THE CHEMICALS OUT and/or clean-up vaccines. The chemicals that can be found in vaccines have made chemist's

370

eyebrows rise off their faces in rational concern and warning. Parents are outraged to learn their children are being exposed to vaccine chemical harm. We as consumers of vaccines should act to stimulate the cleaning up of vaccines and we as, **PARENTS MUST BE FREE TO PROTECT CHILDREN FROM BEING CHEMICALLY COMPROMISED. Many of the chemicals of vaccines are the building blocks of disaster, negatively impacting health; causing Autism. The foundation of CHEMICALIZATION AUTISM is laid by such, chemicals. It would be a tragic parental mistake to be the least dismissive about the unnatural to human biology chemicals that have been found in vaccines or remain in vaccines! You best protect your children from Autism by not compromising their biochemistries!**

The universal laws of chemistry obviously apply to the chemicals pumped into our children's bloodstreams when our children are vaccinated. Just like when children combine chemicals or powders in their chemistry sets, setting off bubbling reactions and concoct smelly, gooey by-products so, is true in our children's bloodstreams when vaccine chemicals combine with other vaccine chemicals or these harmful chemicals readily react with the our once natural pure chemistry of the body. Over the short duration of multiple vaccination exposures children's internal chemistry are being manipulated; transmuting a healthy chemistry INTO ONE THAT SPAWNS AUTISM. Different substances react with one another and combine to create free radicals and unnatural renegade reactants, which interfere with the normal biology of the body and thereby, induce abnormality. Health does not come in a needle! Health comes from the inside-out and is totally dependent upon proper chemistry. Do not adulterate your children's biochemistry and they will become healthy adults.

The estimate of how vaccine elements react within our children's delicate blood chemistry or within the cells of the brain is relatively unknown and injecting vaccine unnatural to the body chemicals must be considered experimental at best. To fear vaccines with its unnatural to the body chemicals is unfortunate however, it is a most rational fear instead, of living in fear let us, assure vaccine safety with the implemention of the TWO STEPS OF CORRECTION. Estimates of harmful results could be off, who knows what ill-health effectors are assembled from vaccines' alien, unnatural to the body chemicals. The body's health integrity is dependent upon a range of chemical reactions. Health is generated, by having the right chemistry and thus, the needed bioreaction whereas, health is degenerated, and sickness and/or abnormality become prevalent by having the wrong chemicals and thus, abnormal bioreactions. Over our evolutionary duration we have evolved to have a certain range of, a biochemical homeostasis that is needed for health. It is not hard to rap your head around the concept that vaccine chemicals disrupt this chemical homeostasis unless; you robotically accept and/or do not question chemicalizations. INJECTING MANMADE CONCOCTIONS OF VACCINE CHEMICALS INTO THE NATURAL BIOLOGICAL SENSITIVE CHEMISTRY IS FRAUGHT WITH RISKS THAT PARENTS MUST BE FREE NOT TO HAVE THEIR CHILDREN TAKE!

The fact that vaccine chemicals are accelerated into motion by injection and upon entering into a constant streaming bloodstream is problematic, in that when a net force of motion is applied to chemicals those chemicals state of inertia and/or the state of accelerated chemicals can cause the chemicals to be even more harmful and/or reactive. Accelerated (energized) unnatural to the body chemicals can cause worse abnormal reaction complexity

and cause more severe to health reactions. Temperature, pressure and motion all have effect upon the elements of a reaction and should be thoroughly studied to access plausible threat to health. Our children should not be used as, human guinea pigs in a vaccine chemicalization experiment or unknown consequence. It is a much safer to assume the worst about chemicals being pumped into the bloodstream. A critical mass, chemical syndrome of abnormal renegade chemical reactions can be reached having monstrous health consequences. **It is impossible to accurately predict what health destroying new compounds may form under these conditions or just how it interferes with the needed normal chemical reactions and/or bioproduction's. Anti-health chemicals must never be in vaccines or be injected!**

If you want the best for your children and I'm sure that you do or want them to have the greatest chance at optimum health and less of a chance of becoming a victim of CHEMICALIZATION AUTISM; you want the most competent chemistry for your children's biology, a chemistry that assures health! Safeguard your children's vital chemistry by making sure it is not chemically denatured or compromised especially, by the injection of alien to the body chemicals! Having unnatural to human biology chemicals in vaccines make it unacceptable to inject. Only consider **SAFER** vaccines for injection! It is difficult to accurately determine the negative consequences of unsafe vaccines, not only over the span of time that they are given but rather, over the lifetime of the vaccine recipient. The cumulative unnatural to the body chemicals from all the multiple shots can react with one another and must react with the once normal biochemistry; this needs to be thoroughly, analyzed, studied and understood! **The list of adverse side-effects and harms from vaccinations continues to grow over time and experience. It is a real sobering thought to realize that the mandated vaccination law is enforcing chemicalization of unnatural to the body chemicals upon our children.** The more our children are being exposed to the multiple vaccinations of non-**SAFER** vaccines; the more of these harmful chemicals will penetrate their vital systems and brain cells. The total consequences and/or harms that result from injecting vaccine chemicals may never be fully understood however; even if the harm it is not yet proven or understood **parents must be FREE to protect their children from such, chemically laced vaccines. The slippery slope of mandated vaccination has resulted in MASS CHILD ABUSE BY CHEMICALIZATION.**

Vaccine advocates are continually proven wrong about vaccination safety. When enforced vaccination was first perpetrated upon the people; vaccine producers and its advocate cohorts were grossly mistaken or had purposely, disseminated a major falsehood that vaccination was "absolutely safe". Time has proved their mistaken **ASS**umption or misleading representation very wrong or an outright lie. Either way, vaccines should never have been mandated under such, a falsehood or lie. Vaccines do cause injury and have been found to have chemicals that are too dangerous to inject. **Biochemists recognize the danger of such, chemicals in vaccines and more importantly, more and more parents do! Certainly, vaccines could be a lot SAFER and parents want what is SAFER for their children and that is why SAFER vaccines' the charity, has as its primary mission the achievement of SAFER vaccines by the TWO STEPS OF CORRECTION. Please, become logic stricken about what chemicals are in vaccines and its danger to your children; protect your children accordingly!**

Big Pharma has become much too big, too powerful; and absolute power corrupts absolutely. If you think the pharmaceutical industry has your back or is looking after your best interest

think again! Just look at the opioid crisis of prescription drugs such as, Vicodin and other even more harmful chemicalizations; 150 people a day are dying from opioid overdoses obtained from pill mills or doctors that do not really examine the patient before giving the drug addict their prescription. Of course, the pharmaceutical companies know where its drugs are being sold or whom is a likely candidate for over dispensing. Most, if not all Big Corporate decisions are based on money; not safety unless the liability exposure is too great! Once again, it is obvious that negligence law must be steadfastly applied, and high awards given to curtail negligence and prevent unneeded injuries. The real epidemics that need to be fought are those created by Big Pharma and its puppet government and that includes the Autism epidemic that is spawned by all the chemicals for profit, not safety, in vaccines. Those same people responsible for or complacent with the opioid epidemic are the same characters responsible for the Autism epidemic or complacent with our babies being injected with unnatural to human biology chemicalizations. Your children need your help to survive! Parents need to be empowered with informed consent/DENIAL to adequately protect their children. Parents need to be freed up to get their children off the slippery slope of mandated vaccinations. We need a total voluntary vaccination system and one that allow parents to choose SAFER vaccines!

The superabundant and redundant competent reports from parents on the bad reactions from vaccines, proximate to their children being vaccinated is an alarm that has been ringing loud and clear for a long, long time; way too long a period for nothing major to be done about it on the part of vaccine producers or its puppet government. No, those responsible for vaccine contents or its ridiculous enforcement are not looking after our best interest. Many doctors are not even reporting when parents claim their children were injured after vaccination. The history of vaccinations shows that vaccines have chemicals that cause signs and symptoms and/or a gamut of health problems. The fact, that the courts have found that vaccines have caused major injuries that called for victims of vaccine induced injuries to be awarded about a **BILLION DOLLARS** (that's right a **BILLION DOLLARS**) is testament to how unsafe vaccines really are. In addition, the fact, that Big Pharma did the unconscionable by manipulating our legal system so, that it does not pay anything when vaccines do injure, is testament that Big Pharma is self-serving, not at all interested in doing what is right and that vaccines are indeed, unsafe and too dangerous to inject. It strongly indicates that vaccines do cause so, many injuries that the profit minded vaccine producers were concerned about its cost to the company for its negligence that it did the unconscionable and unprecedented by manipulating a self-serving total liability shield were tax dollars pay instead, of who should rightfully pay, Big Pharma. **Make no mistake, vaccines injure and CHEMICALIZATION AUTISM is an injury!**

Once abnormal to body, chemically laced vaccines are injected into the body and blood of a baby it **very quickly circulates throughout the entire body; becoming a SYSTEMIC CHEMICAL EXPOSURE that induces biochemical and metabolic disturbances. When these chemicals reach the brain the brain cells are doped with these alien chemicals and it takes its toll on brain cellular metabolism and function. Exposure to multiple vaccination episodes can have a higher probability of causing a chemicalization mass syndrome than a single exposure however, one can be problematic enough and be devastating to one's health; making optimum health impossible and Autism a much higher probability. Biochemical and metabolic alterations deserve the same emphasis as has been assigned to overt**

pathological manifestations. We must be FREE to stop chemicalization of OUR children! To have it that vaccine industry has unfettered power to put whatever, it wants in vaccines and a total liability shield from liability is subject to abuse; like we are seeing by vaccines having unnatural to human biology chemicals. Parents do not want such, chemicals in vaccines or to be injected into babies. This abuse of power must be stopped!

A systemic exposure can elicit adverse responses at the cellular level or tissue functional levels; having deleterious impact. Abnormal chemicalization can impair physiological activities within the cells of the heart, lungs, blood, nerves, **BRAIN** and can negatively impact immune competence. **Abnormal to the body chemicalization should give parents pause, sparking parents to research what chemicals are in vaccines and recognize what injuries can occur from the unnatural chemicalization. Parents should be consumer advocates for SAFER vaccines by insisting that the vaccine producers remove such, chemicals from vaccines and demand the common healthcare requirement and human dignity of informed consent/DENIAL. Before considering injecting any vaccine into your children's vital systems, protect your children by refusing any vaccine that you deem too chemically unnatural to the body and too dangerous. In addition, vaccine producers must become accountable and financially liable for vaccination induced injuries in order, to promote better, SAFER vaccines for the sake of all children's welfare. If we don't keep children from being chemically compromised; health and life itself, can be in the balance.**

There are 3 natural portals of entry into the body; the skin, lungs and the digestive system. However, vaccine chemicals do not enter the body through these normal channels; **they are injected directly into the body**. The body has no inborn design or innate intelligence and/or built in ability to select the good from the bad chemicals that enter in this abnormal way; the body cannot diminish or eliminate the chemicals of harm from the injection of chemicals whereas, chemicals that attempt to penetrate internally from the normal 3 natural portals all have a sort of speak, quality control over what can penetrate and/or become part of the bio-chemistry. For example, digestion slowly breaks down what is in the digestive system and eliminates bad chemicals; chemicals not indigenous or utilized by the body are **defecated and urinated out. Chemicals of vaccines can immediately circulate to the brain cells; its impact is unabated. One should not consider a vaccine if it has unnatural to the body or what you deem to be toxic chemicals! One should only consider a SAFER vaccine for injection!**

There has been no sufficient research study done on the effects of being exposed to multiple vaccinations; not over the short-term nor the long-term. This indicates that children whom undergo multiple vaccine **CHEMICALIZATIONS** are subject to unknown results; like lab rats or guinea pigs in a long-term experiment. The chemicals from one vaccine must react within the body and of course, the chemicals of the multiple injected vaccine **CHEMICALIZATIONS** must react with not only the natural biochemistry of the body but rather, all the of the unnatural to human biology from all other vaccine **CHEMICALIZATION.** How all these chemicals from vaccinations react with the body and with each other over time is a study that desperately needs to be thoroughly investigated. Children deserve the very highest level of safety for vaccines and parents need to assure vaccines contemplated for injection do not have anti-health chemicals. We must prevent the **slippery slope of vaccinations** from violating our Rights and that they do not expose children to injury from chemicalizations. **The SANITY TEST FOR VACCINE SAFETY will help assure children are not**

chemically exposed and secure children's safety. It is negligent to expose children to vaccine injections that are tainted with **chemicals that are unfit for human health. Chemicals that have been found in vaccines are not safe for injection and would not pass the SANITY TEST FOR VACCINE SAFETY and/or parental scrutiny.**

The magnitude of upsetting the intricate, finite, natural balance of the blood and/or brain cell's chemistry is off the scale of health destruction. It does not take a genius to realize the obvious dangers inherent with receiving such, chemically laced vaccines. Even if the hard evidence has not yet been accumulated or our technology is not yet advanced enough to exactly determine all the negative to health impact upon children's delicate systems; parent's Right to protect their children from chemical infiltration must rein supreme. There is no one in the vaccine industry that possesses a gift of being all knowing or has an unprecedented predictive power to determine what is the consequence of injecting chemicals, that are not natural to the chemical make-up of the body or that are alien to the biological chemical reactions of the body. Parents cannot be expected to allow the injection of chemically laced vaccines of unknown consequences or be expected to rely upon vaccine producers. Parents must not have to beg and plead for vaccines that have no unnatural to the body chemicals! Parents must be FREE to refuse unwanted vaccines! Parents need to be FREE to protect their children from chemicalization harm and/or CHEMICALIZATION AUTISM! Vaccines need to have chemicals for health and not have chemicals for profit or be unnatural to human biology chemicalizations. A result of the mandated vaccination law is that we cannot refuse an unwanted vaccine, and this turns our children into chemically injected human guinea pigs by subjecting them to an ongoing chemicalization experiment. It MAKES VACCINES UNSAFE because vaccine producers are free to put whatever chemicals it wants or chemicals for profit in vaccines. It is unjust that you cannot refuse it! Be aware of what is in vaccines; prevent injury! Be a proponent of vaccines having no chemicals for profit in them; consider SAFER vaccines!

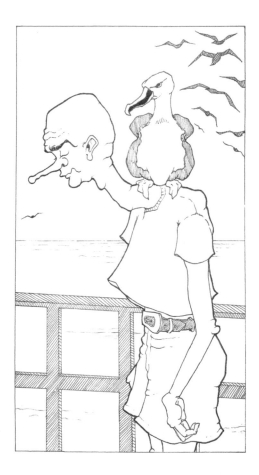

The negative to health adverse effects from being injected with a vaccine containing unnatural to human biology chemicals burdens your vital biochemistry and is like carrying a huge albatross on your shoulders. Abnormal chemicalization = abnormal reactions = ABNORMALITY.

Although, there is a web of causative chemical factors that spawns **CHEMICALIZATION AUTISM**; it is the injected source of chemicals that infiltrate into our babies or children's quickly developing systems that is of primary etiology and concern. There should be biological monitoring performed after vaccination delivery. Specimens routinely used for biological monitoring include blood and urine, saliva and hair. Parents need to be acutely aware to look for the signs and symptoms of injuries from chemicalization. Fever, rash, convulsion, inconsolable crying, starring and the lack of smiling, laughing, playing and loving after vaccination are telltale signs of unnatural to the body chemicalization and/or toxic reaction. Parent's observations of their children's health declining after vaccination needs to be given the importance and significance it warrants. Is it wise and called for, in the face of an epidemic of Autism, to more accurately research the signs and symptoms after vaccination? Clearly, vaccination chemicalization is the main cause of Autism and/or that vaccine chemicalization injections is an **AUTISM PLAGUE** maker. Chemicals of vaccines are not part of the body's **HEALTH EQUATION**. Certainly, the worst of the bad chemicals must be immediately removed! Because there is an Autism epidemic and since, parents are rationally concerned about the consequences of injecting chemically laced vaccines, extensive competent research should be performed regarding the health risks of injecting any vaccine chemicals. Vaccine producers must remove the unnatural to human biology chemicals for profit from vaccines. Vaccine chemicals are a direct hit against health; they enter the blood to immediately interact and upset the normal chemistry of the body and chemically dope the brain cells.

Mandated vaccination proponents' strong efforts to mandate more and more vaccines and to assure everyone must be vaccinated are backfiring. Of course, assuring vaccination compliance equals assurance of money generated from vaccination. The pro vaccination lobbyists have been having such, free rein at mandating more and more vaccinations and at closing down legitimate ways not to be vaccinated that they have been given enough rope to hang themselves; much of the public is so, outraged that a mass movement to rightfully ABOLISH VACCINATION MANDATES is well underway. For example, there is growing outrage over California's recent law that vaccinations are not only mandatory to enter public school but now also, private school. Californians no longer have the option to pay for private school to not subject their children to unwanted vaccine chemicalization that parents deem as, too dangerous to inject. They have no way out of not injuring their children with injected chemicalizations; this is cornering parents to come out swinging to protect their children from unwanted vaccine poisons. People who strongly oppose being chemicalized and violated by the result of this all-inclusive vaccination mandate are in mass becoming awoken; it has woken a wave of parents, a woken sleeping giant of freedom fighters and/or parents that insist upon protecting their children from vaccine chemicalizations. People are left no choice but to right the wrong! No one wants to have to defend themselves however, parents that once chose private school to avoid confrontation or vaccine war are now left no choice but, to right the wrong or injustice by ABOLISHING VACCINATION SLAVERY and protecting children's chemistry.

The slippery slope of mandated vaccination is increasing to a point that non-State entities such as, New York City has slipped in an illegal mandate of a vaccine that the State does not even mandate (the Flu shot). NYC Board of Health and Mental Hygiene's 2015 decree that all children in pre-school and daycare regulated by the City of New York MUST GET ANNUAL FLU SHOTS. Now, this is especially disturbing because Flu vaccines usually have thiomersal, the mercury derivative despite the fact, that Big Pharma and its puppet autocrats know that it has been forbidden to have such, a toxic element, chemical or compound in vaccines. Vaccines for children have been mandated to be produced without mercury however, due to the fact, that the Flu shot was never mandated or considered a childhood vaccination it was not included in the SAFER vaccine mandate that has no mercury. That means the bone head puppet politicians of Big Pharma that rallied to mandate the Flu shots for kids are knowingly exposing our children despite it has already been decreed illegal to do so, with mercury.

If you want to read the bloviation and over pontification of the case surrounding the attempted erroneous Flu mandate it is Garcia v. NYC Board of Health and Mental Hygiene. Thus far attorney Aaron Siri representing a group of parents have prevailed in Supreme Court (New York's lowest court) and in the higher court of the Appellate Division, where Siri won 5-0 that the mandate to suffer preschoolers with a Flu shot is unenforceable. The ruling so far, is that the City cannot impose vaccine mandates in addition to the vaccines mandated by the State. Beware, the slippery slope is attempting to cause our children to be stuck with more needles and injected with chemicalizations; even, vaccines that have the toxin mercury that is totally inconsistent with valid law not to have mercury laden vaccines injected into children. These parents were not asleep at the wheel of caring for children and prevented a disaster of chemicalization harm to all our children! Hold everything, children are still in grave danger because the profiteering-based Flu vaccination advocates stubbornly, had a last chance appeal, to the highest court of New York State, the New York Court of Appeals on 6/6/18. Money may end up dictating after all instead, of common sense, parental rights and keeping children safe from vaccines that are poisonous! It is obvious that the REAL MAIN ISSUE for parents that hired this legal creative strategist is that parents must be FREE to refuse vaccines that that the parents deem are too dangerous to inject and not that the City or a municipality has no Police Power to mandate additional vaccines that are not already mandated by the State. The REAL MAIN ISSUE needs to be litigated to set us FREE and protect all children! So, just to make it abundantly, clear; it is settled law that when it comes to childhood vaccines they must not have mercury and yet, carelessly and callously the Flu shot that often has mercury was erroneously mandated to be injected into all preschool children. Do not let your children slip into unwanted negative to health, unnatural to human biology chemicalizations! Do not let the slippery slope of vaccination slip your child's health away!

What's next, will Big Pharma instigate Flu shots for hospital employees, oh wait a minute; they already have! What's next, you cannot go to the hospital to visit someone unless you carry proof that you had the current (shot in the dark Flu shot) or must wear some horrible mask that will scare the patient that you intended to visit or worse; they will not admit the patient into the hospital because of some Flu mandate and/or that the person in dire need of hospital care is not vaccinated. **The slope is getting so, slimy that people will no longer stand for it**! What's next, will they try to mandate who knows how many vaccine shots including the Flu shot for adults in senior citizen homes. What's next, will Big Pharma attempt to manipulate government officials to assure all places where people gather in numbers that attendees must be vaccinated. Imagine, you go to enjoy a ball game and you must prove you have been vaccinated otherwise, stick your arm out to be injected with the Flu shot or any other vaccine chemicalization concoction they require. "No, no, no", you say, well think again; is the mandating of the Flu shot for perfectly healthy children that gather so, drastically different? Are mandating vaccinations for old people that gather, whom likely have failing health even more appropriate? The real reason why Flu shots are not mandated all over the place for adults is because **adults would not put up with it**; we would consider it an egregious **violation to our most fundamental Right of being in control over our health**. Parents' need to become just as, concerned about the control over their children's health!

They will not be able to convince you; that your tiny baby, your small infant and/or your very young child will not be in placed in danger from alien, unnatural to the body chemicalization! The theorized benefit of vaccination does not erase its known adverse side–effects nor does it ward off all the logical ill-health effects of being subjected to repeated vaccine chemicalizations. **Do not be misled; warding off a theoretical and/or an unlikely severe childhood disease should not deter parents from keeping their children safe from bad for health chemicals. Parents' FIRST concern should be about what chemicals are in vaccines that are being contemplated for injection! Be sure you do the all-important evaluation of what chemicals are in the vaccines.**

Choose SAFER vaccines! If vaccines have unnatural to the body chemicals logically, you should refuse. Parents need to control the health destiny of their children and in doing so have the omnipotent power to deny an unwanted vaccination. Parents' being in ultimate control of children's well-being is the natural order and is required to assure vaccines are safer; this is in the best interest of all our children!

To maintain a completely balanced metabolic system, one that promotes health not Autism, it is necessary to eliminate the injection of unnatural to human biology chemically laced vaccines. Your children stand a much higher chance of not being autistic if not chemically compromised or if you eradicate the net force effects or harmful influence of such, chemicals. The presence of these unnatural body chemicals has physical properties that alter their surroundings and its chemical propensities cause abnormality. Such, vaccine chemicals all have alien to the body molecular and magnetic properties and/or forces that negatively impact one's natural molecular biology and thereby, take its unhealthy toll. The chemical's physical presences and their invisible forces govern how our internal biochemistry interacts; transforming and resulting in abnormality and/or an abnormal metabolism. Vaccine chemicals are an identifiable unnatural to the body chemical source that we can zone in on to remove from vaccines rendering vaccines much SAFER. Parents must be assured that there will no longer be such chemicals in vaccines and should never consider exposing their children to alien to the body chemicalization. Parents must not be coerced or enforced to vaccinate, ABOLISH VACCINATION SLAVERY!

We all have a magnetic signature or magnetic field and the body has a natural magnetic range. Magnetic fields have influence on our cells, tissues, organs and systems. It is wise that the headboard of your child's bed is not against the wall where the main power lines enter the house. Anything that destabilizes the body's natural magnetic field or resonance will cause abnormality. Injecting chemicals that are foreign to the body and/or heavy metals disrupts the needed normal magnetic field. Abruptly, manipulating the magnetic character of the brain tissue through vaccine chemical injection produces a magnetically induced brain fog and/or a magnetic disruption that is destructive to brain function and is an etiology of Autism. Do not let your children's magnetic fields be manipulated by chemicals that should not be in the body. To best protect the health of your babies do not let them wear sleepers that have magnetic closure buttons especially, sleeper magnetic closures adjacent to their heart. Wisely choose traditional buttons or snaps to secure your child's clothing instead of exposing your infant to foreign magnetic field influences. Exposing children to magnets adjacent to the body is not health wise; exposing children to alien to the body magnetic signatures from injected unnatural to the body chemicals is sheer madness.

The accepted concept of attractive forces offers a means by which large objects can build up from smaller moving chemicals and/or particles that float and move in the bloodstream. Each chemical not only has its characteristic molecular attractive and repulsive forces but has a mass that also is a force of attraction. This cumulative force of attraction and/or chemical molecular interactive force from the foreign to the body chemicals of vaccines cause abnormal attraction interactions, forming unhealthy biological reactions. In addition, the natural homeostatic chemicals, normally found in the blood combine with the injected unnatural to the body chemicals to form renegade reactions. We must clean-up vaccines for our children's health sake. **TWO STEPS OF CORRECTION** is required to rid vaccines of chemicals. Parents must never fall asleep at the wheel of control; they must protect their children from **denaturing chemicalization**.

The future healthcare will strongly recognize the importance of electromagnetic forces upon health, in its negative affects upon health and in its positive treatment of disease. The **chemical entanglement** created by the infiltration of unnatural to the body chemicals from vaccine injections dilutes, corrupts and denatures the natural chemistry of the bloodstream and/or the body. The entangled with these chemicals originate from being vaccinated with chemical laced vaccines. **Parents need to take into consideration the electrical and magnetic effects that can be generated by this introduction of these alien to the body vaccine chemicals.**

The injected unnatural to the body chemicals change the normal electric and magnetic field immediately surrounding these chemicals, there also, can be changes more distant from these chemicals. The normal chemistry of the blood and the functions that take place within the bloodstream are disturbed, distorted and/or become abnormal. Each chemical has its own signature electromagnetic resonance and/or electrostatic force, having effect upon its surroundings. There is an electromagnetic wave radiating outward from each alien chemical, like the ripples from a pebble or rock tossed into a pond, these ripples of energy interfere with normal function, production, reactions and/or homeostasis within. British physicist Michael Faraday developed the now widely accepted concept that electric and magnetic forces are intermediaries that enable electric and magnetic forces to be conveyed through space, in the instant case the space is the bloodstream.

As these foreign to the body chemicals travel in the bloodstream they are a **MOVING CHARGE.** The moving charge makes it next to impossible to pinpoint but their impact broadens as they travel throughout the bloodstream. The foreign chemicals move within the flow of blood of the bloodstream **producing abnormal changing electric and magnetic fields throughout the course and space of the bloodstream, disrupting the normal fields of the chemicals, molecules, elements and/or compounds natural to the bloodstream. In the bloodstream an abnormal fluctuating magnetic field result. Changing magnetic fields induce electric fields and creates abnormality and resultant health problems.**

Electromagnetic waves flow from foreign to the body chemical sources, forming an electromagnetic radiation and vibration that is detrimental to health. Electromagnetism acts over an incredible wide range of distances, from the very minute scale of atoms within to the molecules of the blood, to the large proteins that are produced within the body and to the colossal span of the organs and muscles. **Unnatural to the body chemicals infiltrating into children disrupts their endocrine and neurological development. Parents have become inundated with all the vaccine dosages their children are enforced to endure; they are overwhelmed by the sheer magnitude of unnatural to the body chemicalizations and the frequent visits to the doctor's office to subject children to all the chemicalization denaturing's! At all costs, we must halt the slippery slope of vaccinations and GET THE CHEMICALS OUT!**

Chemical entanglement and its electromagnetic radiation induce abnormal changes in the body and **IN THE BRAIN.** It is health wise and health essential to **get the chemicals out of vaccines**. There is no controlling reason to inject children with the chemicals that have been found in vaccines. Children's health must not be placed in jeopardy by injected chemical anti-health agents; there must be safety first in vaccines before a vaccine can be suggested for injection. **The SANITY TEST and safety measure of parents being FREE TO REFUSE an unwanted chemical vaccine injection must rule over vaccinations; this assure safety! To have it that parents cannot refuse what they think is an unsafe vaccine places their children in grave danger of vaccine induced injuries. To have that anyone other than children's parents have the controlling power to decide what is best for their children and/or decide upon the vaccination debacle undermines the well-established RULE OF LAW THAT PARENTS PROTECT THEIR CHILDREN BY DECIDING UPON HEALTHCARE.**

Without question, the safety of our children must permeate in every decision as, to what chemicals are to be in vaccines; the fact, that unnatural to human biology chemicals have routinely been found in vaccines shows beyond a doubt the gross systemic problem that exists in vaccine production and/or in those whom are supposed to be and should be, held accountable and responsible for what our children are injected with. The obvious bias in decision making as, to what chemicals are in vaccines, when it impacts how much money is generated or saved by Big Pharma makes it abundantly, clear that parents who are the natural decision makers for their children's welfare and whom are by the norm rule of law are the healthcare decision makers' must also, be the vaccination decision makers. Only the potential vaccination recipient or the parents of potential recipient children, by natural Right, should be empowered to accept or **DENY** vaccinations! **Chemical entanglement should not be forced upon our children. Freedom of healthcare decision must apply to vaccinations** just as, it evenhandedly is applyied to all other healthcare. Enigmatically, informed consent and/or freedom to refuse healthcare presently, do not apply to vaccinations. **We need to in source not outsource the vaccination decision and/or responsibility; it must be a parental or a family decision! Mandated vaccinations are repugnant to the Constitution and to our fundamental parental Rights and/or authority. We must overcome the oppression of mandated chemical infiltration by becoming absolutely, FREE to protect our children from the vices of medicine! LIBERTY TO PROTECT CHILDREN MUST BE YOURS!**

There is now incontrovertible proof that the claim that vaccinations are good for our children's welfare is fundamentally flawed because of their present unnatural to the body chemical content. Vaccinations can be a gift to mankind if they are cleaned-up and based upon informed consent/ **DENIAL.** The present state of vaccinations alters the normal environment of the bloodstream, which trickles down to a negative to health environment for cells of the body. Each of us has approximately fifty trillion single cells and the single cells and the entire communities of **cells are controlled by their awareness of their environment. Create an abnormal cellular environment and you spawn abnormal cellular activity.** A cell's life is not so, much controlled by its genes but rather, by the cells **chemicals** and energetic environment. The new cutting-edge science fields of **SIGNAL TRANSDUCTION and EPIGENETICS proves genes are turned on and off and/or cells functions are being directed by environmental signals that regulate command and propel life. It is imperative to eliminate alien chemicals from the vaccines injected into children's natural internal environment to assure normal genetic expression.**

Epigenetics has shown that modifications to proteins called histones that hold DNA together turn your genes on by removing a molecule called methyl (carbon-hydrogen molecule) and turn your genes off by adding a molecule of methyl. Exposure to toxins in the environment such as, the vaccine toxins that are injected into the bloodstream can cause these modifications. **Changes to these proteins are called Epigenetics.** The word Epigenetics means on top of the genome. **New study's results indicate that a person's life span can be altered by altering the individual's internal chemical environment** and the health of the individual can also, be manipulated. **Chemical doping of the brain cells by injecting anti-health, vaccine chemicals grossly manipulates the environment in and around the brain cells causing malfunction.**

There is the possibility that mass vaccination with unnatural to human biology chemicals is not just causing immediate harm to the vaccine recipient but rather, could be setting a genetic distortion into motion that can lead to chemicalization Autism becoming genetic. The alien to the body chemicals of vaccines, which are injected into our children's environmentally sensitive blood chemistry abnormally alters the health generating environment that our genes and/or our cells are regulated and/or commanded by and thereby, instigate abnormal and/or unhealthy genetic and/or cellular expression. There is a possibility that the **health and life span** changes that are **triggered by prolonged changes to one's internal environment** can be **transmissible between generations.** Findings suggest that there is **EPIGENETIC INHERITANCE** that is not encoded by the genome that is still **transmissible between generations.** Because Autism is largely caused by the changed environment from vaccine chemicals; it suggests **Autism** may become **transmissible** and/or able to be passed from generation to generation (genetic) and without further exposure to more toxins. We may find that when Autistic couples have children; their children might also, be Autistic.

Signal Transduction science studies the biochemical pathways by which cells respond to their environmental cues. Environmental signals alter gene expression and thereby, control cell function, output and fate. An individual cannot remain optimally healthy when foreign to the body chemicals are placed in the bloodstream and/or cellular or gene environment. The cutting-edge science of Epigenetics studies how **environmental signals control genes**. These new sciences and awareness reveal how **CHEMICAL signals select, regulate and modify gene activity**. Epigenetic insights have revealed how the environment controls gene activity in stem cells, this is of interest because stem cells in a developing human must differentiate normally to be healthy and **vaccines laced with alien, environmentally changing chemicals, interferes with normal stem cell function and/or differentiation. Stem cells differentiate to various kinds of cells as, nature deems necessary in the developing human.** The indoctrination that we are all **helpless victims of our genetic disposition is now been rendered less controlling and is an antiquated theory** by this new leading-edge science. Keeping your internal and external chemical environments as, pure and/or health promoting as, possible has **controlling impact on our genes, cells and overall health. Autism could have a genetic trend, mass exposures to all the multiple vaccines chemical injections overtime; may SET A GENETIC TREND. The slippery slope of vaccination may cause a new genetic weakness abnormality; AUTISM!**

It is intellectual dishonesty to say that it is best for children to be vaccinated when the vaccines that they are injecting expose children to unnatural to human biology chemicalizations. Such, vaccines chemicals morph the blood chemistry and then the cell chemistry and eventually the environment that comes to contact with the genes. Abnormal to human biology chemicals distort the homeostatic environment that regulates our children's genes, manipulating the environment not to be in life's harmony or best interest and thereby, creates a life struggle and/or Autism. The nuts and bolts of life no longer are commanded to build health but rather; cause destructive abnormality. The very foundation of life is upset by injecting alien chemicals that manipulate, alter, morph and/or bastardize our children's internal sacrosanct chemical environment. The vaccination industry must reflect these new science revelations and **GET THE CHEMICALS OUT;** for the sake of public safety. The **TWO CORRECTIVE STEPS** will protect the public from the for profit, vaccination chemical industry and the now antiquated vaccination system; assuring **SAFER** vaccines and no enforcement of unwanted **vaccinations**.

Hopefully there is no Autism gene to speak of at least not as, of yet; there is only an environmental genetic command. Genes get turned on and off by their environment. The more generations that are unwisely exposed to vaccine alien chemicals as, generation after generation have their environment that regulate their genes abnormally manipulated with vaccine unnatural to human biology chemicals, the more at risk and/or the greater likelihood that there will be a creation of an Autism causation gene (Autism gene). What I am alluding to is that Autism may become hereditary if vaccinations continually chemically expose children generation after generation. A genetic Autism weakness can result from mandated, continual vaccination chemicalizations. If a genetic weakness exists in a child that renders one much more susceptible to Autism, then that child will have more of a tendency toward becoming Autistic and the genetic proclivity to be Autistic may need less chemical exposure to render that child Autistic. This is like when diabetes runs in the family; a child does not have to consume tons of sugar to become diabetic. Health wisdom is needed when formulating vaccines; do not chemicalize your babies!

How many generations of exposure must occur for a genetic factor and/or an Autism gene hereditary trait is unknown. If Autistic people breed with Autistic people and in addition, their children are again exposed to alien vaccine chemicals, then the possibility and/or the probability of the creation of an Autism gene becomes more probable or exponential. The bad news is that we have arrived at a point that vaccination chemicals have permeated through the population due the mandated vaccination program and vaccine producer's callous insistence upon using chemicals in their vaccines is the main cause of the chemicalization Autism epidemic. WARNING: Autism has permeated through the masses and now puts Autism on the brink of becoming hereditary. **The good news is that we have become aware that unnatural to the body chemicalization is the enemy and we can act to clean-up vaccinations and not disrupt the health promoting natural environment and thereby, prevent an Autism genetic disposition.**

Once our cellular function has been altered, once our genes have become regulated by the changed environment, once the resultant abnormal processes ensue and/or once Autism has taken root and taken over the individuals' life there is a probability that the Autism may spawn into a genetic trait that can be passed down to other generations. Children of Autistic parents could be what biologists call, **hard wired for Autism**, highly likely, to become Autistic and able to **pass it on to the next generation**. The lesson here is to recognize that injecting vaccine chemicals that are alien to the body causes abnormality and can trigger abnormal genetic expression and that continued generation after generation of abnormal genetic expression will likely cause a genetic mutation and/or genetic producing gene given time. Another factor in producing a genetic Autism tendency is if Autistic couples procreate. The future is shaky on the slippery vaccination slope!

There are some scientists that caution that it is unhealthy to inoculate with fugal poisons known as, mycotoxins. There is evidence mounting that mycotoxins which enter the body can destroy one's good health and even be life threatening. The resulting fungus destroys the integrity of the tissue it infests. Heavy metal residues are examples of a fungal poison and antibiotics are also mycotoxins. Fluids like a vaccine that are injected into the bloodstream can be a vessel for mycotoxins invasion. Parents must be **FREE** to access a vaccine for harmful mycotoxins. If it is not absolutely, sterile, having no mycotoxins; the vaccine is too dangerous. **Refusal of vaccines is part of the basic Right to Self-govern one's health and it assures SAFER vaccines!**

People freak-out when a tiny mosquito is trying to land on them with its little NEEDLE like proboscis perhaps, people should do the same when a comparatively, huge inoculation needle is being pointed at their tiny baby ready to be plunged in to empty its entire vial of contents that include unnatural to human biology chemicalization. What do you want circulating in your babies quickly developing systems? The itch after a mosquito bite (sting) is not the problem that is most concerning; it is what is injected through the mosquito's NEEDLE like proboscis that can cause health problems. It is the unnatural to human biology chemicalization of vaccines that is of monumental concern that causes health problems and is the main cause of the Autism epidemic!

There is the reservation in the People of the conclusive control over one's very own bloodstream. The vaccination delivery system must operate under this guiding principle to grant parents, for the sake of their children, the basic healthcare /Right of informed consent/DENIAL. Furthermore, unless the vaccination production heads acknowledge the truth of what these new sciences offer and thereby, curtail the use of chemicals that are alien and/or that alter the natural internal environment of the body, **the public's confidence in vaccinations will continue to spiral downward** and vaccination compliance will further decline. **With what chemicals have been found in our children's vaccine supply there is a strong propensity for vaccines to be flawed and/or unsafe under the omnipotent supervision of vaccine producers. It is negligent to not have your children under your parental protection.**

You can highly recommend vaccinations and you can speak till you are blue in the face to try to convince someone to vaccinate, if their willing to listen, however, that's as, far as, it can go; there must not be any coerciveness and/or forced vaccinations. A doctor can remonstrate with parents to vaccinate but the vaccination decision must not be over-influenced and needs to always remain the parents for the sake of their children. **A voluntary vaccination program is the only vaccination program that can survive and that can be allowed in a FREE AMERICA. Parents must be FREE to protect their children's natural chemical geometry. Vaccine producers must be held accountable and liable for vaccine induced injuries, made to pay to compensate the injured otherwise, negligence will run amuck and vaccine safety will suffer and/or vaccines will continue to have unnatural to human biology chemicals. We need to end the slippery slope of mandated vaccinations and have an even playing field where parents are not ignored but rather, are in absolute control over their children's vaccination destiny and/or welfare; be FREE to protect children to the best of one's ability!**

We no longer can shut our eyes to the painful truth or deceive ourselves any longer; Autism is primarily caused by the injection of alien, foreign to the body vaccine chemicals and

parents are being abused by an antiquated callous vaccination mandate that enforces vaccinations upon children even though, parents think it too dangerous to inject and vaccines do cause injuries. The People have been programmed to blindly trust that vaccines ae safe under an erroneous and antiquated vaccination mandate or an **ENFORCING** of vaccinations program. **Those who would refuse vaccination are coerced into vaccinating and there are those who acquiesce or blindly vaccinate under mandate**. The vaccination program forces vaccine injections that are realized by many parents as, too dangerous, injurious and main etiology of the Autism Epidemic. **Chemicalization** of children's blood and the doping of brain cells are vaccination consequences that **parents must be FREE to avoid and/or refuse**.

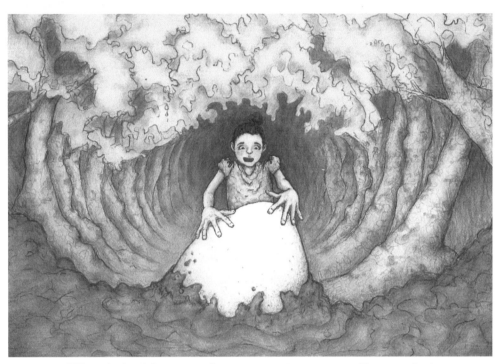

What is inside a vaccine may outrage you. Know what chemicals are in a vaccine before you embrace it.

The People have been ENSLAVED to be vaccinated. No longer stand for involuntary vaccination, demand to be liberated, demand the Right to deny unwanted healthcare; demand to refuse unwanted vaccine chemicalization intervention! We insist that vaccines be manufactured with parent's health concerns in mind and/or that vaccines will no longer be laced with alien, unnatural to the body chemicals. The golden rule of healthcare, that no medical intervention can be administered to a child unless the parents give their TRUE INFORMED CONSENT; must also, be the rule for vaccinations. Moreover, if a parent gives their INFORMED DENIAL; no vaccination can take place and there must be no prejudice or repercussions for the parents whom refuse a vaccination.

Parents need to be FREE to care for their children the way parents individually think best; that means being FREE to deny an unwanted vaccine injection. Vaccination companies need to be legally brought in line with all other producers of consumer goods, taking the precautions to assure vaccine safety otherwise, take on the litigation and expense if they do not. **It is a biological imperative that parents be empowered and/or enabled to protect their children**

from a conceived of vaccination harm. To allow for the supreme natural Right of parental protection the erroneous vaccination mandate laws must fall; and liberty abound!

The People require the unfettered and/or unbridled control over their own and their children's healthcare decisions. What can enter or not enter the bloodstream is entirely up to that individual or the parents of children. Perfectly, healthy adults and the parents of perfectly, healthy children must have control over what or if any vaccine will be permitted to be injected and thereby, be enabled to deny or accept vaccination intervention. The fact, that vaccines have unnatural to human biology chemicals and/or can cause injury makes it that much more abundantly, clear whom should control the vaccination decision. The People's healthcare decisions, especially preventative medical intervention decisions, must be under the absolute control of the individual and their personal healthcare decisions must not be disrespected. People must FREE to control their chemistry; enjoy the fundamental liberty of Self-Determined Healthcare without prejudice or being discriminated against for one's health decisions. Individuals' must never be violated with unwanted vaccine injection CHEMICALIZATIONS; they must be FREE to live undisturbed!

The People are well advised not to expose their children to any alien, foreign to the body chemicals. Chemical exposure leads to chemical reactive chaos within the body and a resultant onslaught of health problems. A person should not chemically alter their internal environment with toxins because not only does the presence of toxins cause abnormal chemical reactions but also, due to the fact, our genes are sensitive to changes in its surrounding environment. Genes can be altered by environmental changes and then our genes can become directors of sickness instead of health; cellular function becomes misdirected. The laws of nature and/or chemistry tell us, that to chemically pollute our children's internal or external environments could be disastrous to health. Do not gamble with your children's welfare; do consider vaccinating but, with only SAFER vaccines. Visit the website SAFERvaccines.ORG or, .COM to learn about SAFER vaccines. There is also, probability that our genes are sensitive to not only the chemicals that are cells are infiltrated with but also, the emotions we experience. It is already scientifically known that emotions can alter one's internal chemistry and hormone and enzyme levels; and that mental stress causes abnormality or unhealth. To suffer vaccination when you fear them or do not want them is also, unhealthy!

At the conception of mandated vaccinations, the politicians that voted to enact the mandate and the public were misled by being told many times that vaccinations were "absolutely safe"; the public is now aware they are too often NOT SAFE due to chemical content and that almost a Billion dollars has been paid by government to those injured by vaccines (and that is with caps on the amounts allowed to be rewarded). This is excellent reason to end the mandating of vaccinations however, there are many reasons to void the mal-mandate. Informed consent/DENIAL and/or being in control of your health destiny is now in the forefront and rules over healthcare delivery. We have become a poison conscious nation; now taking proper precaution not to be exposed to unnatural to the body chemicals. We now have lots of laws to protect the public against hundreds of body poisons; we now need the law to protect us from vaccine abnormal to the body or unnatural to human biology chemicalization. Common sense dictates that we put poisons on the top shelves so that children cannot reach them. Parents go to any extreme to avoid their children encounter poisons. Finally, parents are wising up to what chemicals are in vaccines and they are rightfully concerned over its detrimental impact on their children. Parents do not want their children injected with the slightest amount of toxins and/or unnatural to the body chemicals. Anti-health agents, chemical poisons and/or unwholesome contents should not be in vaccines. Public awareness that vaccines are chemically laced is crucial to the prevention of health problems including, Autism. It is just wrong to eliminate parent's authority to protect children or diminish parental importance; the vaccination mandate does just that and perpetuates UNSAFE vaccines. The mandate renders parents' impotent protectors of children since, they cannot refuse vaccination.

We must see to it that vaccines are cleaned-up, GET THE CHEMICALS OUT and thereby, assure children are not chemically exposed. We must instill vaccine producers and its puppet government to avoid putting chemical poisons in vaccines. We must protect our children from the poisons of vaccines just as, we intelligently and responsibly protect children from all other poisons. When a vaccination needle is being pointed at a child, about to be plunged into a child and injected with chemically laced vaccine contents; it would be very wise for parents not to rely on or ASSume that vaccine producers did not utilize anti-health chemicals and/or that the vaccination will not cause health problems. Proper parenting requires not gambling with their child's health! Be in supreme charge of your children's well-being by being in control of whether the vaccine is administered. Determine if the vaccine is too chemically dangerous to inject. PARENTS MUST BE FREE TO REFUSE ANY CHEMICAL EXPOSURE! Autism is an illness of mainly, chemical origin and parents must be FREE to protect their children from chemical exposures and/or chemical illness. It is imperative o safety that vaccine producers can be named in lawsuits surrounding injuries from vaccinations!

Parents must be in the driver's seat when it comes to protecting their perfectly healthy children; no erroneous mandated vaccination law should dictate otherwise! When a parent determines that a vaccine injection is too dangerous or controversial for injection their decision not to vaccinate must rule and be respected. Parents are ordinary people who occasionally must make major decisions however, THE DECISION IS THEIRS TO MAKE! It is the natural order of things that parents are in charge or rather, it is a perversion and against the natural order that the decision to vaccinate or NOT vaccinate has been taken from parents. Taken, the consequence of the ill-conceived vaccination mandate is that a taking has occurred; children's blood chemistry, their healthcare decision and welfare is not in the caring and loving confines of parents, it has been taken by a profit-based vaccination monopoly. Parents must be adequately, informed about the chemicals in vaccines and be empowered to judge accordingly. Most parents would rather, not risk having their children injected with unwholesome, CHEMICALLY LACED, vaccines. No rational person would want to inject their child with any alien, unnatural to the body CHEMICALS. Parents should not be enforced by an erroneous mandate, to upset the harmonious natural chemical balance of their children's blood, body and/or brain cells!

The body has a chemical balance that it must maintain in order, to be healthy. When conditions are just right the body morphs as, a direct result of the chemicals within. The body undergoes a kind of pleomorphism. Dimorphism in nature shows us that there is a dormant form of a fungi that is not disease causing and there is a virulent form of the same fungi, which has long spindles, that is disease causing. **The chemical condition surrounding the fungi dictate what form the fungi morphs into. The laws of chemistry apply to organic life forms and the unnatural chemicalization of a baby is going to cause abnormality. Pleomorphism indicates that bacteria, viruses and fungi are a single entity that changes forms.** The **chemical** condition must be just right for pleomorphism to occur. **Abnormal chemicalization of the sensitive homeostatic chemical balance alters the chemical condition to cause pleomorphism and/or a virulent form of the pathogens that are in our bodies; causing disease and is a contributing causation of Autism.** The millions of cells that make up our body can promote disease if the conditions, the environment and/or the sensitive normal chemical balance become abnormal; **a type of pleomorphism of our cells. Health is dependent upon what chemicals are inside us; we are a manifestation of the chemicals within us. Vaccine unnatural to human biology chemicals injected into the bloodstream set the stage for the abnormal, morphing what is required to be healthy. The slippery slope of vaccination chemicalization is exposing children to chemical disarray that is much too dangerous!**

We must set the chemical conditions for optimum health by setting the highest level of SAFE vaccine production. MAKE vaccine producers seek first to satisfy the rational safety concerns of parents by applying consumerism to vaccinations; make it a voluntary vaccination system instead, of a tyrannical enforcement of vaccinations. **Strike the proper tone** that rings loudly and clearly **to produce vaccines in their quintessential form; with no negative to health substances within our children's vaccines. In order, to achieve a quintessential form of a vaccine, which is a non-disease generating form of a vaccine; the TWO STEPS OF CORRECTION are required.** The **TWO STEPS** grant the health promoting graces of informed consent/**DENIAL** and hold vaccine manufacturers **FEET TO THE FIRE OF SAFETY** by holding them liable and accountable, when their vaccines cause injury. **Without these essential STEPS in place the conditions remain set for unsafe vaccines or vaccine production negligence and children remain at risk. Let us, prompt much SAFER vaccines!**

There is a biochemical signature of good health and there is biochemical signature between a mother and her child, these biochemical signatures can be interfered with by altering the environment that our cells are exposed to. To inject foreign chemicals into a baby, infant or child is counterproductive to assuring health and can be considered an act of CHILD ABUSE. To be forced to inject such, substances is an assault and battery upon the unwilling individual who is being coerced and/or enforced to withstand the unwanted vaccination. Enforced vaccine injections do cause physical injury and it also, causes emotional distress and/or trauma to the child victim of the unwanted vaccination and to the empathetic parents' whom are victims as, they witness the unwanted vaccine injection.

Mandated and/or enforced vaccination is a plight upon the People. Mandated vaccination is crushing our parental Right to decide what is best for our children and annihilates our basic healthcare liberty. Parents' must be allowed to be what they are supposed to be; protectors of children. How perverse is it that parents are forbidden to protect their children from unwanted and/or perceived of as, too dangerous to inject vaccines? Vaccinations need to be based upon informed consent/**DENIAL and be strictly voluntary! Parents deserve to have the preservation of their parental protection of their beloved children. Liberate your parental**

protection of your children, demand to freely deny or accept your children's vaccinations; implement the TWO STEPS OF CORRECTION!

One of the slimiest of recent attempts on the slippery slope of vaccination is that there has been an attempt to write a Bill into law that allows a school nurse to ask a 9-year young little girl if they want the Gardasil injection and the nurse can over influence the fledgling immature mind into it. The slimy attempt to make money from Gardasil sales totally takes parents out of the equation, it skirts parental input and leaves parents totally ignorant of the fact, that their little girl was injected. Parents not being able to decide what is best for their children and not even being aware of a shot being given is so, dangerous to children that it would be the reckless endangerment of children. Parents will be rendered blind, deaf and dumb that their child was injected, and the reckless endangerment of the child will occur because parents will not be looking for any adverse reactions from the shot. When making money is the priority this is the kind of evil or lunacy that occurs. A 9-year young girl does not know her right hand from her left and certainly, does not understand the pros and CONS of Gardasil. A nine-year-old cannot reasonably, accept or deny vaccination. This is a sham of obtaining informed consent from a child that has no requisite capacity; it truly is a slimy slope of vaccination!

Well, I hope you come away with a possible health and/or lifesaving understanding that the very premise of injecting chemicals that are unnatural to the body and thinking that it is not harmful is wayward. To command that people must accept these chemical injections is to be persistent or obstinate in what is wrong. Proponents of children being commanded and/or placed in bondage, to submit to unwanted injections, have turned away from what's right and/or good for health preservation. The source of this wicked health corruption must be uprooted; the TWO STEPS OF CORRECTION will accomplish this most positive health preservation and righteous end. GET THE CHEMICALS OUT of our children's vaccines must be the priority. The SANITY TEST FOR VACCINES must rule and the TWO STEPS must rule, and the slippery (very slimy) slope of vaccinations must be stopped! Vaccination must be voluntary and not be like stepping off a very high diving board and plunging into the dark unknown of unnatural to the human biology chemicalization. Protect your children to the best of your very fine ability by knowing what chemicals are in vaccines and then decide what is best for your children's well-being. Do consider vaccination however, only consider SAFER vaccines! Visit the websites SAFERvaccines .ORG or, .COM to properly protect your children and learn more. BE FREE TO REJECT INJECTIONS THAT YOU DEEM TOO DANGEROUS TO INJECT!

CHAPTER 12

DIAGNOSIS AUTISM

"DIAGNOSIS AUTISM" is being heard at epidemic proportion, it rocks families like an earthquake magnitude infinity and the chemicals in vaccines are the main cause of the epidemic. We need to make vaccination a more intelligent choice! Vaccinating with vaccines that are laced with unnatural to human biology chemicals is not rational; it distorts the vaccine recipients' homogeneous natural biochemistry needed for optimum health. Choose your vaccines wisely! SAFER vaccines .ORG and .COM are the websites of the charity, SAFER vaccines where you can find out what vaccines are SAFER and learn what vaccines are unsafe due to harboring anti-health agents or having unnatural to human biology chemicals. The charity and its web sites are designed so that you become educated about health and vaccines. The goal is to prevent you from ever hearing "DIAGNOSIS AUTISM". Do not think that you can inject your tiny baby, small infant or child with vaccines that are laced with unnatural to human biology chemicals and it not cause abnormal reactions within. ABNORMAL REACTIONS = ABNORMALITY! GET THE CHEMICALS OUT of vaccines and you do what is needed to help PREVENT AUTISM. There must be unification to stop vaccine producers from putting chemicals for profit in vaccines. Those who dictate children must endure vaccines that are laced with unnatural to human biology chemicalization do a grave disservice to the welfare of children!

The term "chemicalization" is a word that I invented; the word is readily understood as, describing chemicals entering or infiltrating the body at or after exposure to chemicals. A healthy chemicalization is one that is beneficial to health or needed to be healthy such as, vitamins and minerals; involving chemicals that are building blocks of health that are used by the body to make proteins, enzymes and other metabolic requirements of health. An unhealthy chemicalization is one that is not part of the normal biochemistry, not used by the body as a building block for health instead, it stresses the body, is a burden to the body and/or distorts the normal biochemistry and can interfere with needed normal bioreactions or bioproduction's, it can cause abnormal to the body reactions which spawns abnormality; chemicals that are unnatural to human biology that enter the body is an unhealthy chemicalization. Vaccines that have unnatural to human biology chemicals are unhealthy chemicalizations whereas, SAFER vaccines are not!

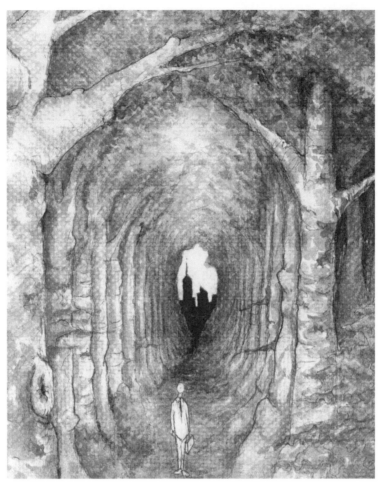

The charity, SAFER Vaccines mission is to **GET THE CHEMICALS OUT** and thereby, achieve much SAFER vaccines for SAFER CHILDREN. Learn how to obtain SAFER vaccines.

CHEMICALIZATION AUTISM is the diagnosis and vaccine chemicalization is the main cause! Chemicalization Autism is a diagnosis signifying the cause of the Autism is chemicalization. The Autism epidemic is mainly a chemicalization manifestation due to vaccination. Today expectant mothers and young children are being exposed to more chemicals than ever before. This increased chemical exposure makes it that more imperative that we safeguard against chemicals especially, the chemicals in vaccines. Injection of chemicals into the delicate blood and systems of children is the worst type of exposure because it quickly circulates in the blood unabated and penetrates through the blood brain barrier to penetrate the brain; doping the brain cells with whatever unnatural to the biology chemicals that are in the vaccine. Children are more susceptible than ever before to injected chemicals because they are more frequently exposed to unnatural to human biology chemicals than ever before from the environment, clothing and tainted foods and therefore, one's chemical tolerance can be challenged or maxed out prior to vaccine **CHEMICALIZATION**. However, make no mistake, Autism is mainly caused by the abnormal to the body chemicals of vaccines; Autism can be an injection away! The **TWO STEPS OF CORRECTION** stated in my book, *SAFER vaccines, SAFER CHILDREN* and reiterated in this book, *PREVENTING AUTISM* will assure SAFER vaccines with no bad for health chemicals. The rate of Autism will rage on until the **TWO STEPS** are implemented.

Everyone has a chemicalization breaking point; where health degenerates. How many non-consented to shots is intolerable depends upon your tolerance for chemical abuse. Your breaking point to no longer blindly obey the erroneous vaccination mandate can depend on if you know someone whose health has been devastated by vaccine chemical injections. It has become much too common to personally know of someone claiming that vaccinations are the cause of their children's Autism; it is an epidemic! Parents know best when their children are injured by vaccinations. Diagnosis Autism is what is being told to multitudes of parents after they submit children for vaccinations and they contemporaneously observe their children's health disintegrate into AUTISM. Preventing chemical exposure is possibly the most important health protection; parents must be FREE TO PROTECT children from vaccine anti-health chemicals. Vaccine producers and those who advocate injecting children with unclean vaccines that have chemicals for strictly profit and not safety; need to learn the lesson of the difference between a laboratory and a lavatory and thereby, stop putting crap in our children's vaccines. We want the safest vaccines possible and no rational person can argue otherwise and only the reckless would allow the chemicals that have been found in vaccines to be in or remain in vaccines. It is staggering at any level that vaccine producers would purposely put certain chemicals in vaccines such as, but not limited to thimerosal (a mercury derivative) or aluminum and thereby throw our children under the bus. Children desperately deserve and need SAFER vaccines that do not compromise their vital to health biochemistry. TWO STEPS OF CORRECTION are needed!

It is difficult to calculate all of the negative to health impact from injecting babies with abnormal to their body or unnatural to their normal biochemistry particulates found in vaccines however, know the egregious injections of multiple chemicalizations are harmful. Parents of children diagnosed with Autism are wise to prevent a progressive or more severe Autism by not chemically compromising the children any further so, consider to never ever again inject them with any vaccine that has any degree of unnatural to human biology chemicals. Children with Autism need their parents to protect them by doing everything they can to rid their children of harmful chemicals and assure that they are not ever again infiltrated by unnatural to the body chemicals. In addition, make their physically and emotionally environments health promoting. Diet should be pure with no harmful chemicals and be charged with the vitamins, minerals and live enzymes which are necessary to promote optimum health. Create an atmosphere for Autistic children of constant affection, love, caring and nurturing. Visualizations and perceptions should strive to become very positive and health promoting. The next chapter entitled, "POSITIVE HEALTH MEASURES" gives more insight on helping Autistic children live a near normal life and recover from being chemically compromised.

All the natural and non-invasive methods of healthcare and healing should be freely sought to improve the health of the Autistic child; one should not be handcuffed to rely or robotically take drugs that chemically compromise you. Taking drug chemicals for every little thing that is wrong is very unwise and children suffering from chemicalization Autism should not be further chemically compromised with drugs that have too long a list of negative to health effects! To make rules or law that people must submit their perfectly healthy children for chemical injections is undemocratic, totalitarian, tyrannical and CHILD ABUSE BY CHEMICALIZATION. Be FREE to do everything you can to protect your children and have the liberty to create a health promoting natural environment for your children and once obtained, preserve it; without governmental interference or commands. To be enforced to chemicalize children with unnatural to human biology chemicals is far beyond unreasonable; it is nothing less than insanity and is tyrannical medical intervention child abuse. Basic liberty requires **PARENTS TO BE IN SUPREME** control over their children's welfare! What will serve best to assure vaccine safety and prevent children from exposure to bad chemicals or unsafe vaccines is for parents to be **FREE** to refuse any vaccine that they think is not chemically safe; there must be **LIBERTY TO REJECT INJECTIONS!** History has shown that vaccines have chemicals that are extremely, objectionable. You need to protect your children and your children desperately need your protection!

To chemically compromise your children by injection is not what parents bargained for when they innocently bring their children in to be vaccinated. There must be full and complete disclosure of all the chemicals in vaccines and parents must have the fundamental liberty to refuse a vaccine if they determine it is not in their children's best interest. Parents' **MUST NOT** acquiesce in being left no choice but to submit their children for unwanted chemical injections. It is in the best interest of children that vaccinations be based upon parental consent and input. Vaccinations must no longer be permitted to intrude upon the parental obligation and responsibility of caring for and/or safeguarding their children. The level of violation to parental Rights is off the scale; the injustice too extreme, and the results are horrific. Children are being injured because parents are not given their fundamental Right to refuse unwanted vaccine chemicalizations and do to the injustice that producers of vaccines cannot be litigated against for vaccine induced injuries. It is a perversion of caring for children to enforce inject babies with chemicals.

Nowhere, in healthcare is medical intervention enforced upon the public as is done with vaccinations; it wrongfully, oppressively and unjustifiably is enforced. These are perfectly healthy children that are being enforced to be injected and chemically compromised. Even if vaccines had no history of adverse reactions or that it was not a fact, that almost a billion dollars have been paid to the vaccine injured after being proven that the vaccine caused injury by the Vaccination Court; the decision to vaccinate should squarely rest with parents as, is all other healthcare decisions for children. The long reach of the profiteering pharmaceutical industry has manipulated a sure way to permanently, make mega-profits. Big government has been overwhelmingly lobbied to make these unjust mandated vaccination laws that assure the mega-profiteering from an enforced vaccination **ENSLAVED** public. Children are in desperate need of their parents informed consent/**DENIAL** protection therefore, **INFORMED DENIAL**/informed consent law must control vaccinations just as, it applies to all types and modes of medical interventions.

Please, recognize that vaccination is big business and that Big Pharma lobbies to keep vaccination mandated to assure profiteering. One should question whether so many vaccinations are needed and raise both eyebrows off your face in bewilderment as to, why any vaccination is mandated under a biased profit-based system or since vaccines can cause injury or that perfectly healthy children can have their vaccination decisions made by parents as is all other children's healthcare decisions. When it comes to making money it too often causes the need for the medical intervention. Practically all surgeons have an inherent financial conflict of interest 'That's because they are paid approximately ten times more money to perform surgery than to manage your problem conservatively.' —James Rickert, MD, an orthopedic surgeon in Bedford, Indiana. In addition, many times the need for vaccination or a diagnosis is very often erroneous. A patient sent his slides to three different pathologists and got three different answers, 'I got very upset on hearing that. Now I never rely on just one pathology exam. If your doctor finds something, ask him to send your slides to a nationally recognized reference lab—not just one or two slides but the whole lot—and get a second interpretation.' —Bert Vorstman, MD, a prostate cancer specialist in Coral Springs, Florida.

Private hospitals push doctors to do more operations and pay them more for doing more procedures. It has been estimated that 25% of operations are unnecessary. The Cleveland Clinic has said, 'this system of paying doctors is so ethically immoral that it started paying its doctors a flat salary no matter how many operations they do.' When it comes to vaccinations doctors are not on the same page in that many think not all are needed and many doctors think that informed consent should rule over vaccinations. Almost all doctors think that SAFER vaccines that have less or no unnatural to human biology chemicals is in the best interest of all children. One of the main reasons why Chiropractors do not have hospital rights is because it prevents back operations and that it helps people recover from aliments without the use of drugs or medical procedures and that means a loss of big money to hospitals. Many doctors and hospitals are ethical; many are not. Your children need your uncompromised, incorruptible, principled decision on vaccinations! If parents control vaccination delivery vaccines will not have chemicals for profit and not safety. The TWO STEPS OF CORRECTION will make all vaccines, SAFER vaccines for children's safety!

The Pharmaceutical industry has so many lobbyists pushing politicians around or to turn a blind eye to vaccine safety requirements that nobody is doing anything to assure vaccine safety measures. The US Department of Health and Human Services (HHS) admitted in a federal court stipulation signed on July 6, 2018 that it never submitted biannual reports to Congress detailing improvements in vaccine safety made by HHS as required by the 1986 National Childhood Vaccine Injury Act (NCVIA) at 42 U.S.C Sec. 300aa-27(c). It is incredulous that there is a total lack of following legal requirements that assure our children's safety. The first report was due in 1989 and was supposed to be followed with reports every two years but, no reports have occurred; not filing required reports indicates no improvements in vaccine safety and not adhering to proving required improvements is the reckless endangerment of our children. The admission was obtained in a lawsuit filed by the Informed Consent Action Network to compel HHS to produce the requested documents (that do not exist). The Informed Consent Action Network was represented by Robert F. Kennedy, Jr. My first book, *STING OF THE MEDICAL MOSQUITO*, was reportedly handed to Robert F. Kennedy, Jr. and hopefully it helped energize him into beneficial action. Apparently, the HHS has fallen susceptible to lobbyists and left our children fall victim to less or no vaccine safety quality control. It is no wonder that unnatural to human biology chemicals have been found in vaccines! The evidence is overwhelming that children need their parents to protect them from the lack of protection by those entities charged with protecting the public; no one is better suited or has better reason to assure children's safety than parents thus, parents must be **FREE to REJECT INJECTIONS that they deem too dangerous to inject and/or have unhealthy chemicals.**

Even though the primary source of unhealthy chemicalization is due to injecting it into the body or blood, all sources of unnatural to the body chemicalization should be best eliminated. Everything the Autistic child eats, or encounters should be analyzed for its chemical content to be sure there are no further foreign to the body chemical exposures. Anti-health chemical agents are the enemy and vaccine chemicalizations are enemy number one; the most dangerous type of chemical exposures because it is injected. Autism can regress, and optimum health can once again resonate! The main key to the prevention of Autism is to assure pure blood chemistry and the main way to recover from Autism is to regain naturally pure blood chemistry. Prevent exposures to unnatural to the body chemicals and do not inject these chemicals. Anti-health chemicals should not be injected. Once Autism is diagnosed begin purification of the blood. Prevention of unnatural to human biology chemical intake is essential to prevent and recover from Autism; it is in your children's best interest.

Parents should be aware of all the various chemical exposure possibilities and immediately eliminate all exposures that are anti-health chemicalizations. Make no mistake, toxic to the body chemicals cause Autism and the injection of these harmful chemicals is the main etiology of Autism and gateway to all kinds of health issues. There are a few surprising sources of chemical toxic exposures like when independent studies found that 38% of 50 retail milk samples collected in 10 major cities were contaminated with sulfa drugs and antibiotics used to treat sick cattle. Consequently, these chemicals have been ingested by babies, infants and children. Sulfa-methazine has also been found in milk and this chemical is a suspected carcinogen. Everyone is susceptible to health problems from unnatural to the body chemicals. There are many sources of contamination however, vaccine injected chemicals are the most common cause of a critical chemical mass syndrome that can lead to Autism. Upset your biochemistry and the life generating bio-reactions faulter; **ABNORMAL BIOCHEMISTRY = ABNORMALITY!** Prevent your children from being chemically compromised and you prevent your children from "DIAGNOSIS AUTISM." Proper parenting requires that you protect your children from harmful chemicalizations; only consider the injection of SAFER vaccines and do make sure it is a SAFER vaccine! Think before you leap into vaccinating with a chemically compromising vaccine. Safeguard your children's vital life-giving blood biochemistry. Be FREE to be the best parents you can be! Think of the consequences of injecting toxic to the body chemicals such as, but not limited to, thimerosal (a mercury derivative and known neurotoxin) and Aluminum, a high magnetic conductor upon the fragile developing systems of your tiny baby, infant or child! To do so, is the reckless endangerment of children and **CHILD ABUSE** by chemicalization.

Abnormal to the body or unnatural to human biology chemicalization has infiltrated our way of life and we are being adversely affected by it. The Autism Epidemic is partially a result of environmental and food toxic chemicalization, but it the main causation are injections of the multiple vaccines with all its alien to the body chemicalizations. There are about 30,000 animal drugs in use today of which their residues can be found in meat, milk and eggs. Many years can elapse between the granting of "emergency" approval to ban veterinary prescription drugs and the end of their use. Use of banned drugs can continue illegally for instance, Chloramphenicol, an antibiotic banned for use in meat animals since 1968 because of its residues can cause a fatal blood disorder in humans, continued to be used for over 20 years after it was banned. Hormonal drugs typically are used in animals to promote growth and of course to assure greater profit; these harmful chemicals find their way into our children's meals. In fact, it is common that hormonal pellets are placed in illegal points or in double dosage in animals that are destined to be eaten by our children. Gentian violet an animal drug is a known carcinogen and yet it is nevertheless continuing to be used as a mold-inhibiting additive to poultry feed. There is a long list of drugs that cause cancer in laboratory animals that the FDA still allows for common use. It is obvious that Drug Companies and/or Vaccine Producers and the FDA do not hold our best interest. With all these chemical exposures; it is that much more imperative NOT TO INJECT VACCINES WITH UNNATURAL BODY CHEMICALS! The FDA and Big Pharma are biased toward one another and too often bounce back and forth landing golden jobs with each other; the conflict of interest is off the scale. If vaccinations were not so unconscionably profitable there would be NO VACCINATION MANDATES.

They put mercury in vaccines as a preservative to stop spoilage; this toxic chemical for profit assures greater profit because the pharmaceutical rep only comes to the doctor's office rarely instead, of regularly and stock piling of huge sales can take place with no risk of returns from spoilage. Most parents or vaccine recipients would rather, have a vaccine without such, toxic chemical preservatives or choose a vaccine that has salt as a preservative or select a vaccine with a short shelf-life without any preservative or poison. Parents must become proactive to protect their family from bad chemicalization exposures! Exposure to chemicals effectuates disease and Autism. Become informed and acutely aware of the long list of chemicals that can enter your children and take affirmative action to prevent all unnatural chemical infiltrations. The next time someone points a vaccine injection at your children with intension to inject; make absolutely, sure it will not be chemically compromising your children and setting the course for AUTISM! If someone unintelligently remarks or presumes that the chemical exposure is insignificant; think about the overall cumulative chemicalization danger and that because vaccines are directly injected into your children's delicate and susceptible blood, it poses a truly ominous threat. The injection of chemically laced vaccines can tip the chemical scale enough to cause a critical mass chemical syndrome and thereby, SPAWN AUTISM.

The TWO STEPS of CORRECTION will GET THE CHEMICALS OUT of vaccines and stop the prevalence of DIAGNOSIS AUTISM. We must take every measure and precaution to make sure the needle puncturing children's skin is clean and the vaccine to be injected is clean! Make sure the vaccine that is about to become systemic is devoid of ALEIN, UNNATURAL TO THE BODY CHEMICALS. Recognize that the origin of Autism is mainly due to foreign chemical infiltrations and resultant abnormal reactions from their toxic presence and/or propensities. Vaccine producers must no longer exploit and use for their profiteering agenda the Police Power of the State to enforce vaccinate. The Police Power must not be used to guarantee profit from mandated or enforced vaccine sales or be used to place our children's health in chemical peril; it must not assure a vaccination monopoly and/or vaccination mandated profiteering! The perversion and injustice of denying parents their fundamental right of Self-determined healthcare and its basic liberty to refuse the unwanted medical intervention of vaccination must end and SAFER vaccines will result!

The degree of harm that chemically laced vaccine injections cause makes the violation of the Police Power that much more egregious. There are different injuries that can take place in life, some injuries are minor, taking merely a short period of time to recover and/or heal while other injuries cut deeper and are much more difficult to recover and/or heal. The type or degree of harm that can come from enforced, no choice but to vaccinate, injections can be devastating to health and plaque the chemicalization victim for life. Make no mistake, chemical exposure is the number one enemy of health, the number one cause of health problems and vaccine chemical injections are the most formidable enemy cloaked in sheep's clothing. There does not need to be a tradeoff that one must suffer unnatural to human biology chemicalization to have the proposed benefit of vaccination. We may need or want vaccination to prevent childhood disease however; we do not need the chemical exposure risk. We must rid vaccines of their chemical harms and trust in a strictly voluntary vaccination program. We also must recognize all sources of chemical exposure and do everything humanly possible to stop it.

The Environmental Protection Agency (EPA) ranked pesticide residues in food as the nation's number 3 environmental cancer risk, right after toxic chemicals exposure in the work place and radon gas exposure in the home. Yes, chemicals introduced into the body disrupt the normal functioning and biochemistry of the body. Pesticides are big business just like chemical vaccinations are. Some pesticides, known as "systemic pesticides" spread throughout the plant and just cannot be rinsed or washed off. United States farmers now use approximately 10 times more insecticide than 50 years ago. Children that are raised on farms which have a high frequency of exposures to pesticides and/or herbicides have a marked increase in the frequency of cancers and birth defects. Chemicals called Neonicotinoids have been banned because it is thought responsible for killing off the Bee population; mass use of chemicals destroy life and mass use of vaccine chemicals destroy health; spawning AUTISM.

Children throughout America are having their unhealthy fill of chemical exposures. The chemical exposure base has been increasing over the generations as we become entrenched in a chemical ridden world and when this is combined with the chemical onslaught of chemically laced vaccinations the possibility of a critical mass chemical syndrome increases exponentially. How many chemicals can a human be exposed to until health is placed in jeopardy or until CHEMICALIZATION AUTISM becomes a reality? How many vaccines of unnatural to human biology chemicalizations can a baby withstand? Perhaps many or perhaps 1 or maybe none! In order, for parents to best protect their children they need to be cognizant of what chemicals their children might be encountering and be vigilant not to expose their children to chemicals that destroy health. An important study that should be performed is to compare the Autism rate among these farm children that have been exposed to a higher degree of chemicals and are also exposed to the enforced vaccinations, as compared, to the general population that does not have the farm related chemical exposures. The farm exposed fully vaccinated group will likely have a higher Autism rate than the general population fully vaccinated group unless the chemical exposure from vaccinations are so significant a cause of Autism that additional source of chemical exposure cannot be detected or register as an additional causation of Autism. If diagnosed with Autism follow the chemical trail to not repeat chemical exposure; it is best to avoid all chemicals that are unnatural to the body and absolutely, avoid further toxic chemical vaccine injections. Become a detective of what caused the health degeneration, seek out the CHEMICAL culprits and you will more than likely discover that vaccinations were the main etiology of Autism. SAVE YOUR CHILDREN FROM AUTISM BY SAVING THEM FROM BAD CHEMICALIZATION!

How many injections of vaccine chemicals in conjunction with all other sources of toxicity that children encounter before a chemical critical mass episode is reached can only be attempted to be quantified. The chemical exposure madness must be stopped at all costs; our children's lives are at stake. The TWO STEPS OF CORRECTION is the giant leap in the right direction to protect children's welfare and is in their best interest. We can no longer stand idle or be expected to endure our children's continual increasing exposures to alien to the body chemicals. The ABOLISHMENT of vaccination SLAVERY is needed to end these chemical exposures and to regain; FREEDOM of SELF-DETERMINED HEALTHCARE and PARENTS' RIGHT TO PROTECT CHILDREN and allow fundamental FAMILY AUTONOMY.

What results from bombarding our bodies with foreign to the body chemicals is an altering of the normal biochemistry that makes for abnormal biological reactions and the prevention of required for health reactions. Consequently, there is now a tremendous amount of people being diagnosed with Dementia and/or Alzheimer's, Cancer, Vision problems, Diabetes and an AUTISM EPIDEMIC. All these health problems continue to be increasing despite modern medicine because ONE CANNOT FIGHT A CHEMICALLY INDUCED PROBLEM BY INTYRODUCING MORE CHEMICALS IN THE FORM OF DRUGS AND/OR CHEMICALLY LAIDEN VACCINES. Our bodies are all sensitive to unnatural to the body chemical exposure and we all have tolerance levels that once reached cause our neurological and endocrine systems to malfunction. Chemical infiltration is the key causation of most of today's health problems. PREVENT CHEMICALIZATION AND YOU PREVENT MOST HEALTH PROBLEMS! Government must not mandate vaccine injections especially injections of any degree of unhealthy chemicals. We must be FREE to self-control what runs throughout our bodies! Be FREE to decide as our children's parents, what is best for our children!

If one is not exposed to harmful chemicals, one has a much greater chance at being healthy and not need to go to the doctor. Compare the quickly growing population of those who have claimed a religious exemption so not to be vaccinated or those that home school to remain unvaccinated to that of the vaccinated population; the numbers of those with Autism reveal that vaccine chemicals are the main etiology of Autism. In addition, compare the unvaccinated with the vaccinated as to, how often the children have had to run to the doctors or have been on antibiotics or had fevers, asthma, petite mal seizures, convulsions, headaches, allergies, skin rashes and missed school days. You will find that the comparison is startling; making it obvious that the injecting of vaccine chemicals, after vaccine chemicals, after vaccine chemicals; are the main etiology of most children's health problems. You must be FREE to protect your children from vaccine chemicalizations and have your healthy, unvaccinated children, enter school; unmolested or prejudiced! **VACCINATION SLAVERY' ENFORCES CHEMICALIZATION CHILD ABUSE!**

Obviously, the laws of chemistry apply to the chemicals inside of our bodies. When you pollute your sensitive internal chemistry; renegade reactions are induced and many of the normal, essential for health reactions are blocked. When a child is suspected of becoming Autistic because of vaccination and parents do not let their other children be vaccinated because of it; a very revealing statistic occurs. What is revealed is that the siblings of the child that was rendered Autistic do not become Autistic; their health remains intact because they were not vaccinated. The fact, that siblings with practically the same genetic makeup are or are not Autistic and the only eye-opening variable is vaccination strongly points to vaccine chemicalization as the cause in fact, of Autism. The genetic causation is proven wrong; the main cause of the child's Autism is that the child was chemically compromised by the vaccine chemicalization. One cannot expect to remain 100% normal and/or optimally healthy when injected with foreign to the body, chemically laced vaccines. Keep clear of chemical exposure and you will not cause health problems. Make vaccine producers clean-up their vaccines and the main reason for the Autism epidemic will cease. Parents must be FREE to keep their children's blood pure!

When the natural range of chemicals are circulating in the blood and feeding the brain and body cells optimum health is possible and highly probable; the normal biochemistry allows for the normal physiology and/or needed biological function. When this natural chemistry range is thrown out of kilter or rendered abnormal by the infiltration of injected anti-health chemicals then the health homeostasis is disrupted, and **AUTISM** can be spawned. You cannot chemically adulterate children's blood **WITH BAD VACCINE CHEMICALS** at such an alarming vaccination schedule and expect children to remain healthy; its illogical. To enforce injections of vaccine chemical insults that alter the normal chemical integrity is a breach of the trust that we have placed in vaccine producers and its puppet government. Parents are well-advised to trust in the laws of chemistry and not in the erroneous vaccination mandate laws. Protect your children's chemistry; keep it natural and pure! Parents' must be FREE to safeguard their children's natural chemical geometry!

One example of just how chemically and/or molecular sensitive we are and the health problems that occur due to the slightest change to our internal chemistry is seizures that can occur in a Diabetic patient. When insulin levels and/or sugar levels become abnormal a seizure can occur. Interestingly, the changes are so slight that modern medicine has a difficult time detecting the changes **UNTIL A SEIZURE IS APPARENT. VACCINE CHEMICALIZATION EFFECTS AND/OR THEIR AFFECTS UPON THE VACCINATION RECIPIENT ARE OFTEN UNDETECTED UNTIL, A FULL-BLOWN AUTISM DIAGNOSIS IS RENDERED.** Look at the signs and symptomology of the Autistic such as, the neurological malfunction or abnormality and realize that when these signs and symptoms first appeared they insidiously began until a full-blown Autism was spawned or another unfortunate vaccine chemicalization of unnatural to human biology chemicals was inoculated. Observing parents have reported that they detected something wrong or was beginning to go wrong or felt or detected the abnormal chemical changes that caused abnormality or unhealth in their children at the time or proximate to a vaccine chemicalization was injected into their child. Perhaps, parents have a special sense or bond with their offspring that alerts them.

In seizures, the subtle body chemical changes can be detected by man's best friend, the dog; dogs can actually warn us to act to either normalize sugar levels and/or insulin levels long before the chemical problem escalates into a terrible seizure. Dog's sense of smell gives them the capability to detect the chemical changes in the person who is heading toward a seizure. What this shows us is that our health is very dependent upon a stable natural chemistry and that the slightest deviation can cause problems and that the chemical alterations that cause abnormality can be detected by dogs and/or felt by parents. Abnormal chemical occurrence or unhealthy chemicalization's effects or affects have a geometric register that is observable and/or detectable! Vaccines' unnatural to human biology chemicals that are injected into the blood and/or body is a definite chemical deviation from the norm. Perhaps dogs can be trained to detect the chemical changes and/or chemical chaos that ensue after alien vaccine chemicals are injected and/or as Autism begins or before full blown Autism occurs. Dog's acute sense of smell or their ability to detect magnetic field or energy changes can be used to alert us to health degeneration subtle health facts before parents hear "DIAGNOSIS AUTISM".

Someday soon, in the not too distant future, dogs will be used for early detection of all kinds of health problems that most humans are incapable or not in tune to detect such as, depression, Cancer or Autism. Dogs have become an extension of ourselves, they can detect things that we cannot and then communicate the alarming fact to us. The spiraling chemical reactive chaos form chemically laced vaccines be told. Dogs that undergo a bad vaccination also, often are dealt health problems. Dogs often exhibit excessive licking at the vaccination site and uncontrollable hyperactivity for long periods of time and on occasion develop permanent trembling, digestive disorders and other health issues. The universal laws of chemistry apply to all life; so, keep your children's biochemistry pure and/or natural and then abnormal reactions and/or abnormality becomes remote! Inject SAFER vaccines to keep the biochemistry pure as, possible. Visit the web-site SAFERvaccines .ORG or .COM to obtain knowledge for SAFER vaccines.

One more revealing bark about man's best friend, all dogs originated from wild, wolfs or coyotes or foxes, that all have a genetic wild, very vicious propensity. Selective breeding and changing the animals ENVIORNMENT has changed the genetic expression of the now, approximate 400 different species of dogs that man has had their hand in creating; to be genetically coded docile and man's best friend. Dogs can be changed back to their ancestry vicious propensity by doing the opposite. Analogously, the creation of a certain negative to health environment triggers our genes to help cause health problems such as, but not limited to Autism. Changing back to a natural chemical environment should over time allow natural, healthy and/or normal, life force once again and therefore end the increasing Autism epidemic. Every 7 years almost all our cells are replaced thus, given time one could become healthy. We must GET THE CHEMICALS OUT of our children and/or OUT OF THE VACCINES that we inject into them!

There was an experiment in Russia, attempting to take the aggressive nature out of wild foxes; it took only 8 generations of selective breeding of allowing only the calmest foxes to breed and a regular nurturing, petting environment, with humans to render the fox genetically domestic and no longer aggressive. What this all points out is that our genes can be turned on or off according to the environment that we are in and perceive. Keeping our natural environment that promotes health and happiness is Nature's lesson. Generations of the vaccinated, with alien, unnatural to the body chemicals can alter cellular and the gene's environment, will likely cause a mutation, an altered state or changed genetic propensities and/or a hereditary form of AUTISM. Diagnosis Autism is from chemically changing the cellular environment and can turn hereditary.

We have been living under the tyranny of enforced vaccination suffering our perfectly healthy children with unnatural to human biology chemicalization by injection with no viable liberty to refuse the vaccination even when the parents are either not convinced of the vaccines safety or are convinced that the vaccine is not safe and/or is too dangerous to inject! Parents have a GOD given supreme Right to care for their children and under this most fundamental and all-important of Rights parents must be completely FREE to decide if a vaccine is or is not in their children's best interest. Parental protection of their offspring from what parents deem is a too dangerous vaccine injection is an invaluable, unalienable Right that cannot legally be taken or diminished or even temporarily shelved. The mandate of vaccination especially, in perpetuity is therefore, illegal and must be stricken down for being so! Vaccines have become too dangerous, being proven to have unnatural to human biology chemicals and have induced or caused many injuries, even death. We have become desensitized to this egregious injustice of mandated vaccination. People who dare question vaccine safety or claim that mandated vaccination is more about profiteering than our children's safety are often punished, threatened with having their children taken or treated prejudicially for speaking up for their liberty or for acting to right what they know is wrong. WE THE PEOPLE are no longer allowed to think for themselves or self-govern our very own bodies and blood chemistry. The mass of pharmaceutical lobbyists has assured mandated vaccination continue in perpetuity for profit and that parents have no part in the vaccination decision; having no adequate ability to protect their children from perceived or actual vaccine induced harm. There is hope for WE THE PEOPLE and for our progeny and that is THE TWO STEPS OF CORRECTION. SAFER vaccines are a direct result of the TWO STEPS and our FREEDOM!

All we need to do collectively, as individuals, one by one, is to stand up for our SUPREME RIGHT OF SELF-PRESERVATION through, informed consent/DENIAL; to deny a vaccination that is suspect or too controversial for injection. Demand to know all the chemicals used in the vaccine's production and act to protect your children from chemical insult. Protect your children with the Self-preservation power to decide what healthcare is in your children's best health interest. Forbid the enforcing of harmful vaccines or vaccination that you deem not in your children's best interest or is too dangerous to inject. Informed consent must steadfastly apply to vaccinations and vaccine producers must be held accountable and liable for vaccine induced injuries, made to compensate those proven injured by vaccination. Extreme caution is recommended to those contemplating a "suspect vaccination". It is your life, it is your body to control and it is your own children that you must be FREE to protect! The present state of chemically laced vaccines and the mandate that enforces VACCINATION SLAVERY is shameful and is really lawlessness. TO ALLOW THE DECENCY AND NATURAL PROTECTION OF PARENTS' ENABLED TO REFUSE VACCINATIONS, WILL HAVE A PROFOUND POSITIVE IMPACT FOR SAFETY; IT WILL PROMPT SAFER VACCINES!

Vaccine producers put all kinds of garbage in vaccines that treat the vaccine recipient like a toxic dump. They had to pushed and prodded into removing thiomersal (mercury) from vaccines and it is so abundantly, obvious that it should not, must not and need not be in vaccines; it is a commonly known neurotoxin. Neurotoxins trigger the faulty release of neurotransmitters causing a neurological hyperactivity. Attention deficit disorders and/or Autism have a main component of hyperactivity and/or inability to relax and be calm when one normally is meant to. When the body is supposed to be at rest either, voluntary or involuntary rest; it is interfered with because of the presence of chemical neurotoxins. Make no mistake, parents would NOT have heard, "DIAGNOSIS AUTISM" but for, the presence of abnormal to the body or unnatural to human biology unhealthy chemicalizations. Chemicals like Aluminum and other commonly found vaccine chemicals abnormalize the biochemistry and must NOT be in vaccines to have SAFER vaccines. Having less not more foreign to the body chemicals in vaccines is quintessential to developing a normal neurological and endocrine system. It is an essential to health understanding that vaccines must not be laced with toxins and/or foreign to the body chemicals. The TWO STEPS OF CORRECTION will push, prompt and force the makers of vaccines to produce vaccines with this essential to health understanding in mind! Chemicals for profit will no longer be in vaccines; making profits will not cloud judgement! The chains that hold children to suffer chemicalization will be broken by the TWO STEPS. Every strong hold on parenting will come down, every limitation will be released, and all the chains will be broken; allowing every fiber of parental protection to be reestablished. Children deserve the full dose of parental protection; they need ABUNDANT PARENTING!

Vaccination chemicals, artificial food additives such as, the food dyes, red dye 40, yellow dye 5 and 6 are just a few of the hurtful chemicals that are neurotoxins that cause synapse problems. Aspartame and other artificial sweeteners also contribute to the Autism spectrum causation. Preventing chemical exposures, which cause expecting mothers to become obese and/or stopping overweight people from continuing their circle of eating foods with harmful chemicals, are factors in Autism prevention. Realize that anything we put on our skin can be absorbed into the bloodstream, so please read the chemical contents and be the wiser for it. Parent's lathering up their babies at the beach with sun block may stop too much sun exposure but, please recognize it is a chemical absorbable source. Taking drugs in the sun is usually not wise however, do the proper amount of sun exposure without drugs can be very beneficial to staying healthy and recovering from health problems. Conventional wisdom tells us to take major precaution and steps to avoid being consumed by all these chemicals that are deleterious neurologically. Since, vaccinations are multiple and injected directly into babies, infants and children, it is of extreme importance, an emergency, that we assure vaccines are produced without unnatural to the body, harmful chemicals. In order, to accomplish this health preservation and/or health assurances' the TWO STEPS of CORRECTION must be taken. Be safe, not sorry when it comes to what is injected into your baby; make sure you only consider SAFER vaccines.

FDA chooses to be toothless; their position on all of these harmful chemicals is not to act to prevent us from exposure to any of these harmful chemicals but instead, merely conclude that all the children affected by these chemical exposures somehow, have a "unique sensitivity". The FDA blame our children for the Autism because they have "unique sensitivity" and not the reality that it is the chemicalization that is the main cause of the Autism epidemic. The prevention of the Autism epidemic could have been realized if only the FDA did not distract attention from the truth. The truth is that all children have sensitivity to vaccine alien, unnatural to the body chemicals; it is a falsehood and distraction to state or attempt to put the blame on children and not the chemicalizations. The FDA blinded the People from the major cause of Autism by pointing the belittling finger at the children and distracting the people from the truth that it is the chemicals. The contention that vaccine chemicals are not at all dangerous and/or harmful but rather, it is merely that there is some unique sensitivity that children have is a gross inaccuracy and an actual misleading. The term "unique" indicates that the FDA is confusing the public into thinking that only certain children are sensitive and that the blame is on the children and not the harmful chemicals. The truth that the chemicals of vaccines are the causative agent of Autism is brushed aside by calling children's weakness into the lime light of distraction.

The so called, "Vaccination Court" where it mis very difficult to bring a case and get awarded damages from the "Master" (NOT A JUDGE AND NO JURY) despite all its shortcomings and inequities the Vaccination Court has awarded mega-millions to vaccine induced injury victims; this clearly shows that vaccines do injure and at an alarming frequency and/or that the injuries are severe. In addition, there is a mounting mass of parents that have witnessed their children's health demise because of vaccinations that never take issue in the Vaccination Court. All of this has been suppressed; the toxic facts about vaccines has not been publicized as, it should. Despite the public not being properly or adequately informed about vaccines' toxic facts, many parents know that vaccines are not safe and want SAFER vaccines for their children.

Deep down in parent's bones is the need to protect their children; parents must be FREE to refuse chemical infiltration injections and/or chemical exposure; this basic liberty will automatically trigger the need for vaccine producers to make SAFER vaccines. Parents must ensure their children's safety and that includes being enabled to refuse vaccination, chemical injections. The mandated vaccination law is in direct conflict with parental protection. Perhaps, the FDA has forgotten the basic laws of chemistry or the rules of chemical engagement or reactions and outcomes and that the injection of unnatural body chemicals into tiny babies, little infants and small children is an inevitable poisoning of their blood and brain cells! It is vastly, important for parents to understand the negative to health propensities of unnatural to the body chemicals and protect their children accordingly! There is certainty that the abnormal to the human biology chemicals injected into children will react once injected and there is the uncertainty principle that can these abnormal reactions reach a level that will cause Autism or permanent abnormality. Parents by mal-law vaccination mandate must not be enforced to compromise children's chemistry.

The truth is all our children have sensitivity to such, chemicals; it is the chemicals that injure that need to be brought into the spotlight of blame and causation. The FDA is too quick to blame children for their so called, "unique sensitivity" perhaps, it is the FDA's obvious bias toward the chemical industry or its close ties with Big Pharma is making the FDA's conclusion; the FDA conclusion is baffling at best. Children are not so inherently, different from each other to have drawn such, an erroneous conclusion. The FDA responses and their steadfast positioning and/or support for the vaccine industry or that the more chemicals the better positioning makes the FDA cohorts of the vaccination and chemical industry. One can conclude the FDA is colluding in a cover-up to stop vaccine chemicalization from being recognized as the true cause of Autism and is continually acting to protect the profiteering from vaccines. The FDA higher ups landing golden jobs at Big Pharma directly after their work at the FDA is a sign that we need to pay attention to! The proper control needs to be in parents hands to assure proper child protection.

The mandated vaccination law is not merely a regulatory support of the vaccine industry; it is an outright creation of guaranteed profiteering from an enslaved people that all must be subjected to suffer their children with vaccination; it is a medical monopoly! This pushed or mal Marshall law monopoly has resulted in UNSAFE vaccines where chemicals for profit, not safety are commonly found in vaccines! Drug Companies/Vaccine Producers and the FDA staff too often have a very close working relationship that can lead to bias or favors. There is a major conflict of interest because select workers for the FDA are offered very high paying jobs, working for the very Vaccine Producers/Drug Companies that they are supposed to police. One is COGNITIVELY CAPTURED to do what is in the best interest of vaccine producers or rather, not in the interest of the public when jobs/cash dangle in front of them; CONFLICT OF INTEREST and negative to safety spawns. The TWO STEPS will give parents back the control of children's welfare; REMEMBER, THEY ARE YOURS TO PROTECT! The mandated vaccination laws enfeeble parenting or parents right or ability to safeguard children, to protect offspring from abnormal to the body chemicalization.

Law must not deter, misdirect or nullify parents from refusing what parents deem too dangerous or too harmful vaccines from being injected into their children. Vaccine concoctions that have been proven to be laced with unnatural to human biology chemicals must not be enforced upon the people. To mandate vaccines that taint one's blood or manipulate one's blood chemistry with abnormal to human biology chemicals is a ruthless disregard of human life. Children's require the cautious guidance of their parents to best safeguard them from unwanted medical intervention or untrustworthy or corrupted by unnatural to human biology chemical vaccines; parental efficacious management best protects children! Parents protection of children's blood chemistry and/or health must not be negatively impacted by mal-law. The vaccination mandate enjoins parents to suffer their children with vaccine chemicalizations that the parents object to and/or have determined are bad for the welfare of their children; it therefore, must be rendered illegal! By the fundamental maxims of true liberty, parents' obligations toward securing the well-being of their children must not be so, interfered with by for profit, mandated vaccinations. We must be forever vigilant not to subvert parents' power of protection of children. Parents need to be completely FREE to secure their children's life-giving natural chemistry. Law and the FDA must secure our liberty of parenting and allow children to benefit from it! Do not come in second place when it comes to protecting your children.

Instead of protecting our children from the transgressions of those who put unnatural to human biology chemicals that harm in vaccines, the FDA callously continues to display slated, one-sided judgments. FDA has a rigid and unbending support of vaccinations on unsound grounds. They are a monstrously deceptive; they do not serve to protect us when they allow unnatural chemicalizations of children. The FDA appears to have a violent prejudice to anything natural or that does not serve to perpetuate profit for the drug industry. Perhaps, knowing that FDA employees have obtained very lucrative jobs and titles or the hope for potential better jobs is influencing judgement to be so, positively biased toward vaccine manufacturers at our children's health expense. Big Pharma provide a whopping 60% of the FDA's drug/vaccine review costs and that means most of the FDA funding comes from those they are supposed to be investigating; this is a huge conflict of interest. The FDA often receives over 700 MILLION FROM Big Pharma per year; the FDA knows who is buttering both sides of its toast. The FDA's conflicts of interest have infiltrated into GMO being treated with unfair pro bias at the public's safety expense for example: Michael Taylor, started as an attorney for Monsanto, then quickly worked for the FDA just long enough to draft the FDA's policies decreeing that GMOs are "generally recognized as safe" and are exempt from labeling, and then went *back* to Monsanto. They are pulling this off in broad daylight however, we are all asleep or stupidly blindly trust in the FDA. The CDC is under the same conflicts of interest; Big Pharma is sure to influence all concerned. Parents need to be in charge of children's vaccination welfare; parents have no such, conflicts! The good news is that we can assure our children have SAFER vaccines for parents to choose.

The FDA beats a loud drum that always beats the same tune and there will always be those that reflexively march to the beat of the same deafening drum. It cannot be denied that expectant mothers and young children are being exposed to more chemicals than ever before. This increased chemical exposure makes it that much more imperative that we assure our children are not exposed to vaccine chemicals which are not indigenous to the body. Injected chemicalization is the worst kind of chemical exposure because it enters the body unabated and quickly circulates to breach the blood brain barrier and thereby, dopes the brain cells with its full chemical payload. Children's chemical tolerance can be challenged prior to vaccination and the FDA needs to take this into account. Human Rights forbid the enforcement of unwanted vaccine CHEMICALIZATIONS. Vaccines should always be works in progress to achieve the highest degree of safety; the TWO STEPS OF CORRECTION applied to vaccination will achieve SAFER vaccines and instill that vaccine producers constantly strive for safety, always being on the verge of excellence. There is no valid excuse for abnormalizing children with unnatural to the human biology chemicals in vaccines such as, but not limited to thimerosal or aluminum; the TWO STEPS will assure such, abnormal to the body chemicals or chemicals for strict profit are not used.

The FDA is WRONGFULLY, being used to stamp out competition for Big Pharma. There is attempting to make vitamins something that can only be prescribed. You no longer will be able to state the truth that vitamins and minerals can be a cure or aide or PREVENT disease because if you do; it automatically subjects it to be categorized as a drug and THAT IS CRAZY. The FDA is trying to regulate that if it claims to cure and/or help in recovering from an ailment or disease, it must be classified as a drug and thereby, can only be prescribed; the public will no longer have free access; vitamins and minerals will no longer be able to be sold in stores. This is utter nonsense, vitamins come from food, in fact, it must be considered food. Vitamins keep you healthy and/or help make you healthy and **PREVENT YOU FROM FAULTERING TO THE POINT THAT YOU HAVE NO CHOICE BUT TO TAKE CHEMICAL DRUGS.** Because vitamins negate the need or decrease the need to spend money on drugs it is being subjected to unfair attacks and unwarranted or unjustified regulation. Important to health; vitamins are naturally utilized by the body whereas; drugs are chemicals are unnatural to the body and all have adverse side-effects. The FDA's true mode of operation is to assure the drug industry's welfare and not ours! We need liberty to access to natural remedies and not be overburdened to obtain needed or wanted vitamins or be forced to needlessly spend time and money go to the doctor to attain them. It is drugs and vaccines that need more FDA oversight; just look at the Big Pharma induced opioid and vaccine **CHEMICALIZATION** epidemics.

When it comes to the cause of Autism; it is **CHEMICALS** that need to be blamed and not our children! **YES,** children all have sensitivity toward toxic chemicals, but children's susceptibility cannot be corrected and is not the causation of Autism or health problems rather, it is the chemicals. What can and needs to be corrected is to stop using alien to human physiology, abnormal to one's biochemistry and unnatural to human biology chemicals in our children's vaccines! **STOP EXPOSING OUR CHILDREN TO CHEMICALS** that all children are sensitive to that cause abnormal reactions and abnormality. Children's chemical geometry must not be manipulated by mandated vaccine **CHEMICALIZATIONS. PARENTS MUST BE FREE TO REJECT INJECTIONS THAT ARE UNWANTED OR DEEMED DANGEROUS; SECURING THEIR CHILDREN'S PERFECTED NATURAL BIOCHEMISTRY!**

Biologically we are not that different from one another; all children are susceptible to **HARMFUL UNNATURAL TO HUMAN BIOLOGY CHEMICALS.** The more natural we keep our children's blood or biochemistry the healthier they will be for it. The less unnatural to human biology chemicals that surge through the bloodstream or distort the natural biochemistry that healthier children will be for it; the **SAFER** our children will be! Although, our children's level of exposure to unnatural chemicals differs; it is a biological accurate fact, that unnatural to the body chemical exposure is negative to the health of all children and that Autism is chemically induced. The level and/or degree of chemical exposure causing the consequential level and/or degree of negative to health results can be the only question. For the FDA to have so quickly and readily concluded that children develop problems from their exposure to chemicals merely because they are "uniquely sensitive" is so off base that it is suspect. It appears to purposely misdirect a proper concern about vaccine chemicals causing Autism; there needs to be laser focus on the chemicals that our children are unwisely, being exposed to. The prevention of chemical exposure of our children will majorly help prevent Autism.

If the FDA were to conclude that the presence of chemicals in the body has anything even remotely to do with Autism the axe would fall, the truth be told, and the revelation revealed of the etiology of Autism; their Drug company cohorts would be in trouble and jog opportunity would disappear. The chemicals from all the vaccines that are pumped by injection into children's delicate blood are the major cause of Autism and a gamut of other health problems. To have allowed children to have been exposed to the mercury derivative thimerosal, a known neurotoxin is scandalous and to continue to allow children to be injected with unnatural chemicals should be considered gross negligence, reckless endangerment of children and/or is toxic corruption. The chemicals of vaccines do cause harm and are the main etiology of Autism! It is all too common after being vaccinated to have a fever and the fever can be very high; this in itself is an alarm ringing loud and clear that the vaccine is causing injury. A high fever by itself could be a contributing factor in **DIAGNOSIS AUTISM** however, a fever in conjunction with unnatural to human biology chemicals from vaccines surging around in the body or blood is too much for a tiny baby, little infant or small child to survive healthy with.

It is that the FDA which has the problematic unique sensitivity to anything that might interfere with its too close relationship with vaccine companies. The FDA appears to be colluding with Big Pharma and seems to with grant vaccine producers an out of jail card and is deaf, dumb and blind to the fact, that vaccines have been found to have toxic chemicals or chemicals which are unnatural to human biology; we should all be very concerned about it. By the FDA stating that children who are "uniquely sensitive" are adversely affected at least gives the public a degree of warning although, not the proper degree. The FDA should have completed their thought by clearly, stating that these children become Autistic. This can be considered definitive proof that the FDA KNOWS vaccination chemicals cause Autism. The truth needs to be told that all children have sensitivity and can be caused Autism; it primarily depends upon the level and frequency of chemical exposure (CHEMICALIZATION). Just as one cannot be half pregnant, one is pregnant or not and so, it is true with chemicals; chemicals either do cause Autism or they do not; and clearly, chemicals do cause Autism. The twisted words of the FDA still confirm that unnatural to the body vaccine chemicals cause Autism; end of story. Do not let them alter your children's internal chemistry unless, you truly think it is in your children's best interest however, do consider vaccinating with **SAFER** vaccines, generated by the **TWO STEPS**. Chemicalization is the enemy; vaccine chemicalization the main cause of Autism.

The FDA has been so inattentive to allow a mercury compound and/or other unhealthy chemicals to be used in vaccines and have hindered the truth that vaccine chemicals are the major cause of Autism; it marks their duplicity and bias. Turning the blind eye toward Big Pharma's purposeful use of unnatural to human biology chemicals in vaccines and FDA's cooperative agenda to limit Big Pharma competition by making natural remedies require a prescription or be categorized as a drug if a vitamin or natural remedy claims to cure anything places collusion at the feet of the FDA. Vaccine producers use of mercury and other chemicals in vaccines destroys the trust we naively, placed in them. In 2001, a U.S. Food and Drug Administration (FDA) study revealed that a 6-month-old receiving the recommended complement of childhood vaccinations was exposed to total levels of vaccine-based mercury **TWICE AS HIGH AS THE AMOUNT CONSIDERED SAFE** by the E.P.A. (Environmental Protection Agency) for diet, it sounds too crazy to be true but, it is true. Vaccine producers conceived and achieved the use of the known neurotoxin mercury in our children's vaccines and that is unforgivable and hopefully unforgettable. Deranged minds, that irresponsibly, place mercury and other harmful chemicals in vaccines, must **NOT** be trusted with our children's welfare. Children need to be protected by parents and to do so, parents 'must be FREE to refuse perceived of as, too dangerous vaccination; the FDA will not protect children as parents do so, parents must control the vaccination decision.

Let me be clear, it should not be said that vaccines cause autism rather, it is the unnatural to human biology chemicals in vaccines that are unhealthy and primary cause of the Autism epidemic. It is the reckless endangerment of children to inject such, chemicals and to mandate the masses of children to be vaccinated with such, vaccine chemicalizations is to mandate mass child abuse by chemicalization. I do not know of one vaccine producer who has lost their job for irresponsibly, putting mercury in our children's vaccines; in fact, they may have received raises for the profits procured. You see, mercury despite its obvious negative to health attributes allows the vaccines a longer shelf-life, allowing the vaccines to sit on doctor's shelves and not spoil and thereby, assures more stock piling and less vaccine returns do to spoilage and that equals greater profit however, it is all at our children's health expense. We must get all the chemicals out; mercury is merely just one of health's stumbling blocks and/or ill-health's building blocks. It is the unnatural to the body vaccine chemicals that build the foundation for Autism. Autism is not idiopathic; it is the result of negative to health chemical infiltration! In order, to stop the prevalence of hearing "DIAGNOSIS AUTISM", the TWO STEPS must be initiated. Parents have every reason to be concerned! Our invaluable Human Right to protect our children and supreme CONSTITUTION need reawakening; the TWO STEPS will do that and more! We do not want to destroy the vaccination compliance; we want to improve vaccine safety by achieving much SAFER vaccines and thereby, make vaccinating a RATIONAL CHOICE.

The charity at SAFER vaccines.org wants to open the eyes of parents to the importance of proper or healthy chemicalization and be properly warned about the dangers of improper or unhealthy chemicalization. It is of ultimate importance to health that health giving biochemical geometry is respected and that the laws of chemistry of t and within the body is not transgressed by vaccine injected unnatural to human biology chemicalization. Contemplate how the chemicals within your baby work to develop health or CHEMICALIZATION Autism, respect and understand how the laws of chemistry apply to either produce health or spawn Autism. Unclean vaccines act to destroy health; we must act to GET THE CHEMICALS OUT to give our children SAFER vaccines! Persevere in securing your children's vital chemistry free of unhealthy unnatural to human biology chemicals and you will not hear, "DIAGNOSIS AUTISM". Be FREE TO REJECT INJECTIONS of bad chemicals. A law is unjust and unworkable if it attempts to SEPARATE WHAT IS INSEPERABLE! The mandated vaccination law acts to separate children from inseparable parental guidance and protection when parents want to protect their children from what parents determine is a too dangerous to inject vaccine injection and are forbidden by mal-mandate to do so. When parents who determine a vaccine is not in their children's best interest and would refuse but for the mal-vaccination mandate acts to separate what is inseparable (the parents' protective decision not to vaccinate with what parents deem a vaccine that is not in their children's best interest). The erroneous mandate fails because in practice it is an impermissible FORFEITURE of parenting, an egregious violation of parental Rights that denies the parental and human trait to protect children from a possible or actual harm.

It would be an extraordinary claim that the injection of unnatural to human biology chemicals such as, but not limited to thimerosal (mercury derivative) and aluminum is harmless without extraordinary proof of it being harmless. The law of chemistry dictates that such, chemicals will take part in the reactions within the body and thereby, spawn abnormal to the body reactions causing **ABNORMALITY** and that is why it is unacceptable for many parents to jeopardize their children with such, vaccines. If you understand the consequences of altering the health or life-giving biochemistry you will want to consider only vaccinating with **SAFER** vaccines. No scholarly, doctor would inject unnatural to the body chemicals into tiny babies, small infants and very young children and have the ignorant state of mind to tell parents, in all good health conscious that it will not cause disharmony with health and/or that it could not possibly contribute to or cause the spawning of Autism. Chemicals are either health's building blocks or stumbling blocks; in the instant case of unnatural to human biology vaccine chemicalization it is the stumbling blocks of health and/or the causation of **CHEMICALIZATION AUTISM.** Again, more evidence that they attempt to put the blame on children instead, of properly putting the blame squarely on vaccine chemicalization is when they infer that people who are pre-disposed to have a mitochondrial dysfunction can develop autistic conditions following vaccination. The current President of Merck's Vaccines Division, Julie Gerberding inferred just that but by doing so, she with the same breath confirmed to CBS News when she was Director of the US Centers for Disease Control that vaccines do cause Autism:

Now, we all know that vaccines can occasionally cause fevers in kids. So, if a child was immunized, got a fever, had other complications from the vaccines. And if you're predisposed with the mitochondrial disorder, it can certainly set off some damage. Some of the symptoms can be symptoms that have characteristics of autism. " **WHAT QUACKS LIKE A DUCK IS A DUCK = WHAT IS CHARACTERISTIC OF AUTISM IS AUTISM! Chemicals dictate health or AUTISM!**

The above statement is an inadvertent confirmation that vaccines cause Autism! However, the statement does attempt to misdirect the causation by stating that the Autistic victim must have a fever and be pre-disposed to whatever; the truth is that **ALL CHILDREN ARE PRE-DISPOSED TO HAVE ABNORMAL REACTIONS AND HAVE ABNORMALITY FROM INJECTECTED VACCINES THAT CONTAIN UNNATURAL TO HUMAN BIOLOGY CHEMICALS.** There is no myth that vaccines cause harm there is only the stark reality that vaccines do cause harm. We can render vaccines to be a much more intelligent choice by commanding **SAFER** vaccines through the **TWO STEPS OF CORRECTION.** Vaccinations being mandated and Big Pharma acting irresponsibly by negligently producing its vaccines with unnatural to human biology chemicals has made vaccination an irrational choice and given parents legitimate fear of vaccination!

When you investigate what chemicals have been found in vaccines or why they got there it becomes abundantly, clear that we should not let our children's health and/or health decisions be dominated by vaccine producers or Big Pharma's puppet politicians. For your information, the EPA recommends that women of **CHILDBEARING** age eat no more than six ounces of albacore per week. Canned (white) tuna has more mercury than canned (light) tuna and swordfish contains the highest level of mercury so, do not eat it. What is interesting

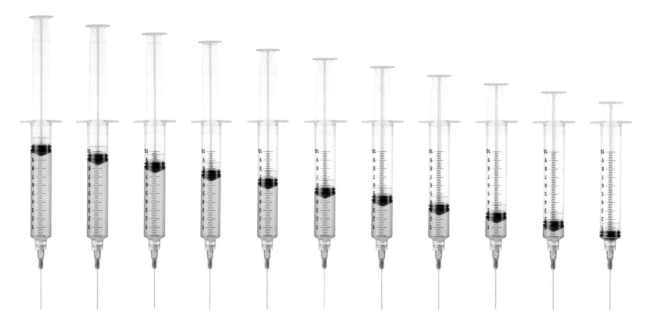

How many chemicalization will induce Autism? The least chemicals in vaccines the better!

here is that the recommendation is directed at potential pregnancies however, the protection is really for the eventual newborns. If the EPA is concerned over mercury exposure for pregnant mother' or rather, newborns; vaccine producers should have the requisite insight and concern. Parents' must have extreme concern over the slightest degree of mercury in vaccines or any unnatural to the body chemical! In fact, the vaccine-based mercury was "twice as high as the amount considered safe by the E.P.A." therefore; the concern should be off the scale and a stopping point for using mercury by vaccine producers. Public outrage and outcry were the main reason why most of the mercury was removed from most vaccines. Parents' of Autistic children upon learning that their children were injected with such, chemicals in vaccines become extremely, upset and many rightfully become outraged. Parents should not put their children's health in profit based, callous, careless, unconcerned, self-serving hands! Be safe not sorry; vaccinate with only SAFER vaccines!

The harm from injected mercury is exponentially worse than the ingestion of it; there is no comparison. When we ingest mercury from tainted food it is much more slowly absorbed and there is a good chance that our digestive and elimination system will to a degree of efficiency and effectiveness eliminate the harmful chemical or minimize its absorption. The full dosage of ingested mercury will not enter the blood whereas, injected vaccines that contain mercury or other unnatural to human biology chemicals go directly into the body or blood and circulates quickly, to one's fragile and all-important brain, doping the brain cells with the unabated full chemical payload; this poses a much greater danger to brain cells and brain function. Vaccine chemicals enter the bloodstream all at once and suddenly with the velocity its injection, wreaking havoc with chemical homeostasis and/or health. Even someone who is not an expert of science can easily recognize that this is a severe danger. These chemicals enter all at once and with nothing to slow the absorption or decrease the amount of chemicals that enter the blood. Parents are wanting this abnormal to the body chemicalization stopped; they no longer are willing to put their children's welfare into the hands of such, chemical folly. Parental responsibility has been awakened as, parents are demanding informed consent/DENIAL. Parents recognize that they need to adequately protect their children so, parents want to hold the vaccine industry liable for vaccine induced injuries and thereby, children can begin to be properly protected! Parents do not want their children injected with unnatural to human biology chemicals.

How many chemical injection exposures will it take to cause Autism? No one can be certain however, the more injections the more the likelihood of Autism and the more toxic the chemicals the less exposure is required to bring about the onset of Autism. By the age of 2 a toddler would have to submit to being injected with 28 doses of vaccines according to the schedule of vaccinations recommended by the Centers for Disease Control and Prevention; this is an unreasonable command since, vaccines place our children in double jeopardy, reacting to the antigens inherent in vaccines and being polluted by the toxic chemicals found in vaccines. Add up all the chemical exposures and its array of chemicals from the 28 vaccines that are all injected by the very young age of 2, which interact to cause chemical chaos within our children and DIAGNOSIS AUTISM becomes a plaque. Gardasil vaccine is yet another chemical insult that will be recommended to be injected and eventually attempted to make mandatory. Parents should do everything in their power to assure vaccines do not expose their children to unwanted, anti-health chemicals; the TWO STEPS OF CORRECTION is that assurance. Demand not to be a VACCINATION SLAVE!

WARNING: A new vibration and/or insight about prenatal ultrasound; a Yale study recently, revealed that prenatal ultrasound can cause brain damage in the developing fetus. During fetal development, neurons of the brain migrate to their correct positions. In a study of 335 mice, the researchers found that the ultrasound waves interfered with the normal migration of the neurons in fetuses. The amount of money being made from ultrasound is staggering; this Yale study is already being suppressed and innocent expecting parents will likely, not be given this potentially life and/or health saving information. It is obvious to me that the energy or magnetic field disturbance and/or the sound waves rippling into fetuses from frequent ultrasounds can cause health problems. As an Autism prevention it is wise not have abundant ultrasounds or limit it to when it is only absolutely warranted; newborns need to have all the neurons in their brain in perfect position for optimum brain function. Vaccine chemicalization of the babies that have had many unneeded disruptive to neuron ultrasounds is more of a sure recipe for Autism. Medical intervention of unnatural to the body chemicalization is the main causation of the Autism epidemic and ultrasounds' is yet, another medical intervention that is an Autism cause. AUTISM IS MAINLY AN IATROGENIC DISEASE (physician induced)!

Most parents find themselves in disbelief that they are so restricted by mandated vaccination regulation that they cannot decide what is best for their own flesh and blood or protect their children from what parents might deem too dangerous to inject vaccines. Parents are becoming logic stricken; they can add 1 and 1 and know that it is unwise in fact, outright wrong and dangerous to the health of their children to inject unnatural to human biology chemicals. People want the benefit of vaccines without being chemically compromised if they undergo vaccination! With all these chemicals in vaccines our children face the danger of a critical mass chemical overload and syndrome with each injection. Autism could be a vaccination away! We must be ever so careful not to alter the normal chemistry of the bloodstream, brain and body and/or tip the chemical scale to its tipping point, the point of creating a critical chemical mass syndrome. Over time the multiple vaccinations can interact spawning abnormal bio mutations. If foreign to the body chemicals continue to be pumped into children's blood the Autism epidemic will not decrease. Stop putting mercury in childhood vaccines was a step in the right direction however, we must not stop there; we must CLEAN-UP VACCINES to achieve SAFER vaccines. Steer clear of chemical infiltration particularly, injected chemicals and you will protect your children from neurological disturbances and prevent hearing "DIAGNOSIS AUTISM". Be vigilant to protect your child's natural geometric chemistry and they will naturally be healthy!

Anyone with basic knowledge of chemistry can understand the danger of injecting unnatural to human biology chemicals. Most, if not all, people who understand the laws of chemistry are in agreement or on the same page, that to inject such, chemicals is hazardous to health. There is even controversy among the experts as to whether it is in children's best health interest to expose them to all the varying vaccine antigens especially, when toddler's immune systems are just starting to come on line. Exposure to vaccine's antigens could severely strain an immature immune system and cause the immune system to malfunction perhaps, permanently. This is analogous to a very young person who foolishly, lifts too much weight in a poorly supervised or unsupervised workout; the under-developed youth could easily become strained, injured or herniated. Just as it is unwise to workout with heavy weight when very young or rather, wiser to slowly build up your ability to lift heavy weights; one could injure the immune system by forcing it to work out or work to concur the antigens of vaccines. One can strain an immature developing immune system with vaccine injected antigens. This onslaught of antigens when combined with the presence of unnatural vaccine chemicalization is much more harmful or problematic. Parents need to be FREE to weigh-out the pros and cons of vaccinations and must not be enforced to vaccinate! When parents detect a danger to injecting the chemicals of vaccines and/or have determined that vaccination is not in their children's best interest; no vaccination should be given or legally can be allowed to be given. Those children that have Autism are chemically compromised and parents must be FREE to stop further VACCINE CHEMICALIZATION; this prevention gives the best chance at recovery!

Life without boundaries is chaos and parents not placing boundaries on what their children can or shall be injected with leads to their children's welfare chaos and/or Autism. Why vaccines manufacturers risk children's welfare or place their health in chaos by putting unnatural to the biology chemicals in vaccines is troubling and raises many questions. When it comes to vaccine contents or its lack of safety there are towering questions- questions too tall for us to see past, even when we stand on tiptoe. Rather, be safe than sorry; do consider vaccinating however, only vaccinate with SAFER vaccines! How many chemical injections can your children withstand? Does 28 doses of vaccines by age 2 concern you? What number of enforced vaccine doses of chemicals is cause for concern to the rational parent is it, 1, 2, 28, 38, 50, 100 or more? How many chemicals would you let your children be exposed to before you COMMAND "STOP" AND TAKE PROTECTIVE ACTION? CHEMICALIZATION Autism can be one injection away! The least toxic chemicals your children are exposed to the lower the chances of hearing, DIAGNOSIS AUTISM. The enforcement of even one injection is outrageous and must be forbidden. Live FREE to reject injections. Protect your children from unwanted chemical exposure; protect them from Autism, as you see fit. One enforced chemicalization is one to many, in the eyes and hearts OF THE FREE. Overzealous vaccination advocates appear to think that if they gave so many vaccines that it replaced one's blood completely that it would be fine and would cause no health problems. Make no mistake, health is dependent upon proper chemicalization (the building blocks of health) and the prevention of unnatural to human biology chemicalization (stumbling blocks)!

Further, excellent reason to demand your fundamental healthcare Right to refuse an unwanted vaccine chemicalization is that many doctors themselves refuse to have it. Doctors are supposedly more in the know, they realize that the benefit of the vaccination are vastly, outweighed by the fact, that vaccines come with multiple risks from the bad CHEMICALS INHERENT. In the February 1981 Journal of the American Association found that 66 percent of pediatricians REFUSED to take the rubella vaccine and an astounding 90 percent of obstetricians REFUSED. Moreover, during interviews with many doctors, who prefer to remain anonymous for fear of being ostracized, they revealed that they have not had their own children vaccinated or completely vaccinated because of the possibility of harm and doctors confessed they falsified immunization records to make their children appear to be vaccinated. In the British Medical Journal, January 27, 1990, a survey of 598 doctors revealed over 50 percent of the doctors REFUSED hepatitis vaccine, despite that they belonged to the high-risk group and were strongly urged to undergo vaccination. It is unjust and inequitable for children to be enforced into vaccine chemicalization especially, when the parents want to refuse it! If doctors were presented with SAFER vaccines, they would less likely refuse. The TWO STEPS of CORRECTION will increase safety and cause less fear of vaccination.

The medical profession itself apparently, thinks vaccinations should not be enforced upon children by a government vaccination mandate. On November 2nd 2000 at their 57th annual meeting in St. Louis, Missouri, members of the Association of American Physicians and Surgeons (AAPS), unanimously passed a resolution, without a single vote against the resolution, calling for, "a moratorium on vaccine mandates and for physicians to insist upon truly informed consent for the use of vaccines." However, even though doctors unanimously do not want vaccinations given without the true consent of parents and that vaccine quality suffers because of the mandate; the big business and deep pockets of Big Pharma commands that children callously continue to be handcuffed to be vaccinated by vaccination mandate. For profit, vaccine manufacturers' want to keep us or rather, our children ENSLAVED to be vaccinated and pave the way for more and more vaccines for profit to be mandated. They want to keep children ENSLAVED to be vaccinated to assure mega profiteering from vaccine sales produced by enforced vaccinations. They want to assure vaccines sales continue to grow undisturbed and uninterrupted. It does not want its profit-making machine to be messed-up by free thinking parents that act to protect children from unwanted vaccine CHEMICAL harm.

The AAPS Executive Director Jane Orient, MD had two statements that are important, the first is "Our children face the possibility of death or serious long-term adverse effects from mandated vaccines that aren't necessary or have very limited benefits." The second is "AAPS believes that parents, with the advice of their doctors, should make decisions about their medical care-not government bureaucrats. This resolution affirms that position." Wow, these ethical doctors put patients' Rights above profiteering; we should salute them! PARENTS' NEED TO RECOGNIZE what these ethical doctors' recognize! Mandated vaccination is at odds with the Parental Right to decide what is best for their children, to protect their children from unwanted or perceived of as too dangerous to inject vaccine chemicalizations and with the entire medical association unanimous voted moratorium on vaccine mandates and for physicians to insist upon truly informed consent for the use of vaccines. If mandated vaccination were not so unconscionably profitable, it would not be mandated; money is overpowering liberty and our safety. If people cannot refuse vaccination there will be a dominate and controlling mechanism to put CHEMICALS FOR PROFIT in vaccines that are not safe for injection; we must be FREE TO REJECT INJECTIONS! Protect your children's vital life giving biochemistry!

People' need to stand up for the Right to protect their children from unwanted chemical injection exposures and assure vaccine quality through informed consent or rather, informed DENIAL; to bring vaccines under reasonable restraints and safety. Let us bring about an equitable and just vaccination delivery system based upon safety first; brought on and secured by PARENTAL DECISION AUTHORITY and SAFETY SATISFACTION COMPULSION! The real reason vaccinations are mandated is not for our children's best interest but rather, for corporate interest. ASSuring vaccine sales with a definite endless market of children's arms to stick millions of vaccination needles into and inject its vaccines means endless mega-profiteering. They want parents to have no Right to refuse any of its chemical vaccine injections so, it can profit without interference or restriction. Corporate lobbyists have infiltrated our legal system, bastardized the legal process by manipulating law-making to serve corporate self-interest and not our children's best interest. IF THERE WERE NO PROFIT TO BE MADE BY MANDATING VACCINATIONS; THERE WOULD BE NO MANDATES! It is in the best interest of children to preserve their natural chemical geometry; corporate greed is at odds with this interest!

WARNING: yet another vaccine mandate is well underway or rather, sick mindedly underway, … in the month of October 2011, the Advisory Committee on Immunizations Practices, that advises the U.S. Centers for Disease Control and Prevention, voted to recommend ROUTINE use of Gardasil in 11 to 12 – year – old BOYS. Previously, the Gardasil vaccine was only recommended for girls; now they are additionally, attempting to profit from injecting boys as well as girls. Parents should think twice before having girls injected and think more than that about having their boys vaccinated with a Gardasil chemical concoction. No one should be mandated to be vaccinated! Injecting boys with more chemical toxins and/or Gardasil vaccine venom is a giant step in the wrong direction. Exposing children to more chemicals while their young bodies are growing and maturing and/or going through rapid cell differentiation and metabolic changes is further recipe for Autism. Children's optimum health is dependent upon the proper natural chemistry; to further manipulate or distort it with more vaccines is too dangerous. Gardasil has unnatural to human biology chemicals in it and is therefore, too dangerous. To end the slippery slope of more and more vaccinations and the epidemic of **DIAGNOSIS AUTISM; the TWO STEPS OF CORRECTION need to be implemented!**

The Gardasil vaccination is part of the ongoing slippery slope of vaccinations as, there is further attempt to turn our children into vaccine pin cushions. It wrongfully assumes our children will need vaccine protection due to mere conjecture of sexual promiscuity. It presumes an increased risk of human papilloma virus from having sex with multiple partners. It totally discounts parental moral teachings and egregiously removes parents from the all-important decision over whether their children will need Gardasil's supposed protection. Parents talking to their children about the birds and the bees or safe sex becomes a moot point. According to Gardasil advocates children will all grow to have sex before marriage and/or have sex with multiple partners. Parental responsibility, authority and/or their Right to raise children and protect children according to one's private and personal beliefs and knowledge is under attack. There is alien, unnatural to the body chemicals in the Gardasil vaccine that parents need to access in deciding what is best for their children. Recommending even more vaccine chemicalizations than the already commanded childhood vaccine chemicalizations is further placing your children in harm's way. Chemically induced health problems and/or **CHEMICALIZATION AUTISM** can be an injection away! To make Gardasil mandated is to take the health disaster created from mandated vaccinations and turn it into more of a catastrophe!

How much vaccine chemical exposure does your child have to be enforced to endure until you say "STOP"? Under what set of circumstances would you demand parental decision authority and satisfaction? Is there a chemical content point that would make you prevent the vaccine chemicalization and demand safety and/or **SAFER** vaccines for your children? In order, to **STOP THE CHEMICALIZATION MADNESS** parents must instill the needed **CORRECTIVE TWO STEPS**. Act to prevent **AUTISM**; do not be **ENSLAVED** to compromise your children's chemical integrity! Be on the alert for any attempted violation of your parental Rights or devaluation of the parent/child relationship. Your vested natural parental responsibilities include protecting your children from chemicalization poisons or yet another egregious mandated vaccine. There is plan that Gardasil can be given not only without parental informed consent permission but also, **WITHOUT PARENTAL KNOWLEDGE.** The Gardasil vaccine will test the publics complacency in allowing their children to be further entrenched into vaccination **SLAVERY** and will take it a giant step further in the wrong direction in that the vaccine is being proposed to be delivered **WITHOUT PARENTAL KNOWLEDGE.** Parents, not government, should decide if any vaccine can be delivered! There must be parental permission to vaccinate. Vaccinations must not be enforced upon us; **IT IS AN ABUSE OF GOVERNMENTAL POWER THAT MUST END!**

Vaccination of children must only be given if the parents are convinced that the vaccination is in the best interest of their children. No harmful chemicals in vaccines means the healthier children will be! Children are much better off not being exposed to unnatural to the body chemicals. Parents must remain on guard, turned on, tuned in and tapped in, being constantly vigilant to assure their children's safety. To best assure children's safety the vaccination decision must be in the caring good hands of parents. Government has failed to get vaccines right or are safe and yet, it still mandates vaccinations. Mandated vaccinations are more for the benefit of Big Pharma than it is in the best interest of our children. Parents need to be enabled to refuse an unwanted vaccination to best protect their children as this enablement will get vaccines right; making sure vaccines are SAFE.

In addition, to the risk of chemical exposure from vaccines, there is major concern that vaccinations are a one size fits all approach. It is the author's strongest opinion that dosage requirements should be determined on an individual basis. It is unwise that gender, age, weight differential or state of health does not factor into vaccine dosage or timing of delivery. Medicine is at its best when it is specific to the patient or the patient's needs and it is at its worst when it does not. Mass vaccination based upon mass general dosages is medicine at its worst; vaccination needs to be individualized to prevent injury. Mandated vaccination is not only the practice of BAD medicine; it is the government practicing medicine without a license. It also, perpetuates less need for quality control and thereby, has produced unsafe vaccines. SAFER vaccines charity takes the darkness of not knowing what negative to health contents are in vaccines or not knowing its ill-health consequences and floods light on it; giving insight on what harmful unnatural to human biology chemicals are in vaccines and how to obtain SAFER vaccines for the safety and well-being of children.

Producers of vaccines do not have the requisite compassion nor motivation to protect our children from chemicalization harm; they care not, do not listen to parental concerns about vaccine's being too dangerous due to unnatural to human biology chemical content. The fact, that vaccines continue to have unnatural to human biology chemicals despite injuries that are vaccine induced and parents' rational concerns and its total disregard for the basic laws of chemistry or how its abnormal to the body chemicals cause abnormality; it is more than evident that Big Pharma, its hoards of lobbyists and its puppet government officials have not and will not protect children properly. Implement the TWO STEPS OF CORRECTION and it will assure SAFER vaccines and arrest parental fear! One thing is certain that parents need to do to safeguard their children and that carefully consider what it is that you are contemplating injecting into their vital blood and body. However, many times even when you think the contents are; it turns out it is harmful. The golden rule or the "SANITY TEST for vaccines is that if it has unnatural to human biology chemicals it must be detrimental to some degree and is likely to be devastating to health!

You never know what you are unleashing from a MASS vaccination CHEMICALIZATION program. In a May 11, 1987, London Times article entitled, 'Smallpox vaccine triggered Aids virus' The World Health Organization is studying scientific evidence that immunization with smallpox vaccine Vaccinia awakened the dormant human immuno defense virus infection (HIV). Throughout the world, the greatest spread of HIV infection coincides with the most intense immunization programs. The MASS chemicalizations from the MASS vaccinations are ruled by the LAWS OF CHEMISTRY thus, MASS reactions and abnormal formations unnatural to the body result. There is also, mounting evidence that vaccines do not protect children as they are drummed up to. It is terrible that vaccines are enforced upon us and this is cause enough to make vaccination strictly voluntary however, the growing evidence that vaccinations do not adequately protect what they are supposed to protect; make the enforcement of vaccinations even more outrageous. In the November 21, 1990, (JAMA), Journal of the American Association had an article that stated, "Although, more than 95 percent of school-aged children in the US are vaccinated against measles, large measles outbreaks continue to occur in schools and MOST CASES in this setting occur among previously vaccinated children." The efficiency and effectiveness of vaccines is called into question; those contemplating vaccination should be made aware of this. Those not exposed to vaccine chemicals are obviously, more resilient; healthier. Freedom of choice and fundamental liberty of deciding what is best for one's children requires that parents be FREE to make an educated decision on a vaccine and BE FREE TO REJECT INJECTION that parents deem not in their children's best interest or is too dangerous to inject.

The Community Disease Centre, UK, reported that in the UK between 1970 and 1990, over 200,000 cases of whooping cough occurred in fully vaccinated children. In the July issue of the New England Journal of Medicine a study revealed that over 80 percent of children less than five years of age who had contracted whooping cough had been FULLY vaccinated. According to, The Lancet, September 21, 1991, in Oman between 1988 and 1989, a polio outbreak occurred amongst thousands of FULLY vaccinated children. The region with the LOWEST attack rate had the LOWEST vaccine coverage. Parents' make the vaccination decision; DO NOT BE enforced and/or ENSLAVED to vaccinate your children. The validity or effectiveness of vaccines is important to the vaccination decision. The less unnatural to human biology chemicals equals the more efficient and effective the biochemistry. It is logical that children who have been chemically compromised by unsafe vaccines are rendered more susceptible to childhood disease because of it. Chemicals within effect health resiliency!

When my auto mechanic asked me why his fully vaccinated infant son got the measles and had all kinds of health problems I explained to him that if the vaccine was not a SAFER vaccine that it had all kinds of unnatural to human biology chemicals in it that mixed with the once pure and natural homogeneous biochemistry and that it caused abnormal reactions; causing abnormality and that one is less resilient to childhood disease because of it. My mechanic understood what I said and compared it to what happens to a car when its brake line fluids or its steering power fluid becomes contaminated; it fails because the brake fluid or the steering power fluid is contaminated with chemicals that are not brake or powering steering fluid chemicals that are part of the chemistry needed to brake or assist steering. The brakes and the powering steering can fail because the chemical makeup of the fluid is altered or abnormalized. This demonstrates a good understanding of the situation; that the law of chemistry applies to function, metabolism and/or if one is to be healthy or is being rendered sick or Autistic! I went to eat at a world-renowned restaurant and when the great chef's creation was served I was overwhelmingly pleased. I spoke to the chef about health and how foreign to the body chemicals in vaccines cause Autism. The chef showed me that he had a clear understanding of what I was saying when he responded with the following, "when I am recreating a meal it requires a set range of ingredients to have the same great taste and palate consistency that my patrons expect and appreciate; if a single ingredient is off or a foreign to the recipe ingredient is mistakenly added the outcome can be disastrous, the meal is not the same, it is unacceptable, ruined." The key to outcome is the chemicals that dictate it; unnatural to the body chemicalization "ruins" health.

There is also evidence of cases of "non-polio paralysis" from over-dosing children, too much polio vaccination or intense immunization practices. In addition, CBS News, February 24, 2014, by Ryan Jaslow, 20 – 25 children became paralyzed and had injury to their spinal columns; eerily similar to polio and with polio like symptoms. The polio vaccination likely, caused the so called, "non-polio paralysis; it is polio, with a new misleading name. Prior to the advent of the polio vaccination; these vastly similar signs and symptoms would be diagnosed, POLIO. We know chemicals cause cancer; we need to also, recognize that chemicals cause AUTISM! It is not to long or high of a bridge to cross to conclude the danger of injecting unhealthy chemicals. Your children need and deserve the needed for health chemicals and the best vaccines possible. With liberty of vaccination decision, we can steer clear of unwanted chemicalization; be protected!

If one is not free to decide to do what he or she will with one's body or parents cannot refuse a needling skin piercing and injection of vaccine chemicalization then we are suffered with VACCINATION SLAVERY! This slavery violates our Right to be left alone and annihilates one's liberty to Self-determine healthcare and has caused vaccines to become dangerous chemicalizations. ABOLISH VACCINATION SLAVERY and it prompts clean vaccines; GET THE CHEMICALS OUT! The universal laws of chemistry apply to all the vaccine chemicals so, let us act to get the unnatural to the body chemicals out. Alien/foreign to the body chemicals of vaccines are contaminants to the bloodstream. The fact that vaccines are injected directly into our children's sensitive body and blood and the exposure is all at once is reason for extreme caution and is excellent reason for the condemnation of vaccines that contain unnatural to human biology chemicals. Liberty to refuse promotes SAFER vaccines!

To prevent parents from ever hearing, "DIAGNOSIS AUTISM", parents must be enabled to weigh-out the risks of not vaccinating as, compared to the inherent risks of vaccinating. If parents are not convinced of the safety of a vaccine or if they determine there is too great a risk of health degeneration or Autism, then parents must be FREE to protect their children by refusing the vaccination. There must be no legal pressure or any coercion to deter parents from protecting their children. In addition, if a child is diagnosed with Autism, Parents must be FREE to seek legal action against the Vaccine Producers when parents accuse it of negligent production of a vaccine that may have caused their child's chemistry to be compromised to any degree and/or caused their child harm and/or Autism.

When you are vaccinated with a vaccine that is laced with unnatural to human biology chemicals you definitely, are faced with the unhealthy chemical distortion or abnormality caused by it whereas, if one is not vaccinated there is good probability that they either will not get childhood disease or that if they do get childhood disease they will completely recover from it or may actually become immunologically stronger for it and at the same time have a lifetime immunity because of it. The best scenario is to have SAFER vaccines to choose when weighing out the pros and cons of vaccinating verses not vaccinating. Facing the very real risks of vaccine chemical exposure verses the conjectural, theoretical or remote risk of incurring childhood disease must be decided by parents; not government. Government should not be making our health decisions. The elements required for optimum health and the factors that destroy health should be considered. Nutrition, chiropractic and other natural healthcare help enable the body to fight off disease or aid in recovery and super antibiotics help prevent childhood disease from being so destructive. There must be freedom to discern the options available and the risks inherent. Mandated vaccination is now antiquated law, unworkable law and has caused vaccines quality to fall to the wayside and/or harbor chemicals for profit, not safety. Law must not enforce chemical injection especially, if parents determine it not in children's best interest.

Parents want their liberty TO DECIDE; to weigh out the remote possibility of a childhood disease injuring their child verses the known and unknown injuries from vaccine chemicalization exposure. The logical negative health consequences of exposing children to the vaccine chemicals and antigens of 28 doses by the age of 2; must be allowed to be taken into SERIOUS consideration. Parents should have the Right to protect their children from contamination and/or deny unwanted suspect vaccinations. The contamination is pertinent to health issues and the infraction of our Rights is pertinent and controlling to the legal issues! Parents need to do what they think is right by their children, do what it is they think is in their children's best interest and refuse anything that might cause "DIAGNOSIS AUTISM".

Before you acquiesce with infiltrating your children with unnatural to the body vaccine chemicalizations realize that not only will the presence of these chemicals disrupt the normal reactions and bio-production of the body but also, the chemical environment in and around your cells can set the agenda for your genes and/or cellular function. Genetic perversion, abnormal function, health degeneration and Autism can result. The chemicals of vaccines can alter genes' behavior. It is far better to safeguard our children's internal environment by not exposing them to chemically laced vaccines. Vaccine Producers must be prompted to not use anti-health chemicals. We must not inject unnatural to the body chemicals. We must be FREE to prevent it. FREEDOM to pursue optimum health by pursuing optimum chemistry requires the LIBERTY to deny unwanted chemicalization! The plague of DIAGNOSIS AUTISM is fueled by injections of unnatural to human biology chemicalizations.

Children are becoming disconnected with nature. Children are induced to think that it is perfectly, natural to take pills or be injected with multiple vaccines and to be totally dependent upon medical intervention. Parents must work hard at protecting their children from the constant media blitz to take drugs for everything. Never have children been prescribed so many medicines and take so many illicit drugs; unchecked prescribed drug taking has increased illicit drug taking. The key to preventing Autism is to prevent chemical exposure especially, injected chemicalizations. The key to Autism recovery is to stop further chemical exposure, rid the body of toxic chemicals and assure the proper levels of vitamins and minerals that are health's building blocks. Not injecting anti-health chemicals prevents Autism. Live FREE to follow your own healthcare agenda and/or live a natural life. To curtail the Autism epidemic and prevent hearing, "DIAGNOSIS AUTISM" we must ABOLISH VACCINATION SLAVERY by instilling the TWO STEPS OF CORRECTION.

It is obvious that what we eat has major health consequences and WHAT WE INJECT HAS EVEN MORE HEALTH CONSEQUENCES! You would not allow your children to eat some of the chemicals found in vaccines so, why allow your children to be violated by injection with the harmful chemicals that have been found in vaccines? Know what chemicals are in the vaccine being pointed at your children for injection and act to protect your children from what is a **CHEMICALIZATION HARM**. Vaccination was made for man, not man for vaccination. Vaccination were created and established as a benefit for people. The advocates of Big Pharma, however, have turned this good gift into a weighty obligation under vaccination mandate. Parents have the sovereign authority to determine how vaccination delivery should be practiced; there must not be mandates that command parents to submit their children to suffer unwanted vaccine chemicalizations or even command wanted vaccinations. I tell you, if you allow your children to be chemically compromised that it will alter their vital biochemistry and thereby, cause abnormal reactions and/or abnormality. A critical mass chemicalization syndrome can spawn **CHEMICALIZATION AUTISM**. There are too many stumbling blocks of health in vaccines that are not **SAFER** vaccines. Perhaps the greatest positive health measures are to assure your children are receiving their needed for optimum health level of vitamins, mineral and pure water (the building blocks of health) and to avoid bad chemicalization especially, the injection of vaccines that carry unnatural to human biology chemicals (the stumbling blocks of health). Prevent Autism by preventing injected chemicalization!

Understanding how the body works and the consequences of injecting into the body vaccines' unnatural to human biology chemicals, illuminates the cause of the Autism epidemic. The atom is the smallest particle (smallest unit of matter) that takes part in a reaction. Atoms combine to form compounds. Chemical compounds can generally be classified into two broad groups: molecular compounds and ionic compounds. Molecular compounds involve atoms joined by covalent bonds and can be represented by a variety of formulas. Ionic compounds are composed of ions joined by ionic bonding. What keeps the atoms together is bonding which is when atoms share electrons. A law of chemistry says that chemical reaction rearranges atoms into a new product. Chemical bonds are made or broken in order to create a new molecule. The presence of unnatural to human biology chemicals in the body can spawn alien to the body products that are not indigenous to human metabolism or physiology or biology. Chemicals change temperature and pH levels, affecting amino acid or enzyme activity or function. It is unwise to have chemicals in vaccines that are not within the biochemistry of the human and it is more unwise for noncarbon chemicals or noncarbon chemical compounds to be in vaccines. If you distort the chemical biosphere of your baby, infant or child expect abnormality! The unnatural injected chemicals will become part of children's cells, enzymes and/or proteins.

Vital bioproduction's of the body and their proper functioning require the proper geometric chemistry! The biochemistry within our cells and the environmental biochemistry surrounding cells is crucial to health and/or the prevention of **CHEMICALIZATION AUTISM**. **The normal biochemistry or original reactants** and final **products** of the chemically dependent bioreactions can be altered by introducing unnatural to human biology chemicals. Chemistry's collision theory is that increased motion of chemicals means more collisions in a system and that means **more combinations** of molecules from bouncing into each other. Because vaccines are injected rapidly into a rapidly flowing circulatory system, the moving unnatural to human biology vaccine chemicals spawn more abnormality as it collides in the circulatory system. If you have unnatural to human biology vaccine chemicals colliding with each other and with the normal to human biology chemicals intrinsic to the body there will be more possible combinations than what is normal; consequently, there is a higher chance that the molecules will complete abnormal to the body reactions, creating renegade or abnormal to human biology production and interference with normal production. The reaction will happen faster which means the rate of these abnormal to the body reactions will increase. Homeostasis is reliant upon maintaining the normal environment of the cells and that includes the chemicals inside and that surround the cells. Metabolism is the total of all the chemical reaction you need to survive and/or be optimally healthy. Abnormalize reactions and abnormalize production and thereby, it spawns abnormality and/or Autism. Be a body detective and seek all sources of unnatural to the body chemicalization to eliminate its exposure to children especially, injected infiltrations of chemical compounds.

The slightest change to your biochemistry can have major impact on health. Just look at what happens when you take prescription drugs; the chemicals have major impact. For example, when you take a steroid chemical formulation it is slowly destroying your internal organs; when you get older, you can have kidney and liver problems and you can even die from overuse. Literally, every chemical drug formulation has adverse side-effects and/or causes health problems. It is understood that unnatural to the human biology chemicals can cause cancer. Be warned: the same type of chemicals which can cause cancer can cause Autism. Injecting unnatural to human biology chemicals from vaccines is the leading cause of Autism. We must be FREE to prevent our children from being abnormally chemicalized; we need SAFER vaccines. Never take drugs to enhance your body. Those athletes are hurting their bodies. They can't see it, because it is slowly destroying their internal organs and not the muscles. Never vaccinate with a vaccine that has unnatural to human biology chemicals; you may not see its negative to health impact immediately, but its negative to health impact is there. Parents rapped in their parental supreme authority and/or constitutional prerogatives have control over whether a vaccine will or will not be injected; trumping any mandated vaccination law or for mere profit regulation! We must not expose children to unnatural to the body chemicals such as, but not limited to, heavy metals because it is a poison to enzymatic activity. Heavy metal ions react with S-H group of cysteine bonds, forming a covalent bond with sulfur atom and displacing the hydrogen ion. This causes the enzyme to lose its ability to catalyze reactions. Vaccines can have heavy metals such as, mercury; and almost all vaccines have aluminum (super conductor.)

It is known that poisons and contaminants can adversely affect enzyme activity, abnormalizing it; vaccines' unnatural to human biology chemicals are abnormalizing! Enzymes are bundles of amino acids. Science has discovered 50 amino acids however, only 20 amino acids are absolutely needed. It is crucial to have a normal biochemistry that produces the twenty amino acids needed to make proteins by humans to survive and be optimally healthy and, the required five nucleotides. Of the 20 amino acids, 9 are defined as essential in adults because an adult can synthesize the others 11 however, children require them all. If reaction controlling or magnetically stronger unnatural to human biology chemicals reactants are in the mix, bioreaction degeneration will result and Autism can be spawned. It would be extremely disturbing if snake venom were in vaccines and it is as, disturbing that heavy metals, mercury derivative (thimerosal), aluminum or other unnatural to the body chemicals are in vaccines. There is no controlling reason to have such, chemical poisons in children's vaccines! If the EPA considers mercury toxic to the environment; CLASSIFY IT TOXIC TO HUMANS! The chemicals that have been found in vaccines are not part of

the cycles that create those biological compounds required for life in fact, the unnatural to human biology chemicals interfere with the cycles that create the needed for health biological compounds. There is no excuse to have such, abusive chemicals in vaccines and to mandate such, vaccine chemicalizations is to **MANDATE MASS CHILD ABUSE BY VACCINE CHEMICALIZATION!**

We have seen to it or allowed it to occur or are blind to the fact, that unnatural to human biology chemicals have infiltrated the water we drink, the food we eat, the air we breathe, our environment and the vaccines we inject. These chemicals are the stumbling blocks of health and the building blocks of disease and/or **CHEMICALIZATION** Autism. The water authority has been closing wells everywhere because they are polluted. We dump batteries and toxins in our landfills that leach poisons into the ground and our water supply and the food that we eat is grown in toxic dirt and watered with toxic content. We are all being chemically compromised and are much more susceptible to cancer and **CHEMICALIZATION** Autism for it. There are those politicians or leaders that despite the clear understanding that such, chemicalization causes cancer and Autism remain blind to it and there are everyday citizens or parents that choose to ignore the truth or be blind to it. The blind that lead the blind will both fall into a bottomless pit of unhealth and despair. The fact, that todays adults and children are chemically compromised is more reason to assure that babies, infants and small children are not further chemically compromised with vaccines that have unnatural to human biology chemicals. We want to freely be able to choose to be vaccinated and obtain the potential benefits from vaccines however, it must be a rational choice therefore, we desperately need as, consumers of healthcare; **SAFER** vaccines. Recognize that chemicalization by injection is by far the worst type or kind of exposure because it is unabated; its chemicals have full impact as, it circulates passing the blood brain barrier to dope the brain cells. This can set you **FREE**; no longer be blind, safeguard yourself and children from chemicalization!

The cycles that make the required for optimum health biological compounds rely upon enzymes and other proteins to move the atoms and molecules. Metabolism is the total of all the chemical reactions we need to survive; vaccine chemicals abnormalize metabolism as its alien to the body chemicals take part in reactions. Make a tree good and the fruit will be good, make a tree bad and the fruit will be bad. Make your children's biochemistry good and pure and their chemical reactions, enzymes, proteins and/or biological compounds will be good, making your children healthy; without **CHEMICALIZATION** Autism. It is true to a large degree that what you eat affects your health; it is true that what chemicals you inject to an exponentially higher degree affects your health. What the body manufacturers is totally dependent upon the chemicals within. Optimize your internalization of chemicals strategy and you optimize your health! Internalize unnatural to human biology chemicals by injecting those chemicals found in non-**SAFER** vaccines and you do not optimize health but instead, optimize the spawning **CHEMICALIZATION AUTISM.**

The body is like a factory, there are thousands of combinations of those twenty amino acids; they are used to make all the proteins in your body. Amino acids bond together to make long chains. Those long chains of amino acids are also called proteins. There are the **Essential Amino Acids:** Histidine, Isoleucine, Leucine, Lysine, Methionine, Phenylalanine, Threonine,

Tryptophan, and Valine. There are the **nonessential Amino Acids:** Alanine, Asparagine, Aspartic Acid, Glutamic Acid. There are the **conditional Amino Acids:** Arginine (essential in children, not in adults), Cysteine, Glutamine, Glycine, Proline, Serine, and Tyrosine. Think about what can go wrong with the biological manufacturing of all the amino acids and its complicated long chains (proteins) when you inject a baby with unnatural to human biology chemicals which are alien reactants that have abnormal to the body chemical reactive propensity and disruptive to reaction magnetic fields. You do not need a study confirming that such, an occurrence causes abnormality; it is too obvious a conclusion. A body with a divergent from normal biochemistry is divided against itself and who's health will be destroyed by it. Certainly, our children's bodies cannot escape the efficiency of the normal biochemical processes going on in each cell, so it is probable that children who are injected with vaccine's unnatural to human biology chemicals cannot escape its chemical influences or processes. **Make sure your children are not held captive to unwanted chemicalization!**

Magnetic fields of unnatural to the human body chemicals found in vaccines resonate the cells and impact biological production within its zone of effect. Such, chemicals have traits that can adversely affect the outcome of bioreaction and its production! Human biology is an intricate and complex working of chemical reactions for production of what is required to be optimally healthy and/or not Autistic. Polar amino acids adjust themselves in a certain direction. Chemical traits allow amino acids to point towards water (**hydrophilic) or away from water (hydrophobic). Growing chains of amino acids can twist and turn when they are being synthesized according to chemical traits and/or under its magnetic field of influence. The balance of biochemistry is very sensitive and altering it with unnatural to human biology chemicals is destructive to health and/or toward human biology and/or physiology and functionality. A study that needs to be done, if it is humanly possible, is to analyze the quantity and quality of the bio products such as, but not limited to, enzymes of a child proximate to being vaccinated and of those proximate to being diagnosed with Autism and compare to an unvaccinated healthy child. Bio productions such as, enzymes will be shown to be abnormalized by quantity and/or quality; enzyme control is lost. Immune cell production levels will be shown to be abnormal etc.**

For one neuron cell to communicate or send an impulse to another neuron cell the synapse between the neurons must have proper chemical geometry and/or normal neurotransmitters need to be present. The presence of unnatural to the body elements have abnormal magnetic fields that can disrupt amino acid production. Putting science aside, the sheer logic of it is overwhelming; you cannot inject substances that you do not require for life and expect health perfection or not expect abnormality. Logic dictates that chemicals play a major role in Autism. Those unvaccinated are not benefiting from vaccination however, they are not being induced to suffer Autism. The Amish people and the Christian scientists who do not vaccinate do not suffer Autism as the vaccinated do. Statistics is food for logical deduction; what does your logic tell you? It is theorized that Autism is partially a protein disorder.

Even our (blood) hemoglobin is a mass complexity of amino acids. Unnatural to human biology chemicalization from vaccination explains why so many types of health problems are reported after vaccination. Even enzymes are proteins (a mass of amino acids). Enzymes are biological proteins that act as catalysts that help complex reactions occur in the body. Enzymes are everywhere in the body and we could not survive without them.

Enzymes are very diversified and designed for specific tasks. Enzymes are very specific catalysts and usually work to complete one type of function. Certain enzymes have certain jobs; there are enzymes for intestine cells that are specific for protein digestion and another enzyme is specific for carbohydrate digestion, there are enzymes specific for neural cells, specific for saliva cells etc. The complexity of problems of someone suffering with Autism indicates that the vaccine chemicalization is abnormalizing amino acid production and its combination. The alien to the body magnetic disruption and the abnormalizing chemical propensities of the vaccine chemicalization is causing children's building blocks of health (amino acids) to become stumbling blocks. Think before you allow such, injection; only consider SAFER vaccines!

The main reason why vaccination is mandated is because it secures profits for Big Pharma and Big Pharma lobbyists are making sure of it. Lobbyist are ruining America by hijacking government. As of 2018 there is an overwhelming 24,000 plus lobbyists and it is over a six (6) BILLION-dollar business. Big Pharma by itself has an outrageous task force of 13,000 lobbyists to push into regulation its self-serving unhealthy agenda and that is why more and more vaccines are mandated, that is why chemicals for profit remain in vaccines and that is why our children's best interest is not being best served and that is why parents must now step up to the plate of parenting in order, to protect their children from all these unamerican antics. Children's welfare is NOT best served under such, a one-sided power and purse of lobbyists. It has ruined our system of government; It is no longer government for the People and by the People instead it is bought and paid for regulation that keeps our innocent and vulnerable children under the oppression of vaccine chemicalization madness. Negative self-serving agenda has permeated every branch of government to the point of total control; our liberty is being destroyed and or safety being placed in danger because of it. We need SAFER vaccines that can only be procured by a FREE and fair market place that is based upon freedom of medical choice!

Big Pharma and its cohorts of lobbyists have seen to it that mandated vaccination violate our Human Right to medical choice; all for the pursuit of unjustly unearned dollars. There is the fundamental Right to have control or self-govern over what can or cannot enter one's very own body. The concept of mandating the injection of whatever vaccines that Big Pharma's lobbyist manipulate into regulation is so wayward to this fundamental liberty that it should no longer be permitted in a freedom-based America. What healthcare to accept or deny for perfectly healthy children is strictly a parental decision and matter of utmost privacy. The unnatural to human chemicals for profit that continue to be in vaccines would not be there if we implement fully the TWO STEPS OF CORRECTION. Some incorrectly argue that the particles are so, small so, finite that it could not be harmful. With the advent of particles with a size inferior to 100 nm non-toxic materials become toxic and carcinogenic when sub-100 nm can become more toxic or carcinogenic. Perhaps, some toxic and carcinogenic materials become innocuous, but the opposite is usually true. For example, titanium was not known to cause health problems until the advent of titanium nanopowders. Vaccines will likely cause more problems with Nano-particles; not less. Parents should be FREE to refuse no matter what size the particles!

How much unnatural to the body chemicals can your baby internalize before the scale of bioreactions are tipped to abnormality? Irresponsibly those who are charged with protecting us have failed horribly to do so, they are hereby, the UNPROTECTORS for allowing bad chemicals to permeate our environment and be in children's vaccines. It was reported on 8/16/18 that Roundup Weed Killer found in Cheerios and Quaker Oats. Glyphosate is the active ingredient in Monsanto's Roundup weed killer, and at high levels, has been linked to cancer; parents must be concerned about what even small amounts are doing to their small children! Lucky Charms was also, found to have too high levels of this poison; how unlucky it is for those children who eat it! There are other foods that this toxin has permeated into and good old incredulous Monsanto's keeps driving its nasty product into our lives for profit. Interestingly, almost simultaneously with the above findings a jury, on 8/10/18, after a trial in a San Francisco Superior Court, returned a verdict in favor of Dewayne "Lee" Johnson, a former groundskeeper whose job required the use of Roundup and Ranger Pro weed killers. The jury rejected Monsanto's arguments that years of 'science' refuted Mr. Johnson's claimed link between Roundup and his terminal cancer diagnosis, (Case entitled: Johnson v. Monsanto Company, San Francisco Superior Court, case number: CGC016-550128). We need litigation liberty in vaccine cases!

Inequitably, parents claiming their children have been injured and/or been induced to be Autistic by vaccines that have toxic chemicals are forbidden to seek compensation or injunctive relief against Big Pharma (vaccine producers) because its lobbyist obtained an unconscionable liability shield that forbids it. Not having redress against Big Pharma is un-American and places Big Pharma above the law. Parents need to be conscious about chemical exposures and protect their children accordingly, do not leave it up to the UNPROTECTORS. How many chemicals will you allow to be injected into your babies highly susceptible systems until you start to refuse it? You can choose to allow your children to eat Roundup breakfast or refuse to let them eat it but, you must allow a vaccine chemiclization; YOU SHOULD BE FREE TO REFUSE ANY UNWANTED CHEMICALIZATION!

Parents need to be FREE to refuse what parents consider a vaccine that is too dangerous to inject; without legal restriction. Vaccination mandates divide parents from their children, severing and nullifying parents' liberty and legal ability to protect children from what parents deem a vaccine that is too dangerous to inject; it is a perversion of justice and renders America upside-down. You cannot strip away parent's authority, power and knowhow of doing what they think best for children and have safer children or a FREE America. One must be FREE to not allow their children to become drunk with unnatural to human biology chemicals; not permitting one's children's brain cells to be doped by injection with objectionable chemicals that could be or are in vaccines. You would be living in reality and be completely accurate and correct to state that unnatural to human biology chemicals are enemy number one to your children's optimum health or welfare. Bad chemicalization causes abnormal bioreactions, abnormality, malfunction, disease proliferation, cancer, abortion and yes, it causes CHEMICALIZATION AUTISM. I will end this chapter repeating the all-important words, VACCINATION WAS MADE FOR MAN, NOT MAN FOR VACCINATION! Do not be a statistic of DIAGNOSIS AUTISM.

There are negative to health consequences after being injected with unnatural to human biology vaccine chemicals that arise from the chemicals' reactive propensities. In addition, there are the negative to health consequences from the strong magnetic resonance of certain chemicals in vaccines as, it rages throughout the circulatory system and when it surrounds or enters cells. In the back of every parents' mind, when in the pediatricians' office, is the possibility of harm from the proposed vaccination. Some parents allow the injection because they do not want the responsibility of the decision and many are coerced into it even though they think it could be to some degree injurious. All children have a degree of anxiety when the doctor comes at them with a vaccination needle and most if not all, children who have any degree of understanding about the controversy or safety concerns over vaccines have high anxiety as they stick out their arm to be stabbed with possible injection pain or harm. The following paragraph is about the mind/body connection and health problems that occur from being injected against your will and/or when you think it can or will cause harm and/or increase the risk of Autism. If the vaccine is or is not dangerous has no relevance to injuries caused by a sure mindset.

Analyzing what mental problems and/or physical problems can occur when parents are enforced or coerced to vaccinate their children against their will or subject their children to it when they or their children are afraid of it or have it in their minds that it is injurious or harmful reveals that to suffer vaccination under such, circumstances can cause harm to that individual because of one's mindset, in what is a result of "NEGATIVE PLACEBO EFFECT"; everyone has heard of the placebo effect; this is what is called a "NEGATIVE PLACEBO EFFECT". The placebo effect is a two-way road; if you think that the action you take will have positive results then there will be a positive placebo effect that will cause positive results despite the level of effectiveness of the drug or action whereas, if you think the action you take is bad for you or that the vaccine will cause negative to health results there will be a NEGATIVE PLACEBO EFFECT that will cause negative to health results despite how the effect of whatever bad chemicals are in the vaccine. When parents are convinced that a vaccine has chemicals that cause health problems and/or if the child that is to be vaccinated is afraid or is witness to their parents fear or anxiety or senses it and/or is afraid themselves then if that child is injected despite it all, that child will likely suffer a NEGATIVE PLACEBO EFFECT. In addition, if actual anxiety is caused it is harmful in that it has adverse effect upon hormones, adrenalin etc. To receive a vaccine chemicalization under these circumstances can only cause more probability of abnormality or harm and/or Autism. It is rational to fear vaccines that are not tested with double or triple blind studies as, all drugs are usually tested; vaccines are rushed through the system and released upon the public. Being fearful when a vaccine is an unnatural to human biology chemicaliztion is totally rational; be extremely concerned!

What is the surest or best way to prevent Autism? Should parents be enabled to stop or prevent their children from being exposed to chemicals that parents think are dangerous? Do you want vaccines not to have unnatural to human biology chemicals such as, the chemicals used as, preservatives in vaccines that give vaccines very long shelf-life? Do parents know what is best for their children or does government? I hope by reading this book that you answer all these questions with confidence and conviction to protect your children from unnatural to human biology chemiclization by injection abuse. The most important question that I hope you can answer with authority after reading this book is the following: Will having vaccines and the vaccination delivery system based upon the **TWO STEPS OF CORRECTION** achieve and/or assure **SAFER** vaccines? Know that **SAFER** vaccines will exponentially decrease the chances of chemiclization Autism!

The mission for **SAFER** vaccines is more centered upon science, law of chemistry and biology than the emotional outcries of those being injured by unsafe vaccines however, the documented injuries from vaccines that are happening all of the time and abundantly, gives clearer perspective of the need for **SAFER** vaccines. Below are decisions of the United States Court of Federal Claims awarding compensation to vaccine-injured clients as reported by Maglio Christopher & Toale, P.A. a competent law firm, through the National Vaccine Injury Compensation Program. The law firms' attorneys have recovered more than $300 million dollars for vaccine injured clients. Trust that your natural biochemistry gives you the best chance at optimum health and trust that to distort the chemistry with vaccine's unnatural to human biology chemicals causes abnormal reactions and that equals abnormality.

Date	Vaccine Name	Illness or Symptoms	
5/22/2018	Influenza	Guillain-Barre Syndrome, Myasthenia Grabis (MG), Death	$245,000
5/17/2018	Tetanus-Diptheria Acellular Pertussis (Tdap)	Guillain-Barre Syndrome	$130,000
4/2/2018	Influenza	SIRVA	$61,014.65
3/7/2018	Influenza	SIRVA	$140,000
3/7/2018	Influenza	SIRVA	$112,500
3/7/2018	Influenza	Transverse Myelitis	$107,000
2/15/2018	Influenza	SIRVA	$88,000
2/5/2018	Influenza	Guillain-Barre Syndrome	$115,000
1/24/2018	Influenza	SIRVA	$122,000
1/11/2018	Tdap	SIRVA	$87,000

Date	Vaccine Name	Illness or Symptoms	
1/2/2018	Tdap Vaccine	Guillain-Barre Syndrome (GBS)	$235,000
11/20/2017	Measles Mumps Rubella (MMR)	Encephalopathy	$101,000
11/13/2017	Tdap and Influenza Vaccines	Guillain-Barre Syndrome (GBS)	$125,000
10/27/2017	Flu Vaccine	Transverse Myelitis	$100,000
10/23/2017	Influenza Vaccine	Guillain-Barre Syndrome (GBS)	$328,638
10/19/2017	Flu Vaccine	Guillain-Barre Syndrome (GBS)	$683,309
10/19/2017	Influenza	SIRVA	$110,000
10/13/2017	Influenza Vaccine	Guillain-Barre Syndrome GBS	$523,454
10/10/2017	Influenza Vaccine	SIRVA	$116,292
9/29/2017	Influenza Vaccine	Neuropathy	$125,000
9/27/2017	Influenza	Guillain_Barre Syndrome (GBS)	$120,000
9/1/2017	Influenza Vaccine	Guillain-Barre Syndrome (GBS)	$140,000
8/25/2017	Influenza Vaccine	Guillain-Barre Syndrome (GBS)	$180,720
8/23/2017	TDaP	Guillain-Barre Syndrome (GBS)	$850,000
8/11/2017	Influenza Vaccine	Guillain-Barre Syndrome (GBS)	$125,000
8/11/2017	Influenza Vaccine	Transverse Myelitis	$100,000
8/8/2017	Flu Shot	Guillain-Barre Syndrome (GBS)	$355,000
8/7/2017	Influenza Vaccine	Guillain-Barre Syndrome (GBS)	$195,000

Date	Vaccine Name	Illness or Symptoms	
8/7/2017	Influenza Vaccine	Guillain-Barre Syndrome GBS	$431,367
7/28/2017	Influenza Vaccine	Transverse Myelitis; Death	$150,000
7/24/2017	Meningococcal Vaccine	Disseminated Encephalomyelopathy ADEM	$115,000
6/29/2017	Influenza	SIRVA	$85,000
6/28/2017	Tdap and Influenza Vaccines	Bell's Palsy	$85,000
6/23/2017	Tetanus Diphtheria (Td)	SIRVA	$85,000
6/20/2017	Tetanus	SIRVA	$133,000
6/16/2017	Tetanus Diphtheria Acellular Pertussis (Tdap)	Guillain-Barre Syndrome	$325,000
6/13/2017	Influenza	Guillain-Barre Syndrome	$193,000
6/13/2017	Influenza	SIRVA	$77,000
6/2/2017	Influenza	SIRVA	$37,500
5/25/2017	Flu Vaccine	SIRVA	$100,000
5/25/2017	Influenza & Tetanus Vaccines	SIRVA	$90,771
5/23/2017	Influenza Vaccine	SIRVA	$82,000
5/22/2017	Influenza Vaccine	Guillain-Barre Syndrome (GBS)	$165,000
5/12/2017	Influenza Vaccine	Guillain-Barre Syndrome (GBS)	$20,000
5/11/2017	Influenza Vaccine	Guillain-Barre Syndrome (GBS)	$150,000

Date	Vaccine Name	Illness or Symptoms	
5/10/2017	Tdap	Guillain-Barre Syndrome (GBS)	$150,000
5/9/2017	Flu Vaccine	Guillain-Barre Syndrome (GBS)	$210,000
5/6/2017	HPV Vaccine	Neuromyelitis Optica	$11.5 Million Over Lifetime
5/5/2017	Influenza Vaccine	SIRVA	$85,000
5/3/2017	Influenza Vaccine	SIRVA	$102,882

The above monetary awards are but a drop in the bucket of the real amount that will be paid to victims of vaccine chemicalization. The Vaccine Court has already paid over $3.7 BILLION in damages to families injured by vaccines with a lot more pending. This is an eye opening figure of monetary awards especially since the CDC estimates at only about 10 percent adverse events are reported. The amount of money awarded gives one strong indication of the harm caused by vaccine chemicalization.

All of this money has been awarded to the approximate 10% of those who suffered vaccine induced injury; leaving 90% out of the grave picture of how vaccines are causing injuries. In addition, the amount of money although staggering, would be a great deal more if it were not for the unfair and unprecedented award caps placed upon recovery awards for injuries caused by vaccination. The sheer number of people being injured by vaccine chemicalization and the telling amount of money awarded clearly indicate the emergency is no longer childhood disease but rather, the danger from vaccine unnatural to human biology chemicalization. This very real emergency is being perpetrated by mandated vaccinations and the unconscionable total liability shield carved out for vaccine producers. This makes the profit based vaccine industry above negligence law as, it acts with impunity when it puts unnatural to human biology chemicals in vaccines.

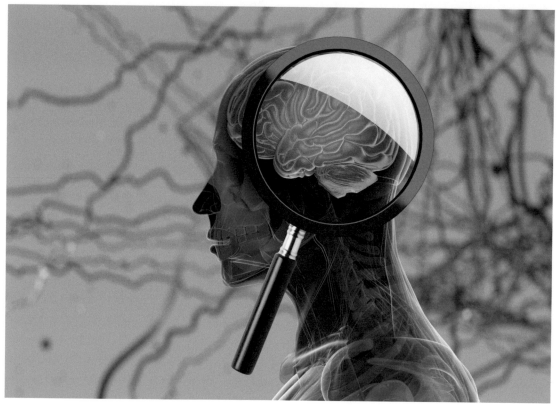

**Unnatural to human biology chemicals cause brain malfunction;
only consider SAFER vaccines for injection.**

Protect your children from becoming a statistic
of vaccine chemicalization child abuse!

Thank you for reading my book and good parenting!

Dr. Robert Caires Esq., inactive in practice but,
very active as a SAFER vaccines advocate.

Dr. Robert Caires commits to donate all royalties and after tax
profits from the sale or proceeds from his book titled, SAFER
Vaccines, Safer Children to the charity SAFER Vaccines, which
is dedicated to achieving SAFER Vaccines for safer children. Dr.
Caires will not make any money from the sale of this book.

I would like to end this book with a prayer that I was inspired to write that is a basis to **LIVE** and **HEAL** by titled, **ABC Prayer**.

ABC PRAYER

HOLY FATHER

Allow the healing of those in need and to heal ourselves
Be always within us, in all we feel, hear and see
Forgive us for our sins, faults and weakness
Protect and guide us in all that we do
Help us to be righteous and strong
Creator of all that is and shall be
Place us on the paths of purity
Heal our bodies and minds
Bring forth all goodness
Shine grace upon us
Purify our souls
Lift our spirits
Enlighten us
Protect us
Bless us
Bestow peace and serenity
Help us to love one another more
Show the way to become one with GOD
The power of GOD is now healing and protecting us
Bless us with Abundant Happiness
Bless us with Brilliant Health
Bless us with Constant love

AMEN

SAFER
VACCINES

Printed in the United States
By Bookmasters